Neonatal Intensive Care Nursing

2nd edition

Thoroughly revised and updated, this new edition of *Neonatal Intensive Care Nursing* is a comprehensive, evidence-based text for nurses and midwives caring for sick newborn babies.

Written by and for nurses, it concentrates on the common problems occurring within the neonatal intensive care unit. This user-friendly text will enable nurses to recognise, rationalise and remedy these problems using both a multi-systems and an evidence-based approach. Individual chapters include:

EVIDENCE-BASED PRACTICE • DEVELOPMENTALLY FOCUSED NURSING CARE • FAMILIES IN NICU • RESUSCITATION OF THE NEWBORN • MANAGEMENT OF THERMAL STABILITY • MANAGEMENT OF RESPIRATORY DISORDERS •MANAGEMENT OF CARDIOVASCULAR DISORDERS • NEONATAL BRAIN INJURY • MANAGEMENT OF HAEMATOLOGICAL DISORDERS • MANAGEMENT OF NEONATAL PAIN • FLUID AND ELECTROLYTE BALANCE • NUTRITIONAL MANAGEMENT IN NICU • NEONATAL INFECTION • DIAGNOSTIC AND THERAPEUTIC PROCEDURES • NEONATAL ANAESTHESIA • NEONATAL SURGERY • NEONATAL TRANSPORT • MEDICATION IN THE NEWBORN • BEREAVEMENT IN THE NICU • ETHICS AND NEONATAL NURSING

Neonatal Intensive Care Nursing will be essential reading for experienced nurses and midwives caring for sick newborn babies within the neonatal intensive care unit, for nurses undertaking qualifications in the specialism of neonatal nursing and for pre-registration students undertaking relevant modules or placements.

Glenys Boxwell (Connolly) is an Advanced Neonatal Nurse Practitioner for Plymouth Hospitals NHS Trust. She was previously a senior lecturer at Homerton College, Cambridge.

Neonatal Intensive Care Nursing

Second Edition

Edited by

■ Glenys Boxwell

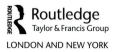

Routledge
Taylor & Francis Group

LONDON AND NEW YORK

First published 2010
by Routledge
2 Park Square, Milton Park, Abingdon, Oxon, OX14 4RN

Simultaneously published in the USA and Canada
by Routledge
270 Madison Avenue, New York, NY 10016

Routledge is an imprint of the Taylor & Francis Group, an informa business

© 2010 Glenys Connolly; the contributors, their chapters

Typeset in Sabon by Keystroke,
Printed and bound in India by
Replika Press PVT Ltd

British Library Cataloguing in Publication Data
A catalogue record for this book is available from the British Library

Library of Congress Cataloging in Publication Data
Neonatal intensive care nursing / edited by Glenys Boxwell. — 2nd ed.
p. ; cm.
Includes bibliographical references and index.
1. Neonatal intensive care.   2. Newborn infants—Diseases—Nursing.
3. Intensive care nursing.   I. Boxwell, Glenys, 1957-
[DNLM: 1. Intensive Care, Neonatal—methods.   2. Neonatal Nursing—methods.
3. Infant, Newborn, Diseases—nursing.   4. Infant, Premature,
Diseases—nursing. WY 157.3 N438 2010]
RJ253.5.N467 2010
618.92'01—dc2   2009034680

ISBN10: 0-415-47755-7 (hbk)
ISBN10: 0-415-47756-5 (pbk)
ISBN10: 0-203-85707-0 (ebk)

ISBN13: 978-0-415-47755-0 (hbk)
ISBN13: 978-0-415-47756-7 (pbk)
ISBN13: 978-0-203-85707-6 (ebk)

Contents

Figures

Tables

Contributors

Anne Aspin has been Nurse Consultant for Neonatal Surgery within the Yorkshire Neonatal Network and Leeds Teaching Hospitals NHS Trust since October 2004.

Dee Beresford is Editor of the *Journal of Neonatal Nursing* and has affiliation with the Neonatal Nurses Association.

Stevie Boyd was a Senior Staff Nurse in the Neonatal Intensive Care Unit, Norfolk and Norwich Healthcare NHS Trust. She was also an editorial adviser to the Journals *Infant* and the *Journal of Neonatal Nursing*.

Liam Brennan is a Consultant Paediatric Anaesthetist at Addenbrooke's Hospital, Cambridge. He trained in paediatric anaesthesia at the Hospital for Sick Children, Great Ormond Street, London. He has published in the areas of pre-operative assessment of children, day case anaesthesia and post-operative nausea and vomiting.

Joan Cameron is a Lecturer in Nursing and Midwifery at the University of Dundee.

Glenys Connolly is an Advanced Neonatal Nurse Practitioner for Plymouth Hospitals NHS Trust.

Liz Crathern has been a Neonatal Nurse since 1980 and in neonatal education since 1992. Her research interests focus on the family in NICU, she is writing up her doctoral study on the experiences of first-time fathers in NICU.

Jackie Dent is a former Nurse Teacher at the University of Nottingham School of Nursing and was Course Leader for the Neonatal Nursing programmes.

Pauline Fellows is Neonatal Project Facilitator (NSC Network and Cambridge) at Cambridge University Hospitals Trust, UK.

Yvonne Freer, Clinical Reader, is the Programme Lead for neonatal nurse education delivered through NHS Lothian, Edinburgh Napier University and Edinburgh University.

Helen Frizell is Lead Educator in Maternal and Child Health at Basingstoke and North Hampshire NHS Foundation Trust. An experienced neonatal and paediatric nurse, Helen's area of specialist interest and knowledge is medical law and the practical application of this to clinical practice.

Beverley Guard is an Anaesthetist with a special interest in paediatric anaesthesia and sedation for paediatric procedures and day surgery.

Anja Hale has been a Registered Nurse working in the Paediatric and Neonatal fields since 1984. She works as a Clinical Nurse Specialist at the Waikato Newborn Intensive Care Unit, New Zealand.

Catherine Hall (Baldridge) is the Associate Lead Medicines Management and Accountable Officer for Controlled Drugs NHS South of Tyne and Wear.

Elizabeth Harling is an Advanced Neonatal Nurse Practitioner in the Neonatal Intensive Care Unit at Liverpool Women's Hospital.

Rachel Homer is a Clinical Fellow in Paediatric Anaesthesia and Intensive Care at Alder Hey Children's NHS Foundation Trust.

Fiona Hutchinson is a Senior Lecturer in Nursing and Midwifery at Northumbria University, UK.

Simone Jollye has worked in the field of neonatology since 1992 and has been an Advanced Neonatal Nurse Practitioner since 2003. She worked at James Cook University Hospital in Middlesbrough until 2009. She is currently working at the Royal Children's Hospital in Melbourne as an ANNP. Her areas of interest are neonatal respiratory care and neonatal resuscitation.

Rosarie Lombard is an Advanced Neonatal Nurse Practitioner in the neonatal unit at University College London Hospitals NHS Foundation Trust. Her interests include developmental care, perinatal brain injury and neuroimaging, and drug administration safety.

Katie McKenna is the Nurse Educator in neonatology at The Children's Hospital at Westmead, Sydney, Australia. She is interested in aEEG monitoring, newborn pain, and issues involving surgical neonates.

Anne Mitchell is an Advanced Neonatal Nurse Practitioner at Simpson Memorial Maternity Pavilion, Edinburgh.

Peter Mulholland's (MRPharmS FCCP) area of expertise is in neonatal paediatrics, where he practises as an independent prescriber. He is currently webmaster for the Neonatal and Paediatric Pharmacists Group (NPPG) website and board member, and practitioner member of the faculty of Neonatal and Paediatric Pharmacy.

Tilly Reid was Senior Lecturer in neonatal nursing at the University of Central Lancashire until June 2008. Since then she has been employed as Research and Development in Cumbria and Lancashire (RaDiCaL) Lead, NHS North West.

Kaye Spence is an Associate Professor and Clinical Nurse Consultant in neonatology at The Children's Hospital at Westmead, Sydney, Australia, and holds an appointment as Honorary Research Fellow in the Faculty of Medicine, Dentistry and Social Sciences at the University of Melbourne. Her research interests include newborn pain, feeding, developmental care and issues involving surgical neonates.

David Summers is a Charge Nurse at the Neonatal Unit of Royal Victoria Infirmary, Newcastle-upon-Tyne.

Sue Turrill is a Lecturer in Neonatal Care at the University of Leeds, UK. Her special interests include quality in education and practice and, in particular, the health outcomes of neonatal care.

Preface

This is the second edition of *Neonatal Intensive Care Nursing*, first published in 2000. In the intervening years since the publication of the first edition, one would probably think that much has changed in neonatal nursing, but, in reality, little has. Newborn infants in the main (approximately 90 per cent) still survive the arduous and challenging processes around the time of birth and escape the 'neonatal intensive care experience'. Unfortunately that leaves the 10 per cent of the newborn population who will require our services. The vast majority of those will be infants in the preterm category, with a smaller proportion being term infants who become compromised around the time of birth.

Without doubt, technology and interventions now allow us to manage certain conditions more effectively, for example, the use of inhaled nitric oxide and improved ventilation techniques in persistent pulmonary hypertension of the newborn. Additionally, diverse therapeutic strategies have been introduced into common practice in the thermal management of infants. The technique of delivering preterm infants into polyethylene bags (a simple yet incredibly effective manoeuvre) has been revolutionary in achieving and maintaining thermal stability in the most premature populations, with the opposite end of the spectrum, that of significant cooling of the compromised term infant, being introduced to minimise brain injury. Aspects of care delivery that are unchanged are those of providing support for parents within the NICU and coping with the ethical dilemmas that nurses face constantly within their daily practice.

Is a second edition of this textbook necessary? Many people are of the view 'by the time a book is published, the information is out of date!' While there may be a degree of truth in that statement, it also has to be said that most published material, if well researched, has credence and can be used as a starting point for a more up-to-date search for information on a particular topic of interest. To that end, each chapter contains a wealth of referenced material so that if further detail is required, then the reader is directed to the relevant reference for further exploration into the subject matter.

There has been a burgeoning development in internet sources of information since the first edition of this textbook which is incredibly useful. However, many practitioners still rely upon resources that are readily available to them, that can be easily accessed, especially for those awful 'two o'clock in the morning moments' just before an exam!

The book could easily have been double in size, at least, if it were to cover all of the conditions and situations that may be encountered within a NICU. That would, I believe, have made it an unwieldy tome and turned it into a less user-friendly book.

As previously, this book has been written by people who care for preterm and sick infants on a daily basis, managing their disease process and their concomitant complications. Hands-on practice is the guide in this volume.

Each chapter author has endeavoured to incorporate the anatomical and physiological basis for the conditions described, along with management strategies based on the most current evidence available. By applying this knowledge to clinical practice, it is hoped that disease processes will be better understood, care will be more effectively delivered and parents more effectively supported.

The philosophy of *Neonatal Intensive Care Nursing* is not only that its content will aid students undertaking courses through the arduous process of finding 'evidence' to support comments made in assignments, but also encourage the process of linking evidence-based theories to everyday nursing practice within the NICU.

Glenys Boxwell (Connolly)
Plymouth
November 2009

Acknowledgements

The rewriting of this book has been a team effort and all the contributors are to be commended for their commitment to writing while engaging in full-time work responsibilities and, no doubt, personal lives. They have withstood my constant badgering about submissions and questions about content with great fortitude!

Additionally, I would like to thank the specialist reader Susanne Symonds, who provided valuable advice on many aspects of the chapter contents, the development team, the proofreader and especially Susan Dunsmore (the copy-editor) who painstakingly read the entire text and identified any production errors.

My thanks finally go to Joe, who has borne the brunt of this project and has been patient and supportive throughout its development.

Glenys Connolly
Plymouth
November 2009

Abbreviations

ABSS	Anderson's state scoring system
A/C	assist control ventilation
ACTH	adrenocorticotrophic hormone
ADH	antidiuretic hormone
ADP	adenosine diphosphate
aEEG	amplitude-integrated electroencephalography
ANNP	Advanced Neonatal Nurse Practitioner
ANNT	aseptic non-touch technique
APIB	Assessment of Preterm Infant Behaviour
ARF	acute renal failure
ASD	atrial septal defect
ATP	adenosine triphosphate
AV	atrioventricular
BAT	brown adipose tissue
BIIP	Behavioural Indicators of Infant Pain
BPD	bronchopulmonary dysplasia
CAF	Contact a Family Directory
cAMP	cyclic adenosine monophosphate
CAVH	continuous arteriovenous haemofiltration
CBF	cerebral blood flow
CDH	congenital diaphragmatic hernia
CFUs	colony-forming units
cGMP	cyclic guanasine monophosphate
CHARGE	Coloboma, Heart, Atresia choanal, Retardation (growth), Genital and Ear anomalies
CHD	congenital heart defects
CHF	congestive heart failure

CLD	chronic lung disease
CMV	cytomegalovirus
CMV	continuous mandatory ventilation
CNEP	continuous negative expanding pressure
CNS	central nervous system
CO	cardiac output
CO	carbon monoxide
CONS	coagulase negative staphylococcus
CPAP	continuous positive airways pressure
CRP	C-reactive protein
CRT	capillary refill time
CSF	cerebrospinal fluid
CVP	central venous pressure
DCT	direct Coomb's test
DDH	developmental dysplasia of the hip
DIC	disseminated intravascular coagulation
DJF	duodeno-jejunal flexure
DSVNI	Distress Scale for Ventilated Newborn Infants
EBF	erythroblastosis fetalis
EBM	expressed breast milk
EBP	evidence-based practice
ECF	extracellular fluid
ECG	electrocardiogram
ECHO	echocardiography
ECMO	extracorporeal membrane oxygenation
EDRF	endothelium-derived relaxing factor
EEG	electroencephalogram
ETT	endotracheal tube
FBM	fetal breathing movements
FFP	fresh frozen plasma
FiO_2	fractional inspired oxygen concentration
FISH	fluorescence in situ hybridisation
FRC	functional residual capacity
GBS	group B beta-haemolytic streptococcus
GCSF	granulocyte colony stimulating factor
GFR	glomerular filtration rate
GMH	germinal matrix haemorrhage
GO/ERD	gastro-(o)esophageal reflux disease
GOR	gastro-oesophageal reflux
HAS	human albumin solution
HDN	haemorrhagic disease of the newborn; also haemolytic disease of the newborn
HFJV	high frequency jet ventilation
HFOV	high frequency oscillation ventilation
HFPPV	high frequency positive-pressure ventilation
HI	hypoxic ischaemic

HIE	hypoxic-ischaemic encephalopathy
HMD	hyaline membrane disease
HUSS	head ultrasound scan
HWM	heated water-filled mattresses
IADH	inappropriate (secretion) of antidiuretic hormone
IM	intramuscular
IMV	intermittent mandatory ventilation
iNO	inhaled nitric oxide
IPPV	intermittent positive-pressure ventilation
ITR	immature to total neutrophil ratio
IUGR	intrauterine growth restriction
IVC	inferior vena cava
IVH	intraventricular haemorrhage
IVIG	intravenous immunoglobulin
LBW	low birth weight
LCPUFA	long chain polyunsaturated fatty acid
LCT	long chain triglycerides
LMA	laryngeal mask airway
LP	lumbar puncture
MAP	mean airway pressure
MAS	meconium aspiration syndrome
MCT	medium chain triglycerides
MDT	multidisciplinary team
MetHb	methaemaglobin
MHRA	Medicines and Healthcare Products Regulatory Agency
MRI	magnetic resonance imaging
MV	minute volume
NBAS	Neonatal Behavioural Assessment Scale
nCPAP	nasal CPAP
NEC	necrotising enterocolitis
NI	nosocomial infection
NICU	Neonatal Intensive Care Unit
NIDCAP	Neonatal Individualised Developmental Care and Assessment Programme
NIRS	near-infrared spectroscopy
NK	natural killer cells
NMC	Nursing and Midwifery Council
NNS	non-nutritive sucking
NO	nitric oxide
OA	oesophageal atresia
OFC	occipito-frontal circumference
OI	oxygen index
$PaCO_2$	partial pressure of carbon dioxide in arterial blood
PaO_2	partial pressure of oxygen in arterial blood
PBE	practice-based evidence
PCA	postconceptional age

PCV	packed cell volume
PD	peritoneal dialysis
PDA	patent ductus arteriosus
PEEP	positive end-expiratory pressure
PFO	patent foramen ovale
PH	pulmonary haemorrhage
PHH	post-haemorrhagic hydrocephalus
PHVD	post-haemorrhagic ventricular dilatation
PICC	peripherally inserted central catheter
PIE	pulmonary interstitial emphysema
PIP	peak inflation pressure
PPHN	persistent pulmonary hypertension
PROM	premature rupture of membranes
PSV	pressure support ventilation
PTV	patient-triggered ventilation
PVH	periventricular haemorrhage
PVHI	periventricular haemorrhage infarction
PVL	periventricular leukomalacia
PVR	pulmonary vascular resistance
RCT	randomised controlled trial
RDS	respiratory distress syndrome
r-HuEPO	Recombinant Human Erythropoietin Therapy
ROP	retinopathy of prematurity
SaO_2	saturation of haemoglobin (oxygen)
SBR	serum bilirubin
SCBU	special care baby unit
SG	specific gravity
SGA	small for gestational age
SIDS	sudden infant death syndrome
SIMV	synchronised intermittent mandatory ventilation
SIPPV	synchronised intermittent positive pressure ventilation
SVC	superior vena cava
SVT	supraventricular tachycardia
TA-GVHD	Transfusion Associated Graft versus Host Disease
TAT	transanastomotic tube
TcB	transcutaneous bilirubinometers
TDM	therapeutic drug monitoring
TEWL	transepidermal water loss
TGA	transposition of the great arteries
THAM	Trishydroxyaminomethylmethane
TINA	Transport of Neonates in Ambulances
TOF	tracheo-oesophageal fistula
TORCH	Toxoplasmosis, Rubella, Cytomegalovirus and Herpes
TPN	total parenteral nutrition
TSE	transmissible spongiform encephalopathy
TSH	thyroid-stimulating hormone

TTN	transient tachypnoea of the newborn
UAC	umbilical arterial catheter
UVC	umbilical venous catheter
VACTERL	Vertebral, Anal, Tracheal, (O)Esophageal and Renal anomalies, plus Cardiac and Limb anomalies
VATER	Vertebral, Anal, Tracheal, (O)Esophageal and Renal anomalies
VC	volume control
vCJD	variant CJD
VILI	ventilator induced lung injury
VKDB	vitamin K deficient bleeding
V/Q	ventilation perfusion
VSD	ventricular septal defect
VT	ventricular tachycardia

Glossary

Selected terms are highlighted in **bold** type in the text on their first occurrence or in key contexts.

abduction   to move (a limb) away from the midline of the body

adduction   to draw (a limb) into the mid-line of the body

adenosine triphosphate (ATP)   organic molecule in body cells responsible for storage and release of energy

aganglionic   without ganglia (innervation)

amniocentesis   removal of amniotic fluid via the maternal abdominal wall for fetal diagnostic purposes

anabolism   building phase of metabolism

anastomosis   a union between two structures

anion   ion carrying one or more negative charges

antecubital   in front of the elbow

anterior   towards the front of the body

anteroposterior   an X-ray view taken using a vertical beam with the patient placed in a supine position

antibody   protein released by plasma cells in response to an antigen

antigen   substance recognised as foreign by the immune system

apoptosis   programmed cell death

aspiration   fluid entering the lungs

atelectasis   alveolar collapse

atresia   a blind-ended tube

auscultation   the process of listening with a stethoscope

autoregulation   the automatic adjustment of blood flow to a particular body area in response to current need

B cells   cells responsible for humoral (antibody-mediated) immunity

baroreceptors   receptors stimulated by pressure change

bradyarrhythmias   slow heart, usually due to extracardiac pathology

bradycardia slow heart rate, less than 80bpm (term) and 100bpm (preterm)

brown adipose tissue (BAT) specialised, strategically placed tissue (fat) which is capable of generating heat

calcaneus heel bone

cardiac output amount of blood pumped from ventricles in one minute

carina the keel-shaped cartilage at the bifurcation of the trachea into the two main bronchi

catecholamines compounds that have the effect of sympathetic nerve stimulation

cation a positively charged ion

caudal relating to the tail end of the body

cell-mediated immunity immunity conferred by activated T cells

cephalad towards the head

cephalhaematoma collection of blood beneath the periosteum of a skull bone

cephalocaudally from the head to the 'tail'

chemoreceptors receptors sensitive to chemical change

choroid plexus CSF producing a capillary 'knot' within a brain ventricle

chromatic related to structures within the cell nucleus which carry hereditary (genetic) factors

cytochrome iron containing proteins found on inner mitochondrial layer which function as electron carriers during oxidative phosphorylation

diaphoresis sweating

diastole relaxation phase of the cardiac cycle

distal further from the attached limb or the origin of a structure, e.g. the elbow is distal to the shoulder

dorsiflexed backward flexion of the hand or foot

dorsum the upper or posterior surface of a part of the body

dynamic precordium visible heartbeat due to PDA

ecchymoses discoloured patch resulting from escape of blood into the tissues just under the skin

embolus (plural emboli) obstruction of a blood vessel by particulate matter, e.g. blood clot or air

epiglottis leaf-shaped cartilage at back of throat, covers the larynx during swallowing

erythropoietin hormone released predominantly by the kidney which stimulates red blood cell production (erythropoiesis)

eventration flattening and non-movement of the diaphragm following denervation – may be congenital or acquired

evidence-based (care) the integration of best available clinical evidence with an individual's expertise

extravasation leakage of fluid from a vessel into the surrounding tissue

extremely low birth weight infant of less than or equal to 999g

facilitated tucking supported positioning of a baby to contain a limb

fistula unnatural connection between two structures or body cavities

flexed   to curl inwards

fundoplication   surgical procedure in which the proximal stomach is wrapped around the distal oesophagus to prevent reflux

gestational age   period of time from the first date of last normal menstrual period to the date of birth. Expressed in number of completed weeks or days

glomerular filtration rate   rate of filtrate formation by the kidneys

gluconeogenesis   formation of glucose from a non-carbohydrate source, e.g. muscle

glycogen   stored carbohydrate predominantly in muscle

glycogenesis   formation of glycogen from glucose

glycogenolysis   breakdown of glycogen to glucose

glycolysis   breakdown of glucose to pyruvate

haemolysis   rupture of red blood cells

Heimlich valve   a one-way blow-off valve

histamine   chemical substance which promotes vasodilatation and capillary permeability

holistic   encompassing all aspects of care

homeostasis   a state of equilibrium within the body

humeral immunity   immunity conferred by antibody production

hydrocephalus   an abnormal increase in the amount of cerebral spinal fluid within the ventricles of the brain

hypertonic   fluids containing a high concentration of solutes, e.g. greater than cells

immunoglobulins   antibodies that bind to specific antigens

inferior   away from the head or towards the lower body or structures

interferon   chemical that provides some protection against a virus

intrathecal   within the subarachnoid space

isotonic   fluids that have the same osmotic pressure as cells

kernicterus   yellow staining of brain stem, cerebellum and hypocanthus with toxic degeneration of nerve cells due to hyperbilirubinaemia

lateral   away from the mid-line of the body

lateral decubitus   lying on one side

lipophilic   substance attracted to fatty tissues

loculated   collected in defined areas or pockets

low birth weight (LBW)   infant of less than or equal to 2499g

lymphocytes   white blood cells arising from bone marrow denoted T or B cells

macrophages   principal phagocytes found at specific sites or within bloodstream

malrotation   anomaly of fetal intestinal rotation and fixation resulting in intestinal obstruction

medial   towards the mid-line of the body

mesenteries   extensions of the peritoneum that support abdominal organs

mitochondria   organelles found in all cells responsible for production of adenosine triphosphate (ATP)

myelination   the formation of a fatty insulating sheath surrounding most nerve fibres

nephrotoxic   damaging to nephrons/kidneys

nociception   the perception by the nerve centres of painful stimulation. The term used in relation to pain perception in neonates

non-shivering thermogenesis   ability to produce heat by activation of BAT

nosocomial   an infection that develops within the hospital environment

oligohydramnios   reduction in liquor volume

oliguria   diminished urine output, e.g. < 1ml/kg/hr

opisthotonus   severe contraction of the back muscles causing the body to arch backwards

opsonisation   process whereby antigens are made more 'attractive' to phagocytes

ototoxic   damaging to the eighth cranial nerve/hearing

petechiae   small haemorrhages in the skin

phagocytes   white blood cells (leucocytes) that destroy pathogens by engulfment

pharmacodynamics   how drugs affect the body

pharmacokinetics   absorption, distribution, metabolism, excretion or what the body does to a drug

phocomelia   congenital anomaly with absence of limbs

plantar   relating to the sole of the foot

pleural effusion   the presence of fluid in the pleural space

pneumoperitoneum   free air in the peritoneal space

pneumothorax   free air in the pleural cavity

polyhydramnios   an excess of amniotic fluid

postconceptional age   current age calculated from date of conception

posterior   towards the back of the body

preterm   less than 37 completed weeks of gestation (259 days). Accounts for 8 per cent of births

primiparous   pregnant for the first time

prokinetic   agent that increases gastric motility

proximal   closer to the body or origin of a structure, e.g. the knee is proximal to the ankle

recidivity   collapsing

situs inversus   major organs (e.g. heart and stomach) are reversed from their normal positions (as seen on X-ray)

situs solitus   normal position of major organs (as seen on X-ray)

small for gestational age (SGA)   infant with birthweight less than the 10th percentile

solute   substance dissolved in solution

stenosis   an abnormal narrowing

stroke volume   amount of blood pumped from the ventricles with each contraction

superior   towards the head or upper part of the body or a structure

supine   lying on back, face upwards

suprapubic   above the symphysis pubis

syncope   fainting, loss of consciousness

systole   contraction phase of the cardiac cycle

T cells   cells responsible for cell-mediated immunity

tachycardia   heart rate greater than 160bpm (term) and 180bpm (preterm) at rest

tension pneumothorax   free air (under pressure) in the chest resulting in a shift in the mediastinum potentially reducing cardiac output

term   from 37 to 42 completed weeks of gestation (259–93 days); see also **preterm**

thermogenesis   production of heat

thoracic vertebrae   the twelve bones of the backbone to which the ribs are attached

thrombus   a clot that develops and persists within a blood vessel

torsion   twisting, e.g. of gut

tracheomalacia   'floppy' trachea

turbidity   clouded with a suspension of particles

vallecula   a depression in an organ (beneath the epiglottis)

very low birth weight (VLBW)   infant of less than or equal to 1499g; see also **small for gestational age**

xiphisternum   the lower part of the breastbone

Chapter 1

Exploring Evidence-based Practice (EBP) in Neonatal Care

Fiona Hutchinson

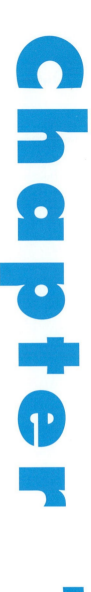

Contents

Introduction

This chapter will explore the concept of evidence-based neonatal nursing care and encourage reflection on differing forms of evidence used in day-to-day practice. Increasingly neonatal nurses are being asked, by peers as well as parents, to provide a rationale for their clinical actions. During nurse training the majority of theoretical evidence is derived from textbooks, journals and lectures. Clinical skills are gained by observing others and receiving support by mentorship. Once qualified, nurses must be accountable for their actions, and must be able to demonstrate that their practice is based on safe and contemporaneous evidence (NMC 2008). The chapter begins by revisiting the concept of evidence-based practice and will explore differing sources of evidence which may be used in practice. The final section of the chapter will discuss how evidence is used in everyday clinical decision-making and explore some sources of evidence which you previously may not have considered.

Exercise 1.1

Think back to the last baby you cared for. Try to recall all the care you provided for the baby and then answer the following questions:

1   What were the sources of knowledge you utilised in order to undertake your actions?
2   Did you verify that the source of your knowledge was reliable and valid?
3   Were your sources up to date?
4   If you feel that your practice was research-based, can you quote which research was utilised and have you critiqued the research yourself?
5   Do you think that your practice was evidence-based?

Exercise 1.1 is intended to make you reflect on differing sources of knowledge utilised to underpin neonatal nursing practice and is useful as a starting point when considering the concept of 'evidence-based practice'.

What is evidence-based practice (EBP)?

No chapter on **evidence-based practice** (EBP) would be complete without first repeating Sackett *et al.*'s well-quoted definition of evidence-based medicine: 'The conscientious, explicit and judicious use of current best evidence in making decisions about the care of individual patients' (Sackett *et al.* 1997, p. 2). As this definition was linked with evidence-based *medicine*, it was, for a while, a common assumption that the only type of evidence was empirical research derived from the quantitative tradition. Much of the momentum sustaining evidence-based medicine (EBM) derives from the Cochrane Collaboration which was designed in 1993 by Cochrane, a physician-epidemiologist interested in the need for evidence to support health care decisions. He worked with Iain Chalmers in formulating an evidence hierarchy which designated the randomised controlled trial (RCT) as the 'gold standard' of evidence (Jennings and Loan 2001). Systematic reviews are the core focus of the Cochrane Collaboration which enables the reader to synthesise the differing results of studies. The frequent interchange between EBM and EBP has led to confusion in identifying the underlying philosophies underpinning evidence. Jasper (2006) describes how evidence-based medicine developed in the early 1990s with evidence-based *practice* becoming popular in the late 1990s. The introduction of evidence-based practice was to extend the original ideas of evidence-based medicine to other professional disciplines such as nursing and midwifery. Evidence-based *nursing* was first recognised in the mid-1990s and resulted in a strong professional response to evidence-based practice within nursing as a result of key government documents. Cluett (2005) describes how evidence-based practice was advocated as a key component for quality midwifery practice and was a core element in several government publications including *The NHS Plan* (DoH 2000) and *Changing Childbirth* (DoH 1993). Whichever terminology is utilised, it is important to remember that evidence is not static as it constantly changes in response to new research and practice-based experience. What may be deemed as 'good or safe practice' today may be consigned to the archives as new evidence emerges. This becomes particularly important when writing neonatal unit protocols, guidelines and procedures as it is essential that these are based on contemporaneous evidence.

In 1999, the United Kingdom Central Council (UKCC) argued that evidence-based practice should be integral to the preparation of nurses (Swinkels *et al.* 2002). Rycroft-Malone *et al.* open their discussion on evidence-based practice by stating that '"evidence" may well be one of the most fashionable words in health care' (2004, p. 82). They suggest that confusion still exists with defining what 'evidence' is and how it differs from 'scientific' research and provide a useful framework for identifying sources of evidence. Rycroft-Malone *et al.* (2004) and Boogaerts *et al.* (2008) identify varying sources of knowledge utilised in evidence-based policy development and practice. These are discussed in more detail in the following section of this chapter.

Propositional knowledge (scientific knowledge)

The Department of Health views scientific research, e.g. RCTs, as the 'gold standard' of evidence and proposes a hierarchy of 'best' evidence placing personal experience at the bottom of the structure. A randomised controlled trial is a study performed with an homogeneous population, controlled variables and specific interventions using a placebo (Girard 2008). Evans (2003) provides an example of the so-called 'hierarchy' of evidence as follows:

1   Systematic reviews, multi-centre studies.
2   Randomised controlled trials, observational studies.
3   Uncontrolled trials with dramatic results, before and after studies, non-randomised controlled trials.
4   Descriptive studies, case studies, expert opinion, studies of poor methodological quality.

The above list is limited in nature as it ignores other forms of evidence which will be discussed later. In this hierarchical structure Evans has given equal status to expert opinion, descriptive studies, case studies and studies of poor methodological quality, whereas other frameworks (e.g. Ellis 2000) distinguish between studies and expert opinions in the hierarchical structure, ranking the former above the latter. Brocklehurst and McGuire (2005), in their review on evidence-based care in perinatal medicine, identify some of the difficulties in undertaking neonatal randomised controlled trials. These are summarised as:

■   limited infrastructure to support studies;
■   large trials needed to detect modest effect sizes;
■   limited funding;
■   limited potential for industrial partnership;
■   trial recruitment undertaken by busy clinicians or carers;
■   informed consent obtained at stressful times;
■   public perception of neonatal research;
■   need for long-term follow-up.

(ibid., p. 36)

There is no doubt that there is a need to evaluate any potential interventions prior to their use in neonatal care. Large multi-centred trials such as the TOBY trial (to determine whether the use of hypothermia as a treatment would reduce mortality and neurodevelopment impairment at 18 months of age) have proved useful in providing evidence to support practice. In view of the difficulties identified above, however, Brocklehurst and McGuire suggest that there should be more perinatal networks for undertaking multi-centre trials as is the case in North America and Australasia. Such collaboration would ensure that competing trials do not occur simultaneously and that parent groups and researchers can prioritise their most important research questions.

Long-term outcomes for very **preterm** babies have been evaluated in an attempt to appraise the effectiveness of perinatal and neonatal care (e.g. Larroque *et al.* 2004). The findings of this particular study (Epipage) concluded that 42 per cent of those born at between 24–28 weeks were receiving special support at 5 years. Of these children, 50 per cent were also receiving care from psychologists or psychiatrists. Studies like these are essential for long-term planning of resources as they remind us that service needs for these children extend long after discharge from the neonatal unit. As with all forms of evidence, however, it depends on how accurate the data are.

Qualitative research is a broad term used to refer to a variety of research traditions originating in philosophy, anthropology, psychology and sociology. It is an inductive approach to discovering or expanding knowledge and is a useful means of generating knowledge about an area that has been little researched previously. Qualitative studies are the best designs to understand experiences, beliefs and attitudes. Wigert *et al.* (2006) undertook a qualitative study of ten mothers in order to find out their experiences of having a baby in a neonatal intensive care unit. This study provided useful evidence for neonatal nurses as the implications for practice established that the mothers in the study felt excluded from the care of their baby and experienced a sense of not belonging to either the maternity care unit or the neonatal unit. The authors concluded by stating that this has implications for maternal–infant attachment and discuss the importance of neonatal nurses developing strategies which support the women in caring for their baby while in the neonatal unit. A systematic review of research into the effectiveness of bereavement interventions in neonatal intensive care was undertaken by Harvey *et al.* (2008). Their findings concluded that qualitative research may be the key to discovering the most effective way of providing bereavement care due to the sensitivity of the subject area and ethical dilemmas of conducting RCTs. Post-bereavement care is an example of a research topic whereby the findings of an RCT may not be applicable to individual circumstances. The 'best' intervention, as elicited from a controlled trial, may not be appropriate for all bereaved parents. Henley and Schott (2008) and Kendall and Guo (2008) provide some good examples of how qualitative research is important in providing evidence of how nursing staff can impact on parents' experiences of bereavement. They argue that this experience has a huge impact on their ability to cope not only at the time of the bereavement but for years afterwards. These examples demonstrate the usefulness of qualitative research in providing evidence to underpin nursing care within the neonatal unit.

Qualitative research, however, is not without its limitations. Bryman (2008) acknowledges that the main criticism of qualitative research are issues surrounding the subjectivity of the researcher, the difficulty in replication of the study, the lack of transparency in the research process, and problems with the generalisation of findings. It would not be an appropriate method for gathering evidence when testing a new pharmacological intervention, for example. What is interesting in Bryman's work, however, is that he lists the similarities between the two methods, suggesting that they are both ways of achieving evidence to underpin practice even though they utilise differing philosophies.

Two differing approaches to obtaining propositional knowledge are described above, each with their strengths and weaknesses. Flemming (2007) argues that while nurses have developed diverse ways of obtaining knowledge for practice, they have predominantly adopted a medical model of evidence by focusing on evidence obtained from RCTs and other quantitative studies as listed above. In specialist areas like neonatal intensive care, this is understandable, as medical interventions which are derived from scientific sources of evidence tend to take priority. She suggests that in order to develop nursing practice in such specialist areas, nurses need to synthesise differing forms of research methods, and provides a very strong case for incorporating mixed research methods in order to inform nursing practice. She argues that the combination of qualitative and quantitative research methods produces findings that can enhance the evidence base for nursing practice. Mulhall (1998) suggests that nurses should primarily focus on designing imaginative research which will improve many aspects of nursing practice. It is important to remember that qualitative studies elicit rich data which can provide valuable insight into parents' experiences of neonatal care (e.g. Wigert *et al.* 2006). This, however, is achieved at the expense of acquiring large sample sizes, thus reducing the ability to generalise the findings. Data such as this are of great importance when considering ways in which to develop an evidence base for (neonatal) nursing practice. It is beyond the scope of this chapter to provide an in-depth discussion on the 'qualitative versus quantitative' debate. A detailed discussion on the differing philosophies underpinning these methodologies can be found in Proctor (1998).

Knowledge gained through practice experience

Mantzoukas (2007) argues that knowledge is inextricably linked with practice and therefore should not be solely derived from the distancing and rigour of scientific research. The most renowned advocate of clinical experience as a source of evidence for practice is Patricia Benner (Benner 1984). Knowledge gained through this way is often tacit (implied without being stated) and intuitive. Estabrooks *et al.* (2005) studied how paediatric and adult intensive care nurses obtained the majority of their practice knowledge. The findings indicate that evidence-based care protocols are often rejected in favour of practices based on their own personal experience. The practitioners felt confident in justifying and defending their actions. Nurses also stated that they gained knowledge for practice from social interactions with peers. The authors conclude the study by stating that social interactions and experience should be given more credence as a source of knowledge than more legitimate sources, for example, research and policies, which reinforces the complexity of differing sources of evidence required for practice.

Personal experience

An example from personal experience provides an illustration of how experience gained through past practice can have a long-lasting impact. As part of my midwifery training I spent several weeks in the neonatal unit. Two babies were being nursed side by side in incubators. One was a male infant born at 28 weeks' gestation weighing 980 grams at birth. The other was a female infant with a birth weight of 1,000 grams at 40 weeks' gestation. I remember how their medical and nursing needs were vastly different even though there was only

20 grams difference in their birth weight. Thirty years later I still use this example when teaching student midwives to illustrate the differences between prematurity and growth restriction. The practical experience gained from observing these two babies and how they were cared for has stayed with me all these years and is an example of how knowledge gained through practice can have long-lasting implications. This experience taught me more about the difference between a premature baby and a growth-restricted baby's medical and nursing needs than any books, lectures or research.

Reflection on and in practice can be considered a process of transforming unconscious types of knowledge and practices into logically articulated ones that can be used in clinical decision-making. If undertaken systematically, utilising an appropriate model, for example, Smyth's double loop model, reflection can evaluate the incident from a theoretical perspective by exploring which nursing theory and social practices have influenced the incident and how these may need to be modified (Greenwood 1998). Much is written about intuitive practice and it is important to remember that intuition can only develop in response to an accumulation of practice knowledge. It has a direct bearing on the analytical processes in patient care as it is often a trigger for reflective practice (King and Appleton 1997).

Knowledge from patients, clients and carers

Knowledge from parents and neonatal nurses can provide an important insight into the lived experience of neonatal care. This may take the form of individual case studies, parents' narratives or empirical research. An example of parents' experiences of neonatal care may be found on the website www.healthtalk online.org (previously known as DipEx). This is a registered charity established in 2001 by two doctors after they had both experienced health care as patients. One particular interview provides a moving account of a mother whose baby was diagnosed with a congenital heart defect. The narrative provides a detailed account of the effect of the experience on her whole family. Rycroft-Malone et al. (2004) describe two types of potential patient evidence. The first is specific to one patient's experience in an episode of care; the second is building up evidence from different patient narratives which could then be utilised to inform policy-making. Lindberg et al. (2008) undertook qualitative research in order to obtain information about the experience of adjusting to being the father of a premature infant. The findings provide an invaluable and honest account of how fathers feel, how they attempted to adjust and gain confidence in becoming a father. Likewise, Fegran and Helseth (2008) studied the parent–nurse relationship in a neonatal intensive care unit and concluded their work by stating that distancing is necessary to maintain professional boundaries, but achieving the right balance between closeness and distance can assist with parents developing independence in caring for their baby. Jasper (2006) argues that while practice should be based on propositional knowledge and clinical experience, it also needs to take into account patient preferences (in the case of neonatal care, parents' wishes). A recently published survey by Bliss (2008) provides a good example of a mixed method research methodology. The survey undertaken in 2008 asked neonatal units about their activity and also included questions for parents relating to their experiences of having a baby in the neonatal unit and their impression of neonatal care. The comments made by parents in the report, in conjunction with the survey data, provide a detailed picture of life in a neonatal unit from the perspectives of both parents and staff. Not surprisingly, one of the major themes identified by both groups was the shortage of nursing staff.

Knowledge from a local context (audit and evaluation)

Audit and evaluation are essential activities for the provision of evidence about current practice (Lindsay 2007). Audits measure practice against a pre-determined standard, while evaluation focuses on measuring current service provision. Current strategies emphasise the importance of involving users (in the case of neonatal care, parents) in the process of audit and evaluation. Lindsay claims that the effectiveness of audit and evaluation as providers of evidence is dependent on factors such as the setting of appropriate standards (for audit), reliable data collection and analysis and clear reporting of findings. Redshaw and Hamilton (2005) surveyed all neonatal units in the UK and received a response rate of 70 per cent (153 neonatal units). Services evaluated included those of neonatal networks, admission and transfer rates, staffing levels and some elements of practice. Data like this are useful in providing an overview of national practices and in highlighting areas for improvement, but, as the authors concur, are solely descriptive in nature.

Three frameworks have been utilised in order to identify differing sources of knowledge used in providing evidence for practice. Two further sources of knowledge not alluded to in the hierarchy previously identified by Evans (2003) are mentioned below as they are utilised by health care professionals, especially when undertaking further study. Some would argue that these are not always contemporaneous or accurate sources of evidence.

1   *Websites*. Most people today have access to the internet and when a mother has a preterm baby, the probability is the first thing she will do is undertake an internet search on 'prematurity'. It is for this reason that neonatal nurses should be aware of the evidence that is available on the internet in order to address any queries that arise. Reviewing some of the available websites, it is evident that some are well meaning but misguided. One site recommended that in order to prevent preterm labour, a woman should not climb the stairs more than twice a day. Conversely, the website mentioned in an earlier section provides a wealth of knowledge about what it is like to give birth to a baby with a congenital heart defect and the effect it has on the whole family structure (www.healthonline.org). Several frameworks are avail-

able for evaluating the reliability and validity of the content of a website; however, the most important questions that need to be asked are:

(a) Does the site cover the topic comprehensively and accurately?
(b) Is the information predominantly fact or opinion?
(c) Can you understand what is being said?
(d) Is it written at the right level for the target audience?
(e) Is the site referenced?
(f) Are the web links well chosen and relevant?
(g) Is the site regularly updated?

(Sing-Ling Tsai and Sin-Kuo Chai 2005)

2   *Books*. Books have their place in providing evidence for practice. Rolfe and Fulbrook (1998) categorise books as a source of scientific theoretical knowledge. While acknowledging that textbooks are of limited use in providing contemporaneous evidence, they are invaluable for providing principles for practice and information that does not have a limited life span, for example, anatomy and physiology. They are also useful in providing information about a specialist area of nursing practice and are listed as key texts in several undergraduate and postgraduate courses.

The use of evidence in clinical decision-making

The next part of this chapter will explore how differing sources of evidence may be used in making decisions about neonatal practice. Clinical decision-making may be defined as 'choosing between alternatives' (Thompson and Dowding 2002). Knowledge utilised to underpin clinical decision-making has been recognised for many years as falling into one of the following categories forming the 'evidence-based nursing jigsaw' as described by Di-Censo *et al.* (1998), and Flemming (2007):

■   clinical expertise;
■   evidence from research;
■   available resources;
■   patient (or in the case of neonatal care, 'family') preferences.

Thompson (2003) claims that the majority of evidence used in day-to-day clinical decision-making is based on experiential knowledge. Reliance on this form of evidence means that nurses must use cognitive shortcuts or heuristics for handling information when making decisions. One of the disadvantages of this is the potential for subjectivity because of previous experiences.

Historically, there have been three main models to assist with decision-making based on differing sources of evidence:

1   *The information processing model* – Rooted in medical decision-making, it uses a hypothetico-deductive (scientific) approach to assist with reasoning.

It is derived from the field of cognitive psychology and involves testing hypotheses and then modifying them on the outcome of the situation being tested (Manias *et al.* 2004). Decision trees can be used to assess potential outcomes, for each decision tree, possible outcomes can be assigned a numerical value and the probability of reaching a specific outcome is assessed. This rule of probability is known as Bayes theorem. This form of analysis is used to calculate the risks of particular problems, for example, the risk of fetal hypoxia following meconium staining of the liquor (Raynor *et al.* 2005).

2   *The intuitive-humanist model (pattern recognition)* – The focus of this model is intuition and the relationship between nursing experiences, the knowledge gained from it and how it enriches the clinical decision-making process. In this model, hypothesis testing is not used as a marker of accurate or inaccurate propositions and reasoning. Critics of this model state that it lacks scientific reasoning and focuses on reasoning based on hunches or intuition. Rew defines intuition as 'the act of synthesizing empirical, ethical, aesthetic and personal knowledge' (2000, p. 95). One drawback of using this model is that initial hunches or cues may be misleading, resulting in an incorrect decision being made. Pattern recognition is the process whereby a judgement is made on the basis of a few critical pieces of information, i.e. it uses 'stored knowledge' from past experiences (heuristics). Decisions are made on representativeness (how it relates to previous experience), availability (how easy it is to recall information) and anchoring adjustment (favouring originally held beliefs, but adjusting them on the basis of new evidence (Cioffi and Markham 1997)). The difference between pattern recognition and intuitive practice is that intuition occurs at an unconscious level whereas pattern recognition occurs at a conscious level (Raynor *et al.* 2005). They are, however, very similar thought processes (Manias *et al.* 2004) and an expert practitioner will have more stored knowledge than a novice practitioner (Benner 1984).

3   *Spur-of-the-moment decision-making* – Neonatal emergencies such as resuscitation decisions are usually 'spur-of-the-moment' decisions as any delay could be detrimental to the well-being of the baby. Because they are made quickly, it does not, however, mean that no thought has gone into them and they are not based on appropriate evidence. They are usually based on written guidelines as a form of evidence where specific steps are followed (e.g. the ABC of resuscitation). Guidelines are usually based on deductive reasoning, not feelings or emotions (the hypothetico-deductive process) and it is for this reason that other sources of knowledge are utilised in practice. Byrne *et al.* (2008), in their narrative on the ethics of delivery room resuscitation, conclude that, in conjunction with agreed guidelines, parents' views should always be included when making decisions about resuscitation of the newborn.

From the discussion above, it is apparent that decisions made in clinical practice are based on several forms of evidence. Payot *et al.* (2007) describe in their qualitative study how parents and neonatologists may work together to engage in decision-making about whether or not to resuscitate extremely preterm infants. The findings conclude that the key to arriving at a consensual decision is based on negotiation and taking into account knowledge in diagnostic information and treatment from neonatologists and knowledge from the families who are experts in their own family history, family roots, philosophy and ways of life.

Practice-based evidence/nursing-based evidence

The above discussion has attempted to reinforce the notion that evidence used to inform clinical decision-making in practice is derived from several sources. Earlier in this chapter the concepts of evidence-based medicine, evidence-based practice and evidence-based nursing were discussed. More recent literature describes two other ways that nurses may gain knowledge to underpin practice.

The first is from Girard (2008) who describes an alternative concept; that of *practice-based evidence* (PBE). This differs from EBM/EBP/EBN in that it recognises the individuality of each patient, stating that not every patient reacts to an intervention or care pathway as anticipated. She argues that while EBP utilises the best evidence to make decisions about care, it does not necessarily include the patient in any care plan. As discussed earlier, the gold standard of EBP is the randomised controlled trial, but Girard warns that it can lead to the conclusion that there is only one best treatment or cure. This is not always the case as, while the intervention may be the most effective in trials, it may not be the most acceptable treatment to the patient because of side effects, etc. Byrne *et al.* (2008) in their study of the ethics of delivery-room resuscitation discuss the problems of decision-making when resuscitating babies, particularly extremely preterm babies on the borderline of viability. They describe the problems with current available evidence and suggest that professionals are not always receptive to taking parents' views into account, tending to rely on statistical data instead even though it is not always accurate and predictive. Shieh (2006) describes turning her day-to-day experiences into evidence by generating ideas directly from practice experience working with women with perinatal drug abuse problems. She demonstrates that by listening to clients' views and narratives of their experiences, practice can be modified and improved health care delivery achieved. She concludes her article by stating that 'research and practice should be intertwined, one complementing the other' (Shieh 2006, p. 378).

The second concept is one offered from the speciality of mental health nursing by Geanellos (2004): *nursing-based evidence*. Geanellos argues that mental health nursing has historically relied on other disciplines to provide knowledge to develop practice. She suggests that nursing needs to establish its legitimacy by articulating a distinct contribution to health care. Comparisons to neonatal nursing can be made here in that there is a tendency to place emphasis on quantitative research derived from medical researchers as a source of evidence to underpin practice. In this paradigm, Geanellos proposes that by using the bio-medical model as a source of evidence in isolation, patients' health care is perceived as a series of problems to be reduced, objectified, researched and cured. An important aspect of neonatal nursing, however, is communicating with families and attempting to provide meaningful care by understanding the 'lived experience' of having a baby in a neonatal unit. This can only be achieved by obtaining knowledge from the families using qualitative research methodologies and learning from previous experience.

Jenicek (2006) provides an interesting summary of variations on a theme of 'evidence-based medicine':

- faith-based medicine (belief and trust in something);
- experience-based medicine (increase in knowledge and skills over time);
- conviction-based medicine (based on firmly held opinions and beliefs);
- big-heart-based medicine (as dictated by the doctor's own compassion and empathy);
- gut feeling-based medicine (as instinctive and intuition-driven understanding and decision-making);
- authority-based medicine (enforced by rules).

Conclusion

This chapter has explored differing forms of evidence used in day-to-day nursing practice. Hierarchies of evidence have been identified and other less utilised sources of evidence discussed. The aim of this chapter is to encourage reflection on where knowledge is obtained to underpin nursing practice and further explore the concept of evidence-based practice in relation to neonatal care. In summary, evidence for practice may be derived from several sources; the most frequently utilised sources are as follows:

- propositional knowledge (e.g. research);
- knowledge gained through practice experience (incorporating intuitive practice and reflecting on practice);
- knowledge from parents and carers (individual narratives or a composition of differing experiences).

Websites and books may also be used as sources of evidence; it is important, however, that the reader checks the writer's source of evidence and acknowledges their strengths and weaknesses. Guidelines and protocols are also to be found in most neonatal units – these too should be underpinned by appropriate evidence and regularly updated. Whatever the source of evidence used for practice, it is essential to be able to critically analyse the material and not take it at face value.

Other chapters in this book will demonstrate how differing forms of evidence are used to inform day-to-day neonatal practice. Scrutiny of each reference list provided will demonstrate how many differing sources of evidence each author has used. I conclude this chapter by reiterating what I stated in the first edition of this publication: 'Neonatal Nurses have a wealth of experiential and personal knowledge which should be utilised and disseminated amongst their peers' (Allan 2000, p. 10). It is hoped that this chapter has demonstrated that this source of evidence is valuable and, if used in conjunction with propositional knowledge, can truly contribute to the package of 'evidence-based neonatal nursing practice'.

References

Allan, F. (2000) 'Advanced neonatal nursing practice', in G. Boxwell (ed.) *Neonatal Intensive Care Nursing*, London: Routledge.

Benner, P. (1984) *From Novice to Expert: Excellence and Power in Clinical Nursing Practice*, Reading, MA: Addison-Wesley.

Bliss (2008) *Baby Steps to Better Care*, Bliss Baby Report (October), London: Bliss Publications.

Boogaerts, M., Grealish, L. and Ranse, K. (2008) 'Policy and practices: exploring tensions to develop practice', *Practice Development in Health Care* 7(1): 49–57.

Brocklehurst, P. and McGuire, W. (2005) 'Evidence-based care', *BMJ* 330: 36–8.

Bryman, A. (2008) *Social Research Methods*, 3rd edn, Oxford: Oxford University Press.

Byrne, S., Szyld, E. and Kattwinkel, J. (2008) 'The ethics of delivery room resuscitation', *Seminars in Fetal and Neonatal Medicine* 13: 440–7.

Cioffi, J. and Markham, R. (1997) 'Clinical decision-making by midwives: managing case complexity', *Journal of Advanced Nursing* 25: 265–72.

Cluett, E. (2005) 'Using the evidence to inform decisions', in M.D. Raynor, J.E. Marshall and A. Sullivan (eds) *Decision-making in Midwifery Practice*, Oxford: Elsevier Churchill Livingstone.

Cranston, M. (2002) 'Clinical effectiveness and evidence-based practice', *Nursing Standard* 16(24): 39–43.

Di-Censo, A., Cullum, N. and Ciliska D. (1998) 'Implementing evidence based nursing: some misconceptions', *Evidence-based Nursing* 1: 38–9.

DoH (1993) *Changing Childbirth: The Report of the Expert Midwifery Group: Baroness Cumberlege*, London: HMSO.

DoH (2000) *The NHS Plan: A Plan for Investment, a Plan for Reform*, London: DoH.

Ellis, J. (2000) 'Sharing the evidence: clinical practice benchmarking to improve continuously the quality of care', *Journal of Advanced Nursing* 32(1): 215–25.

Estabrooks, C.A., Rutakumwa, W., O'Leary, K.A., Profetto-McGrath, J., Milner, M., Levers, M.J. and Scott-Findlay, S. (2005) 'Sources of practice knowledge among nurses', *Qualitative Health Research* 15(4): 460–76.

Evans, D. (2003) 'Hierarchy of evidence: a framework for ranking evidence evaluating health care interventions', *Journal of Clinical Nursing* 12: 77–84.

Fegran, L. and Helseth, S. (2008) 'The parent–nurse relationship in the neonatal intensive unit context: closeness and emotional involvement', *Journal Compilations*, Copyright 2008 Nordic College of Caring Science.

Flemming, K. (2007) 'The knowledge base for evidence-based nursing: a role for mixed methods research?' *Advances in Nursing Science* 30(1): 41–51.

Geanellos, R. (2004) 'Nursing based evidence: moving beyond evidence-based practice in mental health nursing', *Journal of Evaluation in Clinical Practice* 10(2): 177–86.

Gerrish, K. and Lacey, A. (eds) (2006) *The Research Process in Nursing*, 5th edn, Oxford: Blackwell.

Girard, N. (2008) 'Practice-based evidence', *AORN* 87(1): 15–16.

Greenhalgh, T. (2001) *How to Read a Paper: The Basics of Evidence-based Medicine*, London: BMJ Publishing.

Greenwood, J. (1998) 'The role of reflection in single and double loop learning', *Journal of Advanced Nursing* 27: 1048–53.

Harvey, S., Snowdon, C. and Elbourne, D. (2008) 'Effectiveness of bereavement interventions in neonatal intensive care: a review of the evidence', *Seminars in Fetal and Neonatal Medicine* 13: 341–56.

Henley, A. and Schott, J. (2008) 'The death of a baby before, during or shortly after birth: good practice from the parents' perspective', *Seminars in Fetal and Neonatal Medicine* 13: 325–8.

Jasper, M. (2006) *Professional Development, Reflection and Decision-making*, Oxford: Blackwell Publishing.

Jenicek, M. (2006) 'The hard art of soft science: evidence-based medicine, reasoned medicine or both?' *Journal of Evaluation in Clinical Practice* 12(4): 410–19.

Jennings, B.M. and Loan, L.A. (2001) 'Misconceptions among nurses about evidence-based practice', *Journal of Nursing Scholarship* 33(2): 127.

Kendall, A. and Guo, W. (2008) 'Evidence-based neonatal bereavements care', *Newborn and Infant Nursing Reviews* 8(3): 131–5.

King, L. and Appleton, J.V. (1997) 'Intuition: a critical review of the research and rhetoric', *Journal of Advanced Nursing* 26: 194–202.

Larroque, B., Breart, G., Kaminski, M., Dehan, M., Andre, M., Burguet, A., Grandjean, H., Ledesert, B., Leveque, C., Maillard, F., Matis, J., Roze, J.C. and Truffert, P., on behalf of the Epipage study group (2004) 'Survival of very preterm infants: Epipage, a population-based cohort study', *Archives of Disease in Childhood Fetal and Neonatal Edition* 89: 139–44.

Lindberg, B., Axelsson, K. and Ohrling, K. (2008) 'Adjusting to being a father to an infant born prematurely: experiences from Swedish fathers', *Journal Compilations*, Copyright 2008 Nordic College of Caring Science.

Lindsay, B. (2007) *Understanding Research and Evidence-based Practice*, London: Routledge.

Manias, E., Aitken, R. and Dunning, T. (2004) 'Decision-making models used by "graduate nurses" managing patients' medications', *Journal of Advanced Nursing* 47(3): 270–8.

Mantzoukas, S. (2007) 'A review of evidence-based practice, nursing research and reflection: levelling the hierarchy', *Journal of Clinical Nursing*. Journal Compilation. Copyright Blackwell Publishing Ltd. Doi: 10.1111/j.1365-2702.2006.01912.x.

Mulhall, A. (1998) 'Nursing research and evidence', *Evidence-based Nursing* 1(1): 6. Downloaded from www.ebn.bmj.com on 24 September 2008.

National Institute for Health and Clinical Excellence (2005) *A Guide to NICE*. Available at www.nice.org.uk.

Nursing and Midwifery Council (2008) *The NMC Code of Professional Conduct: Standards For Conduct, Performance and Ethics*, London: NMC.

Payot, A., Gendron, S., Lefebvre, F. and Doucet, H. (2007) 'Deciding to resuscitate extremely premature babies: how do parents and neonatologists engage in the decision?' *Social Sciences and Medicine* 64: 1487–500.

Proctor, S. (1998) 'Linking philosophy and method in the research process: the case for realism', *Nurse Researcher* 5(4): 73–90.

Raynor, M.D., Marshall, J.E. and Sullivan, A. (2005) *Decision-making in Midwifery Practice*, Oxford: Elsevier-Churchill Livingstone.

Redshaw, M. and Hamilton, K. (2005) *A Survey of Current Neonatal Units Organisation and Policy* (commissioned by BLISS), London: NPEU Publications.

Rew, L. (2000) 'Acknowledging intuition in clinical decision-making', *Journal of Holistic Nursing* 18: 94–108.

Rolfe, G. and Fulbrook, G. (1998) *Advanced Nursing Practice*, Oxford: Butterworth-Heinemann.

Rycroft-Malone, J., Seers, K., Titchen, A., Harvey, G., Kitson, A. and McCormack, B. (2004) 'What counts as evidence in evidence-based practice?' *Journal of Advanced Nursing* 47(1): 81–90.

Sackett, D.L., Rosenberg, W.M., Gray, J.A., Haynes, R.B. and Richardson, W.S. (1996) 'Evidence based medicine: what it is and what it isn't', *British Medical Journal* 312: 71–2.

Shieh, C. (2006) 'Practice-based evidence', *The Association of Women's Health, Obstetric and Neonatal Nurses* 10(5): 375–8.

Sing-Ling Tsai and Sin-Kuo Chai (2005) 'Developing and validating a nursing website evaluation questionnaire', *Journal of Advanced Nursing* 49(4): 406–13.

Swinkels, A., Albarran, J.W., Means, R.I., Mitchell, T. and Stewart, M.C. (2002) 'Evidence-based practice in health and social care: where are we now?' *Journal of Interprofessional Care* 16(4): 335–47.

Thompson, C. (2003) 'Clinical experience as evidence in evidence-based practice', *Journal of Advanced Nursing* 43(3): 230–7.

Thompson, C. and Dowding, D. (2002) *Clinical Decision-making and Judgement in Nursing*, London: Churchill Livingstone.

Wigert, H., Johansson, R. and Berg, M. (2006) 'Mothers' experiences of having their newborn child in a neonatal intensive care unit', *Scandinavian Journal of Caring Science* 20: 35–41.

Website

www.healthtalkonline.org/InterviewTranscript.aspx?interview=763&Clip=0 (available online, accessed 6 November 2008).

Chapter 2

Developmentally Focused Nursing Care

Tilly Reid and Yvonne Freer

Contents

Introduction

The term 'developmental care' is used to describe broadly those interventions which support and facilitate the stabilisation, recovery and development of infants and families undergoing intensive care, and beyond, in an effort to promote optimal outcome. The theoretical basis for current understanding stems from both animal and clinical studies. Animal studies provide evidence of positive and negative early experiences altering the structure and function of the developing brain (Anand and Scalzo 2000), while clinical studies show that infants admitted to a Neonatal Intensive Care Unit (NICU) are at increased risk of medical complications, neurological impairment and a range of more subtle cognitive and behavioural deficits (Fasting 1995; Perlman 2001; Ment *et al.* 2003; Salt and Redshaw 2006). The increasing survival of **low birth weight** (LBW) infants and particularly those at the limits of viability has created new challenges and there remains an urgent need to explore strategies which support optimal outcome.

While illness and treatments may have adverse effects on the rapidly developing brain, the environment of care, e.g. the neonatal intensive care unit, is in itself a source of stress for **preterm** infants and their families. Although it is accepted that fetal development and in-utero experience may not be the appropriate theoretical model for our understanding of the newborn environment and the delivery of care, it seems appropriate to mimic the uterine environment where practically possible in infants born preterm. However, delivering critical care in such circumstances is complex and it is important to acknowledge the difficulties of combining the 'art' and 'science', the technological treatments and the humanitarian acts of nurture and how they can be combined to best effect. Apart from the management of the infant, psychosocial support of the parents and extended family/friends can be seen in the ways we deliver family-centred care, for example, promoting breastfeeding, parent–infant attachment and dealing with anxiety, depression or hostility (Harrison 1993).

It is difficult to determine the effects of the environment, treatments, pathology and particular intervention strategies in a straightforward cause and effect way. So far, the evidence from large-scale trials is scarce and equivocal (Symington 2006), yet it is generally agreed that efforts to nurture, comfort, protect and advocate for fragile patients are worthwhile. This has implications for investment in training, environmental modification, equipment and other resources. Developmental care is thus viewed as an expansion of neonatology in which evolving infant and family systems interface with the biological, environmental and psycho-emotional risks of preterm birth.

Theoretical approaches to developmentally focused care

Developmental support programmes/interventions have been guided by different theoretical models, and approaches have varied from single interventions to initiatives based on observations or assessment (Goldson 1999). They have generally aimed to deliver one or more of the following outcomes:

- interventions which counteract sensory overload or deprivation, for example, reducing stress responses or promoting positive sensory experiences;
- interventions which aim to help parents to resolve the emotional crisis of preterm birth and promote maternal–infant attachment;
- interventions that help parents to be more sensitive and responsive to their infant's behaviour and improve social interactions, practical care-giving or confidence;
- interventions aimed at infants and families with diagnosed developmental delay or chronic illness.

Sensory overload/deprivation

One approach views the infant as an 'extra-uterine fetus' with the assumption that after birth, development is likely to progress as it would prior to birth. From this perspective, the NICU is seen as being overly stimulating compared to the natural uterine environment. To limit the effects of the NICU, proponents of this approach advocate minimal handling and reduced sensory input. This protection from potential hazard, for example, loud sound and bright lighting, is thought to reduce the stress response and thus promote greater stability and increased tolerance of handling. An alternative approach is that the infant's developmental trajectory differs considerably after birth and progress is inherently and inevitably different, regardless of gestation. As the infant is deprived of appropriate in-utero sensory input, additional stimulation is provided in an effort to improve outcome. Some studies have used a single intervention: auditory (maternal voice, heartbeat sounds), tactile (massage, stroking), visual (mobiles, facial presentation), or vestibular (oscillating cot, waterbed, rocking) while others have used a combination of strategies (Liu *et al.* 2007).

Applying the findings from these studies is difficult due to the variations in sample size and distribution, the wide range of interventions and the different short- and long-term outcomes. A systematic review of developmental care by Symington and Pinelli (2006) highlighted small improvements in the severity of chronic conditions in experimental groups, but the findings were inconclusive regarding cognitive improvements.

The developmental needs of preterm infants are complex, as they attempt to balance their lack of fetal experiences with the hazards of treatments necessary for survival. Current understanding would suggest that both approaches have merit depending upon the individual infant's medical condition, age and developmental agenda, and the environment of care.

Key point

In practice, while modifications to the environment may be generally beneficial, their appropriateness in individual circumstances must be continually assessed.

Parent–infant attachment

The feto-maternal and maternal–infant relationship is also in deficit and requires consideration from a developmental perspective. Maternal role development depends upon self-esteem and mastery of natural mothering behaviours and these are unlikely to proceed appropriately in the circumstances of having a sick newborn infant and the ensuing period of intensive care (Reid 2000; Fenwick *et al.* 2001). Family-centred models of care have considerably improved the situation of parents who were often excluded from care-giving and care planning decisions, but there is still much that can be done to support the development of healthy relationships which are crucial to the success of newborn intensive care and the goal of optimal outcomes in the longer term. Parental education on how to support their infant's emerging developmental agenda is increasingly regarded as an essential component of developmentally focused care (Melnyk *et al.* 2006). By understanding infant behaviour, parents can observe more closely the individuality of their infant, become able to 'reset' their own expectations of infant behaviour and development and thus offer more infant-led support.

Brazelton (1973) was among the first to note the highly organised term infant's abilities to be active participants and social partners who affect care-giving behaviours. Als (1982) observed that preterm infants, although less organised, were similarly competent for their stage of development. She proposed a dynamic model for preterm infant behavioural organisation, known as the synactive theory of development, which identified subsystems (autonomic, motor, state, attention-interactional and regulatory) of functioning which interact with each other and are influenced by the infant's internal and external environment. This model provides a basis with which to understand preterm infant behaviour, assess subsystems functioning and thus identify the emerging developmental goals. Utilising the synactive theory improves the scope for facilitative parent teaching, as parents learn to understand the individuality of their infant and ways in which they can offer support which promotes stability and development.

In order to incorporate developmentally focused care, practitioners must have knowledge of preterm infant developmental theory, be able to assess behaviours and interpret their meaning in the context of internal and external factors. In addition, it is essential that practitioners are able to determine and deliver an appropriate plan of care, have the resources to deliver the required strategy and the ability to evaluate its effectiveness.

Key point

With increased understanding of developmental theory and systematic behavioural assessment, the emphasis of developmental care moves towards a more individualised and holistic approach, rather than the general introduction of developmentally supportive initiatives, such as modifying the environment or the provision of positioning aids. Nevertheless, both approaches are important; there are many initiatives of a general nature which will facilitate developmental stability, but individualised assessment will highlight the emerging agenda for the infant and enable care to be delivered according to infant cues. Advocacy is a fundamental principle of nursing care, and the ability to communicate effectively with parents, the extended family and friends is an essential component.

Behaviour

The following themes identified from the literature and various practical initiatives are likely to support the goal of improved medical and developmental outcomes for infants undergoing intensive care, or enhance parent–infant interaction and subsequent psychosocial relationships:

- behavioural assessment;
- recognition and appropriate management of distress and pain;
- the reduction of environmental hazard;
- the promotion of contingent handling;
- postural support;
- family-centred, developmentally focused models of care.

Well **term** newborns have stable autonomic and motor systems function and rapidly acquire distinct state system organisation. Sleep and drowsy states predominate, but term infants can achieve quiet and active alert states as well as fussy, irritable and lusty crying states. They can be readily consoled and satisfied and are able to 'shut out' stimulation for rest and sleep. The emerging task of the term newborn is for increasing time in alert states with growing differentiation and responsiveness. An active and responsive social partner is essential to support this development which should be rewarding and stimulating for both participants and supportive of an increasing interest in the external world. The capacity of the infant for active participation in developing and maintaining a relationship with others and thus affecting his social environment and his emerging developmental agenda is described by Brazelton and colleagues (1973, 1984; Brazelton and Nugent 1995).

Als (1982) was among the first to assert that preterm infants also had distinct behavioural patterns and that it was possible to assess and interpret them. Preterm infants, while driven by the similar goals of stability and organisation, are at a stage of development which is more concerned with their internal world. They have immature systems organisation and their behaviours are consequently more diffuse and less stable. The autonomic subsystem, demonstrable through respiratory, cardiovascular and digestive function, often requires support to enable stable functioning and this stability is likely to be under duress when challenged by handling, environmental disturbance, pain and illness. Stability and organisation in all other subsystems depend upon autonomic stability and in this model it can be viewed as the basis for more complex, hierarchical developmental tasks. The motor system, demonstrable through muscle tone, posture and movements, is the second emerging subsystem. Preterm infants have reduced muscle bulk and power and an immature central nervous system which inhibits smoothness and purposefulness of movement and may result in a flattened and extended posture.

Sleeping and waking states represent a level of maturity of the central nervous system, the infant's relationship with the external environment and the ability to regulate and stabilise underlying internal systems. By 24 weeks' gestation, cycling between sleeping and waking can be identified by EEG (Hellstrom-Wetas *et al.* 1991) and by 28 weeks, these states are distinct (Holditch-Davis 1990). Prior to 36 weeks' gestation, there is poor co-ordination between states and with decreasing gestation, behaviours which demonstrate particular states are increasingly difficult to identify, even by trained observers. State transitions are diffuse, erratic and more easily influenced by internal and external stressors. Preterm newborns spend greater amounts of time in light sleep or drowsy states and have difficulty in achieving deep sleep. Deep sleep and quiet alertness, when infants are socially responsive, are rarely observed in NICU conditions and require facilitation from contingent handling and environmental manipulation. The active alert state which is usually generated by care-giving regimens may result in hyper-alertness and arousal followed by system collapse/compromise.

Two additional subsystems, the attention-interactional and the regulatory subsystems, are the final components of the synactive theory of development (Als 1982). Attention and interaction are assessed when the infant is in alert state and regulation is an assessment of the infant's success in achieving a balance in the subsystems. Each subsystem can be described independently but it is the processes of subsystems' interaction or synaction combined with the infant's interaction with their environment which completes the developmental theory. With experience and reflection, practitioners can begin to assess the attention-interactional and regulatory abilities of infants, but careful assessment of the autonomic, motor and state subsystems can provide sufficient knowledge of an individual's developmental agenda to determine appropriate interventions in most practical situations.

Reflective exercise

Note the infant in light sleep who, upon handling, immediately becomes hyper-alert and agitated with extensor postures and 'panicked' facial expression. Note also the difficulty in achieving quiet, alert state with responsive and animated facial expression. The observer has the additional problem of being unable to detect distinct states due to the infant's immature behaviours and the environment in which the infant is unlikely to give his best performance.

Sleep–wake state scoring systems

There are several sleep–wake scoring systems, based on careful observations of term and preterm infants (see Table 2.1). The Neonatal Behavioural Assessment Scale (NBAS) (Brazelton 1973) catalogued detailed definitions of infants' behavioural states. The scores are used to determine predominant states, transitions between states and the quality of alertness. It has the advantage of being widely used in research and clinical practice and is relatively easy to use due to the distinct definitions (Brazelton and Nugent 1995). However, due to the small number of states described, it fails to capture the indeterminate and transitory qualities of preterm infant behavioural states.

Thoman's revised state scoring system (1990) is more sensitive and has inter-rater and test–retest reliability with preterm infants (Holditch-Davis 1990). There are ten states which differentiate state-related behaviours in preterm infants and those with perinatal complications. This system is more difficult to learn and training is not readily available, but it has been shown to have predictive validity with later developmental outcome.

Anderson's state scoring system (ABSS) was devised following earlier work with preterm infants and was used to demonstrate a relationship between heart rate, energy consumption and behavioural state (Ludington 1990). Gill *et al.* (1988) used the scale to show the effects of non-nutritive sucking on behavioural state. There are few published studies using this scale, so its reliability and validity are not well established; however, it was constructed specifically for preterm infants and was based on extensive observations of their behaviours. Although similar to other scales, it is more complex, as it takes into account physiological parameters and thus is derived from a different theoretical base (Holditch-Davis 1990). It is likely to be a useful instrument for quantitative studies into the relationships between interventions and infant state, but its use as a clinical instrument is not yet clearly defined.

Als (1982) defines behavioural state in greater detail in the Assessment of Preterm Infant Behaviour (APIB) which is a modification of the NBAS (Brazelton 1973, 1984). This scale more closely describes the state-related behaviours of preterm infants' responses to their internal and external environments and can be used with infants of very low gestational ages. The scale has been expanded to account for the immature and diffuse nature of emerging preterm state-related behaviours. As the scale is based on the NBAS, it is more familiar to researchers and clinicians, but training and supervision in its use are essential. The advantage of the system is that it is used as part of a holistic assessment and care planning programme, where state functioning is an important consideration. According to the synactive theory of development (Als 1982), stability and organisation in autonomic and motor function can support and facilitate state system stability, thus enabling the infant to engage with the external world or settle into better quality sleep states. Sleep–wake state is more difficult to assess because of the subtle definitions described; nevertheless it is essential to recognise the current functioning of this subsystem in order to protect the infant from stressors and to facilitate and support emerging competencies.

Table 2.1 Sleep–wake state scoring systems

Brazelton (1973)	Thoman (1990)	Anderson (Gill et al. 1988)	Als (1982)	Reid (2000)
1. Deep sleep	1. Quiet sleep	1. Quiet sleep, regular respiration	1B. Very still deep sleep	1. Very quiet sleep, regular respiration
2. Light sleep	2. Active–quiet transitional sleep	2. Quiet sleep, irregular respiration, slight movement	1A. Deep sleep	2. Quiet sleep, irregular respirations, slight movement
3. Drowsy	3. Active sleep	3. Active sleep, irregular respiration, movement	2B. Light sleep	3. Restless sleep, unsettled, some movement
4. Alert	4. Sleep–wake transition	4. Very active sleep, whole body movement	2A. Noisy light sleep	4. Drowsy, inattentive, some movement
5. Considerable motor activity	5. Drowsy	5. Drowsy	3A. Drowsy with activity	5. Quiet awake, calm, focused attention
6. Crying	6. Daze	6. Alert, slight movement, fixated eyes	3B. Drowsy	6. Restless awake, irregular respirations, suck searching, some movement
	7. Alert	7. Quiet awake, no movement	4A. Quiet awake or hyperalert	7. Fussing, grunting, increased movement
	8. Non-alert waking	8. Awake, some movement	4B. Bright alert	8. Crying, facial grimace, tongue or jaw tremor
	9. Fuss	9. Awake, whole body movement	5A. Active	
	10. Crying	10. Fussing, prolonged exhalation	5B. Considerable activity	
		11. Crying	6A. Crying	
		12. Hard crying, clenched fists	6B. Lusty crying	

A modified sleep–wake assessment which has practical validity and 95 per cent inter-rater reliability with experienced nurses has been developed by Reid (2000). Although it is less sensitive than other preterm sleep–wake assessments, it can be readily utilised in general practice with minimal training and supervision.

Behavioural assessment

Behaviours fall into two categories: stress or avoidance signals, where the stimulation is beyond the infant's capacity to assimilate and approach, or stability signals, where the behaviours demonstrate organisation or self-regulatory activity (Table 2.2). Approach signals inform the observer of the infant's current stable functioning and point to the next level of developmental goals.

Behaviours should be assessed before, during and following handling activity. It is important to take note of the context of the intervention, including the responses of the infant to care-giving and the influences of the environment. A developmental review should therefore consist of observations of infant behaviour, an assessment of the current level of functioning and recommendations which support stability within the infant's immediate environment of care. Wider developmental issues such as modifications to the environment at large, education of staff and parents, and institutional awareness, all have an impact on the ability to integrate developmentally focused care, but careful, systematic observation is pivotal to its success.

Reflective exercise

Consider the fetal environment: consistent temperature, gravitational support and containment, attenuated light and sound, and subtle nutritional, hormonal and psychological influences Now consider the postnatal environment.

The NICU environment

The birth of any infant presents a dramatic change in environment. The well full-term infant is ready for the transition to extra-uterine life and quickly adapts with increasing interest in it (Trevarthen 2004). In contrast, the immaturity of physiological systems in the preterm infant makes this transition difficult and consequently the complex environment of the NICU becomes overly stimulating, creating a state of sensory overload in the infant.

While there are several sources of stress, of particular concern are non-contingent or aversive handling events and the effect of sound and light on the

Table 2.2 Stress and stability signals

Stress signals	Stability and organisation signals
Autonomic system	**Autonomic system**
Respiratory pause, tachypnoea, gagging, gasping or sighing	Stable heart rate, respiratory rate, oxygenation and colour
Colour, vascular and visceral changes	Tolerance of enteral feeds
Tremor, twitch or startle	
Posit, vomit or hiccough	
Bowel strain	
Cough, sneeze or yawn	
Motor system	**Motor system**
Flaccidity of trunk, extremities or face (gape face)	Smooth, well-modulated movements
Hypertonicity – extension of legs, arms, head and neck, fingers, trunk arching, facial grimace, tongue extension	Relaxed postures and tone, with increasing flexion towards mid-line
Hyperflexion – trunk, limbs, fists, feet, neck	Mobility and efficient self-regulatory activity, e.g. ■ hand and foot clasping ■ hand-to-mouth activity ■ grasping and handholding
Protective manoeuvres – hand on face, salute, high guard arm position	
Frantic, diffuse activity	Suck searching and sucking
Fixed, stereotypical postures	
State system	**State system**
Diffuse, oscillating sleep–wake state, whimper or high-pitched cry	Clear, robust sleep states
Strained or irritable fussiness or cry, lack of consolability	Clear, robust, rhythmic cry
	Ability to self-quiet or to be consoled
Eye floating or staring, lack of facial expression, strained or panicked alertness Active averting	Alert, intent or animated facial expression
	Focused wide-eyed alertness

sensory modalities of hearing and vision which are particularly immature in the preterm infant. The greater the degree of immaturity, the more injurious the physical environment may be, leading to undesirable fluctuations in heart rate, respiratory rate, blood pressure, motor and state systems stability (Blackburn and Vandenberg 1993) and possible maladaption. The goal of nursing care then is to create a physical environment and approach to care-giving interventions that support the infant's physiological and neurodevelopmental needs.

There are recommendations for newborn intensive care unit design, including the structure, lighting, noise control, infection control, family space and other considerations (White 2006). In general, these suggest that there are many practical ways in which subdued calmness and appropriate care-giving can be achieved without making structural changes. The general atmosphere of a unit can be gradually modified as practitioners become more aware of infant reactions, but this requires a reflective and creative approach by both medical and nursing staff; for example, Slevin et al. (2000) showed that introducing a 'quiet period' modified staff behaviour and reduced ambient noise levels. These changes, however, had little effect on the infant's physiological state but there was an increase in infant restfulness.

Sound hazard

Sound is heard in two dimensions: pitch (frequency) and loudness (decibels). The timing of auditory maturation does not appear to be altered by preterm birth (Graven 2000); however, unlike the fetus, the NICU infant is not protected by the maternal tissues and amniotic fluid which significantly attenuate both high and low frequency sounds. The auditory experience is therefore very different, and greater care is needed to protect infants.

Concerns in the preterm infant relating to sound exposure are: repeated arousal of the infant causing problems with physiological stability and an inability to achieve relaxed sleep and alertness (Morris et al. 2000), alteration in the recognition and integration of sound (Therien et al. 2004), damage to the cilia of the developing cochlea and the increasing susceptibility to hearing loss in infants exposed to both continuous loud sound and **ototoxic** drugs, for example, aminoglycosides (Graven 2000). While the literature focuses on immediate and medium-term effects of sound, there is little evidence on consequences of sound on long-term development or on the optimal sound level for stability (Morris et al. 2000; Barreto et al. 2006). Graven (2000) advocates that sound levels should be kept to 50dB or less and with the co-operation of the whole team it is possible to modify sound bursts over this level. However, careful monitoring and audit are needed and there also needs to be a commitment to amend the physical environment where required.

Equipment manufacturers are taking into consideration incubator and alarm noise, and bins with softly closing lids are available. Telephones and nursing stations should be located outside the immediate clinical vicinity. Large, sparsely furnished rooms tend to be more resonant but these can be modified by the use of thick curtaining, clinical grade carpeting and noise-absorbent ceiling tiles. Soft furnishings have the advantage of appearing more home-like and less clinical, which will help to alleviate parental anxieties (Padden and Glenn 1997). Smaller nurseries with four to six cots per room have lower activity levels than larger rooms and can provide a more intimate and private atmosphere for parents and staff. A separate admission area may prevent other infants from being subjected to frequent bursts of activity.

The provision of auditory stimulation in the form of a softly modulated voice when the infant is receptive can help to promote alertness. Parents have described seeing their infant respond to their voice by turning, eye opening, calming or becoming animated as a powerful emotional event, which helps them to feel closer to their infant (ibid.). Other forms of auditory stimulation such as musical toys can be inappropriate, particularly if left inside the incubator to be switched on by staff who are not vigilant about contingent stimulation. Graven (2000) suggests that recorded sound should not be used in NICU.

Light hazard

Light is measured in two ways: illuminance (the amount of light measured in lux), and irradiance (the kind of light measured in $\mu W/cm^2/nm$). In NICUs, lighting levels are variable with some units providing continuous high-intensity light and others reduced levels with diurnal patterning. Infants may also be exposed to additional amounts of light from their proximity to windows and the use of medical equipment and procedural lamps.

While there are no studies showing adverse long-term effects of exposure to variable levels of lighting. it does have an impact on physiological stability and circadian rhythm development. Bright lighting conditions in the NICU appear to affect the sleep–wake state, causing arousal and producing stress-like responses in the infant (Mann et al. 1986; Blackburn and Patteson 1991; Shogan and Schumann 1993). Preterm infants are unable to shut out stimulation for rest and sleep and are unable to achieve wide-eyed alertness unless environmental conditions are modified. If sleep–wake state is carefully observed under dimmed lighting conditions, it becomes apparent that this environment can improve the quality of sleep and promote alert states. Under bright and constant lighting, infants' autonomic and motor systems are likely to be aroused and they may remain in transitional states with closed eyes, neither deeply asleep nor available for social contact.

The lighting of clinical areas is an important environmental consideration. Practitioners need to balance the need for soft lighting to promote rest and sleep and support alertness with the need for close observation of the infant. Bright, overhead lighting is inappropriate for the needs of fragile preterm infants who are unable to shut out the stimulation if they remain unprotected. Dimmer switches should be fitted to overhead lights to modify lighting conditions. Spotlights or anglepoise lighting can be utilised to illuminate a particular cot space, which prevents other infants in the nursery from being exposed.

Wall-mounted up-lighters can provide ambient lighting while improving the clinical atmosphere and appearance of the nursery.

There are inevitable limits to the extent of environmental modification, particularly if it is not possible to make structural changes. It is possible, however, to focus on the immediate cotspace to reduce the impact of the clinical environment in vulnerable infants. Incubator hoods or blankets can be used to absorb noise and attenuate lighting conditions. Thick, soft blankets and quilts around the mattress have a dual purpose of promoting comfort and absorbing incubator and tubing noise. Cycled lighting appears to promote physiological stability, improved growth, increased sleep time and earlier entrainment of circadian rhythms (Mann *et al.* 1986; Shiroiwa *et al.* 1986; Brandon *et al.* 2002; Graven 2004; Rivkees 2004).

Activity, sound and lighting are reduced in order to enable infants to rest and sleep. A gradual lengthening of this period may be possible if infant behaviour is noted to improve as a result of the reduced activity. The quality of sleep and alert states should be monitored, as well as physiological parameters which suggest more stable autonomic functioning. Improved motor system stability may also be observed; tremor, startle, frantic diffuse or extensor activity should be replaced by more relaxed postures, tone and movements with self-regulatory activity.

Reflective exercise

Observe the reactions of infants in different environmental conditions. Note the circumstance which supports the infants' efforts to quieten and relax or reach alertness. Observe infant behaviour during periods of high activity and note the stress responses. Compare state system stability in relation to the environment of care.

Handling

Handling is the most direct source of stress for infants in NICU; it is a well-known hazard to which experienced nurses are well attuned. The majority of handling episodes are inevitably unpleasant, stressful or painful, and for the most vulnerable infants these experiences dominate. The more robust infants make efforts to regulate themselves by grasping, sucking and boundary searching, but the more fragile infants are unable to mount the resources needed to stabilise and organise their behaviour.

Contingent care

Handling can also be the most effective source of comfort and pleasure. Human contact, particularly parental contact, can be both stimulating and stabilising, provided that it is appropriate and the surrounding environment is conducive. The introduction of positive handling experiences is important at every stage of the infant's progress, but it is important to monitor their tolerance. Even low-key, gentle handling can cause distress if not delivered in the context of the environment or with consideration to the schedule of care. For example, it may be unreasonable to expect an infant to respond to parental contact following practical care-giving such as nappy change or feeding, when resources are depleted. Yet between the care-giving schedule, the infant may be lying quietly alert and socially available. Parents' expectations of social contact generally revolve around practical care-giving, but this may not be the most appropriate time for promoting alert and animated interaction. Lighting, sound and activity levels as well as infant preparedness must be taken into consideration prior to social handling if parent–infant interaction is to be optimised. Parents should be encouraged to spend time observing their infants, to become accustomed to their individuality, as an important first step towards contingent interaction. With guidance, many parents could develop observational skills which would support practical care-giving, and similarly, parents who are unable to provide direct care can still have an important role to play, being better equipped to advocate for their infants. Parents may be more sensitive to their infant's needs, which is a sound basis for better quality interaction, and may help to improve maternal self-esteem.

Handling stress can be reduced by incorporating measures to stabilise the infant's status and minimising the risk of overloading their capacity to assimilate events. Infants frequently demonstrate less stress responses in contained, flexed postures as motor stability is achieved and underlying physiological stress responses are minimised. Autonomic and motor stability can be supported by hands-on containment, concave nests with deep boundaries or swaddling and by maintaining flexed, mid-line postures and head support while performing cares. These techniques provide greater opportunity for the infant to tolerate the intervention without aversion, stress or total systems collapse. In the most fragile infants undergoing hazardous interventions, it may be necessary for two people to perform the intervention: one to maintain flexed containment, and one to deliver the treatment or care. This approach to handling can have a marked effect on systems' stability and reflecting on the comparative outcomes of different handling techniques is a worthwhile exercise.

Autonomic stability can be supported by gently introducing the handling episode through voice and soft touch, in order to prevent immediate stress responses; this may also help to prevent the infant from remaining in a constant state of partial arousal or exhaustion.

The environment and schedule of care are also important for the more mature and robust infants; consider, for example, oral feeding. The organisation and energy required for feeding success are considerable and infant efforts can be considerably supported by ensuring that they are in optimal readiness. Any source of stress, for example, vigorous handling or background activity, can provoke failure as the behavioural organisation fails to cope with the additional demands.

In order to support the infant's responsiveness to social handling, it is essential that we schedule care which is realistic for the infant's abilities and which supports the parents' needs. This will often require teaching parents to adjust their expectations and to understand their infant's need for low-key, unimodal interaction.

Postural support

Preterm infants are unable to counteract the effects of gravity and without support will develop imbalance between active and passive muscle tone, stereotypical head, shoulder and hip flattening which in turn, leads to problems with mobility (de Groot *et al.* 1995; Monterosso *et al.* 2002). This results in an inability to engage in self-regulatory behaviours such as exploration of the face and mouth, hand and foot clasping, boundary searching and flexion and extension of the limbs. Thus persistent flattened postures cause a cycle of reduced mobility, inhibiting opportunities for self-regulation and developmental exploration (Fay 1988; Hunter 1996). Suboptimal movement and activity may result in abnormal neuronal connectivity and poor or delayed motor system development. The development of crawling, walking and fine motor skills may be directly influenced by mobility in the neonatal period (Fay 1988).

Furthermore, infants who are unable to maintain flexed postures or summon protective manoeuvres may remain in autonomic arousal at a cost to their energy and oxygen expenditure and systems' stability. The goals of postural support are therefore multidimensional:

- to support physiological stability;
- to prevent **abduction** or rotated postures of shoulders and hips and flattening of the head;
- to prevent pressure damage from persistent stereotypical or favoured positions;
- to promote mobility and motor systems' stability and development;
- to facilitate protective manoeuvres and self-regulatory behaviours.

It is essential to support the infant in a range of positions in order to promote optimum outcome. Flexed, mid-line containment in side-lying and **supine** postures is ideal, and some form of hip and shoulder elevation in prone positions will help to reduce flattening. Various commercial products are available for swaddling, nesting and stabilising positions, but 'home-made' resources can be equally effective (Figure 2.1).

(a)

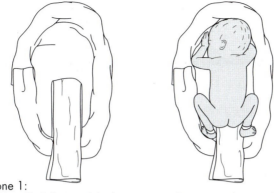

Prone 1:
Softly rolled sheet or blanket positioned in a complete circle. One smaller softly rolled sheet placed over the sheet circle and cover sheet, folded to support pelvic and thoracic lift. Arms and shoulders can be elevated to improve lung function, or fixed and tucked under the thorax. An additional cover may be needed to tuck under the nesting sheet. This serves to draw the nest closer into the infant, supporting flexed containment.

(b)

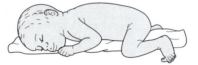

Prone 2:
Nappy roll length-wise under the body from head to hips. This may require additional rolls or blankets across the baby. The head can be supported at an oblique angle, if tolerated.

(c)

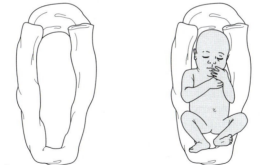

Supine 1:
Soft blanket or sheet rolled into a nest encourages flexion of lower limbs, brings shoulders forward and keeps the head in mid-line. If this continues round the contours of the head it may promote comfort. A small degree of neck flexion, if tolerated, can provide greater stability.

Figure 2.1 **Postural support: (a, b) prone position; (c) supine position (continued overleaf)**
Source: Redrawn from positioning chart provided by the Edinburgh Sick Children's NHS Trust, courtesy of Maureen Grant, Superintendent Physiotherapist

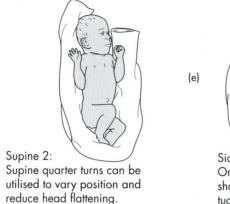

(d)

Supine 2:
Supine quarter turns can be
utilised to vary position and
reduce head flattening.

(e)

Side-lying:
One firmly rolled blanket in a 'U'
shape. May need to be supported by
tucked covers. Note the opportunity
for tactile and visual stimulation in this
position.

Figure 2.1 (d) supine position; (e) side-lying position
Source: Redrawn from positioning chart provided by the Edinburgh Sick Children's NHS Trust,
courtesy of Maureen Grant, Superintendent Physiotherapist.

Key point

Physiological stability is the prime goal of nursing the acute or chronically ill
infant and any postural intervention should be considered not only for its
intrinsic value but also for optimising this subsystem stability.

Equipment

Many infants also benefit from a soft head boundary. When in supine postures,
the head can be supported to enable occipital lying, the only position which
helps to reduce the incidence and severity of head flattening (Cartlidge and
Rutter 1988). This can be achieved by the use of a soft roll or small sheet closely
contouring the head, but loose enough to ensure some mobility. The use of neck
rolls should be avoided as they may damage the delicate vessels at the back of
the neck and may cause neck extension and may alter cerebral blood flow. The
sheet can be fixed in position by gently tucking it under the shoulders. This
elevation will help the shoulders to fall naturally into mid-line and support
mobility of the upper limbs. Cushioned mattressing or gel pillows will provide
a 'nesting' effect; the gentle indentation supports flexion and containment, and
reduces the gravity effect on pressure areas.

Prone position

Prone positions are frequently utilised when infants are undergoing respiratory support or recovering from respiratory illness as oxygenation and lung expansion are optimised (Mendoza *et al.* 1991; Heimler *et al.* 1992). As infants recover, prone positions are normally replaced in accordance with the recommendations for reducing the risk of sudden infant death syndrome by supine or side-lying postures. In prone postures, gravity has its greatest effect. The head is always on one side or the other, and hips are forced into abduction and rotation as the infant cannot maintain elevation or lower limb flexion under the pelvis. Shoulders are forced into the mattress, particularly if there is any pelvic elevation and the mattress is flat. Although the lower parts of the limbs can mobilise, mobility is considerably reduced without postural support in the prone position. If the mattress is elevated to aid respiratory function, it can reduce the pressure effects on the shoulders, neck and head. However, it also forces the infant to slide down the cot where lower limbs are cramped against the fixed cot boundary. Support around the buttocks can help to fix the infant in a stable prone position.

Pelvic elevation has been advocated by Downs *et al.* (1991) to prevent hip abduction and rotation and promote lower limb flexion. However, care must be taken to ensure that the infant's weight is not transferred to the femur and knee, as this may cause other problems with hip development (Dunn 1991). Hip slings have been used to fix the lower body in position and provide some degree of pelvic elevation, but they do not prevent hip abduction. Small pillows or rolls can be placed under the infant's pelvis and trunk to elevate the hips and thus enable some protraction of the lower limbs. It is important to ensure that the elevation does not cause respiratory embarrassment, that the infant appears relaxed and comfortable, the weight of the body is evenly distributed and limbs are mobile. Small pillows or gel mattresses can also be used to elevate the upper trunk to allow for some shoulder and hip protraction around it. Similarly, simply elevating the shoulders from the mattress gives some scope for supporting the head and neck at an oblique angle to prevent persistent side-lying.

Supine position

Although supine lying with mid-line occipital support is the position which best promotes mobility, it is associated with decreased ventilation and increased energy expenditure in some early studies, and is therefore more frequently utilised in the mature and stable infant (Martin *et al.* 1979; Masterson *et al.* 1987). These studies should be interpreted with some caution as supine positions were frequently unsupported; that is, infants were not necessarily supported in centralised flexed postures as would be the case today. This position requires some degree of 'nesting' around the infant boundary in order to maintain head, shoulders, pelvis and limbs in mid-line flexion. A small degree of hip and shoulder elevation from the boundary will promote limb mobility, support mid-line alignment and facilitate self-regulatory behaviours such as hand-to-mouth activity. This can be achieved by a combination of nesting into soft bedding, and the use of close, flexible boundaries around the infant's entire body. The lower limbs should be supported in flexed postures, but as limb mobility is facilitated in this position, opportunities for stretching and extending should be provided. Often limbs can be found draped over the boundary, but this does not mean that they no longer need boundary support. They are, in fact, being supported well enough to flex and extend at will while utilising some degree of shoulder and pelvic support. The effects of gravitational pressure are more evenly distributed in the supine mid-line position, and the pressure on the occipital region should ensure a more rounded head shape.

Side-lying position

Side-lying postures tend to minimise hip and shoulder rotation and abduction. Limbs should be adducted and flexed towards the mid-line axis (**adduction**). This posture can be maintained by swaddling in soft, flannelette sheeting. The infant's back should be rounded, and may require some boundary support from a small rolled sheet or towel.

It is essential that boundaries are flexible to closely follow the contours of the body. **Anteriorly**, the infant may benefit from the placement of a soft toy or filled silicone glove within reach of the hands but away from the face. This will provide an opportunity for grasping and tactile stimulation and may encourage flexion towards the object. Side-lying can also be used to treat unilateral lung disease with better oxygenation being achieved by positioning the 'good' lung uppermost (Heaf *et al.* 1983).

Key point

Attention to detail in positional care is crucial to the dual goals of prevention of postural deformity and the facilitation of self-regulation and mobility. It is important to ensure that side-lying and supine postures are utilised and position changes are planned to incorporate a varied range of positions (see Figure 2.1). It is also essential to assess the effectiveness of the intervention by ensuring that the infant tolerates the new position and that it supports both mobility and comfort.

Developmental models of care

In order to fully utilise developmental knowledge, it is essential to incorporate theoretical concepts and practical skills into the model of care. This will ensure that experienced practitioners convey their values to less experienced team members and developmental practice is regarded as an essential component of neonatal nursing care. Effective documentation will ensure that care-planning decisions are based on careful assessment, and implementation is continued over shift changes. Issues such as mobility, sensory, comfort and communication needs are thus considered to be as important as physiological needs and developmental considerations become fundamental to neonatal care. As these issues are incorporated into practice, it is important to evaluate the outcomes, for both individuals and populations. Documentary evidence of the effects of the implementation of a particular strategy, such as reference to more stable functioning, provides the justification for its continuation in a plan of care. Audit of longer-term outcomes such as ventilator days, days on oxygen, days to full feeds and days to discharge, may provide the evidence which will support further investment and practice development in a wide range of strategies and interventions.

The support of parent–infant relationships is perhaps the most important developmental intervention of all, as it is this relationship which will have the greatest impact on long-term developmental outcome. Developmental models of care must therefore place the emotional and educational needs of parents at the centre of practice. This means going beyond the practical care-giving approach and providing structured support for behavioural observation and contingent handling skills development. Parents should be encouraged to actively contribute to care-planning decisions and be fully informed and supported as partners in care. In addition, mothers of infants undergoing intensive care are known to suffer from particular psycho-emotional difficulties associated with loss of self-esteem, guilt, anger and blame (Padden and Glenn 1997). Many may need help to express these feelings in order to recover and proceed with the tasks of caring for their infant, while at the same time resuming daily responsibilities (see p. 48).

Communicating with parents is clearly an important aspect of nursing care and a developmentally focused model should ensure minimal levels of communication are routinely incorporated and documented, for example, teaching plans, interaction support, crisis interviews, practical and social problems and discharge planning. Semi-formal interviews with parents can reveal many underlying difficulties, but these are unlikely to be revealed if communication consists of opportunistic conversation at the cotside, with the multitude of distractions and lack of privacy. This model of care therefore advocates a prearranged meeting with parents on a regular basis, where information giving, decision-making and evaluation can take place with nurses who are familiar with the infant and family.

It can be seen that infant and family are at the centre of this model (Figure 2.2). However, some of the considerations apply to the infant and educational issues clearly apply only to parents. Sensory and comfort needs and emotional and communication needs can apply to both. All should be assessed to see if they require intervention, then planned, implemented and evaluated according to individual requirements.

The model does not have to differentiate between a need, problem or potential problem if they are regarded as systematic considerations. All aspects

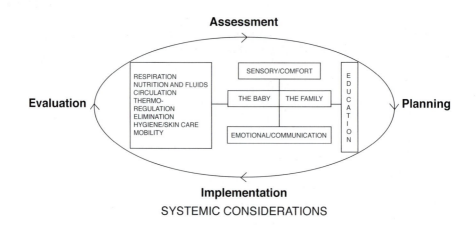

Assessment

RESPIRATION
NUTRITION AND FLUIDS
CIRCULATION
THERMO-
REGULATION
ELIMINATION
HYGIENE/SKIN CARE
MOBILITY

SENSORY/COMFORT

THE BABY | THE FAMILY

EMOTIONAL/COMMUNICATION

EDUCATION

Evaluation

Planning

Implementation

SYSTEMIC CONSIDERATIONS

Figure 2.2 **Family-centred developmental model of care**

must be assessed and the appropriate strategy devised to meet the need, deal with the problem or prevent a potential problem from developing.

Documentation to support the developmental aspects of the model can be devised in the same way that clinical assessments and plans are devised. Charts can record sleep–wake state, postural support, parent interaction and teaching plans. Care plans can record behavioural assessment, interventions and evaluations. Developmental progress can thus be submitted for audit in order to evaluate the effectiveness of developmentally focused care over time and make resource decisions which will influence the future direction of practice development.

Conclusion

In summary, developmental interventions have the potential to enhance the effectiveness of neonatology by supporting traditional medical and nursing care. Although research has demonstrated the potential to improve outcome and reduce health care expenditure, there is no prescriptive approach and there are few conclusive solutions which apply in general, although modification to the environment is likely to benefit all infants and parents experiencing intensive care.

An understanding of developmental theory and knowledge of behavioural assessment will serve to promote a creative approach to individualised holistic family-centred care which reflects the fundamental values and beliefs of neonatal nursing.

References

Als, H. (1982) 'Towards a synactive theory of development: promise for the assessment of infant individuality', *Infant Mental Health Journal* 3: 229–43.

Anand, K.J.S. and Scalzo, F.M (2000) 'Can adverse neonatal experiences alter brain development and subsequent behavior?' *Biology of the Neonate* 77: 69–82.

Barreto, E.D., Morris, B.H., Philbin, M.K., Gray, L.C. and Lasky, R.E. (2006) 'Do former preterm infants remember and respond to neonatal intensive care unit noise?' *Early Human Development* 82(11): 703–7.

Blackburn, S. and Patteson, D. (1991) 'Effects of cycled lighting on activity state and cardiorespiratory function in preterm infants', *Journal of Perinatal and Neonatal Nursing* 4(4): 47–54.

Blackburn, S. and Vandenberg, K. (1993) 'Assessment and management of neonatal neurobehavioral development', in C. Kenner, L.R. Gunderson and A. Brueggemeyer (eds) *Comprehensive Neonatal Nursing Care: A Physiologic Perspective*, Philadelphia, PA: W.B. Saunders, pp. 1094–33.

Brandon, D.H., Holditch-Davis, D. and Belyea, M. (2002) 'Preterm infants born at less than 31 weeks' gestation have improved growth in cycled light compared with continuous near darkness', *Journal of Pediatrics* 140(2): 192–9.

Brazelton, T.B. (1973) *Neonatal Behavioural Assessment Scale*, London: Heinemann.

Brazelton, T.B. (1984) *Neonatal Behavioural Assessment Scale*, 2nd edn, Philadelphia, PA: J.B. Lippincott.

Brazelton, T.B. and Nugent, J.K. (1995) *Neonatal Behavioral Assessment Scale*, 3rd edn, London, Mac Keith Press.

Cartlidge, P.H.T. and Rutter, N. (1988) 'Reduction of head flattening in preterm infants', *Archives of Disease in Childhood* 63: 755–7.

De Groot, L., Hopkins, B. and Touwen, B. (1995) 'Muscle power, sitting unsupported and trunk rotation in preterm infants', *Early Human Development* 43: 37–46.

Downs, J., Edwards, A., McCormick, D. and Stewart, A. (1991) 'Effect of intervention on the development of hip posture in very preterm babies', *Archives of Disease in Childhood* 66: 797–801.

Dunn, P.M. (1991) 'Commentary: postural deformation of the newborn', *Archives of Disease in Childhood* 66: 801.

Fasting, U. (1995) 'The new iatrogenesis', in B. Lindström and N. Spencer (eds) *Social Paediatrics*, Oxford: Oxford University Press, pp. 259–70.

Fay, M.J. (1988) 'The positive effects of positioning', *Neonatal Network* 8: 23–8.

Fenwick, J., Barclay, L. and Schmeid, V. (2001) 'Struggling to mother: a consequence of inhibitive nursing interactions in the neonatal nursery', *Journal of Perinatal and Neonatal Nursing* 15(2): 49–64.

Gill, N.E., Behnke, M., Conlon, M., McNeeley, J.B. and Anderson, G.C. (1988) 'Effect of nonnutritive sucking on behavioral state in preterm infants before feeding', *Nursing Research* 37(6): 347–50.

Goldson, E. (1999) *Nurturing the Premature Infant: Developmental Interventions in the Neonatal Intensive Care Nursery*, Oxford: Oxford University Press.

Graven, S. (2000) 'The full term and premature newborn: sound and the developing infant in the NICU: conclusions and recommendations for care', *Journal of Perinatology* 20: S88–S93.

Graven, S.N. (2004) 'Early neurosensory visual development in the fetus and newborn', *Clinics in Perinatology* 31: 199–216.

Harrison, H. (1993) 'The principles for family-centered neonatal care', *Pediatrics* 92(5): 643–50.

Heaf, D.P., Helms, P., Gordon, I. and Turner, H.M. (1983) 'Postural effects of gas exchange in infants', *New England Journal of Medicine* 308: 1505–8.

Heimler, R., Langlois, J., Hodel, D., Nelin, L. and Sasidharan, P. (1992) 'Effects of positioning on the breathing pattern in premature infants', *Archives of Disease in Childhood* 67: 312–14.

Hellström-Westas, L., Rosén, I. and Svenningsen, N.W. (1991) 'Cerebral function monitoring during the first week of life in extremely small low birthweight (ESLBW) infants', *Neuropediatrics* 22(1): 27–32.

Holditch-Davis, D. (1990) 'The development of sleeping and waking states in high-risk preterm infants', *Infant Behavior and Development* 13(4): 513–31.

Hunter, J.G. (1996) 'The neonatal intensive care unit', in J. Case-Smith, A. Allen and P. Pratt (eds) *Occupational Therapy for Children*, 3rd edn, St Louis, MO: Mosby, pp. 583–631.

Liu, W.F., Laudert, S., Perkins, B., MacMillan-York, E., Martin, S. and Graven, S. (2007) 'The development of potentially better practices to support the neurodevelopment of infants in the NICU', *Journal of Perinatology* 27: S48–S74.

Ludington, S.M. (1990) 'Energy conservation during skin-to-skin contact between premature infants and their mothers', *Heart and Lung: Journal of Acute and Critical Care* 19(5), Pt. 1: 445–51.

Mann, N.P., Haddow, R., Stokes, L., Goodley, S. and Rutter, N. (1986) 'Effect of night and day on preterm infants in a newborn nursery: randomized trial', *British Medical Journal* 293(6557): 1265–7.

Martin, R.J., Herrell, N., Rubin, D. and Fanaroff, A. (1979) 'Effect of supine and prone positions on arterial oxygen tension in the preterm infant', *Pediatrics* 63(4): 528–31.

Masterson, J., Zucker, C. and Schulze, K. (1987) 'Prone and supine effects on energy expenditure and behavior of low birth weight neonates', *Pediatrics* 80(5): 689–92.

Melnyk, B.M., Feinstein, N.F., Alpert-Gillis, L., Fairbanks, E., Crean, H.F., Sinkin, R.A. Stone, P.W., Small, L., Tu, X. and Gross, S.J. (2006) 'Reducing premature infants' length of stay and improving parents' mental health outcomes with the Creating Opportunities for Parent Empowerment (COPE) neonatal intensive care unit program: a randomized controlled trial', *Pediatrics* 118: e1414–e1427.

Mendoza, J., Roberts, J. and Cook, L. (1991) 'Postural effects on pulmonary function and heart rate of preterm infants with lung disease', *Journal of Pediatrics* 118: 445–8.

Ment, L.R., Vohr, B. and Allen, W. (2003) 'Changes in cognitive function over time in very low birth weight infants', *Journal of the American Medical Association* 289(6): 705–11.

Monterosso, L., Kristjanson, L. and Cole, J. (2002) 'Neuromotor development and the physiologic effects of positioning in very low birth weight infants', *Journal of Obstetric Gynecology and Neonatal Nursing* 31(2): 138–46.

Morris, B., Philbin, M.K. and Bose, C. (2000) 'Physiological effects of sound on the newborn', *Journal of Perinatology* 20: S54–S59.

Padden, T. and Glenn, S. (1997) 'Maternal experiences of preterm birth and neonatal intensive care', *Journal of Reproductive and Infant Psychology* 15(2): 121–39.

Perlman, J.M. (2001) 'Neurobehavioural deficits in premature graduates of intensive care: potential medical and environmental risk factors', *Pediatrics* 108(6): 1339–48.

Reid, T. (2000) 'Maternal identity and preterm birth', *Journal of Child Health Care* 4(1): 23–9.

Rivkees, S.A. (2004) 'Emergence and influences of circadian rhythmicity in infants' *Clinics in Perinatology* 31: 217–28.

Salt, A. and Redshaw, M. (2006) 'Neurodevelopmental follow up after preterm birth; follow up after 2 years', *Early Human Development* 82: 185–97.

Shiroiwa, Y., Kamiya, Y., Uchibori, S., Inudai, K., Kito, H., Shibata, T. and Ogawa, J. (1986) 'Activity, cardiac and respiratory responses of blindfold preterm infants in a neonatal intensive care unit', *Early Human Development* 14: 259–65.

Shogan, M.G. and Schumann, L.L. (1993) 'The effect of environmental lighting on the oxygen saturation of preterm infants in the NICU', *Neonatal Network* 12(5): 7–13.

Slevin, M., Farrington, N., Duffy, G., Daly, L. and Murphy, J.F. (2000) 'Altering the NICU and measuring infants' responses', *Acta Paediatrica* 89(5): 501–2.

Symington, A. and Pinelli, J. (2006) 'Developmental care for promoting development and preventing morbidity in preterm infants', *Cochrane Database of Systematic Reviews*, Issue 2.

Therien, J.M., Worwa, C.T., Mattia, F.R. and O de Regnier, R.A. (2004) 'Altered pathways for auditory discrimination and recognition memory in preterm infants', *Developmental Medicine and Child Neurology* 46(12): 816–24.

Thoman, E.B. (1990) 'Sleeping and waking states in infants: a functional perspective', *Neuroscience and Biobehavioral Reviews* 14: 93–107.

Trevarthen, C. (2004) 'Learning about ourselves from children: why a growing human brain needs interesting companions?' *Research and Clinical Centre for Child Development* 2002–2004. Available at: *www.perception-in-action.ed.ac.uk/PDF_s/ Colwyn2004.pdf.*

White, R.D. (2006) 'Recommended standards for newborn NICU design', *Journal of Perinatology* 26(S3): S2–S18.

Chapter 3

Families in NICU

Sue Turrill and Liz Crathern

Contents

Introduction

One of the most challenging aspects of caring in the NICU is the management and support of parents and families. The emergence of neonatal care brought with it little recognition of the unique role families could play in the recovery of their infant, and the importance of providing opportunities for bonding and attachment. This has presented a myriad of challenges for neonatal staff, not least the juggling act of balancing parental hope for the future with the realism of the present (Crathern 2004).

This chapter will explore this balancing act by addressing the psychosocial impact of having an infant admitted to NICU both from historical and current perspectives and, in doing so, increase the understanding of the internal and external factors which influence this unique family picture. While recognising that this aspect of family care is in itself complex, particular emphasis will be given to facilitating a participative role for both parents.

This may appear to assume the family unit is always one of two happy parents. Experience of families in NICU also shows a picture of 'broken' units, e.g. single or estranged parents, those with intellectual impairment or parents with specific problems of drug misuse. However, the scope of this chapter does not allow for detailed discussion of every family structure or circumstance, so relies on the ability of nurses in practice to apply the concepts discussed to individual situations they face every day.

Historical context of family involvement

The historical basis of caring for families in neonatal units is not one most neonatal nurses of today will be familiar with. From the 1930s, when the first Special Care Baby Unit in the UK was opened (Crosse 1957), through the post-war era, there developed a social trend for hospital rather than home delivery, with care surrounding birth being directed from a medical rather than family perspective (Dunn 2007). Importantly the social acceptance of doctors' authority at this time inhibited a questioning culture from both nurses and parents, either into the specifics of care or their roles as care-givers. This had a huge impact on the role of parents in SCBU.

In a pre-antibiotic era parents were seen as potential carriers of disease and consequently were almost always discouraged from visiting the nursery, and if permitted into the nursery were banned from physical contact (Davis *et al.* 2003). Principles of care where driven by a genuine concern for the vulnerable infant and focused on sterility and cleanliness (Crosse 1957). Fear of death from infection was an overriding driver in the policy of exclusion, and despite improving survival rates of preterm infants, the separation of mothers from their infants increased (Davis *et al.* 2003). As a result, the 1960s saw many special care units permitting parents access to their babies only through the glass windows of viewing corridors, these being built to prevent families from entering the unit while still allowing them to 'see' their baby. Many parents, who were living further distances from increasingly specialised centres, may not have touched their infant for the first time until they were allowed to take them home from hospital. This was to have consequences beyond the neonatal period. The phenomena of 'failure to thrive' and abuse among infants separated from their parents in this way started to emerge with evidence of physical and emotional neglect (Klaus and Kennell 1976).

Throughout the 1960s and 1970s, the volume of research findings stressing the importance of a secure infant attachment continued to have an influence on practice in NICU, and encouraged nurses to promote a greater parental participation in care (Thomas 2008). During the 1970s, the arrival of Neonatal Intensive Care Units (NICUs), with increasing numbers of babies receiving respiratory support, heralded a rapid change in technology and supportive therapies. With this increased level of medical interventions and the consequent lengthening of hospital stay for smaller, sicker babies came the start of further integration of parents, a practice now regarded as necessary for future family functioning (Figure 3.1).

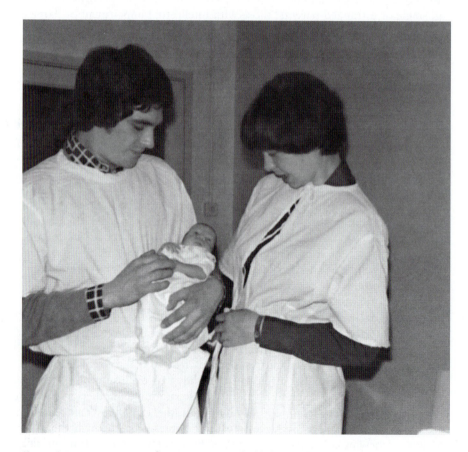

Figure 3.1 Parents required to 'gown up' to hold their baby, circa 1970

The 1980s saw the emergence of social developments in health care such as consumer and maternity pressure groups – the latter promoting the importance of support for the mother and breast feeding in the neonatal period. This also contributed to the recognition of a need to humanise the environment (Davis 2003). In the 1990s, developmental research had contributed to the introduction of both family-centred and developmental approaches to care within many neonatal units, promoting not only physical care but also the family as a central aspect of that care (Raeside 1997; Davis *et al.* 2003). These models of care had a basis in family well-being. Barriers, both physical and emotional, that had previously been created by health care professionals, and assumed to be appropriate by parents, started to be broken down with further integration of families. This involved professionals relinquishing control, while encouraging wider family participation. The Audit Commission (1997) recommended a maternity service that valued women and recognised the importance of communication with the professionals looking after them.

More recently, infants' psychological outcomes have become the focus of attention in research highlighting the importance of 'nurturing' and stability. This recognises the critical role parental love and attachment have in shaping the baby's brain and the effect this has on later psychological functioning. Gerhardt argues this is where the baby's social brain begins to develop. She cautions 'when these influences are less than benign, the groundwork is laid for a variety of later social and emotional difficulties' (2004, p. 3).

The environment

A neonatal intensive care unit is not a normal environment to begin family life. Parents feel strange and out of place in this alien world of alarms and machinery. It has been described as resembling a large fish bowl, designed to enable *staff* to have 100 per cent sight and access to the babies in their care (Drew 2006). Liljeblad (1993) captures the parents' perspective well, describing the experience as one of a 'cacophony of sounds, a plethora of machinery and stifling heat'. The practitioners appear very busy, sometimes frenetic, an atmosphere which can at times create a feeling that a crisis could occur at any moment. Mothers report feeling intimidated, like outsiders, tolerated at best (Liljeblad 1993; Raeside 1997; Heermann *et al.* 2005). Fathers report feeling alienated and out of control (Jackson *et al.* 2003). In the midst of this lies their infant, small, weak, vulnerable and inaccessible, surrounded by technology, wires and machinery.

In order to care for their infant both parents have to adapt to this strange uninvited environment which creates strong feelings of inadequacy (Vandenberg 2000; Fowlie and McHaffie 2004; Franck *et al.* 2005; Hall 2005; Hynan 2005). Importantly, the great paradox of birth and potential death occurring alongside each other means families are exposed to a myriad of emotions. It would seem clear that neonatal nurses are in the prime position to provide support through this time of crisis (Turrill 1999; Crathern 2009). However, 'despite a plethora of literature and research that stresses a major role parents and families have on neonatal outcomes, [the environment is] still largely medically and technically focused' (Davis *et al.* 2003: 284). Nurses must recognise that institutional constraints within their health care systems may curtail their ability to integrate family-focused research into practice. Nevertheless, neonatal nurses have an important pivotal role in alleviating the impact of this environment and in trying to shift the balance towards the needs of the family.

Becoming a parent

Becoming a parent for the first time is a mixture of joy and stress for both the mothers and fathers. It cannot be underestimated how the arrival of a new baby is, for most couples, one of the single most important events in their lives and is normally viewed as very positive (Gross *et al.* 2004; Hall 2005). It signifies the end of one single relationship as a couple (dyad) and the beginning of multiple relationships (dyads and triads) to adjust to in terms of family functioning (Whyte 1997).

Learning to understand their baby's behaviours, cries and grimaces is all part of the way parents begin developing the individual bond they have with their infant. This process takes time and closeness to develop and with healthy babies there is rarely a need to separate the parents from their newborn child. Physical and emotional needs are provided for in a relationship that, while including adjustment and disruption of previous norms, allows for healthy attachment processes to begin.

Both mothers and fathers have unique, individual roles that contribute as a whole in developing the family unit (Jackson *et al.* 2003). These roles are different between couples, and include the diversity of culture, spirituality and economy. Traditionally mothers are seen as carers with fathers taking on the role of provider. Although these roles have become more blurred, the symbiotic nature of the two remains very important. Understanding each other's roles within a couple is part of the strength of that couple. Consequently the breakdown of one role can lead to the unit falling apart. The birth of a sick or preterm infant represents a time of major stress for both parents. Parenting in NICU is likened to a crisis with reactions and anxieties similar to those seen in acute and post-traumatic stress disorders (Ringland 2008; Crathern 2009). It is therefore important to consider the different and specific effects on both mothers and fathers of babies admitted to NICU to understand further the pressure this may have on the successful functioning of each parent and their ability to cohesively create a strong family unit.

Being a mother in NICU

The concept of motherhood has a basis in contact rather than separation. The interaction between mother and baby begins during pregnancy and, with the birth of a normal, healthy baby, the development of this attachment is strengthened by the physical contact immediately following delivery. In addition to this, the experience of attachment can be affected in different ways by each mother's individual situation:

- health during pregnancy;
- type and experience at delivery;
- social and family support network;
- work commitments;
- self-identity;
- relationships with 'significant others'.

(Aagaard and Hall 2008)

For the mother of a healthy baby, transition to motherhood is complex. New mothers are having to establish their role at a time when they feel fragile and unsure, and experience disempowerment at a time when they most need to be in control (Francis 2002). Analysing the concept of transition to motherhood in the unfamiliar environment of NICU, Shin and White-Taut (2007) found that new mothers hovered around the edge of 'motherhood' and, as a consequence of this, feelings associated with becoming a mother were delayed.

There are recognised factors which have a dramatic impact on the planned trajectory to 'normal' motherhood following admission to NICU, causing a sudden change in expectations and a need to renegotiate a 'new kind of mothering' (Wigert *et al*. 2006):

- *Separation*. Being unable to take important first steps to attachment is seen as the most difficult aspect of having a baby in NICU for mothers (Wigert *et al*. 2006). Feelings of exclusion where their infant is cared for by experts with the consequent reduced physical contact, loss of identity as a mother, and not feeling a sense of belonging to either NICU or the maternity wards, leads to feelings of inadequacy. The need to start again in redefining their role to include separation from their baby can be too difficult for many mothers and leave them floundering in a state of 'limbo'.
- *Feelings of guilt and shame*. Pregnant women develop expectations of delivering a normal, healthy baby to add to their family. Once this picture is broken, they feel shame at not meeting their own, and what they perceive to be others', expectations including their partners, parents and society. In addition to this, feelings of guilt appear as they feel they have caused the unwanted situation their child is in the midst of.
- *Loss and grief*. This cannot be underestimated and should not be associated only with the death of a baby. Once a baby is admitted to NICU, the parents lose the baby they had dreamt of. Images of taking the baby home, holding, feeding, and changing nappies have all gone (Dyer 2005). While this is not a tangible loss, it nevertheless carries with it the same degree of sadness and grief to process and come to terms with. This is complicated by a real concern and worry that the infant will not survive, or if they do, will be handicapped in some way.

In conjunction with these personal barriers to healthy attachment, mothers have identified the lack of empowering information, contradictions from different health care professionals and omission of information as compounding their feelings of lack of control (Hurst 2001a, 2001b). They also have to cope with sharing the care of their baby with another person – the normal mother–infant dyad becomes a three-way mother–infant–nurse relationship due to the inevitability of the infant's needs. In order to regain this authority over their baby's care, mothers have been shown to feel the need to 'work hard' with health care staff to learn about the routines and rules which surround their baby (Fenwick *et al.* 2008). In other words, mothers become torn between caring for their baby and impressing professionals about their ability to do so.

Being a father in NICU: role transition and role identity – the forgotten parent

Transition to fatherhood is also a complex phenomenon. It is now viewed as an emotional, physical and financial challenge (Belsky and Kelly 1994) and can be a major upheaval in a man's life. Some have described this event as 'destabilising, decentring and disturbing' and interrupting a man's sense of purpose (Henwood and Proctor 2003). Fathers of well, healthy newborn infants find this transition and conforming to a 'new fatherhood' role more difficult and distressing than they had anticipated before the birth. They also take a 'back seat' to the needs of mothers during the antenatal and early postnatal period (Barclay and Lupton 1999; Bradley *et al.* 2004).

In comparison to mothers, there is a paucity of research on fathers' experiences of becoming a parent in NICU, with many findings having emerged as an addition, or an afterthought, to mother-focused studies (Crathern 2009). Yet, over 25 years ago, Paludetto *et al.* (1981) stressed the importance of both parents having unrestricted access to caring for their infant, and emphasised the many benefits to the mother of a supportive father in NICU. Concerns were later raised that if men became even more marginalised from the women's world of childcare, then the family unit may suffer (Ribbens 1994). Fathers, like mothers, experience feelings of isolation, fear and stress. They hover on the edge of fatherhood and are confused about their role in NICU.

Three specific aspects of the changing roles that fathers have experienced have been identified: those of 'financial burden', 'supporting the mother' and 'suppressing feelings'.

Fathers' changing roles

Financial burden – balancing paid work and family commitments

Many new fathers have to manage the stress and strain of new parenthood while working outside the home (Burgess and Bartlett 2004). Paid work equates with an identity in society – for some men it represents stability and familiarity. For others it becomes a burden to 'deal with' where the financial needs of the changing family have to be addressed by taking on extra work during and immediately after pregnancy. A recent study looked at new fathers who tried to combine parenting a baby in NICU with paid work. The fathers valued their paid employment with a new intensity because it gave them a unique way to provide for their new baby financially. However, this pressure led some to feel useful at work and useless in NICU and this created feelings of intense discomfort when visiting their baby (Pohlman 2005).

Fathers' supporting role

As early as the 1980s, it was recognised that fathers of premature infants have an increased role in care-giving, being more active both in the hospital and the home (Jeffcoate *et al.* 1979; Parke 1981).

A woman's ability to cope with the ongoing demands of new motherhood is enhanced by the stable and supportive relationship of the father (Burgess and Bartlett 2004; Pleck and Masciadrelli 2004). However, this situation is not an easy one for all fathers. Some men are motivated to attend the birth out of a desire to support the mother and a concern for their unborn child while others may feel coerced into a supportive role during labour, and feel unable to voice their concern for fear of being perceived as non-supportive (Mander 2004).

The birth of a preterm or sick baby becomes even more complex. While in NICU, supporting the mother is a difficult role for the father as both parents feel anxious and stressed and, despite all efforts, the environment can continually exert a damaging effect on parents' attachment to their offspring (Franck *et al.* 2005; Pohlman 2005).

There is convincing evidence that 'involved' fathers impact positively on a mother's health and well-being after the birth of their baby, and furthermore gain considerable benefit from this. However, they also require help and support to be successful (Goodman 2005; Fisher 2007). This positive impact is seen particularly in mothers of low birth weight infants, improving their overall well-being and confidence.

Suppressing feelings

Fathers of very ill neonates consistently experience feelings of being 'out of control' with the situation they find themselves in. This, coupled with the need to support their partner, has led some fathers to suppress their own feelings, thus appearing 'in control', as a way of helping their partners cope with the continual stress of living with a baby in NICU. The ongoing negative impact of this was compounded as fathers were less likely to receive consistent information due to the nature of their visiting patterns and therefore found decision-making for their baby both stressful and difficult (Jackson *et al.* 2003; Arockiasamy *et al.* 2008).

Change does appear to be happening in the UK with a noticeable shift in the publication of health-related literature specifically aimed at fathers (see resource section). The Fatherhood Institute (an institute set up to tackle the imbalance of childrearing research and discussion from a father's perspective) suggests that men are keen to talk about their life experiences, though they are seldom asked to do so.

In order to respond to the dynamic changes occurring for parents both during and following admission, nurses must first consider the stressors and coping strategies that may be exhibited by both parents in response to this traumatic, 'out of control' situation.

Signs of parental stress and coping

The psychological impact of having a baby admitted to NICU cannot be underestimated. Figure 3.2 shows some of the descriptors highlighted by parents of babies admitted to neonatal units over the past 20 years. Shaw et al. (2006) explored parenting stress in more detail, specifically acute and post-traumatic stress disorder in NICU, and concluded that both NICU parents exhibit acute stress disorder similar to parents of other critically ill children. Importantly families with an underlying level of conflict and those who tried to suppress feelings seemed to develop yet more stress. During admission the increasing levels of stress can be seen by staff as parents exhibit some of the following signs:

- being unable to process information and requiring repetition of facts;
- difficulty thinking clearly and problem-solving; being unable to prioritise;
- mastering tasks becomes impossible and frustrating, leading to feelings of ineffectiveness as a person;
- increasingly missing cues due to shutting off from the environment;
- withdrawal or irritability.

(Shaw et al. 2006; Hazinski 2009)

Parents exhibit recognisable stages in their initial coping strategies. These can be seen progressively as part of the 'vulnerable child syndrome' (Shaw et al. 2006, p. 210) with immobility on entering NICU; performing a visual survey of machinery and layout; withdrawal from the environment and staff; over-protectiveness; hyper-vigilance and focusing on small things, e.g. tapes, blood stains on sheets or clothing. They move on to try to intellectualise reality, e.g. understanding how machinery works, trying to interpret blood results or showing a greater interest in the pathology of diseases (Pinelli 2000; Hazinski 2009).

Having utilised initial and early coping strategies, some parents do start to feel more confident in being a part of their baby's care and will begin to negotiate care with health care professionals by taking a lead. This has been described in two ways; as moving from an outsider to partner position and from alienation

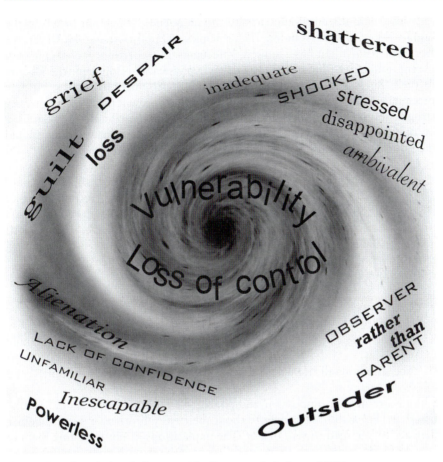

Figure 3.2 The whirlpool of parents' feelings on admission to NICU

to familiarity (Jackson *et al.* 2003; Heermann *et al.* 2005). In addition to this, they will increase their support networks by building relationships with other parents in similar situations and gather support from their immediate family and friends.

Family nursing and support: caring for the whole family

It would seem from this picture that the onus lies with the parents to adapt to this strange world. While the situation itself cannot be changed, the anticipation and management of these all too familiar responses could alleviate their impact dramatically and take some of this pressure away from them.

The purpose of caring for the family is to provide, maintain and restore family health and is primarily concerned with the interactions within and between the family (Friedman 2003). Understanding the influence of the family on each individual infant's development, and the uniqueness the infant brings to the family, is key to understanding the principles of family nursing. However, the sick or preterm infant has a limited, unrecognisable repertoire in engaging with parents and carers due to the level of their physical development, the severity of their illness and the constraints of their environment. This in itself may precipitate a lack of emotional attachment and investment from parents as they struggle to understand their infant. The impact that these limitations can have on developing family relationships should not be underestimated, nor should the positive way family nursing strategies can influence the situation.

Central to successful family nursing are the skills nurses portray in being able to step aside from personal judgements and values and accept the family unit. The notion of families having individual strengths and personal resources, rather than deficits, should be the starting point when planning a tailored approach to family care. It is important to recognise that families span several generations and these multigenerational relationships can be a source of strength for all family members. Bengston (2001, p. 1) suggests three reasons why these relationships are important:

1   The demographic changes of population ageing resulting in longer years of shared lives between generations.
2   The increasing importance of grandparents and other kin in fulfilling family functions.
3   The strength and resilience of intergenerational solidarity over time.

Siblings are also an important component of the family and should not be ignored. They will have concerns about their baby brother or sister whether they are encouraged to visit or not. The implications of not including them in care planning could have longer-term repercussions on family dynamics and function.

A family nursing perspective challenges nurses to adopt an even more collaborative approach to care. The emphasis is on using a style which reflects a whole family's strengths, and assists them in finding solutions to the problems they themselves identify. In doing so, responsibility and therefore ownership of the situation increase for the family, which in turn improves their sense of control. Families who are negatively judged in terms of their lack of ability to either care for, or understand the care being given to their infant can quickly become alienated and feel misunderstood (Feeley and Gottlieb 2000).

Eggenberger and Nelms (2007: 1618), in assessing families in critical care settings, recognised that: 'Being a family unit is what gives most families the ability to endure the emotional upheaval and suffering that come with the critical illness experience.' It requires a skilled approach to look beneath the surface of 'apparent coping' and create the opportunities for families to demonstrate their capabilities and identify their strengths. The foundations of this understanding for nurses are based on the concept of family systems and how the diverse complexities of family dynamics can both hinder and support family well-being.

Family systems and assessment

Each individual, while complete on their own, is an element of the whole family system. The system contains subsystems as pairs or multiples, e.g. the partnership of parents, mother and child, father and child, sibling groups. Using 'family systems' can be a way of describing how parts of a family relate to each other and in so doing it becomes easier to understand the whole. These principles include:

■ One part of the family cannot be understood in isolation from the rest of the system.
■ Family functioning is more than just the sum of the subsystems.
■ A family's structure and organisation are important in determining the behaviour of family members.
■ Communication and feedback mechanisms between family members are important in the functioning of family systems.

Positive family systems include the ability of family members to adapt to a new situation, managing feedback from others and recognising family boundaries. While boundaries between elements of a family are very important to the successful functioning of the whole, there may be situations where a boundary becomes intimidating, i.e. between the family and its environment – in this case, the NICU and its staff. Boundaries can be open or closed. An open boundary welcomes input into the system by welcoming new ideas, information, resources and opportunity. It reaches out for help and utilises support networks. A closed boundary resists input and views change as threatening. The family in this situation become suspicious of support and therefore resist outside influences, attempting to be self-sufficient and deny help (Whyte 1997; Friedman 2003).

Individual family assessment is a fundamental component of all family nursing strategies. It requires a skilled practitioner to assess the particular needs of each individual family and each individual within a family. This includes an understanding of:

■ identifying the structural, developmental and functional needs of the family (Whyte 1997);
■ physical, intellectual, emotional and social needs (Henson 2000);
■ family strategies (maintenance, coherence, change) and individualisation (stress, coping and adaptation) (Friedman 2003).

Importantly, each neonatal unit is also unique with individual challenges and populations. While it is possible to present some generic prescriptors to include in assessment, it is up to each individual unit to integrate these meaningfully.

Strategies for support: anticipating and reducing stress

General principles

In addition to the increased understanding of the ways in which families function successfully, practical guidelines are important to help nurses provide consistent, appropriately focused care.

Simple and easily implemented strategies for including parents in their baby's care have become part of practice guidelines for most neonatal units in the UK today. These start with the first suggestion that their baby may need intervention from specialist services. These general principles can be applied to all families who either have an infant at risk of being admitted, or who have already been admitted to a neonatal unit. The methods detailed in Table 3.1 all relate to creating opportunities for parents to feel included and start to develop attachments with their baby.

Table 3.1 General principles of support

Practicalities for increasing family inclusion

Prior to admission	Visit to parents on the antenatal ward or delivery suite by senior neonatologist and nurse to explain what is likely to happen at, and immediately after, delivery
	Parents visit the neonatal unit prior to admission. Mum may need to be on a bed or in a wheelchair and should be accompanied by a midwife she knows. Attention is paid to: ■ environment ■ machines ■ staff
	Introduction to staff – what the uniforms mean, staff photo board, opportunity to talk to a senior nurse and ask questions
	Written information about visiting – unit, parents' booklet in languages appropriate to the local population
	Parents' sitting room/quiet area, parents' bedrooms or overnight facilities for 'rooming-in'
At the time of admission	Photos of the baby taken for both parents Dad given the opportunity and support to visit on his own if the parents wish
	Mum to visit baby as soon as possible on her bed/chair
	Simple explanation of baby's condition and plans for care
	Talk about infant's unique attributes such as 'tiny toes', vigour, hair colour, etc.

Table 3.1 Continued

	Opportunity to talk to consultant or most senior medical person familiar with the baby's status
Ongoing support	Open visiting
	Access to consultants
	Access to a dedicated parents' telephone line
	Encourage parents to ask questions and offer information if not requested
	Written details of conditions/treatments available in languages appropriate to local population
	Understand the need for repetition and consistency of information
	Explain machinery and purpose
	Suggest unique toys/photos of siblings to put on the side of the incubator to promote a sense of individual identity
	Encourage breast milk expression – provide equipment for this
	Keep postnatal staff updated about baby's condition
	Unit parent support groups
	Overnight visiting accommodation
	Liaison with other health care professionals, e.g. health visitor

More specific strategies

Successful methods used to support families in NICU anticipate the known pathway of stress, vulnerability and perceived lack of control parents experience on admission. Strategies which can be included in individualised family support policies have a basis in empirical research studies undertaken with parents of babies in NICU (e.g. Brazy *et al*. 2001; Jackson *et al*. 2003; Jones *et al*. 2007; Reid *et al*. 2007; Arockiasamy *et al*. 2008). These revolve around positive communication and education and can also include specific intervention programmes.

Specific intervention programmes

More specific intervention programmes have been shown to have positive outcomes for families by reducing the symptoms of trauma and parental stress, and increasing their confidence and competence in caring for their baby (Jotzo and Poets 2005; Kaaresen *et al.* 2006, 2008; Turan *et al.* 2008). In essence, each strategy has the following in common:

■ Parents are central to the well-being of the infant.
■ Verbal and written support of information allows individual and consistent information giving.
■ Acknowledging the emotional turmoil associated with the loss of 'normality' and giving parents tools to learn the new 'normal' is the starting point for increasing feelings of control.
■ Positive interactions between parents and their baby have long-term benefits for both parties.
■ Understanding the differing behaviour of babies in NICU who are either sick or preterm will influence these interactions.
■ Open channels of communication must exist between parents and health carers.
■ Parent education is vital and should be ongoing throughout admission and preparation for discharge.

While neonatal care in the past focused on maintaining physiological stability it would seem appropriate now to include a well-designed intervention strategy to prevent families from experiencing some of the negative feelings and traumatic outcomes associated with admission.

One specific programme which involves minimal increase in resources is the COPE programme (Creating Opportunities for Parent Empowerment) (Melnyk *et al.* 2004, 2006). Not only has this been shown to increase the involvement of fathers in care and reduce anxiety and depression in mothers, it also structures specific activities for parents at a rate to suit their needs in a simple and useful way. The use of audiotaped information, while alien to most health care practitioners, meets the needs of parents in providing consistent information in a clear format to accompany written booklets. This may also address the differing abilities some parents may have in deciphering written language. Table 3.2 outlines the principles of this intervention programme.

Communication

The art of open communication is a skill which develops with experience and time and should not be underestimated when planning the holistic care of families in NICU. The development of a meaningful relationship between parents and health care professionals must be based on honesty and trust. In order for this to exist and continue throughout admission, a positive communication approach needs to be taken from the start. The following are factors to consider in any parent–staff communication policy:

■ *Information giving* – explanation, repetition and consistency of information are vital to the understanding that parents are able to achieve about their

Table 3.2 **COPE (Creating Opportunities for Parent Empowerment) intervention programme for reducing parental stress and improving parent–infant relationships**

COPE: A four-phase educational/intervention programme

Common to all four phases is the following:
- ■ Audiotaped and written information for parents based on the appearance and behaviour of their baby, how parents can meet their baby's needs and improving their baby's development.
- ■ Parent activities to utilise and implement based on the information given in the tapes and leaflets.

Phase I: 2–4 days after admission:
- ■ Taped and written information given to parents relating to simple infant behaviour patterns and the roles of parents.
- ■ Activity – Identify the unique characteristics of their baby and start to keep a diary of their milestones.

Phase II: 2–4 days later:
- ■ Taped and written information that reinforces major points in the initial tape and gives more detailed information on behaviour and infant development. Also further suggestions as to how parents can participate in care.
- ■ Activity – Identify specific characteristics of their baby and start to recognise stress cues, and also cues that show the baby is ready for interaction.

Phase III: 1–4 days before discharge:
- ■ Taped and written information about infant states, appropriate timing of interactions, parent roles in smoothing the transition to home, and how to continue positive parent–infant interaction.
- ■ Activity – Continue to recognise cues and help parents to use strategies that reduce infants' stress.

Phase IV: 1 week after discharge:
- ■ Taped and written information relating to preterm and term infant development, suggestions to foster positive parent–infant interactions.
- ■ Activities – Identify specific activities to perform which foster positive cognitive development.

Source: Melnyk (2004, 2006)

baby's clinical condition. Conflicting terminology and opinions at any stage only add to the stress and anxiety parents feel. This in turn will affect their perception of their level of involvement in care and decision-making. By ensuring a team approach (nurses and doctors together) when speaking with parents, coupled with careful documentation of discussions, the likelihood of confusion and misinterpretation on both sides will be reduced.

Nursing knowledge of both the physical status and care of the baby, and the emotional state of the family becomes vital at this point if parents are to learn to trust nurses looking after their baby. It is equally important that all nurses admit their limitations of knowledge and refer parents to other more experienced staff within the nursing team to avoid confusion and breakdown of relationships. Bialoskurski and colleagues (2002), when looking at relationships in NICU, found that 90 per cent of mothers described the most important aspect of information giving as facts relating to their infant's condition.

Written information, either from hospitals or web-based sites, are also used by parents (Brazy *et al.* 2001). Providing written leaflets and details of appropriate websites for parents to access will help reduce inconsistency of information, often cited by parents as increasing stress and reducing their confidence in neonatal staff.

- *Time spent listening and responding to queries and concerns* – Responses from parents will be diverse and based on each individual's emotional stability at any given time. Time spent engaging with parents on their level, at the speed they can respond to, expressing reassurance and care, will instigate trust and confidence from parents.

  Parents also value communication that is informal or 'chatty' as well as information giving. Showing an interest in parents' lives outside the immediacy of the unit is seen as nurturing and allows parents to express their emotions (Jones *et al.* 2007).

- *Equal partners in caring* – In recognising the need for parents to develop a 'new' role centred around their baby the initial goal for both parents and nurses is the partnership of being equal carers. Feelings of interaction affirm parents' views of being 'important' and build their confidence in the nurses providing care (Wigert *et al.* 2006).

Being able to understand the changing expectations of families as their baby's condition unfolds is crucial to the success of open communication. Parents will travel on an upward trajectory from complete naivety and fear to a position of authority, necessary for them to be able to confidently and happily take their baby home.

Effective communication strategies can be summarised as:

- Nurses changing their behaviour to reduce 'social distance' – recognising behaviour in themselves that is respectful and reassuring, while still professional and friendly; treating parents as equals; not being too formal or demanding.
- Using understandable language – giving clear, direct and consistent information in easily understood terms, rather than vague or inadequate information; checking parents' level of understanding.
- Encouraging contribution to conversations – asking parents questions, encouraging expression of their opinions; avoid dominating the conversation or belittling and disregarding parents' answers.

Education

The education of parents exists alongside all aspects of good communication, but in this context is primarily about equipping parents with the skills to understand and carry out tasks confidently and competently. The ultimate goal for all concerned is for them to take their baby home safely when that time arrives.

Teaching parents about handling, nappy changing and feeding not only instils confidence in parents' ability to care for their baby physically but also supports the parents in developing their unique relationship with their baby. Growing feelings of confidence and control when caring for infants are greatly enhanced as mothers learn to connect with their baby through physical contact. Women described this as becoming a 'real mother' (Fenwick *et al.* 2008).

Another aspect of parent education that nurses are in a prime position to initiate is the recognition of infant behaviour patterns. Knowing when and how to respond to the sick or preterm baby forms the basis of future successful parent–infant relationships. These behaviour cues will be very different to those of the healthy term baby and parents are unlikely to have experienced this difference before. Prompting parents when responding to their baby's cues underpins the sense of uniqueness and belonging they crave at a time when closeness and contact are at a premium.

Creation of an individual, collaborative plan of education with short- and long-term goals can be successful once an assessment of current knowledge and abilities has been made. Parents will have a variety of needs based on their previous experience of childcare, culture and roles within the family. This type of assessment, if used to inform this element of the nurse–parent partnership, can reduce the stress experienced by some parents when faced with the prospect of caring (Turan *et al.* 2008). However, once a plan of learning has been set, they will all need time, practice and positive reinforcement to achieve their goals.

Conclusion

It is undeniable that families experiencing the whirlpool of emotions on entering NICU are existing in a state of extreme pressure, stress and strain. Both parents must quickly learn to adapt to this overwhelming environment to be able to develop the confidence and competence to both care for their vulnerable baby and eventually take control of the situation, thus successfully completing their transition to this different parenting role. Neonatal nurses are in the prime position to orchestrate this multifaceted scenario in order to assist the family in achieving their potential as a strong unit.

Recognising the infant's uniqueness and the family's individual entity and strengths is a vital start to this important process. This begins with the acknowledgement of both parents as individuals and as part of the caring team, taking into account their own stressors and emotional burden. In addition to this, the wider family network spanning the generations from siblings to grandparents must also be considered as having a key role in the dynamic family unit. The infants themselves play a part in this altered structure as their behaviour and responses need to be learnt and reinforced to allow parents to accept their new role as parents in critical care.

Being able to anticipate and plan for the differing responses of parents, and the effect of interactions between family members and nurses, by understanding both the concept of family systems and the practicalities of family nursing, is a skill to be developed to ensure families receive the complex level of support they need.

Case study: stressful time for parents

Jenny is a preterm infant born at 28 weeks' gestation following spontaneous labour. She is now two weeks old and remains on CPAP for respiratory support although this is gradually being weaned. Jenny's condition is quite stable and there are no other specific concerns for her health at the moment.

Mark and Emily are Jenny's parents and are both 22 years old. Jenny is their third child with an older brother, James, aged 4 years and sister, Charlotte, aged 3 years. Jenny's parents have only recently moved into their own home together as they have been living with Emily's parents while they saved up for a deposit for their flat.

Today the nurse looking after Jenny and her family is concerned that something may be worrying Emily as she seems withdrawn. She talks with Emily and Mark about Jenny's progress and discovers that their son James has been diagnosed at school with learning difficulties. Emily has also become very anxious about Jenny's prognosis and concerned about how she will cope with caring for Jenny and dealing with James's special needs. Mark tries to reassure his partner that everything is going to be okay but this seems to increase the tension between them.

Emily's parents have always been very supportive and are expected to visit soon.

With reference to the key points within the chapter, consider the following questions:

Q.1. What were the immediate challenges Emily and Mark had to cope with when Jenny was born?

Q.2. How could you identify Emily and Mark's strengths as a couple?

Q.3. How would you assess the potential family strengths and challenges?

Q.4. Which key family members do you need to engage with and why?

Q.5. How can the staff support the family unit during their time on the neonatal unit?

Q.6. Which other health care professionals should be involved in supporting the family and how would you initiate their involvement?

Devise a family support plan. Identify key issues and methods you would employ, giving clear rationale for your decisions. What potential situations may occur that might mean you will need to revise your plan?

Case study: family cultural issues

Abdul and Sofi are third-generation British Muslims who have become the proud parents of a baby boy called Karim. He was born at 23 weeks' gestation and is now six hours old. He is on maximum ventilation and oxygenation and his prognosis is poor. This is the first boy for Abdul and Sofi; they have three girls aged 7, 5 and 3 years. They are all healthy. Sofi has had complications following the birth and is still in the delivery suite. Abdul has just arrived at the neonatal unit to visit his son. He is very distressed.

With reference to the key points within the chapter, consider the following questions:

Q.1. What are the immediate challenges Abdul and Sofi will have to cope with?

Q.2. What are the immediate needs of the father? How would you respond to these specifically?

Q.3. What are the immediate needs of the mother? How would you respond to these specifically?

Q.4. Are there any cultural issues the family may need support with? How would you negotiate these into your care?

Q.5. How can the staff support the family during this time? Identify the most appropriate roles for all members of the team.

Devise a family support plan for both the immediate period and the following 24 hours, thinking of all potential outcomes. Identify the key issues for the family and give rationale for your priorities in your plan.

Web-based resources for parents

- *BLISS* www.bliss.org.uk Offers support for premature and sick babies across the UK. The website includes a specific section for parents including information about local support groups; downloadable information leaflets relating to specific conditions and treatment; a message board for parents questions; parents stories. There is also a helpline available for parents.
- *Child Bereavement Charity* www.childbereavement.org.uk The CBC exists to support all those affected when a baby or child dies. Its website includes helping families organise practicalities following a baby's death, family stories and links to articles and leaflets relating to all aspects of child bereavement from each family member's perspective.
- *Contact a family* www.cafamily.org.uk This charity offers, via its website, advice, information and support to families of disabled children. This includes a free helpline, understanding the benefits system and accessing the right educational support.
- *SANDS* www.uk-sands.org.uk SANDS supports anyone affected by the death of a baby by offering practical information for families as well as emotional support and understanding. Its website includes, for example, how and when to talking about emotions and feelings, a useful publications list, and stories of personal experiences from bereaved parents.
- *SCOPE* www.scope.org.uk SCOPE will offer support and advice for families with a child with cerebral palsy, helping to identify and address barriers to inclusion.
- *SPRING* www.springsuport.org.uk SPRING offers a counselling service providing support to parents and relatives who have suffered the loss of a baby before or around birth including miscarriage, still birth and termination for fetal anomaly.
- *The Fatherhood Institute* www.fatherhoodinstitute.org This is a charity aiming to engage fathers in the lives of children, to promote an inclusive approach to family policies through the encouragement of father-focused research. The website includes help and advice for all fathers and provides specific information, for example, for young fathers, parenting education, vulnerable families, Muslim fathers.

Acknowledgements

The authors would like to thank Bruce Holliday, Multimedia Developer, University of Leeds for his vision and help in designing the pictorial representation of 'The whirlpool of parents' feelings'.

References

Aagaard, H. and Hall, E.O.C. (2008) 'Mothers' experience of having a preterm infant in the Neonatal Care Unit: a meta analysis', *Journal of Pediatric Nursing* 23(3): e26–e36.

Aroackiasamy, V., Holsti, L. and Albersheim, S. (2008) 'Fathers' experiences in the Neonatal Intensive Care Unit: a search for control', *Pediatrics* 121(2): e215–e222.

Audit Commission (1997) *A First Class Delivery: Improving Maternity Services in England and Wales*, London: Audit Commission.

Barclay, L. and Lupton, D. (1999) 'The experiences of new fatherhood: sociocultural analysis', *Journal of Advanced Nursing* 29(4): 1013–20.

Belsky, J. and Kelly, J. (1994) *The Transition to Parenthood: How a First Child Changes Marriages*, New York: Delacorte Press.

Bengston, V.L. (2001) 'The Burgess Award Lecture: beyond the nuclear family: the increasing importance of multigenerational bonds', *Journal of Marriage and the Family* 63(1): 1–16.

Bialoskurski, M.M., Cox, C.L. and Wiggens, R.D. (2002) 'The relationship between maternal need and priorities in a neonatal intensive care environment', *Journal of Advanced Nursing* 37: 62–9.

Bradley, E., Mackenzie, M. and Boath, E. (2004) 'The experiences of first time fatherhood: a brief report', *Journal of Reproductive Psychology* 22(1): 45–7.

Brazy, J.E., Anderson, B.H.M., Becker, P.T. and Becker, M. (2001) 'How parents of premature infants gather information and obtain support', *Neonatal Network* 20(2): 41–8.

Burgess, A. and Bartlett, D. (2004) *Working with Fathers*, London: DES Fathers Direct.

Crathern, L. (2004) 'Walking the tightrope: experiences of nurses caring for extremely small neonates', *BLISS Newborn News* Spring: 12–13.

Crathern, L. (2009) 'Dads matter too: a review of the literature focussing on the experiences of fathers of preterm infants', *MIDIRS Midwifery Digest* 19(2): 159–67.

Crosse, V.M. (1957) *The Premature Baby*, 4th edn, London: Churchill.

Davis, L., Mohay, H. and Edwards, H. (2003) 'Mothers' involvement in caring for their premature infants: an historical overview', *Journal of Advanced Nursing* 42(6): 578–86.

Drew, D. (2006) 'Mark', *MIDIRS* 16(2): 257–8.

Dunn, P.M. (2007) 'The birth of perinatal medicine in the UK', *Seminar on Fetal Neonatal Medicine* 12(3): 227–38.

Dyer, K.A. (2005) 'Identifying, understanding and working with grieving parents in the NICU, part 1: identifying and understanding loss and the grief response', *Neonatal Network* 24(3): 35–46.

Eggenberger, S.K. and Nelms, T.P. (2007) 'Being family: the family experience when an adult member is hospitalized with a critical illness', *Journal of Clinical Nursing* 16: 1618–28.

Feeley, N. and Gottlieb, L.N. (2000) 'Nursing approaches for working with family strengths and resources', *Journal of Family Nursing* 6(1): 9–24.

Fenwick, J., Barclay, L. and Schmied, V. (2008) 'Craving closeness: a grounded theory analysis of women's experiences of mothering in the Special Care Nursery', *Women and Birth* 21: 71–85.

Fisher, D. (2007) *Including New Fathers: A Guide for Maternity Professionals*, London: Fathers Direct.

Fowlie, P. and McHaffie, H. (2004) 'Clinical review: ABC of preterm birth: supporting parents in the neonatal unit', *BMJ*, available at: http://www.bmj.com/cgi/content/full/329/7478/1336.

Francis, T.C. (2002) 'Transition to motherhood: the neonatal nurse's perspective', *Journal of Neonatal Network* 8(2): 52–5.

Franck, L.S., Cox, S., Allen, A. and Winter, I. (2005) 'Measuring neonatal intensive care unit: related parental stress', *Journal of Advanced Nursing* 49(6): 608–15.

Friedman, M. (2003) *Family Nursing: Research, Theory and Practice*, 5th edn, New Jersey: Pearson Education.

Gerhardt, S. (2004) *Why Love Matters: How Affection Shapes a Baby's Brain*, New York: Routledge.

Goodman, J.H. (2005) 'Becoming an involved father of an infant', *JOGNN* 34(2): 190–200.

Gross, H. and Van den Akker, O. (2004) 'Editorial: the importance of the postnatal period for mothers, fathers and infant behaviour', *Journal of Reproductive and Infant Psychology* 22(1): 3–4.

Hall, E.O.C. (2005) 'Being in an alien world: Danish parents' lived experiences when a newborn or small child is critically ill', *Scandinavian Journal of Caring Science* 19: 179–85.

Hazinski, M.F. (2009) *Nursing Care of the Critically Ill Child*, 3rd edn, New York: Mosby.

Heermann, J.A., Wilson, M.E. and Wilhelm, P.A. (2005) 'Mothers in the NICU: outsider to partner', *Pediatric Nursing* 31(3): 176–81.

Henson, C. (2000) 'Family support', in G. Boxwell (ed.) *Neonatal Intensive Care Nursing*, London: Routledge.

Henwood, K. and Proctor, J. (2003) 'The good father', *British Journal of Psychology* 42(3): 337–55.

Hurst, I. (2001a) 'Mothers' strategies to meet their needs in the newborn intensive care nursery', *Journal of Perinatal and Neonatal Nursing* 15: 65–82.

Hurst, I. (2001b) 'Vigilant watching over: mothers' actions to safeguard their premature babies in the newborn intensive care nursery', *Journal of Perinatal and Neonatal Nursing* 21: 23–60.

Hynan, M.T. (2005) 'Supporting fathers during stressful times in the nursery: an evidence-based review', *Newborn and Infant Review* 5(2): 87–92.

Jackson, K., Ternestedt, B-M. and Scholin, J. (2003) 'From alienation to familiarity: experiences of mothers and fathers of preterm infants', *Journal of Advanced Nursing* 43(2): 120–9.

Jeffcoate, J.A., Humphrey, M.E. and Lloyd, J.K. (1979) 'Role, perception and response to stress in fathers and mothers following preterm delivery', *Society, Science and Medicine* 13a: 139–45.

Jones, L., Woodhouse, D. and Rowe, J. (2007) 'Effective nurse–parent communication: a study of parents' perceptions in the NICU environment', *Patient Education and Counseling* 69: 206–12.

Jotzo, M. and Poets, C.F. (2005) 'Helping parents cope with the trauma of premature birth: an evaluation of a trauma-preventive psychological intervention', *Pediatrics* 115(4): 915–19.

Kaaresen, P.I., Ronning, J.A., Ulvund, S.E. and Dahl, L.B. (2006) 'A randomized, controlled trial of the effectiveness of an early-intervention program in reducing stress after preterm birth', *Pediatrics* 118(1): e9–e19.

Kaaresen, P.I., Ronning, J.A., Tungy, J., Nordhov, S.M., Ulvund, S.E. and Dahl, L.B. (2008) 'A randomized controlled trial of an early intervention program in low birthweight children: outcome at 2 years', *Early Human Development* 84: 201–9.

Klaus, M.H. and Kennell, J.H. (1976) *Maternal–infant Bonding*, St Louis, MO: Mosby.

Liljeblad, C. (1993) 'Neonatal nurse practitioners: paving the way for case management of chronically ill infants and their families', *Journal of Perinatal and Neonatal Nursing* 10(1): 72–8.

Mander, R. (2004) *Men and Maternity*, London: Routledge.

Melnyk, B.M., Alpert-Gillis, L., Feinstein, N.F., Crean, H.F., Johnson, J., Fairbanks, E., Small, L., Rubenstein, J., Slota, M. and Corbo-Richert, B. (2004) 'Creating opportunities for Parent Empowerment: program effects on the mental health/coping outcomes of critically ill young children and their mothers', *Pediatrics* 113(6): e597–e607.

Melnyk, B.M., Feinstein, L., Alpert-Gillis, Fairbanks, E., N.F., Crean. H.F., Sinkin, A., Stone, P.W., Johnson, J., Small, Xin Tu and Gross, S.J. (2006) 'Reducing premature infants' length of stay and improving parents' mental health outcomes with the Creating Opportunities for Parent Empowerment (COPE) Neonatal Intensive Care Unit program: a randomized, controlled trial', *Pediatrics* 118(5): e1414–e1427.

Nelson, D.B. and Edgil, A.E. (1998) 'Family dynamics in families with very low birth weight and full term infants: a pilot study', *Journal of Pediatric Nursing* 13(2): 95–103.

Paludetto, R., Faggiano-Perfetto, M., Asprea, A.M., Curtis, D.E. and Margara-Paludetto, P. (1981) 'Reactions of sixty parents allowed unrestricted contact with infants in a neonatal intensive care unit', *Early Human Development* 5: 401–9.

Parke, R.D. (1981) *Fathering*, London: Fontana.

Pinelli, J. (2000) 'Effects of family coping and resources on family adjustment and parental stress in the acute phase of the NICU environment', *Neonatal Network* 19(6): 27–37.

Pleck, J.H. and Masciadrelli, B.P. (2004) 'Paternal involvement: levels, sources and consequences', in M.E. Lamb (ed.) *The Role of the Father in Child Development*, 4th edn, Chichester: Wiley.

Pohlman, S. (2005) 'The primacy of work and fathering preterm infants: findings from an interpretative phenomenological study', *Advances in Neonatal Care* 5(4): 204–16.

Raeside, L. (1997) 'Perceptions of environmental stressors in the neonatal unit', *British Journal of Nursing* 6(16): 914–23.

Reid, T., Bramwell, R., Booth, N. and Weindling, M. (2007) 'Perceptions of parent–staff communication in Neonatal Intensive Care: the findings from a rating scale', *Journal of Neonatal Nursing* 13: 64–74.

Ribbens, J. (1994) *Mothers and Their Children: A Feminist Sociology of Child Rearing*, London: Sage.

Ringland, C.P. (2008) 'Post traumatic stress disorder and the NICU graduate mother', *Infant* 4(2): 14–17.

Shaw, R.J., Ikuta, L. and Fleisherm, B. (2006) 'Acute stress disorder among parents of infants in the neonatal intensive care nursery', *Psychomatics* 47: 3.

Shin, H. and White-Taut, R. (2007) 'The conceptual structure of transition to motherhood in the neonatal intensive care unit', *Journal of Reproductive and Infant Psychology* 17(3): 408–14.

Thomas, L.M. (2008) 'The changing role of parents in neonatal care: a historical review', *Neonatal Network* 27(2): 91–9.

Turan, T., Basbakkal, Z. and Ozbek, S. (2008) 'Effects of nursing interventions on stressors of parents of premature infants in neonatal intensive care', *Journal of Clinical Nursing* 17: 2856–66.

Turrill, S. (1999) 'Interpreting family-centred care within neonatal nursing', *Paediatric Nursing* 11(4): 22–4.

Vandenberg, K. (2000) 'Supporting parents in NICU: guidelines for promoting parent confidence and competence', *Neonatal Network* 19(8): 63–4.

Whyte, D.A. (1997) *Explorations in Family Nursing*, New York: Routledge.

Wigert, H., Johansson, R., Berg, M. and Hellstrom, A.L. (2006) 'Mothers' experiences of having their newborn child in a neonatal intensive care unit', *Scandinavian Journal of Caring Sciences* 20: 35–41.

Chapter 4

Resuscitation of the Newborn

Glenys Connolly

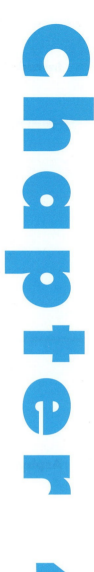

 Contents

Introduction

Resuscitation at birth is a relatively frequent occurrence. Approximately 10 per cent of newborns will require help to establish breathing at birth, with 1 per cent requiring more extensive resuscitation (ILCOR 2006). These numbers suggest that most of these infants will respond to good airway and ventilatory management, but that a small proportion will go on to require further interventions of chest compressions and resuscitative drugs.

Neonatal nurses, as either the lead practitioner or assistants, are often involved in the resuscitation of high-risk infants in the delivery room and infants in their care on NICU. In order to comply with Code of Conduct and Performance (NMC 2008), it is imperative that they deliver care based upon best evidence and practice available and that they keep their knowledge and skills up to date. This chapter examines the current available literature to establish what are effective practices in the resuscitation situation. While it will focus upon delivery room management, the techniques and interventions outlined can be applied in the intensive care unit situation.

Infants who require resuscitation at birth fall into two broad categories: those who have undergone a period of hypoxic stress in utero, and those who are prone to hypoxaemia in the immediate postnatal period due to inadequate pulmonary development, airway obstruction or congenital malformations. Significant hypoxia will lead to asphyxic tissue damage, so anticipation of the need for resuscitation prior to delivery is of great importance.

Asphyxia

Asphyxia before, during or after birth is an important cause of perinatal mortality and morbidity (Williams *et al.* 1993). Asphyxia is literally defined as 'without pulse', but Levene's (1995) definition of 'impairment of placental or pulmonary gas exchange resulting in hypoxia, hypercapnoea and acidosis' is perhaps more reflective of the perinatal situation, as it is this series of events that leads to circulatory compromise and collapse.

Relative oxygen depletion is part of the normal process of labour, with the healthy fetus being equipped with several protective mechanisms that will prevent hypoxic damage to vital organs. The high affinity for oxygen of fetal haemoglobin supports the flow of oxygen to the tissues. This mechanism allows oxygen extraction at tissue level to increase by almost 100 per cent during hypoxaemic events as it shifts the haemoglobin oxygen dissociation curve to the right (decreased affinity), which enhances oxygen extraction delaying the development of hypoxic damage (Bocking *et al.* 1992; Talner *et al.* 1992). The fetal heart rate is a major determinant of **cardiac output**. It is four times greater than that of an adult per kilogram body weight, as it is the combined output of right and left ventricles, with 50 per cent of the output directed to the placenta (Cohn *et al.* 1974). The combination of these mechanisms allows a wide safety margin of adequate oxygen delivery during labour.

In short-duration hypoxaemic events, the heart rate of the mature fetus will fall, but as it is associated with an increase in arterial blood pressure, myocardial contractility is increased and cardiac output is maintained. This is due to vascular resistance changes in the fetal gut and carcass, which divert the blood supply to the heart, brain and adrenals (Cohn *et al*. 1974). This autoregulatory process is modulated at cellular level via metabolic feedback regulation of the calibre of the arterioles and capillary sphincters (Grainger *et al*. 1975, cited in Talner *et al*. 1992). The heart and brain are efficient at **autoregulation** and can maintain their blood flow over a wide range of perfusion pressures and oxygen contents. Hypoxaemic events of this type are intermittent during labour, and the ability of the fetus to quickly redistribute oxygenated blood is very important.

When there is no stress, the fetal and newborn heart is working at close to capacity merely to satisfy normal demands of tissues and growth (Talner *et al*. 1992); therefore any increased output requirement to satisfy suboptimal tissue oxygen demand cannot be sustained for long and myocardial contractility will fail. So while the fetus can make circulatory adjustments to compensate for the rigours of labour, under severe conditions these adaptive mechanisms will be overwhelmed, the shunting of the blood towards vital organs and cerebral oxygen delivery will reduce as the blood pressure and cardiac output fall.

The ability of an organ to maintain aerobic metabolism is dependent on the amount of energy (**adenosine triphosphate, ATP**) needed to maintain functional activity, the amount of oxygen delivered to the tissue and the amount of oxygen extracted by the tissue. The variation in response during labour is related to maturity, with immature fetal tissue being generally more robust. The smaller body mass to placental size gives a larger oxygen reserve to the premature fetus (Greene and Rosen 1995). As the ventricular pressure falls there is a corresponding decrease in cerebral blood flow (CBF). During severe asphyxia CBF is directed to the brain stem rather than the cerebrum, which increases the likelihood of damage to the cerebrum and cortex (Williams *et al*. 1993). When organ blood flow and oxygen delivery are severely compromised, increased tissue extraction of oxygen will not be able to compensate fully for the decrease in oxygen delivery. This will result in aerobic metabolism becoming compromised, and anaerobic metabolism becoming a supplementary mechanism to maintain cellular energy stores.

Anaerobic **glycolysis** produces approximately one-fifteenth of ATP produced aerobically and is consequently a short-term emergency measure. In this state, glucose can only be oxidised to pyruvate and lactate. As the lactate accumulates in the blood and tissues, there is a gradual progression towards a metabolic acidaemia (see p. 136). ATP is required to maintain the ion gradient of sodium and calcium across the cellular membrane. Failure of this mechanism leads to an influx of sodium and calcium into the cells, which allows for an influx of water, leading to intracellular swelling. This acute swelling creates cytotoxic cerebral oedema, which may contribute to brain injury (see p. 191).

The sequence of events that occurs following intrauterine hypoxia has been well documented since the work of Dawes in the 1960s (which is recommended reading for all involved in neonatal resuscitation) and will not be further described. As asphyxia is arguably the most common cause of perinatally acquired severe brain injury in the full-term infant (Levene 1995), practitioners working within the field of neonatal care have a responsibility to be able to ameliorate its potentially devastating effects by prompt and skilled resuscitation. This is true also in management of the preterm infant who, if neglected in the first few minutes of life, is more likely to succumb to hypoxic and thermal stresses that will undoubtedly adversely affect that infant's outcome.

Anticipation

On arriving in the delivery room several factors should be elicited prior to the delivery: the gestation of the infant, any known problems, e.g. congenital anomaly, the presence of multiples, liquor status, e.g. presence of meconium, and risk factors for infection such as prolonged rupture of membranes. If time permits, a more detailed history can be taken (maternal illness or drug use) but the above will enable a plan to be formulated quickly as to whether the infant may need early intubation or whether more help may be needed in the case of multiple births.

Wherever possible, the parents should be spoken to regarding what is likely to happen following the delivery (for example, immediate removal of the infant to the resuscitation platform), so that they are aware of the situation and prepared as much as possible as to why these interventions may be necessary. This is not always possible, of course, when an infant is born unexpectedly compromised. Neonatal resuscitation events are unique in that there are usually other persons in the immediate vicinity who are not directly (practically) involved with the situation. While debate may remain around the presence of relatives in adult resuscitation scenarios and accident and emergency departments (Mitchell and Lynch 1997; Stewart and Bowker 1997), the situation is not up for discussion during delivery room resuscitation events, as the parents are most certainly present and witnessing the events as they occur. This has implications for the professionals' demeanour and the support of the parents both during and after the resuscitation event. The resuscitation situation within the NICU can be further compounded when other parents are in the vicinity. This is particularly pertinent when the parents of the 'collapsed' infant are not present. This situation requires thought and sensitivity surrounding the issues of support and reassurance of the witnesses, while working within the remit of patient confidentiality, and ultimately the support of the actual parents when they are informed of events.

The equipment and environment in the delivery room should be also prepared so that everything that may be required is close to hand and infant heat loss is minimised. While it may appear obvious that equipment is checked, and be sufficient for the task in hand, failure of this simple procedure is implicated in a proportion of neonatal deaths reported annually in the UK (Maternal and Child Health Research Consortium 1995).

Careful attention to thermal homeostasis cannot be overemphasised during a resuscitation event. While practitioners are mindful of its importance, this intervention is often only partly achieved, with the infant being partially dried, with wet hair, and left in contact with damp towels, while other interventions take precedence.

Thermal stability must be maintained. The intrauterine environment is approximately 1.5°C greater than the maternal temperature. A newborn infant's temperature is approximately 37.8°C (range 37–39°C) (Mann 1968, cited in Rutter 1992). Heat losses by convection, radiation and evaporation are high. **Very low birth weight** infants are at an even greater risk of cold stress due to their unfavourable surface to mass ratio. The core temperature of a wet, asphyxiated infant can drop by as much as 5°C in as many minutes (Milner 1995). Cold stress is associated with hypoxia and acidosis, factors which inhibit surfactant production in the newborn and should be avoided (see p. 97). The room should be warm (approximately 25°C if possible), with doors and windows closed to prevent draughts and convective heat losses. A switched-on radiant heat source and several warm towels should be available for immediate use following delivery (see p. 99). As premature infants have been shown to have increased mortality and morbidity if allowed to become hypothermic at delivery (Costeloe *et al.* 2000), they can benefit from being placed, without drying, into polyethylene wrapping or a polythene bag under the radiant warmer (Lyon and Stenson 2004; Vohra *et al.* 2004), the head dried and hat applied, and any further interventions undertaken with the infant's body remaining in the wrapping.

The ABC (D and E) of resuscitation

As soon as the infant delivers, start the clock and assess the situation. This assessment process is crucial. Most healthy mature infants have spontaneous onset of respiration by 10 seconds (Milner 1995); therefore no further assistance is required other than keeping warm by careful drying, followed by skin-to-skin contact with the mother, with any exposed surfaces covered by dry, warm towels. This point is made to reinforce the point that many infants, even those in the 'high-risk' categories, are born in good condition and require minimal interventions. Research indicates that the presence of a paediatrician at such deliveries increases the incidence of unnecessary intubation (Kroll *et al.* 1994), a procedure that is not without potential complications (see p. 353).

An infant born in less than optimal condition requires further assessment. Place this infant on to a warmed padded surface underneath a radiant heat source, and dry off. Immediately remove the wet towels and cover extremities, especially the head, as it accounts for 25 per cent of the infant's surface area and is consequently a site for massive heat loss (Daze and Scanlon 1981). This intervention has the dual effect of reducing heat loss and providing tactile stimulation, which may be enough to induce gasping and onset of respiration.

Airway

Airway management is the next consideration if the infant has failed to cry or is not breathing. The infant should be in the supine position, with the head in a neutral position. As the newborn infant has a prominent occiput, the neutral position can be maintained effectively by the use of a 2cm thickness pad under the shoulders (Zideman *et al.* 1998).

Breathing

The spontaneously gasping infant who has central cyanosis and/or a heart rate around 100 beats per minute may require facial free-flow oxygen, by mask. While this intervention will provide cold stimulus for breathing to occur, it can lead to significant cooling which is counterproductive. These infants may benefit from external stimulation such as rubbing the soles of the feet and trunk to encourage crying and establish spontaneous regular respiration.

Apnoea, pallor or a heart rate less than 100 indicates the necessity for intermittent positive-pressure ventilation (IPPV) via a mask; adequate inflation pressures may stimulate the infant to make spontaneous inspiratory efforts by invoking Head's paradoxical reflex (Milner 1995) and encourage the infant to establish regular respiration. Two systems are commonly available: the self-inflating bag and the T-piece system. If a self-inflating bag system is utilised, the bag volume should be 500ml. Bag volumes less than 300ml rarely produce ventilation greater than the anatomical dead space (Field *et al.* 1986), so are inadequate in creating an adequate functional residual capacity (FRC). This bag should incorporate a pressure-limiting device preset to 30cm H_2O, to avoid inadvertent over-distension of the lungs leading to **pneumothorax**. This limiting device should, however, have the facility to be overridden, as some infants may require generation of greater pressures to achieve appropriate tidal volumes and FRC. Slow compression of the bag is required for the first five breaths so that an inflation time of around 2–3 seconds is achieved. This technique is said to achieve a better formation of FRC (Vyas *et al.* 1981), although this is not easily achieved with some systems.

T-piece resuscitation systems have had a resurgence within neonatal resuscitation in both delivery room settings, and within NICU. With these systems, the first five inflation breaths may be held for up to 2–3 seconds, at a pressure of 30cm of water, observing the chest for movement and auscultating the chest for an increase in heart rate (Resuscitation Council UK 2006). Following establishment of chest movement with these first few slow breaths, a regular ventilation rate of 40–60 per minute should be given. The T-piece system should also have preset pressure limits in order to prevent over-inflation, and the development of air leaks.

Many of these systems also have the ability to give positive end-expiratory pressure (PEEP). The application of PEEP, at resuscitation, may have several benefits for the premature infant. It is thought not only to optimise alveolar expansion and conserve and prolong the effectiveness of surfactant (Wyszogrodski *et al.* 1975; Froese *et al.* 1993), but also attenuate the potential damaging effects of high inspiratory pressures (Carlton *et al.* 1990). A recent study (Arjan *et al.* 2007) suggests that a prolonged inflation breath followed by CPAP alone was effective in establishing FRC and respiration in infants <33 weeks' gestation.

Whichever system is being used (bag or T piece), a soft edge mask, of an appropriate size, should be used to maintain a good seal around the nose and mouth, and prevent trauma to the infant's eyes or skin.

Most infants will respond favourably to mask ventilation (Arya *et al.* 1996), but a proportion will require further intervention of endotracheal intubation (see p. 353), due to extreme prematurity, severe asphyxia, altered anatomy or poor response to bag and mask ventilation. Additionally, mask ventilation is contraindicated in infants with diaphragmatic hernia (Harjo and Jones 1993); therefore in antenatally diagnosed cases a practitioner skilled in endotracheal intubation should be in attendance.

Air or oxygen?

In the past, 100 per cent oxygen was recommended for newborn resuscitation (BMJ Working Party 1997; Chameides and Hazinski 1997; Zideman *et al.* 1998); however, it is now recognised that not only is this unnecessary, it may well have potentially damaging effects. The term 'oxygen-free radical disease' has been introduced into neonatology in recent years, with the main emphasis being its association with retinopathy of prematurity, bronchopulmonary dysplasia, necrotising enterocolitis and persistent ductus arteriosus (Saugstad 1998) in the premature population. There are, though, other considerations to be made in the use of high concentrations of oxygen during resuscitation of both premature and term infants.

Lundstrom *et al.* (1995) measured cerebral blood flow on preterm infants resuscitated with either room air or 80 per cent oxygen. They reported a persistent cerebral vasoconstriction in the high oxygen group which, they concluded, may make the brain more susceptible to hypoxic episodes or ischaemia which may increase the risk of cerebral damage in the newborn period.

In the term asphyxiated population, high oxygen concentrations may also be damaging due to hypoxic reperfusion injury. Animal studies suggest that restoration of blood supply containing a high concentration of oxygen is more detrimental than restoration of the circulation alone, as it appears to create radical oxygen metabolites which lead to further pathological changes (Rootwelt *et al.* 1992; Raivio 1996).

Ramji *et al.* (1993) suggest that room air is no less effective in resuscitation of asphyxiated newborns than 100 per cent oxygen, and Svenningsen and colleagues (1989) have long suggested that 30–40 per cent oxygen will appropriately treat the preterm infant in the delivery room.

While the prevention of hypoxia must remain a high priority during neonatal resuscitation, the indiscriminate use of oxygen needs careful consideration in order to prevent potential long-term adverse sequelae. Studies suggest that some infants initially resuscitated in air will actually go on to require oxygen (Tan *et al.* 2005); therefore if air is the initial gas chosen, oxygen should be readily available for infants who do not respond adequately.

Circulation

The heart rate should be assessed by auscultation using a stethoscope. While palpation of the cord or over the heart may be undertaken, the rate felt may be reflective of the operator's pulse rather than the heart rate of the infant. The most frequent cause of an inadequate heart rate is ineffective ventilation, and once this is established, most heart rates will increase. A rate of less than 60 beats per minute, or less than 80 beats per minute despite effective ventilation, requires prompt initiation of chest compressions (American Heart Association 2006).

There are two techniques described for chest compression in the newborn. The optimal technique is for the operator's hands to encircle the thorax, with the thumbs, pointing **cephalad**, placed side by side over the lower third of the sternum (David 1988; Menegazzi *et al.* 1993). The sternum is then compressed to approximately one-third of the thorax depth (Chameides and Hazinski 1997; Zideman *et al.* 1998; American Heart Association 2006). It is important that this rate is not exceeded, as too rapid chest compression will not allow for the relaxation phase of the technique, which will hinder its effectiveness. Each compression should have an equal pressure and relaxation phase. To be most effective, the compressions should be interposed with a ventilation breath every third compression, as simultaneous chest compression may hinder ventilation. This 3:1 ratio will give 120 cycles per minute, for example, 90 cardiac compressions to 30 breaths.

The alternative technique is to place the index and middle finger on the lower third of the sternum and press at the same depth and rate as previously described. This technique may be more appropriate in the extremely low birth weight population due to the size of the thorax or when umbilical venous access needs to be gained but, as it is recognised as being less effective in creating coronary artery perfusion pressures and mean arterial blood pressure, its application should be limited (Menegazzi *et al.* 1993). Compressions should be briefly stopped every 30 seconds to check actual heart rate. Once the infant's spontaneous rate is above 80 and rising, compressions may stop.

In Perlman's (1995) study, chest compression (or drugs) as part of neonatal resuscitation was administered in only 0.12 per cent of 30,839 newborn infants (cited in Ginsberg and Goldsmith 1998), but in the unlikely event that the infant's heart rate is still not improving following adequate ventilation and good-quality compressions, drug therapy needs to be considered.

Drugs

Drugs are not a first-line action in neonatal resuscitation and should only be considered when one is certain that effective ventilation is in operation in that the chest is moving, and the heart rate is still not increasing despite chest compressions.

Drug therapy during resuscitation is one of the most controversial areas, with arguments raging as to which are the most appropriate and most effective agents, dosages, routes of administration and speed of delivery. These controversies are, in part, due to many of the drug dosages being extrapolated from adult data. Also, when the anatomical and physiological differences in the neonate are considered, for example, the presence of lung fluid, right to left shunts, and the susceptibility of the neonatal brain to haemorrhage, these extrapolations may be inappropriate (Ginsberg and Goldsmith 1998). Indeed, the use of drugs at all in certain groups of infants may in itself be inappropriate, as their necessity seems to be associated with an extremely poor outcome (Sims *et al.* 1994).

This section will attempt to rationalise which drugs are the most effective in neonatal resuscitation.

Adrenaline

Adrenaline (epinephrine) is used to stimulate the failing heart during resuscitation in both adults and infants. It is an endogenous **catecholamine** which has both alpha- and beta-adrenergic effects. Its major benefit during resuscitation is the alpha-mediated vasoconstriction which increases the aortic diastolic pressure increasing the coronary perfusion pressure, and myocardial blood flow (Burchfield 1993).

The recommended route of administration is via the central intravenous route but it can be administered via the endotracheal tube. Lindemann (1984) was the first to suggest endotracheal instillation in the delivery room and neonatal intensive care setting. Utilising the same dose as for the intravenous route (0.1ml/kg of 1:10000), he reported the positive response of return to normal heart rate within 5–10 seconds of instillation. Previous to this, adult work had suggested a tenfold increase in the dose to gain net effect if the tracheal route was to be used (Roberts 1978, cited in Burchfield 1993). In the neonatal population, the theoretical risk of intracranial haemorrhage, especially in the highly vascular germinal matrix of the preterm infant, following the acute hypertensive response to the drug, excludes this dose increase from routine recommendation (Nadkarni *et al.* 1997).

Mullett *et al.* (1992) suggest that there may be a delay in diffusion of tracheal adrenaline during the first week of life due to thicker epithelial linings of the respiratory bronchi, alveoli and pulmonary vascular walls, suggesting that infants collapsing after the first week of life may respond more effectively to tracheal adrenaline than those immediately after birth.

The tracheal route should only be used as a first route of administration to 'buy time' while vascular access is being gained (Barber and Wyckoff 2006) for repeated doses or as a route for other drugs that may need to be administered. If the first dose of adrenaline (0.1ml/kg of 1:10,000 strength) does not have the desired therapeutic effect, then a second dose (0.3ml/kg of 1:10,000 strength) can be given after 3–5 minutes (Resuscitation Council UK 2006).

As metabolic acidaemia and hypoxia will attenuate the action of adrenaline (Preziosi *et al*. 1993), the failure of repeated doses may be due to the acidotic state of the infant. Ideally the base deficit should be determined by blood sample analysis, as is the case in the intensive care setting, but in extreme situations, for example, prolonged resuscitation in the delivery unit where the infant is not responding to the above interventions, the use of buffering agents needs consideration.

Buffers

During cardiopulmonary collapse, gaseous exchange in the lungs ceases while cellular metabolism continues in an anaerobic environment. This produces a combination of respiratory and metabolic acidosis. As previously described, acidaemia decreases myocardial contractility, diminishes blood pressure by vasodilatation and decreases the heart's responsiveness to catecholamines.

The correction of this state, then, is not only rational, it is imperative, if recovery is to be achieved. While management of the respiratory component is, without question, good ventilatory support, the management of the metabolic component is at the very least contentious!

Spencer *et al*. (1993) suggest that it is difficult to determine infants with severe metabolic acidaemia clinically, and that by one hour of age a pH as low as 6.99 will be corrected spontaneously by the infant's own compensatory mechanisms.

Koster and Carli (1992) also claim the best buffer agent is 'the return to a spontaneous circulation'. Continued cardiac depression following good ventilation and adrenaline administration may indicate that acidaemia is a contributory factor and that a more expedient return to normal pH is indicated rather than hoping the infant will 'self-correct' if left.

The use of alkaline buffers for correction of metabolic acidosis has a long tradition in cardiopulmonary resuscitation and several drugs are available for clinical use. Wherever possible, the base deficit should be ascertained. This may well be achievable within a resuscitation situation within the NICU but this is not usually feasible within a delivery unit.

Bicarbonate

Sodium bicarbonate has long been the most commonly used buffer for correction of metabolic acidosis of differing aetiologies, as well as acidosis seen at cardiac arrest (Bjerneroth 1998).

In the normal situation, carbon dioxide entering the blood as a result of metabolism in the tissues initially exists as a simple solution. Some of it though will react with water to form carbonic acid, which dissociates to hydrogen and bicarbonate due to the action of carbonic anhydrase in the red blood cells. Most of the carbon dioxide in the body is transported this way. For example:

$$H_2O + CO_2 \Leftrightarrow H_2CO_3 \Leftrightarrow H^+ + HCO_3$$

The reverse set of reactions occurs in the lungs. As the carbon dioxide level declines, bicarbonate ions re-enter the red blood cells and bind with hydrogen to form carbonic acid which is then cleaved by carbonic anhydrase to release carbon dioxide and water for elimination during expiration. This maintains the correct ratio of hydrogen and bicarbonate in the blood to maintain the acid base balance:

$$H^+ + HCO_3 \Leftrightarrow H_2CO_3 \Leftrightarrow H_2O + CO_2$$

Several authors (Howell 1987; Burchfield 1993; Hein 1993; Bjerneroth 1998; Ginsberg and Goldsmith 1998) cite Ostrea and Odell's work of 1972 when describing the use of bicarbonate in correcting metabolic acidosis. They describe it as functioning as a physiological buffer only in an 'open system', in which the carbon dioxide created can be transported to the lungs and blown off. Thus, in inadequate ventilatory situations (during resuscitation) a 'closed system' occurs and the carbon dioxide created shifts the equation to the left, leading to a worsening of the acidaemia. In addition, the tissue and venous side of the circulation probably act also as a 'closed system', in that carbon dioxide cannot be appropriately eliminated due to poor tissue perfusion from the diminished cardiac output (Hein 1993). Thus, bicarbonate will only serve as an effective buffer in balancing the hydrogen–bicarbonate in the presence of adequate ventilation, otherwise the metabolic acidosis will be replaced by respiratory acidosis. Moreover, since the increased carbon dioxide diffuses more rapidly into the cells than the bicarbonate, paradoxically it may actually worsen intracellular acidaemia. Therefore indiscriminate administration of bicarbonate during resuscitation may make matters worse (Howell 1987).

Other potential complications associated with bicarbonate administration are within its hypertonicity. Undiluted bicarbonate contains 2000mOsmol and 1mEq of sodium; as a consequence, it is highly implicated in the development of hypernatraemic states and intraventricular haemorrhage in the preterm infant (Howell 1987; Ginsberg and Goldsmith 1998).

Other buffering solutions may be considered. Trishydroxyaminomethyl-methane (THAM) was initially suggested by Gomori in 1962 (cited in Bjerneroth 1998) for pH control. An organic buffer, THAM is a weak base that acts as a proton acceptor which increases pH and reduces carbon dioxide (Bowman and Rand 1980: 28.25). While it was regarded as a promising alternative to bicarbonate, it has been recognised as having several toxic effects, including hypoglycaemia, severe vasospasm leading to phlebitis and thrombosis, and with extravasation injuries resulting in necrosis. More importantly, it has been demonstrated that it induced arterial vasodilatation, decreasing aortic diastolic pressure and drastically lowering coronary artery perfusion, thereby reducing the success in cardiopulmonary resuscitation (Kette *et al.* 1991, cited in Bjerneroth 1998). In the light of these findings, THAM cannot be recommended during acute emergency resuscitation situations.

The correction of metabolic acidaemia with bicarbonate is undoubtedly controversial with a recent Cochrane review (Beveridge and Wilkinson 2006) unable to find evidence to support or refute its use. Despite this lack of evidence, slow intravenous administration (over 2 minutes) via the umbilical venous catheter of 1–2mmol/kg of a 4.2 per cent bicarbonate solution is thought to be useful in well-ventilated and oxygenated infants who are unresponsive to adrenaline (Burchfield 1993; Zideman *et al.* 1998; Resuscitation Council UK 2006).

Colloid and crystalloid

The use of albumin during resuscitation has become less prevalent in neonatal practice and is no longer recommended following a number of studies that have challenged its efficacy. Roberton (1997) reviewed the use of albumin in neonatal resuscitation and suggests that albumin has little value in the correction of acideamia *per se*, unless it is due to volume depletion. He further states that it is 'physiologically unsound', and that it may actually do further harm by overloading an already failing myocardium. Dixon *et al.* (1997) reported that while both albumin and bicarbonate raised the pH and reduced base excess, bicarbonate appeared to have a superior effect.

The efficacy of albumin as volume replacement has been further challenged (Osborn and Evans 2004; The Albumin Reviewers 2004) with isotonic saline being just as effective in raising the blood pressure (So *et al.* 1997). This is probably due to the infant requiring volume rather than a protein load as it is also questionable whether albumin has any value in the correction of hypoalbuminaemia (Jardine *et al.* 2004). Additionally, as a blood product, albumin carries a higher risk of infection to the recipient and is more expensive than normal saline.

It has to be remembered that volume overload is particularly hazardous in the preterm population contributing to bronchopulmonary dysplasia, necrotising enterocolitis, patent ductus arteriosus, and intraventricular haemorrhage (Roberton 1997), so careful assessment and judicious use of volume replacement are imperative. In an infant where there is evidence of acute blood loss, pallor persisting following oxygenation, poor pulses with an adequate heart rate and a poor response to otherwise adequate resuscitation attempts, isotonic saline 10ml/kg (Resuscitation Council UK 2006) should be given as a bolus via the umbilical venous catheter and repeated if necessary.

Dextrose (glucose)

Whether to use glucose during resuscitation of an asphyxiated infant is yet another unresolved issue, due to inconsistencies in research findings. Glucose is the predominant metabolic fuel for the immature brain, with hypoglycaemia being associated with poorer developmental outcome (Lucas *et al*. 1988). During anaerobic metabolism, glucose stores are rapidly turned over, so it would appear sensible to administer intravenous glucose during prolonged resuscitation events to prevent the development of hypoglycaemia. Several animal studies (Myers and Yamaguchi 1977; Lundy *et al*. 1987) report an increased mortality and morbidity when dextrose was administered during resuscitation, although Vannucci and Mujsce (1992) suggest that an elevated glucose level prior to an asphyxial event appears to be protective. Studies of glucose administration post asphyxial injury are equally contradictory, with benefits and damage being reported equally (Hattori and Wasterlain 1990; Sheldon *et al*. 1992).

Anatomical and physiological differences between the mature and immature brain also seem to have a bearing on this situation. Levene (1995) suggests the immature brain handles glucose differently to the mature (adult) brain. Differences in the blood–brain barrier, rate of consumption of glucose and enzyme release restrict anaerobic metabolism of glucose to concentrations of lactic acid which are not neuro necrotic. It is clear that hypoglycaemia following asphyxia is not beneficial (Salhab *et al*. 2004), but the administration of high concentrations of dextrose solutions during resuscitation cannot be recommended as good practice. Resuscitation Council UK (2006) suggests that 2.5ml/kg of 10 per cent dextrose should be administered if there is no response to adrenaline and bicarbonate.

Extras

Naloxone (Narcan) is, as its tradename suggests, a *narc*otic *an*tagonist, and subsequently has no role in resuscitation of the hypoxic, asphyxiated infant. Its only use is in the reversal of opiate analgesia that has been given to an infant directly, or to a fetus via its mother. At birth, an infant with a good heart rate and respiratory depression may benefit from a dose of 100μg/kg. Naloxone should NEVER be given to an infant of a known (or suspected) opiate-addicted mother, as the withdrawal effects may be severe.

Calcium gluconate has been given in the past during resuscitation as it increases myocardial contractility and excitability. It is also a potent constrictor of the coronary vessels and may invoke asystole if given rapidly. It is no longer recommended in neonatal resuscitation.

Atropine is used to block the inhibitory effects of the vagus nerve, thus speeding up the heart rate. While this may be of benefit in avoiding reflex **bradycardia** during intubation and surgical procedures, it has no place in the correction of hypoxia-induced bradycardia in neonatal resuscitation settings.

Meconium stained liquor

Meconium stained liquor occurs in 10–20 per cent of pregnancies at term (Halliday 1992). While this incidence is high, the incidence of **aspiration** is said to be 5 per cent of infants in the USA (Cleary and Wiswell 1998) and 0.2 per cent of infants in the UK (Greenough 1995). Meconium in the liquor may be an 'innocent' finding due to fetal maturational processes, often associated with post-term deliveries and often described as 'thin' meconium. It may, however, be 'thick' meconium, which is viewed as a marker of fetal hypoxia, the hypothesis being that in-utero hypoxia increases intestinal peristalsis and relaxation of the anal sphincter tone.

Meconium passage is rare in preterm deliveries, and its apparent presence before this time should be viewed with caution as it may be representative of different pathology, such as chorioamnionitis.

Meconium stained liquor, whether thin or thick, requires the presence of someone who is competent at intubation at the delivery in case this intervention is required, remembering that thin meconium may become thick during the latter stages of labour. Manoeuvres such as cricoid pressure, epiglottal blockage and thoracic compression to prevent inhalation are not recommended as they are not scientifically tested, and are potentially dangerous as they can cause vagal stimulation, trauma and deep aspiration due to chest recoil when the encircling hands are released. Suctioning of the infant oro pharynx prior to the delivery of the shoulders is neither thought to confer any benefit and should not be undertaken.

The management of the infant following delivery is dependent on its condition. In the infant who delivers through meconium stained liquor but is vigorous and crying, intubation should not be attempted but gentle oro pharyngeal suction may be of benefit if meconium is visible in the mouth (Halliday and Sweet 2001). Forcing cord visualisation and/or intubation in these infants is more likely to cause trauma or bradycardia and will not improve the outcome.

The infant who is obviously compromised, floppy, with no respiratory effort and low heart rate, requires immediate intervention of direct vision of the vocal cords, and tracheal suction using a wide bore catheter to remove any particulate matter. These interventions should take place under a radiant heat source to curb potential massive heat loss, but *prior* to drying and stimulation in order to prevent invoking any reflex gasping respiration. Repeated intubation and suction may be necessary in order to clear the airways prior to instigation of IPPV. The heart rate will determine how many times this can be undertaken before oxygenation by IPPV should commence.

The infants who are more controversial are the ones who fall between these two situations. In these infants, astute clinical assessment is required; if the infant is less than vigorous and occasionally gasping, visualisation of the cords and suction are probably judicious, prior to initiation of inflation breaths.

There is no evidence to suggest that saline lavage is beneficial in the acute management of MAS as it may dilute the meconium, creating easier dispersal throughout the lung and worsening lung function (Cleary and Wiswell 1998).

The use of surfactant as a pulmonary lavage has been investigated as a potential early treatment option as it increases retrieval of meconium and increases oxygenation (Revak *et al.* 1997; Wiswell *et al.* 2002). The administration of surfactant as a management strategy post resuscitation is thought to be of benefit in reducing severity of respiratory illness and reducing the need for ECMO (El-Shahed *et al.* 2007).

Meconium aspiration syndrome remains an important cause of neonatal mortality and morbidity (Ibrahim amd Subhedar 2005). As a consequence, its active and sometimes rather aggressive management at the time of delivery continues to be justified. See p. 129 for further management.

Evaluation of resuscitation

The prognosis of the term infant following prolonged resuscitation is difficult to determine in the delivery unit and can only really be predicted when there has been a full neurological assessment on the neonatal unit, and the degree of injury (if any) has been determined.

Infants born apparently dead can be successfully resuscitated and have a normal outcome. Casalaz *et al.* (1998) reported a 36 per cent intact survival rate in a series of 42 unexpected stillbirths, with a further 16 per cent reported to have 'equivocal outcome' with mild motor development problems but with no developmental delay. Prediction of outcome in asphyxiated infants is of obvious importance to parents, and the information needs to be given as clearly and honestly as possible. The information given to parents can be more clearly and accurately given if the appearance of the infant at birth and resuscitation manoeuvres are clearly documented. The use of the numerical Apgar score alone is of little value. Infants with the same scores can have vastly differing aetiologies and therefore vastly different outcomes. Full written descriptors should accompany the scoring system if it is to be of any clinical value. Following a resuscitation event, however minor or extensive, the interventions undertaken should be carefully and accurately documented (NMC 2008).

Within documentation the use of the term 'asphyxiated at birth' should be avoided, as an infant who fails to breathe spontaneously immediately at birth may not have undergone a hypoxic-ischaemic insult and use of the term may cause controversy in the long term, both medically and legally (Donn 1998).

In the very low birth weight population, the incidence of resuscitation increases to 80 per cent (Leuthner *et al.* 1994). Several studies indicate that infants in this category who require the full range of interventions, including chest compressions and drugs, in the first few days of life have a very poor prognosis, and use of such interventions may signal a cessation of active management (Lantos *et al.* 1988; Sood and Giacoia 1992; Sims *et al.* 1994; Barr and Courtman 1998). These works have to be taken on balance and on an individual basis. Ginsberg and Goldsmith (1998) suggest that vigorous attempts at resuscitation are mandated in all but a few situations, as a wait and see approach can result in an infant sustaining damage from cold stress, hypoglycaemia, hypotension and hypoxia.

How long should resuscitation continue?

Most hospitals will have their own policies to determine when resuscitative efforts should be abandoned. Recommendations suggest that it may be justifiable to stop resuscitation if an infant has no signs of life after 10 minutes of continuous and adequate resuscitative efforts (ILCOR 2006) or if there is no respiratory effort by 30 minutes, when other factors for respiratory depression, e.g. opiate depression or neuromuscular disorders, have been eliminated (Milner 2005, p. 238). The final decision to abandon resuscitation should be made by the most senior neonatologist or paediatrician available at the time.

Conclusion

Resuscitation events around the time of birth and within NICU are relatively frequent events, but practitioners must not become complacent because of this and feel that they are competent to practise effectively in any given situation. Studies suggest that deskilling occurs over time (Broomfield 1996; Duran *et al.* 2008) and mandatory updating sessions should be undertaken by all members of the team in order to maintain and improve practitioner skills and consequently infant outcomes.

Case study: management of a delivery unit resuscitation

You are asked to assist at the delivery of a 26-week gestation infant.

Q.1. What are your immediate priorities to prepare for the birth?

A boy is delivered weighing approximately 800 grams. He gasps but remains blue and floppy with a heart rate less than 100.

Q.2. What is the immediate management of this infant?

The decision is made to intubate and ventilate prior to transfer to NICU.

Q.3. What are your actions during this procedure?

Following the intubation, the heart rate is less than 60bpm.

Q.4. What should you be looking for at this point?

Q.5. Should drugs be prepared and given in this circumstance?

References

American Heart Association (2006) '2005 American Heart Association Guidelines for cardiopulmonary resuscitation and emergency cardiovascular care of pediatric and neonatal patients: neonatal resuscitation guidelines', *Pediatrics* 117(5): 1029–38.

Arjan, B., te Pas, M.D. and Walther, F.J. (2007) 'A randomised controlled trial of delivery room respiratory management', *Pediatrics* 120: 322–9.

Arya, R., Pethen, T., Johanson, R.B. and Spencer, S.A. (1996) 'Outcome in low risk pregnancies', *Archives of Disease in Childhood: Fetal and Neonatal Edition* 75: F97–F102.

Barber, C.A. and Wyckoff, M.H. (2006) 'Use and efficacy of endotracheal versus intravenous epinephrine during neonatal cardiopulmonary resuscitation', *Pediatrics* 118(3): 1028–34.

Barr, P. and Courtman, S.P. (1998) 'Cardio pulmonary resuscitation in the newborn intensive care unit', *Journal of Paediatrics and Child Health* 34: 503–7.

Beveridge, C.J.E. and Wilkinson, A.R. (2006) 'Sodium bicarbonate infusion during resuscitation of infants at birth', *Cochrane Database of Systematic Reviews* (1): CD004864.

Bjerneroth, G. (1998) 'Alkaline buffers for correction of metabolic acidosis during cardiopulmonary resuscitation with focus on Tribonat – a review', *Resuscitation* 37: 161–71.

BMJ Working Party (1997) *Resuscitation of Babies at Birth*, London: BMJ Publishing Group.

Bocking, A., White, S.E., Homan, J. and Richardson, B.S. (1992) 'Oxygen consumption is maintained in fetal sleep during prolonged hypoxaemia', *Journal of Developmental Physiology* 17: 169–74.

Bowman, W.C. and Rand, M.J. (1980) *Textbook of Pharmacology*, 2nd edn, Oxford: Blackwell Scientific.

Broomfield, R. (1996) 'A quasi-experimental research to investigate the retention of basic cardiopulmonary resuscitation skills and knowledge by qualified nurses following a course in professional development', *Journal of Advanced Nursing* 23(5): 1016–23.

Burchfield, D.J. (1993) 'Medication use in neonatal resuscitation: epinephrine and sodium bicarbonate', *Neonatal Pharmacology Quarterly* 2(2): 25–30.

Burchfield, D.J. (1996) 'Neonatal and fetal resuscitation', in N.A. Paradis, H.R. Halperin and R.M. Nowack (eds) *Cardiac Arrest: The Science and Practice of Resuscitation Medicine*, Baltimore, MD: Williams & Wilkins.

Carlton, D.P., Cummings, J.J., Scheerer, R.G., Poulain, F.R. and Bland, R.D. (1990) 'Lung overexpansion increases pulmonary microvascular protein permeability in young lambs', *Journal of Applied Physiology* 69(2): 577–83.

Casalaz, D.M., Marlow, N. and Speidal, B.D. (1998) 'Outcome of resuscitation following unexpected apparent stillbirth', *Archives of Disease in Childhood: Fetal and Neonatal Edition* 78: F112–F115.

Chameides, L. and Hazinski, M.F. (1997) *Pediatric Advanced Life Support*, Dallas, TX: American Heart Association.

Cleary, J.M. and Wiswell, T.E. (1998) 'Meconium stained amniotic fluid and the meconium aspiration syndrome: an update', *Pediatric Clinics of North America* 45: 511–29.

Cohn, H.E., Sacks, E.J., Heymann, M.A. and Rudolph, A.M. (1974) 'Cardiovascular responses to hypoxia and acidaemia in fetal lambs', *American Journal of Obstetrics and Gynecology* 120: 817–24.

Costeloe, K., Hennessy, E., Gibson, A.T., Marlow, N. and Wilkinson, A.R. (2000) 'The EPICure study: outcomes to discharge from hospital for infants born at the threshold of viability', *Pediatrics* 106: 659–71.

David, R. (1988) 'Closed chest cardiac massage in the newborn infant', *Pediatrics* 81: 552–4.

Dawes, G.S. (1968) *Foetal and Neonatal Physiology*, Chicago, IL: Year Book Medical Publishers.

Daze, A.M. and Scanlon, J.W. (1981) *Code Pink: A Practical System for Neonatal/Perinatal Resuscitation*, Baltimore, MD: University Park Press.

Dixon, H., Hawkins, K.C. and Stephenson, T.J. (1997) 'Randomised controlled trial of human albumin solution versus sodium bicarbonate to treat neonatal metabolic acidosis', Abstract presented at the Neonatal Society, London.

Donn, S.M. (1998) 'Risk management in neonatal practice', Abstract presented at 6th Annual Neonatal Conference, Middlesbrough.

Duran, R., Aladag. N., Vatansever, U. *et al* (2008) 'Proficiency and knowledge gained and retained by pediatric residents after neonatal resuscitation course', *Paediatrics International* 50(5): 644–7.

El-Shahad, A.I., Dargaville, P., Ohlsson, A. and Soll, R.F. (2007) 'Surfactant for meconium aspiration syndrome in full term/near term infants', *Cochrane Database of Systematic Reviews* (3): CD0002054.

Field, D., Milner, A.D. and Hopkin, I.E. (1986) 'Efficiency of manual resuscitators at birth', *Archives of Disease in Childhood* 61: 300–2.

Froese, A.B., McCulloch, P.R., Matasoshi, S., Vaclavic, S., Possmayer, F. and Moller, F. (1993) 'Optimising alveolar expansion prolongs the effectiveness of exogenous surfactant therapy in the adult rabbit', *American Review of Respiratory Disease* 148: 569–77.

Ginsberg, H.G. and Goldsmith, J.P. (1998) 'Controversies in neonatal resuscitation', *Clinics in Perinatology* 25(1): 1–15.

Greene, K.R. and Rosen, K.G. (1995) 'Intrapartum asphyxia', in M.I. Levene and R.J. Lilford (eds) *Fetal and Neonatal Neurology and Neurosurgery*, Edinburgh: Churchill Livingstone.

Greenough, A. (1995) 'Meconium aspiration syndrome: prevention and treatment', *Early Human Development* 41: 183–92.

Halliday, H.L. (1992) 'Other acute lung disorders', in J.C. Sinclair and M.B. Bracken (eds) *Effective Care of the Newborn Infant*, Oxford: Oxford University Press, pp. 359–84.

Halliday, H.L. and Sweet, D. (2001) 'Endotracheal intubation at birth for preventing morbidity and mortality in vigorous meconium stained infants born at term', *Cochrane Database of Systematic Reviews* (1): CD000500.

Harjo, J. and Jones, M.A. (1993) 'The surgical neonate', in C. Kenner, A. Brueggemeyer and L.P. Gunderson (eds) *Comprehensive Neonatal Nursing*, Philadelphia, PA: W.B. Saunders Co., pp. 903–12.

Hattori, H. and Wasterlain, C.G. (1990) 'Post hypoxic glucose supplemental reduces hypoxic ischaemic brain damage in the neonatal rat', *Annals of Neurology* 28: 122–8.

Hein, H.A. (1993) 'The use of sodium bicarbonate in neonatal resuscitation: help or harm?', *Pediatrics* 91(2): 496–7.

Howell, J.H. (1987) 'Sodium bicarbonate in the perinatal setting – revisited', *Clinics in Perinatology* 14(4): 807–17.

Ibrahim, C.P. and Subhedar, N.V. (2005) 'Management of meconium aspiration syndrome', *Current Paediatrics* 15(2): 92–8.

ILCOR (2006) 'The International Liaison Committee on resuscitation consensus on science with treatment with treatment recommendations for pediatric and neonatal patients: neonatal resuscitation', *Pediatrics* 117(5): 978–88.

Jardine, L.A., Jenkins-Manning, S. and Davies, M.W. (2004) 'Albumin infusion for low serum albumin in preterm newborn infants', *Cochrane Database of Systematic Reviews* (3): CD004208.

Koster, R. and Carli, P. (1992) 'Acid–base management', *Resuscitation* 24: 143–6.

Kroll, L., Twohey, L., Daubeney, P.E.F., Lynch, D. and Ducker, D.A. (1994) 'Risk factors at delivery and the need for skilled resuscitation', *European Journal of Obstetrics and Gynaecology and Reproductive Biology* 55: 175–7.

Lantos, J.D., Miles, S.H., Silverstein, M.D. and Stocking, C.B. (1988) 'Survival after cardiopulmonary resuscitation in babies of very low birth weight. Is CPR futile therapy?', *New England Journal of Medicine* 318(2): 91–5.

Leuthner, S.R., Jansen, R.D. and Hageman, J.R. (1994) 'Cardiopulmonary resuscitation of the newborn: an update', *Pediatric Clinics of North America* 41(5): 893–907.

Levene, M.I. (1995) 'Management and outcome of birth asphyxia', in M.I. Levene and R.J. Lilford (eds) *Fetal and Neonatal Neurology and Neurosurgery*, Edinburgh: Churchill Livingstone.

Lindemann, R. (1984) 'Resuscitation of the newborn: endotracheal administration of adrenaline', *Acta Paediatrica Scandinavica* 73: 210–12.

Lucas, A., Morley, R. and Cole, T. (1988) 'Adverse neurodevelopmental outcome of moderate neonatal hypoglycaemia', *British Medical Journal* 297: 1304–8.

Lundstrom, K.E., Pryds, O. and Greisen, G. (1995) 'Oxygen at birth and prolonged cerebral vasoconstriction in preterm infants', *Archives of Disease in Childhood: Fetal and Neonatal Edition* 73: F81–F86.

Lundy, E.F., Kuhn, J.E., Kwon, J.M., Zelenock, G.B. and D'Alecy, L.G. (1987) 'Infusion of five percent dextrose increases mortality and morbidity following six minutes of cardiac arrest in resuscitated dogs', *Journal of Critical Care* 2(1): 4–14.

Lyon, A.J. and Stenson, B. (2004) 'Cold comfort for babies', *Archives of Disease in Childhood: Fetal and Neonatal Edition* 89: F93–F94.

Maternal and Child Health Research Consortium (1995) *Confidential Enquiry into Stillbirths and Deaths in Infancy*, London: Maternal and Child Health Research Consortium.

Menegazzi, J.J., Auble, T.E., Nicklas, K.A. *et al.* (1993) 'Two thumb versus two finger chest compression during CPR in a swine infant model of cardiac arrest', *Annals of Emergency Medicine* 22(2): 112–15.

Milner, A.D. (1995) 'Resuscitation at birth', in M.C. Colquhoun, A.J. Handley and T.R. Evans (eds) *ABC of Resuscitation*, 3rd edn, London: BMJ Publishing Group, pp. 36–9.

Milner, A.D. (2005) 'Resuscitation of the newborn', in J.M. Rennie (ed.) *Roberton's Textbook of Neonatology*, 4th edn, London: Elsevier.

Mitchell, M.H. and Lynch, M.B. (1997) 'Should relatives be allowed in the resuscitation room?', *Journal of Accident and Emergency Medicine* 14(6): 67–71.

Mullett, C.J., Kong, J.Q., Romano, J.T. and Polack, M.J. (1992) 'Age related changes in pulmonary venous epinephrine concentration, and pulmonary vascular response after intratracheal epinephrine', *Pediatric Research* 31(5): 458–61.

Myers, R.E. and Yamaguchi, S. (1977) 'Nervous system effects of cardiac arrest in monkeys: preservation of vision', *Archives of Neurology* 34: 65–74.

Nadkarni, V., Hazinski, M.F., Zideman, D. *et al.* (1997) 'Paediatric life support', *Resuscitation* 34: 115–27.

NMC (2008) 'The code: standards of conduct, performance and ethics for nurses and midwives', *Nursing and Midwifery Council*, London: NMC.

Osborn, D.A. and Evans, N. (2004) 'Early volume expansion for prevention of morbidity and mortality in very preterm infants', *Cochrane Database of Systematic Reviews* (2): CD002055.

Preziosi, M.P., Roig, J.C., Hargrove, N. and Burchfield, D.J. (1993) 'Metabolic acidaemia with hypoxia attenuates the hemodynamic response to epinephrine during resuscitation in lambs', *Critical Care Medicine* 21(12): 1901–70.

Raivio, K.O. (1996) 'Neonatal organ damage due to ischaemia reperfusion', *Biology of the Neonate* 69: 170–1.

Ramji, S., Ahuja, S.,Thirupuram, S. *et al.* (1993) 'Resuscitation of asphyxic newborn infants in room air or 100 per cent oxygen', *Pediatric Research* 34(6): 809–12.

Resuscitation Council (UK) (2006) *Newborn Life Support*, 2nd edn, London: Resuscitation Council (UK).

Revak, S.D., Cochrane, C.G. and Merritt, T.A. (1997) 'The therapeutic effect of bronchoalveolar lavage with surfactant KL_4-surfactant in animal models with meconium aspiration syndrome', *Pediatric Research* 41: 265A.

Roberton, N.R.C. (1997) 'Use of albumin in neonatal resuscitation', *European Journal of Pediatrics* 156: 428–31.

Rootwell, T., Loberg, E.M., Moen, A. *et al.* (1992) 'Hypoxaemia and reoxygenation with 21 per cent or 100 per cent oxygen in newborn piglets: changes in blood pressure, base deficit, and hypoxanthine and brain morphology', *Pediatric Research* 32(1): 107–13.

Rutter, N. (1992) 'Temperature control and its disorders', in N.R.C. Roberton (ed.) *Textbook of Neonatology*, 2nd edn, London: Churchill Livingstone.

Salhab, W.A., Wyckoff, M.H., Laptook, A.R. and Perlmann, J.M. (2004) 'Initial hypoglycaemia and neonatal brain injury in term infants with severe fetal academia', *Pediatrics* 114: 361–6.

Saugstad, O.D. (1998) 'Oxygen radical disease in neonatology', *Seminars in Neonatology* 3: 231–8.

Schierhout, G. and Roberts, I. (1998) 'Fluid resuscitation with colloid or crystalloid solutions in critically ill patients: a systematic review of randomised trials', *British Medical Journal* 316: 961–4.

Sheldon, R.A., Partridge, C. and Ferriero, D.M. (1992) 'Post ischemic hyperglycaemia is not protective to the neonatal rat', *Pediatric Research* 32: 489–93.

Sims, D.G., Heal, C.A. and Bartle, S.M. (1994) 'Use of adrenaline and atropine in neonatal resuscitation', *Archives of Disease in Childhood: Fetal and Neonatal Edition* 70: F3–F10.

So, K.W., Fok, T.F., Ng, P.C. *et al.* (1997) 'Randomised controlled trial of colloid or crystalloid in hypotensive preterm infants', *Archives of Disease in Childhood: Fetal and Neonatal Edition* 76: F43–F46.

Sood, S. and Giacoia, G.P. (1992) 'Cardiopulmonary resuscitation in very low birthweight infants', *American Journal of Perinatology* 9(2): 130–3.

Spencer, J.A.D., Robson, S.C. and Farkas, A. (1993) 'Spontaneous recovery after severe metabolic acidaemia at birth', *Early Human Development* 32: 103–11.

Stewart, K. and Bowker, L. (1997) 'Resuscitation witnessed by relatives might lead to a complaint for breach of confidentiality', *British Medical Journal* 314: 145.

Svenningsen, N.W., Stjernqvist, K., Stavenow, S. and Hellstrom-Westas, L. (1989) 'Neonatal outcomes of extremely small low birthweight liveborn infants below 901g in a Swedish population', *Acta Paediatrica Scandinavica* 78: 180–8.

Talner, N.S., Lister, G. and Fahey, J.T. (1992) 'Effects of asphyxia on the myocardium of the fetus and newborn', in R.A. Polin and W.W. Fox (eds) *Fetal and Neonatal Physiology*, Philadelphia, PA: W.B. Saunders.

Tan, A., Schulze, A. and O'Donnell, C.P.F. (2005) 'Air versus oxygen for resuscitation of infants at birth', *Cochrane Database of Systematic Reviews* (1): CD002273.

The Albumin Reviewers (2004) 'Human albumin solution for resuscitation and volume expansion in critically ill patients', *Cochrane Database of Systematic Reviews* (4): CD001208.

Tomlin, M. (1997) 'Albumin use on intensive care', *The Pharmaceutical Journal* 259: 856–9.

Vannucci, R.C. and Mujsce, D.J. (1992) 'Effect of glucose on perinatal hypoxic–ischaemic brain damage', *Biology of the Neonate* 62: 215–24.

Vohra, S., Roberts, R.S., Zhang, B., James, M. and Schmidt, B. (2004) 'Heat loss prevention (HeLP) in the delivery room: a randomised controlled trial of polyethylene occlusive wrapping in very preterm infants', *Journal of Pediatrics* 145(6): 750–3.

Vyas, H., Milner, A.D., Hopkin, I.E. and Boon, A.W. (1981) 'Physiologic response to prolonged and slow-rise inflation in the resuscitation of the asphyxiated newborn', *Journal of Pediatrics* 99: 635–9.

Williams, C.E., Mallard, C., Tan, W. and Gluckman, P.D. (1993) 'Pathophysiology of perinatal asphyxia', *Clinics in Perinatology* 20(2): 305–25.

Wiswell, T.E., Knight, G.R., Finer, N.N. *et al.* (2002) 'A multicentre randomised controlled trial comparing Surfaxin (Lucinactant) lavage with standard care for treatment of meconium aspiration syndrome', *Pediatrics* 109(6): 1081–7.

Wyszogrodski, I., Kyei-Aboahye, K., Taeusch, J.R. and Avery, M.E. (1975) 'Surfactant inactivation by hyperventilation: conservation by end expiratory pressure', *Journal of Applied Physiology* 38(3): 461–5.

Zideman, D.A., Bingham, R., Beattie, T. *et al.* (1998) 'Recommendations on resuscitation of babies at birth', *Resuscitation* 37: 103–10.

Chapter 5

Management of Thermal Stability

Pauline Fellows

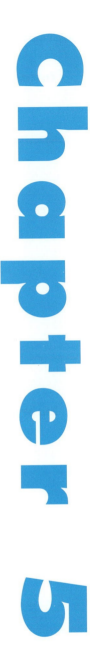

Contents

Introduction

Thermal control has to be initiated by the infant at birth. When born early or in poor condition, the physiological pathways necessary to commence heat production are not fully established or functioning. In the preterm infant, there are insufficient reserves to maintain thermal stability without compromising other body systems. To manage this situation successfully, the neonatal nurse must have knowledge of the systems involved in initiating and maintaining thermal stability, as well as understanding how to assist the infant in the vital transition time after birth. The role of the neonatal nurse is crucial in limiting heat loss at birth and in establishing a suitable environment in which the infant is cared for. This caring begins before the infant is delivered by ensuring the necessary facilities are available in the delivery suite, that all equipment is ready for use to speed any resuscitative measures and that ample warmth is provided (see p. 68). In the neonatal unit, expertise is essential in choosing the right thermal environment for the infant whatever the gestation.

Although the main focus is the thermal management of the preterm infant, it is also important to provide adequate thermal support to the infant born at or near term, who can also be subject to heat loss with all its potential sequelae.

Embryology

The fetus becomes viable (with intensive support) at 23–24 weeks (Nuffield Council on Bioethics 2006), as the lungs become capable of supporting gas exchange. The nervous system has matured enough to direct breathing movements and assist in the control of body temperature. **Myelination** of the peripheral nerve fibres starts in the late fetal period (Hasegawa *et al.* 1992; Bruska and Piotrowski 2004) and assists the transmission of nerve impulses, such as the reaction to cold stimulus and pain. The fore brain divides into the epithalamus, thalamus and hypothalamus at 5–6 weeks and acts as a relay station to conduct impulses to and from the cerebral cortex. Hypothalamic function matures between 5 and 35 weeks' gestation and is involved with the regulation of temperature control, as well as regulating the hormones of the pituitary gland, which in turn secretes thyroid-stimulating hormone (TSH) which can be detected at 10–12 weeks (Moore and Persaud 2003a).

The hormonal mechanisms of thyroxine (T_4) and Triiodothyronine (T_3) are present from 22 weeks and by term are similar to maternal levels. Thyroxine stimulates the enzymes involved with glucose oxidation and so is related to the production of heat. The thyroid gland secretes type II iodothyronine 5' deiodinase, which converts T_4 to T_3, a process that is active by 25 weeks though T_3 levels remain low until 30 weeks (Blackburn 2003a). Infants born before 36 weeks' gestation are likely to have low levels of TSH which will impact on their ability to produce and maintain heat (Clemente *et al.* 2007; Carrascosa *et al.* 2008).

Brown adipose tissue (BAT) has been found to contain mitochondrial uncoupling protein (UCP1) thermogenin – the rate-limiting component of heat production – which is present in increasing amounts between 25 and 40 weeks (Housetek *et al.* 1993). Moore and Persaud (2003a) state that brown fat is being formed at 20 weeks, primarily found in the root of the neck and in the perirenal region. Biopsy of the brown fat of preterm infants aged 25–27 weeks gestation demonstrated that it is thermogenetically active at this stage of development (Zancanaro *et al.* 1995). Rapid activation of UCP1 at the time of birth in conjunction with leptin and prolactin secretion (cytokine hormones) ensures a large increase in heat production (Stephenson *et al.* 2001).

Heat loss is controlled by the release of noradrenaline. The adrenal medulla arises from the neural crest and is part of the sympathetic nervous system (Marieb 1995). The fetal adrenal gland by 4 months' gestation is larger than the kidney (Challis and Thorburn 1976) and it secretes cortisol in response to adrenocorticotrophic hormone (ACTH) by day 50–60. This response is lost in mid-gestation but returns near term (Challis *et al.* 1990), which is an important fact to remember when the infant is delivered before term.

Mechanisms of heat gain

Non-shivering thermogenesis

The newborn infant has limited capabilities to produce heat by shivering, and when the infant is born early, poor muscular development means the neonate has no means of changing position to preserve heat. The infant has more sweat glands than an adult but the ability to use them as a form of heat reduction is limited as they are regulated by the hypothalamus via the nervous system, which is poorly myelinated. The primary source of heat in the newborn is **non-shivering thermogenesis**, which involves the use of brown adipose tissue to produce heat.

Thermogenesis is initiated by three different mechanisms: (1) cutaneous cooling; (2) oxygenation; and (3) separation from the placenta. An increase in oxygen content of blood with increased flow is needed for the initiation of the system. Separation from the placenta when the cord is cut plays a pivotal role in maximising non-shivering thermogenesis (Gunn and Gluckman 1989). The mechanisms of non-shivering thermogenesis include the metabolism of brown adipose tissue, the secretion of noradrenaline and the release of thyroxin (see Figure 5.1).

Brown adipose tissue (BAT)

The majority of brown fat is located around the neck, between the scapulae, across the clavicle line and down the sternum. It also surrounds the major thoracic vessels and pads the kidneys. Brown fat cells contain a nucleus, glycogen and mitochondria. The mitochondria are numerous and provide energy for metabolic conversion (Brueggemeyer 1993). Brown fat contains a high concentration of stored triglycerides and the presence of thermogenin

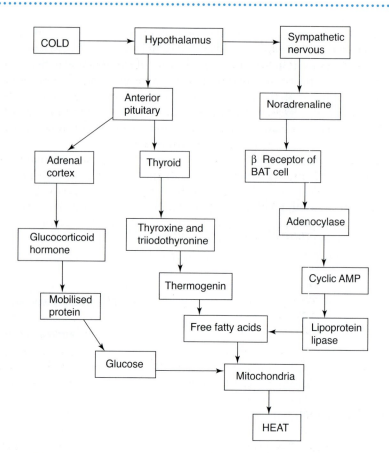

Figure 5.1 The mechanisms of non-shivering thermogenesis

means that when fat is oxidised, heat is produced rather than energy (Sauer 1995). Micheli (1995) suggests that glucose is the main energy substrate in the very low birth weight infant, providing it has entered the cells. Glucose cannot enter the cells if there are low amounts of amino acids, and where these are reduced, insulin production is also lowered, leading ultimately to glucose intolerance and intracellular failure. In Sauer *et al.*'s study (1994), it was apparent that only part of the glucose infused on the first day is oxidised and that half the energy expenditure is provided by fat oxidation by days 7 and 28.

Glycerol and fatty acids, both metabolic products of lipolysis, are good indicators of non-shivering thermogenesis (Power 1998). Some fatty acids enter the blood and provide metabolic fuel for a more prolonged thermogenesis.

Gluconeogenesis

Non-shivering thermogenesis is dependent on a source of energy from glucose and fatty acids; therefore, if the body is unable to generate new glucose, this source of heat production will be affected. **Gluconeogenesis** is the process that converts proteins and lipids into glucose for utilisation. Corticotrophin released from the anterior pituitary stimulates the release of glucocorticoid hormone from the adrenal cortex, to free proteins within the cells for metabolism into glucose. In the preterm or small-for-dates infant the stores may be depleted, thus inhibiting gluconeogenesis. Hormonal levels may also be inadequate, such as TSH and ACTH, which influence thyroxine and the adrenal cortex and assist in gluconeogenesis (Brueggemeyer 1993).

Insulin

Insulin acts in the liver and muscles to increase glycogen synthesis, and in the adipose cells it increases glucose uptake and the conversion of carbohydrate to fat. It decreases lipolysis and increases the uptake of free fatty acids. There is rapid **glycogenolysis** after birth, subsequent to falling levels of insulin. There is a response from glucagon stimulating the sensory nervous system to release catecholamine which frees hepatic cyclic adenosine monophosphate (cAMP). Surges of glucagon and cAMP help to change the activity of the liver from glycogen to glucose production (Blackburn 2003b).

Noradrenaline

Non-shivering thermogenesis is controlled by the release of noradrenaline. Infants born before term have a substantially reduced adrenal medulla, which leaves them potentially adrenal-deficient. Cord blood **catecholamines** are low and the infant's ability to withstand cold stress is reduced. Noradrenaline binds to $beta_1$-receptors increasing (cAMP) by releasing adenosine triphosphate (ATP) from adenocyclase. This increase in cAMP causes the release of kinase which, in turn, leads to a breakdown of the triglycerides in BAT which releases fatty acids to be combusted by the mitochondria (Nedergaard and Cannon 1992). The fatty acids are readily available on the outer membrane of the mitochondria (Nichols and Locke 1984).

The thyroid

The thyroid-stimulating hormone (TSH) which stimulates thermogenesis (Endo and Kobayashi 2008) is released by the anterior pituitary. Free fatty acids and thermogenin accelerate heat production. Thermogenin increases with gestation (Housetek *et al.* 1993) so although there may be sufficient T_4 at 25 weeks, the thermogenin available to convert it is low. Serum concentrations of TSH increase rapidly for 10 minutes after delivery, then gradually fall over 48 hours, which is thought to indicate the acute use of stored pituitary TSH. Where infants were cooled due to a drop in room temperature, there was a significant increase in TSH secretion (Fisher and Odell 1969).

The levels of T_4 (thyroxine), free T_4 and T_3 (triiodothyronine) are significantly low in sick infants (Chen 1994). Where the thyroid receptor alpha gene is lacking, more energy is expended in generating thermogenesis, it is less fuel-efficient and more fat is burned (Pelletier *et al.* 2008) so the preterm infant already with a limited ability to produce heat is further challenged by the extra energy demands. Low stores of thyroglobulin may contribute to the ability to initiate thermogenesis (Bendon 2004).

Thermal receptors

Unmyelinated nerve endings penetrate the basal layer of the epidermis. These contain numerous **mitochondria**, which provide energy for a temperature-sensitive Na^+/K^+ pump changing the cold stimulus into an electrical signal. Deep body thermistors are sited in the pre-optic area and the anterior hypothalamus, which contain both warm- and cold-sensitive cells (Bruck 1992).

In the infant, the hypothalamus reacts to cold stimulus by causing vaso-constriction of the cutaneous blood vessels via the sympathetic nervous system (though this is limited) and increases the metabolic rate by releasing nor-adrenaline, and enhancing thyroxine release (Marieb 1995).

Vasoconstriction

Where there is a layer of subcutaneous fat, peripheral vasoconstriction can result in some reduction in heat loss, especially in full-term infants. However, in the very preterm, this layer of fat is very thin and therefore there is little or no reduction in heat loss through vasoconstriction (Okken 1995).

Thermoneutrality

Thermoneutrality is defined as the environmental temperature at which minimal rates of oxygen consumption or energy expenditure occur (Roncoli and Medoff-Cooper 1992). In setting standards for neutral temperature, Sauer *et al.* (1984) describe the temperature at which infants can maintain a core temperature at rest of between 36.7 and 37.3°C with a change of only 0.2–0.3°C per hour from the core and skin temperatures. Even if an infant has an apparently normal temperature, this alone does not indicate thermoneutrality as the infant may have had to increase his metabolic rate and BAT metabolism to achieve it – so temperature alone does not indicate thermoneutrality (Blackburn 2003b).

Widening of the skin–core gap may be indictaive of a decrease in perfusion pressure or sepsis.

Mechanisms of heat loss

As well as understanding the physiology of heat production, it is important to be aware of the means external to the infant by which heat is gained or lost. Insulation will reduce any transfer of heat. There are two forms of insulation – internal and external. Internal insulation is provided by the layer of sub-cutaneous fat, which starts developing from 26 to 29 weeks' gestation. Fat is a poor conductor of heat and its depth will contribute to its effectiveness. The smaller infant has had less chance to develop this layer of insulation. External insulation is provided by the still air boundary and coverings (Thomas 1994). Transfer of heat between the environment and the infant occurs by conduction, convection, radiation and evaporation. The amount of heat transfer is influenced by the surface area of the infant and the proportions of the body in direct contact with the mattress/clothing (Sedin 1995). The amount of heat lost from convection, radiation and evaporation can exceed the infant's metabolic production, and where this occurs, the infant will remain cold in a warm environment.

Radiation

Radiation involves transfer of radiant energy from the surface of the body to surrounding surfaces that are not in contact with the infant. Up to 60 per cent of heat can be lost this way. It is proportional to the difference between these surface temperatures but independent of the temperature and speeds of the intervening air (Rutter 1992). More heat is transferred if the surrounding surfaces are cold. This process is also reversed where a radiant heat source is used to warm the infant.

Loss through radiation can be limited by making sure that infants are not placed near to cold exterior walls or windows, ensuring that the delivery room is at least 25°C and the use of double-walled incubators. Overheating should be avoided by careful monitoring of the infant's temperature if under a radiant heat source.

Evaporation

Evaporation is the insensible water loss from the skin's surface and the respiratory mucosa dependent on air speed and relative humidity (Roncoli and Medoff-Cooper 1992). Mature infants have the capacity to increase their evaporative heat loss in response to a warm environment by sweating. Evaporative losses account for up to 25 per cent of total heat loss immediately after delivery or during bathing (Blackburn 2003b).

Under normal conditions in a term infant, evaporative heat loss is about a quarter of the resting heat production. However, the preterm infant has much higher evaporative losses as a consequence of transepidermal water loss, which is up to six times higher per unit surface area in an infant of 26 weeks' gestation (Rutter 1992).

Evaporative losses can be minimised by drying immediately after delivery of term infants. For infants born at ≤30 weeks wrapping in polyethylene at delivery and humidifying the incubator will eliminate/reduce evaporative losses.

Convection

Convection involves heat loss due to the movement of air on the skin surface. The amount of loss can be 15 per cent but it will depend on the speed of the airflow, the air temperature and the surface area of the infant that is exposed (Blake and Murray 2006). Therefore, it is important to protect the infant from draughts, wrapping them to reduce exposure of the skin surface. Low birth weight infants should be nursed in incubators with warm air circulating. Delivery of oxygen – if used for more than a short period – should have added warmth because the cool gas is exchanged for warm expired carbon dioxide.

Conduction

Conduction involves the transfer of heat from one object to another when they are in contact with each other, such as the infant being placed on a cool surface (Brueggemeyer 1993). It can also refer to heat conducted from the core of the body to the cool surface. Losses by conduction (approximately 3 per cent) can be minimised by use of warmed blankets, pre-warmed clothing, pre-warmed incubators and resuscitaires, warm coverings for scales and X-ray plates.

Heat exchanged through the respiratory tract

Expired air is more humid than inspired air. This results in an evaporative loss of water and heat from the respiratory tract. There is also a small amount of convective heat transfer. As a result of the alternate inspiratory warming and expiratory cooling of the air, the convective heat exchange depends on the temperature of the inspired air (Sedin 1995).

Surface area

The newborn infant has a large surface area compared to its mass. There is an imbalance in the smaller neonate between the heat-producing ability (mass) and the heat-loss potential (surface area). This large surface area to body mass requires a high calorific intake to support temperature balance (Thomas 1994). Experiments have shown that heat loss increases with an increase in the ratio of body surface area to body mass (Elabassi *et al*. 2004); therefore the very low birth weight infant will have greater potential for heat loss.

Immature skin

The infant of 26 weeks has developed a keratinised stratum corneum but the epidermis is only two or three cells thick. It is thought that transfer from the intrauterine aquatic environment to the external atmospheric environment stimulates and accelerates the maturation of skin (Kuller and Tobin 1990). Rutter (1989) considered that at whatever gestation the infant is born, by the time the infant is two weeks, the skin is similar to an infant born at term. Later work showed that in the very immature infant the development of a fully functional stratum corneum can take significantly longer than four weeks (Kalia *et al*. 1998). Histological analysis has shown that epidermal development is complete in utero at 34 weeks' gestation and infants of 30–32 weeks have a barrier function comparable to adults.

Preterm skin is more gelatinous and transparent than at term. The stratum corneum, the outer horny layer of the epidermal barrier, conserves the body contents, resists noxious agents and protects against trauma. The immaturity of this layer means that the risk of percutaneous absorption of drugs or chemicals is increased. Immaturity also means that the skin is permeable to gases, allowing for the passive diffusion of oxygen in and carbon dioxide out along a concentration gradient (Rutter 1996).

Gestational age has a profound effect on transepidermal water loss in infants less than 30 weeks. It can reach as high as $100g/m^2$ per hour in a 24-week infant on the first day of life (Nachman and Esterley 1971). The skin of a preterm infant comprises up to 13 per cent of its body weight compared to 3 per cent in an adult.

Transepidermal water loss (TEWL)

TEWL is a physical process dependent on the epidermal barrier, the temperature, air speed and humidity. A high air speed can increase TEWL in low birth weight infants and yet when 100 per cent humidity is added, TEWL is stopped. Radiant warmers increase the TEWL by a factor of 0.5–2.0 (Rutter 1989).

TEWL can be as much as five times higher in infants born at 25 weeks compared to those born at term (Sedin *et al*. 1983) (see Figure 5.2). Agren *et al*. (1998) showed that at 24–25 weeks' gestation, when nursed in 50 per cent ambient relative humidity (RH), TEWL was still high immediately after birth and decreased slowly but at a slower rate than more mature infants. However, this addition of humidity to reduce TEWL may actually delay the maturation

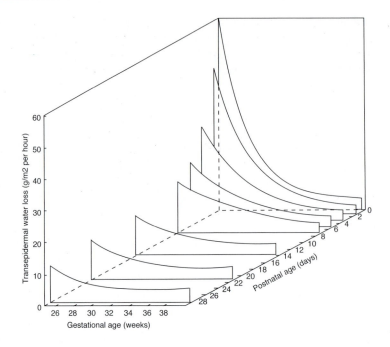

Figure 5.2 **The regression of transepidermal water loss at different postnatal ages**
Source: Hammarlund *et al.* (1983), with permission of Wiley Blackwell Publishers.

of the epidermis, as it has been shown that there is more rapid barrier function of the skin at lower RH (Agren *et al.* 2006).

Baumgart (1985) demonstrated that infants of 31 weeks' gestation (and who already had a developed stratum corneum) who were nursed under radiant heat lost most of their heat through convection, exceeding their loss from evaporation. These losses greatly exceeded the rate of metabolic heat production.

Doty *et al.* (1994) developed a model for predicting TEWL in which it was found that the predicted losses were more accurate at <28 weeks, indicating the thin layer of the stratum corneum. For each millilitre of water lost, there are 560 calories of heat removed. Water loss diminishes with postnatal age as well as the loss of heat through evaporation (Sedin 1995).

Hypothermia

The sick newborn infant is more prone to hypothermia, especially where respiratory disease is problematic. Non-shivering thermogenesis requires the presence of oxygen to metabolise the brown fat. If the infant suffers a degree of hypoxia, the limited ability to produce heat is further diminished.

Preterm and small-for-gestational-age infants are at increased risk from hypothermia (Johanson and Spencer 1992; Blake and Murray 2006). Lyon *et al.* (1997) found that infants less than 1000g have poor vasomotor control at birth but start to develop vasomotor tone in the first few days of life. The cardiovascular responsiveness of growth-restricted infants is absent in the first few days of life, which impairs their ability to mount a thermal response (Jahnukainen *et al.* 1996).

The effect of post-delivery care in an observational study showed that 85 per cent of infants had temperatures lower than 36°C at 2 hours of age and 50 per cent still were below 36°C at 24 hours, with 14 per cent of these still under 35°C. Interventions (kangaroo care, oil massage or plastic swaddler) undertaken after drying were all found to be equally effective and only 38 per cent of infants had temperatures less than 36°C at 2 hours and only 18 per cent were still below 36°C by 24 hours, with none below 35°C (Johanson *et al.* 1992).

Hypothermia is known to be linked to both morbidity and mortality in preterm infants; therefore it is very important to address their temperature requirements as a priority. The results of the Project 27/28 (CESDI 2003) indicated that a significant number of infants admitted to the neonatal unit had temperatures below the standard 'above 36°C' (BAPM and RCPCH 1992).

Cold stress

Infants lose heat during birth, resuscitation and transportation. Cold stress affects oxygenation by increasing the pulmonary artery resistance and reducing surfactant production. Poor perfusion causes an increase in anaerobic metabolism leading to a worsening acidosis. Acidosis itself will increase the pulmonary artery pressure, decreasing the amount of flow through the lungs leading to hypoxia (Lyon and Pushner 1995). Surfactant production decreases and its ability to act as a surface tension lowering agent is impaired if the temperature drops below 35°C (Gandy and Roberton 1987), which will give rise to atelectasis, thereby worsening the hypoxia.

The extra utilisation of glucose caused by increased metabolism can lead to hypoglycaemia, which worsens the acidosis and reduces energy available for growth. An increase in acidosis can lead to the displacement of unconjugated bilirubin from albumin binding sites causing an increase in the risk of kernicterus (Lyon and Pushner 1995) (see Figure 5.3).

Loughead *et al.* (1997) reviewed a sample of 100 very low birth weight infants at a tertiary centre and found that 45 per cent of them were hypothermic on admission and that this group of infants were significantly more likely to be acidaemic than normothermic infants.

Prolonged hypothermia with its resultant poor cardiac output and flow to the central nervous system also has an effect on the intestinal blood flow. It can cause prolonged ischaemia to the gut, which can lead to the development of necrotising enterocolitis (Powell *et al.* 1999). Pulmonary haemorrhage can be a complication of hypothermia due to left ventricular failure and damage to the pulmonary capillaries leading to fluid and cells leaking from the alveoli (Gandy and Roberton 1987) (see p. 127).

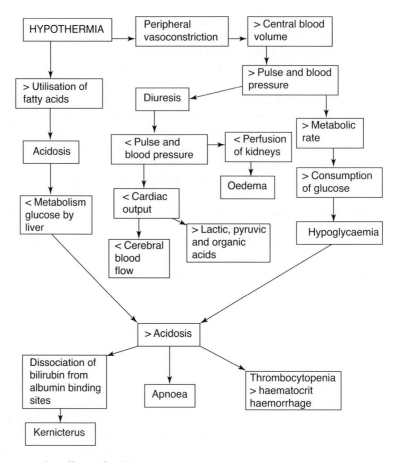

Figure 5.3 The effects of cold stress
Source: Based on data from Brueggemeyer (1993)

Neonatal cold injury

This occurs after a period of extreme hypothermia (below 32°C), where a small drop in the temperature will cause a profound metabolic change. The infant appears a bright red colour due to the dissociation of haemoglobin at low temperatures (Klaus and Fanaroff 1986). The consequences of profound hypothermia are a cascade of acidosis, hypoxia, clotting disorders leading to pulmonary haemorrhage and shock with decreased cardiac output (Gomella 1994).

Re-warming in severe hypothermia

Historically, it was thought preferable to undertake gradual re-warming of the deeply hypothermic infant. Bauer and Versmold (1995) report on studies investigating re-warming techniques that using rapid re-warming (>2° increase per hour) results in a similar or decreased mortality. Tafari and Gentz (1974) showed that those infants who received 20ml/kg of normal saline before re-warming by whatever method had a better outcome. Racine and Jarjouri (1982) reported that during one very cold winter 38 infants were admitted with a rectal temperature of less than 33°C. Re-warming by the gradual method had a lethality of 70 per cent, whereas in those who received rapid re-warming, the death rate decreased to 33 per cent. Thompson and Anderson (1994) reported the case of a profoundly hypothermic 5-hour-old infant in cardiac arrest who had been in a freezer for approximately 4 hours. She had a temperature of 16.2°C. Active internal and external warming methods were used and by 3 hours her temperature was 30.5°C. At 49 minutes into the resuscitation she was in sinus bradycardia and by 53 minutes she moved both upper arms. By 4 months of age she had a normal neurological assessment.

One of the most successful methods of re-warming used in paediatrics has been the use of an extracorporeal membrane oxygenation (ECMO) (see p. 133) as this provides rapid internal warming, and allows volume replacement and oxygenation; however, this procedure is only available in a limited number of centres (Corneli 1992).

Hyperthermia

Hyperthermia in the neonate is unusual and except when the infant has a pyrexia due to sepsis, it is most likely due to inappropriate environmental situation. That is why it is important that all sick infants should have their temperatures closely monitored. In sepsis there will be a large difference in the core and peripheral temperatures. Overheating can make the infant become less active or, in the case of the term infant, restless (Brueggemeyer 1993). The same factors that are responsible for hypothermia can also give rise to hyperthermia – large surface area, limited insulation and limited ability to sweat (Thomas 1994). Sweating can occur in the term infant in response to overheating, which is most readily seen on the forehead and temple (Rutter 1992). Hypotension can occur secondary to the vasodilatation, and dehydration follows an increase in insensible water loss (Blake and Murray 2006) (see p. 168).

Management of thermal stability at delivery

In utero the infant temperature is at least one degree higher than that of the mother to allow a gradient to offload heat from the fetus to the mother via the placenta (Blackburn 2003c). There is evidence that in utero the fetal ability to generate heat is limited by prostaglandins and adenosine via the placenta and that non-shivering thermogenesis is only instigated if the cord circulation is occluded (Schröder 1997). The umbilical circulation allows the fetus to transfer 85 per cent of its heat to the maternal circulation and the remaining 15 per cent is dissipated through the fetal skin to the amnion (Asakura 2004). Therefore, the drop in ambient temperature at delivery is even more marked when the wet infant is delivered into a cool environment. It has been shown that keeping the mother warm with forced air-warming blankets has no advantage on conventional methods of warming on the temperature of their newborn infant after delivery by Caesarean section (Fallis *et al.* 2006); therefore it is the environment that the infant is delivered into that should be at a temperature designed to reduce heat loss.

The recommendation is for delivery room temperature of at least 25°C which should be increased dependent on the gestation of the infant being delivered (WHO 1997) and yet it is apparent that delivery room temperatures rarely meet the basic standard (Knobel *et al.* 2005a).

The healthy infant

The healthy newborn infant is faced with a substantial drop in environmental temperature at birth and will react by increasing heat production. However, if left naked and wet in a temperature of 25°C, the infant's heat loss will exceed heat production. This healthy infant, if dried and wrapped or dried and placed on the mother's abdomen covered in a blanket in a room temperature of 26°C, will be able to maintain its temperature adequately whether born at term or near term (Christensson *et al.* 1992; Bergman *et al.* 2004; Charpak *et al.* 2005). A woollen hat will reduce or even prevent heat loss (Lang *et al.* 2004). Early establishment of feeding will also ensure that the infant has nutrition to support thermogenesis.

Delivery by Caesarean section

It is known that infants delivered by section are more likely to encounter problems with respiration and thermoregulation because they have not undergone the normal processes associated with vaginal delivery. To test the hypothesis that healthy full-term infants delivered by section have more difficulty establishing homeothermic status compared to their vaginally delivered counterparts, a comparative study was undertaken. This showed that axilla and skin temperatures were significantly higher in the infants delivered vaginally and that overall they were slightly warmer in the first 90 minutes after birth (Christensson *et al.* 1993).

The infant with birth suppression

In the case of the potentially suppressed infant, who has the potential for being more vulnerable to heat loss, further measures will be required. A pre-warmed radiant heat source is ideal for short-term use during resuscitation, but longer-term management will be guided by the infant's condition and neurological status where total body cooling may be the regime adopted (Azzopardi *et al.* 2008) (see p. 194).

Meconium stained liquor

The infant who is delivered following meconium staining or aspiration may also have suffered a degree of asphyxia; therefore, along with all important airway management, attention should be paid to reducing heat loss. Remove all wet towels from contact with the infant and ensure that there are warm, dry towels for the infant to lie on under a radiant heat source. However, any drying should be withheld until the status of aspiration has been ascertained. Covering the infant with a warm, dry towel should suffice until the airway is cleared (see p. 78). Where hypoxia is problematic, these infants may go on to develop persistent pulmonary hypertension of the newborn (see pp. 131 and 170), which will impact on their ability to generate further heat.

Infants with congenital anomalies

Certain conditions – such as gastroschisis, exomphalus and mylomeningocele – have increased surface areas for heat loss and increased evaporative loss, and management strategies should be geared to preventing hypothermia (see p. 410).

The vulnerable infant, e.g. preterm or VLBW

This group of infants face many problems (Figure 5.4) and are the most likely to become hypothermic because most delivery rooms are not an optimal thermal environment for them. Commonly the room temperature is low, there may be draughts which increase convective heat loss, the air surrounding the infant has low humidity and there is usually no source for warmed gas (Bauer and Versmold 1995). The body temperature of an exposed 1kg infant can fall at the rate of 1°C every 5 minutes (Rutter 1992). Therefore, the first measure is to ensure a warm delivery room/theatre by setting the temperature to reflect the gestation of the infant about to be delivered, i.e. >25°C for infants <27 weeks gestation (Kent and Williams 2008). Ensuring that all windows and doors are shut at the time of delivery will reduce the air current passing over the infant. The radiant warmer is set to its maximum output with warmed towels to limit heat loss.

All infants who are delivered at less than 30 weeks' gestation should be wrapped in polyethylene skin wrapping at delivery to prevent heat loss (Resuscitation Council 2005). They should be placed immediately into the bag without drying, covering the back of the head (which can be a major source of heat loss), adding a hat but leaving the face free and allowing clear sight of the

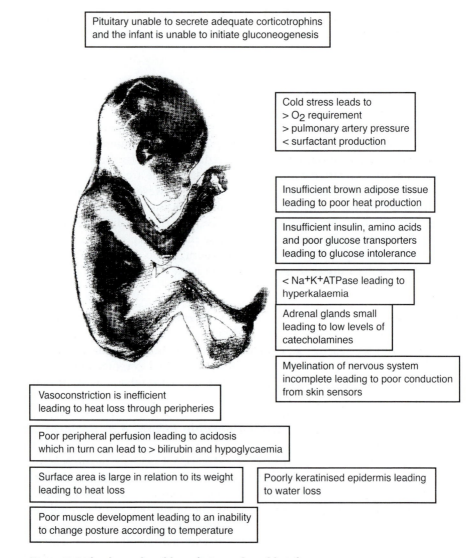

Pituitary unable to secrete adequate corticotrophins and the infant is unable to initiate gluconeogenesis

Cold stress leads to
> O_2 requirement
> pulmonary artery pressure
< surfactant production

Insufficient brown adipose tissue leading to poor heat production

Insufficient insulin, amino acids and poor glucose transporters leading to glucose intolerance

< $Na^+K^+ATPase$ leading to hyperkalaemia

Adrenal glands small leading to low levels of catecholamines

Myelination of nervous system incomplete leading to poor conduction from skin sensors

Vasoconstriction is inefficient leading to heat loss through peripheries

Poor peripheral perfusion leading to acidosis which in turn can lead to > bilirubin and hypoglycaemia

Surface area is large in relation to its weight leading to heat loss

Poorly keratinised epidermis leading to water loss

Poor muscle development leading to an inability to change posture according to temperature

Figure 5.4 **The thermal problems facing vulnerable infants**

chest (Koch 1995; Bjorkland and Hellstöm-Westas 2000; Vohra *et al.* 2004; Bredemeyer *et al.* 2005; Knobel *et al.* 2005b; McCall *et al.* 2008). This simple tool has been proven to be effective both at limiting/preventing heat loss (by 30–40 per cent) but also at reducing TEWL in the very low birth weight infant (Belghazi *et al.* 2006).

However, careful monitoring of the infant's temperature is necessary as a significant number of infants nursed in skin wrap after delivery are hyperthermic on admission to the unit, demonstrating the ability of the wrap to even maintain pre-delivery in-utero temperatures (Bredemeyer *et al.* 2005; Smith *et al.* 2005);

these infants can be iatrogenically heated even further unless care is taken to maintain normothermia.

Management of thermal stability in NICU

Once the infant has been transferred to NICU, it is vital that the correct thermal environment is provided. The neonatal nurse has responsibility to ensure that heat loss is minimised and that the thermal conditions are stable for the infant. In order to provide this, there are various well-developed warming devices but it is important that the equipment is used appropriately.

Radiant warmers

Radiant warmers limit heat loss during interventions because of ease of access and rapid radiant warmer responsiveness (Seguin and Vieth 1996). During the stabilising period the infant may be subjected to many interventions which may involve the infant being covered with sterile drapes or the head of the operator may prevent the heat output reaching the infant, so it is a priority to ensure that these procedures are carried out as rapidly as possible to prevent heat loss. If hypothermia is worsening, a period where the infant can recover will be necessary.

Metabolic rates are higher under radiant heat due to the increased rate of evaporative and convective losses. Therefore, although an open radiant warmer can warm an infant more quickly, the heat losses in the low birth weight infant are much higher and overall more fluctuant (Koch 1995).

Radiant warmers can increase insensible water loss and metabolic rate as the infant tries to produce thermal neutral conditions (Baumgart 1995). This is more often seen in the low birth weight infant of low gestational age who has a poorly developed stratum corneum. It is essential to provide supplemental humidity and shielding to counteract water loss and prevent hypernatraemic dehydration.

Incubators

Incubators have the advantage of providing an enclosed space in which the infant is protected from external noise and the excesses of handling. Most modern incubators are double-walled, which reduces the heat lost through radiation from the infant. Modern incubators are able to surround the infant with a curtain of heat, and endeavour to maintain warmth even with the doors open. Incubators are equipped with safe and efficient humidity systems which mean that prevention of TEWL can be effectively managed.

Temperature control with an incubator is either by skin servo-control or setting an air temperature. Servo-control self-adjusts according to the readings from a skin probe attached to the infant, whereas using the air temperature mode, settings are manually changed according to the infant's monitored temperature. Some early work showed that skin-servo provided a less stable environment than air temperature control (Ducker *et al.* 1985) but later reviews indicate that either methods are effective at maintaining the skin temperature at 36°C (Sinclair 2002).

Ducker *et al.* (1985) state that infants nursed with the air control mode of incubator show less variance in abdominal and peripheral temperatures than those nursed in servo-control mode as the response time of the incubator is slow. Small infants expend a large amount of energy with servo-control in order to maintain temperature, whereas the air control method allows the infant to use energy resources for growth rather than heat production (Boyd and Lenhart 1996).

Radiant warmers vs. incubators

A survey of regional practice indicates that there is no universal approach as to whether low birth weight infants are nursed in radiant warmers or incubators (Seguin and Hayes 1997) but it is apparent from the studies in Table 5.1 that there may be more problems with the use of the radiant warmer even though it has been shown to give more rapid warming.

Seguin (1996) studied infants (range 24–31 weeks with a mean birth weight of 913g) under radiant warmers. All infants were covered in a plastic heat shield with supplemental humidity. Radiant heat did limit heat loss during interventions but in order to achieve these interventions the humidity was removed, which in its turn increased the TEWL. Evaporative heat loss in infants born after 26 weeks is three to five times higher than in the infant born at 31–32

Table 5.1 Comparison of incubators and radiant warmers

Author	Topic	Finding
LeBlanc (1982)	Incubator one day, then radiant warmer the next	Oxygen consumption 8.8 per cent greater under a radiant warmer
Davenport (1992)	Handwashing	More interactions between nurse and infant nursed in radiant warmers
Meyer *et al.* (2001)	Clinical comparison 30 infants in incubator (INC) 30 infants in radiant warmer (RW)	Temperature slightly lower on day 1 in INC group Fluid intake higher in RW group More needed phototherapy in RW group
Flenady and Woodgate (2003)	RW versus INC	A review of eight studies RW increased insensible water loss

weeks (Sauer 1984). An ambient temperature of 37–39°C may be necessary to minimise heat loss through convection and radiation.

So in selecting the environment for the infant it is important to consider the gestational age and likely TEWL, the day of life and current thermal status of the infant.

Handling and temperature

Mok *et al.* (1991) studied 25 preterm infants for temperature changes during care interventions and showed that the core temperature dropped by 0.7°C and the peripheral temperature by 1.3°C. The difference widened by 0.6°C after interventions. Thomas (2003) investigated temperature changes during care-giving interventions and found that the infant's temperature was better maintained if in skin-servo control, so consideration should be given to changing to servo-control for cares. In Montes *et al.*'s study (2005) of thermal stability during hygiene interventions, where the toe and core temperatures were monitored, extremely low birth weight infants demonstrated a sharp fall in both core and peripheral temperatures, with a temperature difference indicative of prolonged thermal stress in spite of measures taken to minimise heat loss. Therefore consideration should be given to the length of any care-giving intervention and the methods used to ensure extra heating to reduce heat losses.

Humidity

Humidity has been shown to reduce skin water loss and improve the maintenance of body temperature (Harpin and Rutter 1985). In contrast, infants nursed without humidity are known to become hypothermic in very high incubator temperatures. A method of coping with TEWL is to increase the fluid load in order to maintain normal serum sodium (Na) concentrations. However, this is known to precipitate sequlae such as patent ductus arteriosus (Bell *et al.* 1980), necrotising enterocolitis (Grosfeld *et al.* 1996), intraventricular haemorrhage (Simmons 1974; Han *et al.* 1997) and can increase the incidence of bronchopulmonary dysplasia (Tammela and Koivisto 1992). Preterm infants may lose up to 13 per cent of their body weight as TEWL in the first day of life when nursed in 50 per cent humidity and their losses can still be significant at four weeks of age (Sedin *et al.* 1985).

Older incubator systems relied on passive humidification, which led to airborne aerosols on which bacteria could grow. Today most incubators are equipped with an active source of humidity, which heats and evaporates water separately from the circulating air and then adds it to the incubator canopy which prevents bacterial growth (Ducker and Marshall 1995). Servo-control allows precise levels of humidity and, because it is an active system, when the portholes are opened, the recovery response is minimal as the vapour is continuously added to the circulating air (Marshall 1997).

Providing humidity via an incubator is a relatively easy task; however, it is difficult to create the same environment using a radiant warmer. Kjartansson *et al.* (1995) studied the comparative rates of evaporation in term and preterm infants in incubators and radiant warmers. This study showed that the evaporation rates of the preterm infants were higher than the term infants when nursed in an incubator at 50 per cent humidity and four times higher when nursed under radiant heat.

There have been a variety of methods to establish a micro-environment providing humidity when using radiant warmers, which involve plastic tunnels, polythene sheeting, bubble wrap, etc., usually with an adapted ventilation humidity system. This can limit the radiant heat transfer to the infant and therefore requires more heat generation. It also makes it difficult to have simple access to the infant. Every time the coverings are removed for observation and attention, the infant is subjected to large swings in TEWL as the infant is suddenly subjected to direct heat and high convective heat loss (Marshall 1997). Such systems make it very difficult to establish a constant level of humidity or to measure it. It requires a flow of 10 litres and a humidifier set at 38°C to achieve a maximum of 74.5 per cent RH (Seguin and Hayes 1997) (Table 5.2).

However humidity is delivered, it is important to remember that although the humidity is essential to reduce water loss and improve temperature control, it will influence the speed at which the skin matures, being a more rapid rate if the relative humidy is low (Agren *et al.* 2006).

TEWL and phototherapy

It is important to note that TEWL can increase by 26.4 per cent during the delivery of phototherapy whether by halogen spotlight or more conventional methods, with the most significant increases in the cubital fossa and groin.

Table 5.2 Guidelines for humidity settings

26 weeks' gestation or less	27–30 weeks' gestation
80 per cent humidity for at least 4 weeks may require higher percentage to cope with raised serum sodium levels (Agren *et al.* 1997; Mitchell 2005)	80 per cent humidity for at least 2 weeks
The infant's skin should have keratinised fully at the end of this period; therefore the humidity can be gradually reduced, as tolerated to maintain an axilla temperature within the normal range (Chiou and Blume-Peytavi 2004).	
Reduce the humidity gradually according to the infant's temperature (70 per cent–60 per cent–50 per cent) until 20–30 per cent is reached before discontinuing.	

Therefore, close monitoring of electrolyte levels is essential and fluid replacement considered (Maayan-Metzger *et al.* 2001; Grünhagen *et al.* 2002).

Skin

The very preterm infant has skin that is very fragile, liable to break down easily and absorb substances as well as allowing large water losses with consequent heat loss. Many methods have been investigated to cover the skin in some way to reduce water loss, e.g. using a paraffin mixture, which reduced water loss by 40–60 per cent (Rutter and Hull 1981). A later study showed that twice-daily application of preservative-free ointment significantly reduced water loss in the first 6 hours of life and reduced bacterial colonisation in the axilla with fewer positive blood and CSF cultures (Nopper *et al.* 1996). However, practical application of any topical mixture is limited in the infant who needs intensive support with lines and monitoring, and care is needed to find a substance that would not be absorbed through the skin.

A further approach to reducing water loss is to cover the skin with a semi-permeable membrane. A study by Donahue *et al.* (1996) showed that semi-permeable dressings caused no skin damage compared to those areas left exposed, though this did not make a significant difference to fluid or electrolyte status. However, dressings can harbour or encourage bacterial growth (Strickland 1997).

Monitoring lead electrodes and their adhesives that are used to care for these small infants can cause trauma, and care is needed to avoid damage on removal. Lund *et al.* (1997) demonstrated an increase in TEWL after removal of adhesive plastic tape and the pectin barrier, though the skin recovered in 24 hours. There was less trauma associated with the removal of hydrophilic gel.

Heated water-filled mattresses

Heated water-filled mattresses (HWMs) have become a useful adjunct to caring for the healthy preterm infant in the nursery. They can help mothers overcome their anxieties about their infants more easily and encourage bonding, compared to the experience of mothers of infants nursed in incubators (Sarman *et al.* 1993). Sarman (1992) showed that resting oxygen consumption and heart rate were lower and the time to cooling of the foot during cares was also reduced in those infants on a HWM compared to those nursed in an incubator. HWMs have also proved useful in re-warming preterm infants (Sarman *et al.* 1989). Where HWM has been compared to incubator care, it showed that mean body temperatures were similar, with no significant differences in the incidence of cold stress, weight gain or morbidity (Gray *et al.* 2004). HWMs have also proved a useful tool to prevent and treat hypothermia in the delivery room (Boo and Selvarini 2005).

Thermal status during transport

Many studies have shown that a significant feature of neonatal transfers is hypothermia in the low birth weight infant (Hood *et al.* 1983; Valls *et al.* 1986; Hals *et al.* 1990; Smith *et al.* 1990; Lundstrom *et al.* 1993). Bowman and Roy (1997) showed that although the incidence of hypothermia has been reduced, there is, however, a constant rate of 3 per cent hypothermia seen in infants.

Holt and Fagerli (1999) showed that when the retrieval team attended the delivery, the after-transfer temperature was significantly higher, indicating that an early request for the team to attend the delivery may impact on the outcome. Moving the sick or small neonate involves some inevitable heat loss due to moving between incubators at both ends of the journey.

A probe should be securely placed in a skin-to-mattress site (intrascapular) and peripheral temperature should be monitored. Where possible, any existing hypothermia should be corrected before the return journey.

Humidification systems designed for transport ventilators will reduce respiratory water loss and airway reactivity. The incubators themselves do not have humidification and the small infant is at risk of high evaporative heat losses unless wrapped in polyethylene. If transferring a surgical infant, this technique can also be used to limit heat and water loss.

There may be some heat loss through radiation unless the walls of the incubator are double-walled (Sedin 1995).

Transwarmer mattresses are a useful adjunct to transferring the hypothermic infant and have been shown to be effective at stabilising temperatures, though they should be between 19 and 28°C at the point of activation to ensure optimal heat output and the infant's temperature should be monitored constantly while they are cared for on the mattress (L'Herault *et al.* 2001; Carmichael *et al.* 2007).

Temperature measurement

Continuous monitoring

Clinical assessment of hypovolaemia in sick, preterm infants is difficult and can be improved by monitoring core and peripheral temperatures (Lambert *et al.* 1998). Monitoring core and peripheral temperature (c–pT) can be particularly useful in giving an early indication of cold stress in this group, who have poor vasomotor control at birth (Lyon *et al.* 1997). Lemburg (1995) states that it is important to record a two-point measurement as less problems of care occur when using this continuous assessment. Low core temperatures can indicate significant thermal stress. A wide c-pT (>2–3°C) is abnormal and might be caused by hypovolaemia, cold stress, catecholamine infusions, infection or patent ductus arteriosus (McIntosh *et al.* 1995). Mayfield *et al.* (1984) found that preterm infants with their lower levels of body fat had less variation in temperature suggestive of a smaller core–surface gradient.

Dollberg *et al.* (1994) investigated the use of zero heat flow temperature sites. The principle relies on the fact that any body has an internal heat-producing component and has a continual heat flow to its surface as long as the surface is cooler than the heat-producing component. Zero heat flux mimics the rectal temperature closely, and is suggested as an appropriate site for measuring core temperatures. Skin-to-mattress (intrascapular) temperature measurement was the most useful site for measuring the core temperature since it is non-invasive and there is no gradient to the oesophageal temperature (Lemburg 1995).

Axillary temperatures alone give a poor indication of brown fat activity and those infants that are compensating through non-shivering thermogenesis may not get the environmental support needed (Bliss-Holtz 1993).

Intermittent temperature recordings

Intermittent temperature recordings traditionally were performed with a mercury thermometer, which was known to be hazardous (Pazart *et al.* 1997; Smith *et al.* 1997; Thigpen and Sexson 1997). Infrared sensors work on the basis that solid objects emit an intensity of infrared radiation, which corresponds to specific temperatures. Pyroelectric sensors detect the heat flow and give a very quick reading (Thomas 1993). This technology is used widely in tympanic thermometers in adults and paediatrics and has been introduced for use in the neonate but studies have shown that the measurements vary depending upon the environment in which the infant is nursed (radiant warmer, incubator or cot) (Hicks 1996; Cusson *et al.* 1997). Therefore it is important to assess the likely environmental effects when choosing the method of measurement and to pay particular attention to the size of the infant on which it is used.

The axillary infrared device has been specifically designed for use in neonates (O'Toole 1998) and appears to give an accurate, quick assessment of the axillary temperature but will still need comparative studies.

The rectum had been considered the ideal site for measuring the core temperature in neonates, but the procedure is not without risks (Fonkalsrud and Clatworthy 1965; Merenstein 1970; Fleming *et al.* 1983) and has been shown not always to reflect a true core temperature (Lemburg 1995).

Therefore intermittent temperature readings should be taken in the axilla and, although this is considered less invasive than the rectal temperature, it has been shown that infants do not tolerate this method any better than the rectal route. The infant has to be disturbed in order to gain access to the axilla and this does cause changes to physiological parameters so should only be performed when necessary (Roll *et al.* 2000).

Hypothermia as a treatment for neonatal encephalopathy

Hypothermia is usually viewed in a negative context, with neonatal nurses devoting a great deal of attention to keeping infants warm. Research (Thoreson and Wyatt 1997; Gunn *et al.* 1997) indicates that for the infant who has received an asphyxial insult there may be a therapeutic use for hypothermia (see p. 194).Trials to date (Gluckman 2005; Shankaran 2005) have indicated that cooling has a significant effect on infants with moderate to severe electro-encephalographic changes and, on the strength of these, the ILCOR (International Liaison Committee on Resuscitation) has recommended that therapeutic hypothermia should be introduced into routine clinical practice prior to the publication of the results of the current trials, e.g. TOBY, ICE and the induced hypothermia trial from the European neo.nEuro Network (Hoehn 2008).

Conclusion

The neonatal nurse needs to have a working awareness of embryology and physiology in relation to thermoregulation, especially when caring for the very preterm infant. In the infant born early, the systems that are involved in thermal regulation are limited and poorly functioning. Knowledge of the mechanisms of heat production and losses will enable the nurse to choose the most appropriate way of providing a thermally stable environment for an infant in their care whatever its gestation.

Nursing practice should be evidence-based and current research should be incorporated into the care delivered; this has been most recently demonstrated in the context of thermal care by the introduction of the polyethylene wraps for the very preterm infant at delivery. This relatively simple manouvre has dramatically improved temperature stability in this particularly vulnerable population.

Case study: effects of temperature instability

Infant born at 27 weeks, one of MCDA twins by emergency LSCS weighing 760g. He was placed in a polythene bag on the resuscitaire with the heat output at maximum. He had poor Apgar scores and needed resuscitation including cardiac massage. By the time he was admitted to the neonatal unit, his temperature was 38°C.

Q.1. Why was he placed in a plastic bag?

Q.2. Why is his temperature 38°C on arrival in the unit?

Following line insertions and initial blood tests/X-rays, he is removed from the polythene bag and humidity is added to the incubator at 80 per cent and temperature montoring has been established.

Q.3. Why has humidity been added to the incubator?

Q.4. How long should the humidity be maintained?

Q.5. How is his temperature monitored?

Case study: effects of cold temperature

Male infant born at 38 weeks by elective LSCS weighing 3.4kg, cried at delivery and after drying and an initial cuddle with his mother has been placed in a cot. At 2 hours of age he has been found grunting and cool to the touch.

Q.1. Why might this infant be cold?

Q.2. Why might he be grunting?

The infant is taken to the neonatal unit in his cot for assessment. The nurse unwraps him from several blankets and towels and finds that the towel closest to him is wet. His temperature is 36°C, RR 84, saturation level 92 per cent and blood sugar level 2.1mmol/L.

Q.3. What will the nurse's first action be?

Q.4. Why is his blood sugar low?

Q.5. Is this infant going to need help with his breathing?

References

Agren, J., Sjörs, G. and Sedin, G. (1997) 'Transepidermal water loss in extremely preterm infants', *Pediatric Research* 42(3): 404.

Agren, J., Sjörs, G. and Sedin, G. (1998) 'Transepidermal water loss in infants born at 24 and 25 weeks of gestation', *Acta Paediatrica* 87(11): 1185–90.

Agren, J., Sjörs, G. and Sedin, G. (2006) 'Ambient humidity influences the rate of skin barrier maturation in extremely preterm infants', *Journal of Pediatrics* 148(5): 613–17.

Asakura, H. (2004) 'Fetal and neonatal thermoregulation', *Journal of Nippon Medical School* 71(6): 360–70.

Azzopardi, D., Brocklehurst, P., Edwards, D., Halliday, H., Levene, M., Thoresen, M. and Whitelaw, A. and The TOBY Study Group (2008) 'The TOBY Study Group: whole body hypothermia for the treatment of perinatal asphyxial encephalopathy: a randomised controlled trial', *BMC Pediatrics* 30: 17.

Bauer, K. and Versmold, H. (1995) 'Prevention of neonatal hypothermia in the delivery room', in A. Okken and J. Koch (eds) *Thermoregulation of Sick and Low Birth Weight Neonates*, Berlin: Springer, p. 219.

Baumgart, S. (1985) 'Partitioning of heat losses and gains in premature newborn infants under radiant warmers', *Pediatrics* 75(1): 89–99.

Baumgart, S. (1995) 'Treatment of sick newborns under radiant warmers', in A. Okken and J. Koch (eds) *Thermoregulation of Sick and Low Birth Weight Neonates*, Berlin: Springer, p. 153.

Belgazi, K., Touneaux, P., Elabassi, E.B., Ghyselen, L., Delanaud, S. and Libert J.P. (2006) 'Effect of posture on the thermal efficiency of a plastic bag in neonate: assessment using a thermal "sweating" mannequin', *Medical Physics* 33(3): 637–44.

Bell, E.F., Warburton, D., Stonestreet, B. and Oh, W. (1980) 'Effect of fluid administration on the development of symptomatic patent ductus arteriosus and congestive heart failure in premature infants', *New England Journal of Medicine* 302(11): 598–603.

Bendon, R.W. and Coventry, S. (2004) 'Non-iatrogenic pathology of the preterm infant', *Seminars in Neonatology* 9(4): 281–7.

Bergman, N.J., Linley, L.L. and Fawcus, S.R. (2004) 'Randomized controlled trial od skin-to-skin contact from birth versus conventional incubator for physiological stabilization in 1200 to 2199gram infants', *Acta Paediatrica* 93(6): 779–85.

Björkland, L.J. and Hellstöm-Westas, L. (2000) 'Reducing heat loss at birth in very preterm infants', *Journal of Pediatrics* 137(5): 739–40.

Blackburn, S.T. (2003a) 'Pituitary, adrenal and thyroid function', in *Maternal, Fetal and Neonatal Physiology*, 2nd edn, St Louis, MO: W.B. Saunders.

Blackburn, S.T. (2003b) 'Carbohydrate, fat and protein metabolism', in *Maternal, Fetal and Neonatal Physiology*, 2nd edn, St Louis, MO: W.B. Saunders.

Blackburn, S.T. (2003c) 'Thermoregulation', in *Maternal, Fetal and Neonatal Physiology*, 2nd edn, St Louis, MO: W.B. Saunders.

Blake, W.W. and Murray, J.A. (2006) 'Unit two: support of the neonate. "Heat balance"', in G.B. Merenstein and S.L.Gardner (eds) *Handbook of Neonatal Intensive Care*, 6th edn, St Louis, MO: Mosby.

Bliss-Holtz, J. (1993) 'Determination of thermoregulatory state in full-term infants', *Nursing Research* 42(4): 204–7.

Boo, N.Y. and Selvarini, S. (2005) 'Effectiveness of a simple heated water-filled mattress for the prevention and treatment of neonatal hypothermia in the labour room', *Singapore Medical Journal* 46(8): 387–91.

Bowman, E.D. and Roy, R.N. (1997) 'Control of temperature during newborn transport: an old problem with new difficulties', *Journal of Paediatrics and Child Health* 33(5): 398–401.

Boyd, H. and Lenhart, P. (1996) 'Temperature control: servo versus nonservo – which is best?', *Neonatal Network* 9(7): 37–40.

Bredemeyer, S., Reid, S. and Wallace, M. (2005) 'Thermal management for premature births', *Journal of Advanced Nursing* 52(5): 482–9.

Bruck, K. (1992) 'Neonatal thermal regulation', in R.A. Polin and W.W. Fox (eds) *Fetal and Neonatal Physiology*, Vol. 1, Philadelphia, PA: W.B. Saunders, p. 676.

Brueggemeyer, A. (1993) 'Neonatal thermoregulation', in C. Kenner, A. Brueggemeyer and L. Porter Gunderson (eds) *Comprehensive Neonatal Nursing*, Philadelphia, PA: W.B. Saunders.

Bruska, M. and Piotrowski, A. (2004) 'Development of the myelin sheath of the hypogastric nerves in human foetus aged 23 weeks', *Folia Morphologica (Warsaw)* 63(3): 289–301.

Carmichael, A., McCullough, S. and Kempley, S.T. (2007) 'Critical dependence of acetate thermal mattress on gel activation temperature', *Archives of Disease in Childhood Fetal and Neonatal Edition* 92(1): F44–5.

Carrascosa, A., Ruiz-Cuevas, P., Clemente, M., Salcedo, S. and Almar, J. (2008) 'Thyroid function in 76 sick preterm infants', *Thyroid*, 21(3): 237–43.

CESDI (2003) *Project 27/28*, London: The Stationery Office.

Challis, J.R.G. and Thorburn, G.D. (1976) 'The fetal pituitary–adrenal axis and its functional interactions with the neurohypophysis', in R.W. Beard and Z. Nathaniels (eds) *Fetal Physiology and Medicine*, London: W.B. Saunders.

Challis, J.R.G., Jacobs, R.A., Riley, S.C., Akagi, K., Yang, K., Tanga, S., Berdusco, E. and Brocking, A.D. (1990) 'Hormonal adaptation by the fetus', in G.S. Dawes, F. Borruto, A. Zacutti and A. Zacutti Jr. (eds) *Fetal Autonomy and Adaptation*, Chichester: John Wiley & Sons.

Charpak, N., Ruiz, J.G., Zupan, J., Cattaneo, A., Figueroa, Z., Tessier, R., Cristo, M., Anderson, G., Ludington, S., Mendoza, S., Mokhachane, M. and Worku, B. (2005) 'Kangaroo mother care: 25 years after', *Acta Paediatrica* 94(5): 514–22.

Chen, J.Y. (1994) 'Thyroid function in healthy and sick neonates', *Chung Hua I Hsueh Tsa Chih (Tapei)* 54(1): 51–6.

Chiou, Y.B. and Blume-Peytavi, U. (2004) 'Stratum cornmeum maturation', *Skin Pharmacology and Physiology* 17(2): 57–66.

Christensson, K., Siles, C., Cabera, T., Belaustequi, A., de la Fuente, P., Lagercrantz, H., Puyol, P. and Winberg, J. (1992) 'Temperature, metabolic adaptation and crying in healthy full-term newborns cared for skin-to-skin or in a cot', *Acta Paediatrica* 81: 488–93.

Christensson, K., Siles, C., Cabera, T., Belaustequi, A., de la Fuente, P., Lagercrantz, H., Puyol, P. and Winberg, J. (1993) 'Lower body temperatures in infants delivered by cesarean section than in vaginally delivered infants', *Acta Paediatrica* 82(2): 128–31.

Clemente, M., Ruiz-Cuevas, P., Carrascosa, A., Potau, N., Almar, J., Salcedo, S. and Yeste, D. (2007) 'Thyroid function in preterm infants 27–29 weeks of gestational age during the first four months of life: results from a prospective study comprising 80 preterm infants', *Journal of Pediatric Endocrinology and Metabolism* 20(12): 1269–80.

Corneli, H.M. (1992) 'Accidental hypothermia', *Journal of Pediatrics* 120(5): 671–9.

Cusson, R.M., Madonia, J.A. and Taekman, J.B. (1997) 'The effect of environment on body site temperatures in full-term neonates', *Nursing Research* 46(4): 202–7.

Davenport, S.E. (1992) 'Frequency of hand washing by registered nurses caring for infants on radiant warmers and in incubators', *Neonatal Network* 11(1): 21–5.

Dollberg, S., Atherton, H.D., Sigda, M., Acree, C.M. and Hoath, S.B. (1994) 'Effect of insulated skin probes to increase skin-to-environmental temperature gradients of preterm infants cared for in convective incubators', *Journal of Pediatrics* 124(5–1): 799–801.

Donahue, M.L., Phelps, D.L., Richter, S.E. and Davis, J.M. (1996) 'A semipermeable skin dressing for extremely low birth weight infants', *Journal of Perinatology* 16(1): 20–6.

Doty, S.E., McCormack, W.D. and Seagrave, R.C. (1994) 'Predicting insensible water loss in premature infants', *Biology of the Neonate* 66: 33–44.

Ducker, D.A., Lyon, A.J, Russell, R., Bass, C.A. and McIntosh, N. (1985) 'Incubator temperature control: effects on the very low birth weight infant', *Archives of Disease in Childhood* 60: 902–7.

Ducker, D.A. and Marshall, N. (1995) 'Humidification without risk of infection in the Drager incubator 8000', *Neonatal Intensive Care* July/August: 44–6.

Elabassi, E.B., Belgazi, K., Delanaud, S. and Libert, J.P. (2004) 'Dry heat loss in incubator: comparison of two premature newborn sized manikins', *European Journal of Applied Physiology* 92(6): 679–82.

Endo, T. and Kobayashi, T. (2008) 'Thyroid-stimulating hormone receptor in brown adipose tissue is involved in the regulation of thermogenesis', *American Journal of Physiology: Endocrinology and Metabolism* 295(2): E514–18.

Fallis, W.M., Hamelin, K., Symonds, J. and Wang, X. (2006) 'Maternal and newborn outcomes related to maternal warming during cesarean delivery', *Journal of Obstetrics, Gynecology and Neonatal Nursing* 35(3): 324–31.

Fisher, D.A. and Odell, W.D. (1969) 'Acute releases of thyrotropin in the newborn', *Journal of Clinical Investigation* September: 1670–7.

Fleming, M., Hakansson, H. and Svenningsen, N.W. (1983) 'A disposable new electronic temperature probe for skin temperature measurements in the newborn infant nursery', *International Journal of Nursing Studies* 20(2): 89–96.

Flenady, V.J. and Woodgate, P.G. (2003) 'Radiant warmers versus incubators for regulating body temperature in newborn infants', *Cochrane Database*. doi.wiley.com/10.1111/j.1651–2227.2004.tb02952.

Fonkalsrud, E. and Clatworthy, H.W. (1965) 'Accidental perforation of the colon and rectum in newborn infants', *New England Journal of Medicine* 272: 1097–100.

Gandy, G.M. and Roberton, N.R.C. (1987) *Lecture Notes on Neonatology*, Oxford: Blackwell Scientific.

Gluckman, P.D. (2005) 'Selective head cooling with mild systemic hypothermia after neonatal encephalopathy: multicentre randomised trial', *Lancet* 365(9460): 663–70.

Gomella, T.L. (1994) 'Temperature regulation in the neonate', in T.L. Gomella, M. Cunningham Douglas and F.G. Eyal (eds) *Neonatology*, 3rd edn, Englewood Cliffs, NJ: Prentice-Hall.

Gray, P.H., Paterson, S., Finch, G. and Hayes, M. (2004) 'Cot-nursing using a heated, water-filled mattress and incubator care: a randomized clinical trial', *Acta Paediatrica* 93(3): 350–5.

Grosfeld, J.L., Chaet, M., Molinari, F., Engle, W., Engum, S.A., West, K.W., Rescoria, F.J. and Scherer, L.R. 3rd (1996) 'Increased risk of necrotizing enterocolitis in premature infants with patent ductus arteriosus treated with indomethacin', *Annals of Surgery* 224(3): 350–5.

Grünhagen, D.J., de Boer, M.G., de Beaufort, A.J. and Walther, F.J. (2002) 'Transepidermal water loss during halogen spotlight phototherapy in preterm infants', *Pediatric Research* 51(3): 402–5.

Gunn, A.J., Gluckman, P.D. and Gunn, T.R. (1998) 'Selective head cooling in newborn infants after perinatal asphyxia: a safe study', *Pediatrics* 102(4 Part 1): 885–92.

Gunn, A.J., Gunn, T.R., de Haan, H.H., Williams, C.E. and Gluckman, P.D. (1997) 'Dramatic neuronal rescue with prolonged selective head cooling after ischemia in fetal lambs', *Journal of Clinical Investigation* 99(2): 248–56.

Gunn, T.R. and Gluckman, P.D. (1989) 'The endocrine control of the onset of thermogenesis at birth', *Baillières Clinics in Endocrinology and Metabolism* 3(3): 869–86.

Hals, J., Bechensteen, A.G., Lindenmann, R. and Buxrud, T. (1990) 'Transportation of newborn infants: a 6-year case load', *Tidsskrift Nor Laegeforen* 110(12): 1501–5.

Hammarlund, K., Sedin, G. and Stromberg, B. (1983) 'Transepidermal water loss in newborn infants', *Acta Paediatrica Scandinavica* 72: 721–8.

Han, B.K., Lee., M. and Yoon, H.K. (1997) 'Cranial ultrasound and CT findings in infants with hypernatremic dehydration', *Pediatric Radiology* 9: 739–42.

Harpin, V. and Rutter, N. (1985) 'Humidification of incubators', *Archives of Disease in Childhood* 60: 219–24.

Hasegawa, M., Houdou, S., Mito, T., Takashima, S., Asanuma, K. and Ohno, T. (1992) 'Development of myelination in the human fetal and infant cerebrum: a myelin basic protein immunohistochemical study', *Brain Development* 14(1): 1–6.

Hicks, M.A. (1996) 'A comparison of the tympanic and axillary temperatures of the preterm and term infant', *Journal of Perinatology* 16(4): 261–7.

Hoehn, T., Hansmann, G., Bührer, C., Simbruner, G., Gunn, A.J., Yager, J., Levene, M., Hamrick, S.E.G., Shankaran, S. and Thoresen, M. (2008) 'Therapeutic hypothermia in neonates: review of current clinical data, ILCOR recommendations and suggestions for implemenation in neonatal intensive care units', *Resuscitation* 78: 7–12.

Holt, J. and Fagerli, I. (1999) 'Air transport of the sick newborn infant: audit from a sparsely populated county in Norway', *Acta Paediatrica* 88(1): 66–71.

Hood, J.L., Cross, A., Hulka, B. and Lawson, E.E. (1983) 'Effectiveness of the neonatal transport team', *Critical Care Medicine* 11(6): 419–23.

Housetek, J., Vizek, K., Pavelka, S., Kopecky, J., Krejcova, E., Hermanska, J. and Cermakova, M. (1993) '"Type II iodothyronine 5"-deiodonase and uncoupling protein in brown adipose tissue of human newborns', *Journal of Clinical Endocrinology and Metabolism* 77(2): 382–7.

Jahnukainen, T., Lindqvist, A., Jalonen, J., Kero, P. and Valimaki, I. (1996) 'Reactivity of skin blood flow and heart rate to thermal stimulation in infants during the first postnatal days and after a two-month follow-up', *Acta Paediatrica* 85(6): 733–8.

Johanson, R. and Spencer, A. (1992) 'Temperature changes during the first day of life in the North Staffordshire maternity hospital', *Midwifery* 8(2): 82–8.

Johanson, R.B., Spencer, S.A., Rolfe, P., Jones, P. and Malla, D.S. (1992) 'Effect of post-delivery care on neonatal body temperature', *Acta Paediatrica* 81(11): 859–63.

Kalia, Y.N., Nonato, L.B., Lund, C.H. and Guy, R.H. (1998) 'Development of skin barrier function in premature infants', *Journal of Investigative Dermatology* 111(2): 320–6.

Kent, A.L. and Williams, J. (2008) 'Increasing ambient operating theatre temperature and wrapping in polyethylene improves admission temperature in premature infants', *Journal of Paediatric and Child Health* 44(6): 325–31.

Kjartansson, S., Arsan, S., Hammerlund, K., Sjors, G. and Sedin, G. (1995) 'Water loss from the skin of term and preterm infants nursed under a radiant heater', *Pediatric Research* 37(2): 233–8.

Klaus, H.H. and Fanaroff, A.A. (1986) 'The physical environment', in *Care of the High Risk Neonate*, Philadelphia, PA: W.B. Saunders, Chapter 5.

Knobel, R.B., Vohra, S. and Lehmann, C.U. (2005a) 'Heat loss prevention in the delivery room for preterm infants: a national survery of newborn intensive care units', *Journal of Perinatology* 25: 514–18.

Knobel, R.B., Wimmer, J.E. Jr, Holbert, D. (2005b) 'Heat loss prevention for preterm infants in the delivery room', *Journal of Perinatology* 25(5): 304–8.

Koch, J. (1995) 'Physical properties of the thermal environment', in A. Okken and J. Koch (eds) *Thermoregulation of Sick and Low Birth Weight Neonates*, Berlin: Springer.

Kuller, J.M. and Tobin, C.R. (1990) 'Skin care management of the low-birthweight infant', in L. Porter Gunderson and C. Kenner (eds) *Care of the 24–25 Week Gestational Age Infant*, Petaluma: Neonatal Network.

Lambert, H.J., Baylis, P.H. and Coulthard, M.G. (1998) 'Central-peripheral temperature difference, blood pressure and arginine vasopressin in preterm neonates undergoing volume expansion', *Archives of Disease in Childhood: Fetal and Neonatal Edition* 78(1): F43–F45.

Lang, N., Bromiker, R. and Arad, I. (2004) 'The effect of wool vs. cotton head covering and lenth of stay with mother following delivery on infant temperature', *International Journal of Nursing Studies* 41(8): 843–6.

LeBlanc, M.H. (1982) 'Relative efficacy of an incubator and an open radiant warmer in producing thermoneutrality for the small premature infant', *Pediatrics* 69(4): 439–45.

Lemburg, P. (1995) 'Thermal monitoring of very preterm infants: which temperature should be measured?', in A. Okken and J. Koch (eds) *Thermoregulation of Sick and Low Birth Weight Neonates*, Berlin: Springer.

L'Herault, J., Petroff, L. and Jeffrey, J. (2001) 'The effectivenss of a thermal mattress in stabilizing and maintaining body temperature during the transport of very low-birth-weight newborns'. *Applied Nursing Research* 14(4): 210–19.

Loughead, M.K., Loughead, J.L. and Reinhart, M.J. (1997) 'Incidence and physiologic characteristics in the very low birth weight infant', *Pediatric Nursing* 23(1): 11–15.

Lund, C.H., Nonato, L.B., Kuller, J.M., Franck, L.S., Cullander, C. and Durand, D.J. (1997) 'Disruption of barrier function in neonatal skin associated with adhesive tape removal', *Journal of Pediatrics* 131(3): 367–72.

Lundstrom, K.E., Veiergang, D. and Peterson, S. (1993) 'Transportation of sick newborn infants', *Ugeskr Laeger* 155(1): 8–11. In Danish.

Lyon, A. and Pushner, P. (1995) *Thermomonitoring . . . a Step Forward in Neonatal Intensive Care*, Berlin: Dragerwerk.

Lyon, A.J., Pikaar, M.E., Badger, P. and McIntosh, N. (1997) 'Temperature control in very low birth weight infants during the first five days of life', *Archives of Disease in Childhood: Fetal and Neonatal Edition* 76(1): F47–F50.

Maayan-Metzger, A., Yosipovitch, G., Hadad, E. and Sirota, L. (2001) 'Transepidermal water loss and skin hydration in preterm infants during phototherapy', *American Journal of Perinatology* 18(7): 393–6.

Marieb, E.N. (1995) *Human Anatomy and Physiology*, 3rd edn, San Francisco: Benjamin Cummings.

Marshall, A. (1997) 'Humidifying the environment for the premature neonate', *Journal of Neonatal Nursing* 3(1): 32–6.

Mayfield, S.R., Bhatia, J., Nakamura, K.T., Rios, G.R. and Bell, E.F. (1984) 'Temperature measurement in term and preterm neonates', *Journal of Pediatrics* 104(2): 271–5.

McCall, E.M., Alderdice, F.A., Halliday, H.L., Jenkins, J.G. and Vohra, S. (2008) 'Interventions to prevent hypothermia at birth in preterm and/or low birth weight infants', *Cochrane Database Systematic Review* (23): CD004210.

McIntosh, N., Wilmhurst, A. and Hailey, J. (1995) 'Experiences with thermal monitoring, influence of neonatal care and how it should be monitored', in A. Okken and J. Koch (eds) *Thermoregulation of Sick and Low Birth Weight Neonates*, Berlin: Springer, p. 69.

Merenstein, G. (1970) 'Rectal perforation by thermometer', *Lancet* 1: 1007.

Meyer, M.P., Payton, M.J., Salmon, A., Hutchinson, C. and de Klerk, A. (2001) 'A clinical comparison of radiant warmer and incubator care for preterm infants from birth to 1800grams', *Pediatrics* 108(2): 395–401.

Micheli, J.L. (1995) 'Body temperature in sick neonates, diseases and chemical disturbances', in A. Okken and J. Koch (eds) *Thermoregulation of Sick and Low Birth Weight Neonates*, Berlin: Springer, p. 37.

Mitchell, A. (2005) Edinburgh: Protocol for humidity for babies less than 30 weeks gestation (personal communication).

Mok, Q., Bass, C.A., Ducker, D.A. and McIntosh, N. (1991) 'Temperature instability during nursing procedures in preterm neonates', *Archives of Disease in Childhood* 66: 783–6.

Montes, B.T., de la Fuente, C.P., Iglasias, D.A., Brescos, C.C., Quilez, C.P., Madero, J.R., Garcia-Alix, P.A. and Quero, J.J. (2005) 'Effect of hygiene interventions on the thermal stability of extremely low-birth-weight newborns in the first two weeks of life', *Annals Paediatric (Barcelona)* 63(1): 5–13.

Moore, K.L. and Persaud, T.V.N. (2003a) *The Developing Human: Clinically Oriented Embryology*, 7th edn, Philadelphia, PA: W.B. Saunders.

Moore, K.L. and Persaud, T.V.N. (2003b) *Before We Are Born*, 4th edn, Philadelphia, PA: W.B. Saunders.

Nachman, R.L. and Esterley, N.B. (1971) 'Increased skin permeability in preterm infants', *Journal of Pediatrics* 79(4): 628–32.

Nedergaard, J. and Cannon, B. (1992) 'Brown adipose tissue: development and function', in R. Polin and W.W. Fox (eds) *Fetal and Neonatal Physiology*, Philadelphia, PA: W.B. Saunders, p. 478.

Nichols, D.G. and Locke, R.M. (1984) 'Brown fat', *Physiological Reviews* 64(1): 1–64.

Nopper, A.J., Horii, K.A., Sookdeo-Drost, S., Wang, T.H. and Mancini, A.J. (1996) 'Topical ointment therapy benefits premature infants', *Journal of Pediatrics* 128(5 Pt 1): 660–9.

Nuffield Council on Bioethics (2006) 'Critical care decisions in fetal and neonatal medicine: ethical issues', London: author.

Okken, A. (1995) 'The concept of thermoregulation', in A. Okken and J. Koch (eds) *Thermoregulation of Sick and Low Birth Weight Neonates*, Berlin: Springer, p. 3.

O'Toole, S. (1998) 'Temperature measurement devices', *Professional Nurse* 13(11): 779–86.

Pazart, L., Devilliers, D., Boute, C., Aho, S., Rupin, C. and Gouyon, J.B. (1997) 'What alternatives to rectal temperature recording with a mercury thermometer?', *Revues d'Epidemologie Santé Publique* 45(6): 516–26.

Pelletier, P., Gauthier, K., Sideleva, O., Samuarut, J. and Silva. J.E. (2008) 'Mice lacking the thyroid receptor alpha gene spend more energy in thermogenesis, burn more fat and are less sensitive to high-fat diet-induced obesity'. Endocrinology. August 21. [Epub ahead of print].

Powell, R.W., Dyess, D.L.. Collins, J.N., Roberts, W.S, Tacchi, E.J., Swafford, A.N. Jr., Ferrara, J.J. and Ardell, J.L. (1999) 'Regional blood flow response to hypothermia in premature, newborn and neonatal piglets', *Journal of Pediatric Surgery* 34(1): 193–8.

Power, G.C. (1998) 'Indicators of thermogenic response', in R. Polin and W.W. Fox (eds) *Fetal and Neonatal Physiology*, 2nd edn, Philadelphia, PA: W.B. Saunders, p. 671.

Racine, J. and Jarjouri, E. (1982) 'Severe hypothermia in infants', *Helvetica Paediatrica Acta* 37(4): 317–22.

Resuscitation Council (UK) (2005) *Newborn Life Support Guidelines,* London: author.

Roll, C., Horsch, S., Husing, J. and Hanssler, L. (2000) 'Small premature infants do not tolerate axillary temperature measurement any better than rectal measurement: study of the effect of axillary and rectal temperature measurement on vital parameters and cerebral hemodynamics and oxygentation', *Zeitschrift für Geburtshilfe und Neonatologie* 204(5): 193–7 [Abstract].

Roncoli, M. and Medoff-Cooper, B. (1992) 'Thermoregulation in low-birth weight infants', *NAACOG's Clinical Issues* 3(1): 25–33.

Rutter, N. (1989) 'The hazards of an immature skin', in D. Harvey, R.W.I., Cooke and G.A. Levitt (eds) *The Baby under 1000 g*, Sevenoaks: Wright.

Rutter, N. (1992) 'Temperature control and its disorders', in N.R.C. Roberton (ed.) *Textbook of Neonatology*, 2nd edn, Edinburgh: Churchill Livingstone, p. 217.

Rutter, N. (1996) 'The immature skin', *European Journal of Pediatrics* 155(Suppl. 2): S18–S20.

Rutter, N. and Hull, D. (1981) 'Reduction of skin water loss in the newborn. I. Effect of applying topical agents', *Archives of Disease in Childhood* 56: 669–72.

Sarman, I. (1992) 'Thermal responses and heart rates of low-birth-weight premature babies during daily care on a heated, water-filled mattress', *Acta Paediatrica* 81(1): 15–20.

Sarman, I., Can, G. and Tunell, R. (1989) 'Rewarming preterm infants on a heated, water-filled mattress', *Archives of Disease in Childhood* 64(5): 687–92.

Sarman, I., Tunell, R., Vastberg, L., Carlquist, U., Can, G. and Toparlak, D. (1993) 'Mothers' perceptions of their preterm infants treated in an incubator or on a heated water-filled matress: a pilot study', *Acta Paediatrica* 82(11): 930–3.

Sauer, P.J.J. (1995) 'Metabolic background of neonatal heat production, energy balance, metabolic response to heat and cold', in A. Okken and J. Koch (eds) *Thermoregulation of Sick and Low Birth Weight Neonates*, Berlin: Springer, p. 9.

Sauer, P.J.J., Dane, H.J. and Visser, H.K.A. (1984) 'New standards for neutral thermal environment of healthy very low birth weight infants in week one of life', *Archives of Disease in Childhood* 59: 18–22.

Sauer, P.J.J., Carnielli, V.P., Sulkers, E.J. and van Goudoever, JB. (1994) 'Substrate utilization during the first weeks of life', *Acta Paediatrica* (Suppl.) 405: 49–53.

Schröder, H.J. and Power, G.G. (1997) 'Engine and radiator', *Experimental Physiology* 82(2): 403–14.

Sedin, G. (1995) 'Neonatal heat transfer, routes of heat loss and heat gain', in A. Okken and J. Koch (eds) *Thermoregulation of Sick and Low Birth Weight Neonates*, Berlin: Springer, p. 21.

Sedin, G. and Fridblom, K.H. (1995) 'Transport of sick newborns in a cold environment', in A. Okken and J. Koch (eds) *Thermoregulation of Sick and Low Birth Weight Neonates*, Berlin: Springer.

Sedin, G., Hammarlund, K. and Stromberg, B. (1983) 'Transepidermal water loss in full-term and pre-term infants', *Acta Paediatrica Scandinavica* (Suppl.) 305: 27–31.

Sedin, G., Hammarlund, K., Nilsson, G.E., Stromberg, B. and Oberg, P.A. (1985) 'Measurements of transepidermal water loss in newborn infants', *Clinics in Perinatology* 12(1): 79–99.

Seguin, J.H. (1997) 'Relative humidity under radiant warmers: influence of humidifier and ambient relative humidity', *American Journal of Perinatology* 14(9): 515–18.

Seguin, J.H. and Hayes, J. (1997) 'Thermal equipment usage patterns in neonatal intensive care units: interunit variability and intraunit consistency', *American Journal of Perinatology* 14: 267–70.

Seguin, J.H. and Vieth, R. (1996) 'Thermal stability of premature infants during routine care under radiant warmers', *Archives of Disease in Childhood: Fetal and Neonatal Edition* 74(2): F137–F138.

Shankaran, S. (2005) 'Whole-body hypothermia for neonates with hypoxic-ischemic encephalopathy', *New England Journal of Medicine* 353(15): 1574–84.

Simmons, M.A., Adcock, E.W. and Bard, H. (1974) 'Hypernatremia and intracranial haemorrhage in neonates', *New England Journal of Medicine* 291: 6.

Sinclair, J.C. (2002) 'Serv-control for maintaining abdominal skin temperature at 36°C in low birth weight infants', *Cochrane Database of Systematic Reviews* (1): CD001074.

Smith, C.L., Quine, D., McCrosson, F., Armstrong, L., Lyon, A. and Stenson, B. (2005) 'Changes in body temperature after birth in preterm infants stabilised in polythene bags', *Archives of Disease in Childhood: Fetal and Neonatal Edition* 90: F444–F446.

Smith, S.C., Clarke, T.A., Matthews, T.G., O'Hanrahan, D., Gorman, F., Hogan, M. and Griffin, E. (1990) 'Transportation of newborn infants', *Irish Medical Journal* 83(4): 152–3.

Smith, S.R., Jaffe, D.M. and Skinner, M.A. (1997) 'Case report of metallic mercury injury', *Paediatric Emergency Care* 13(2): 114–16.

Stephenson, T., Budge, H., Mostyn, A., Pearce, S., Webb, R. and Symonds, M.E. (2001) 'Fetal and neonatal adipose maturation: a primary site of cytokine and cytokine-receptor action', *Biochemical Society Transactions* 29(2): 80–5.

Strickland, M.E. (1997) 'Evaluation of bacterial growth with occlusive dressing use on excoriated skin in the premature infant', *Neonatal Network* 16(2): 29–35.

Tafari, N. and Gentz, J. (1974) 'Aspects on rewarming newborn infants with severe accidental hypothermia', *Acta Paediatrica Scandinavica* 63(4): 595–600.

Tammela, O.K. and Koivisto, M.E. (1992) 'Fluid restriction for preventing broncho-pulmonary dysplasia? Reduced fluid intake during the first weeks of life improves the outcome of low-birth-weight infants', *Acta Paediatrica* 81(3): 207–12.

Thigpen, J. and Sexson, W.R. (1997) 'Mercury toxicity awareness in the nursery', *Journal of Perinatology* 17(2): 140–2.

Thomas, K. (1993) 'Instruments in neonatal research: measurement of temperature', *Neonatal Network* 12(2): 59–60.

Thomas, K. (1994) 'Thermoregulation in neonates', *Neonatal Network* 13(2): 15–22.

Thomas, K.A. (2003) 'Preterm infant thermal responses to caregiving differ by incubator control mode', *Journal of Perinatology* 23(8): 640–5.

Thompson, D.A. and Anderson, N. (1994) 'Successful resuscitation of a severely hypothermic neonate', *Annals of Emergency Medicine* 23(6): 1390–3.

Thoreson, M. and Wyatt, J. (1997) 'Keeping a cool head: post-hypoxic hypothermia – an old idea revisited', *Acta Paediatrica* 86(10): 1029–33.

Valls, I. Soler, A, Castro, C., Centeno, C., Cotero, A. *et al.* (1986) 'Regional organization of a neonatal transportation system', *Anales Españoles de Pediatria* 25(6): 417–23. In Spanish.

Vohra, S., Roberts, R.S., Zhang, B., Jens, M. and Schmidt, B. (2004) 'Heat loss prevention (HeLP) in the delivery room: a randomised control trial of polyethylene occlusive skin wrapping in very preterm infants', *Journal of Pediatrics* 145(6): 720–3.

World Health Organisation (1997) *Thermal Protection of the Newborn: A Practical Guide*, New York: WHO.

Chapter 6

Management of Respiratory Disorders

Simone Jollye and David Summers

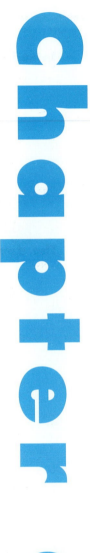

Contents

Introduction

The most common cause of admission to the neonatal unit is due to respiratory problems often resulting in the need for mechanical ventilation (Greenough and Milner 2005). In this chapter, the most common respiratory disorders in the newborn will be presented, incorporating the pathophysiology of the conditions and the strategies that can be utilised in their management. Mechanical ventilation of the neonate is a complex situation and not without risk and complications. As the respiratory support now available is more varied, an overview of ventilation techniques is also included.

The development of the respiratory system

The fetal lung has to develop sufficiently in utero in order that it will be able to support gas exchange that is necessary for the baby following delivery. According to Bhutani (2006), lung development can be divided into seven stages. There are five fetal stages which will be briefly discussed below, a neonatal period of approximately two months to full lung development by approximately 8 years:

1 The embryonic stage (0–7 weeks' gestation). During this stage the laryngotracheal groove develops from the foregut and a septum begins to form which separates the trachea from the oesophagus. Primitive bronchi also begin to develop.

2 The pseudoglandular stage (8–16 weeks' gestation). During this stage a network of narrow tubules develops, airway division commences and terminal bronchioles are formed. Connective tissue, muscle and blood vessels also start to develop.

3 The canalicular stage (17–27 weeks' gestation). During this stage respiratory bronchioles continue to branch and develop. A rich vascular supply is evident with arteries and veins developing alongside the respiratory airways. By approximately 24 weeks pulmonary gas exchange is theoretically possible (Greenough and Milner 2005). Type I and Type II pneumocytes can be identified. Type I cells are flattened and form approximately 90 per cent of the gas exchange surface of the mature lungs. Type II cells are cuboidal secretory cells containing surfactant (Rooney 1998).

4 The saccular stage (28–35 weeks' gestation). During this stage the terminal air sacs multiply and their surface epithelium thins. This allows closer contact with the capillary bed promoting greater gaseous exchange.

5 The alveolar stage (>36 weeks' gestation). This stage involves the further development of air sacs and the formation of true alveoli. This continues after birth and throughout early childhood.

Fetal lung fluid and fetal breathing movements

During fetal life the lungs are full of fluid which increases from 4–6mls/kg during the mid-trimester to 30mls/kg towards term. This fluid is important for cell maturation and development. It also helps to determine the size and shape of the developing lungs (Bland 1998) and its volume is equivalent to the lung fluid's functional residual capacity (FRC) in the early postnatal period. Fetal breathing movements are evident from approximately 12 weeks' gestation with strength and frequency increasing as the fetus matures. It is thought that fetal lung fluid and fetal breathing movements assist in the development of the diaphragm and chest wall muscles. Conditions such as oligohydramnios are associated with a decrease in fetal breathing movements and can lead to pulmonary hypoplasia (Sherer *et al.* 1990). With the onset of labour, fetal lung fluid production ceases and fluid absorption begins, probably as a result of an increase in the production and release of adrenaline.

Surfactant

Surfactant is produced by the alveolar type II cells. It is a complex mixture of phospholipids, neutral lipids and proteins and its function is to reduce the surface tension in the lungs, aiding gaseous exchange. Surfactant prevents the alveoli from collapsing completely (**atelectasis**) at the end of expiration and helps to reduce the work of breathing for the infant. The synthesis and secretion of surfactant are regulated by a series of enzymes and hormones, e.g. glucocorticoids appear to accelerate the normal pattern of lung development. This illustrates the rationale for giving antenatal steroids to women at risk of a premature delivery (Crowley 1999). **Catecholamines** also increase surfactant production. In the infant who is **small-for-gestational-age**, catecholamine response is increased, which explains why, despite their size, many of these infants do not develop respiratory problems (Rooney 1998). Insulin, however, inhibits the production of surfactant and as a consequence infants of diabetic mothers are at an increased risk of developing respiratory distress syndrome (ibid.). Hypothermia and acidosis can also inhibit surfactant production so the importance of keeping babies within an appropriate thermal neutral range, particularly around the time of delivery, cannot be overemphasised. Acidaemic states should be recognised early and have immediate correction.

Respiratory changes at birth

The predominant stimuli for initiating the first breaths are:

- clamping or obstructing the umbilical cord which results in an 'asphyxial' event;

■ cooling – with the sudden drop from intra-uterine temperature;
■ physical discomfort from touching and drying.

(Resuscitation Council 2006)

During the process of labour the lungs start to 'de-water', mediated, probably, by the release of adrenaline (Strang 1991). According to Bland (1988), the average 3kg term baby will clear approximately 100ml of fluid from their airways following the initiation of respiration (approximately 30ml lung fluid/kg). A healthy term infant generates high intrathoracic negative pressures to draw air into the lungs. This pressure is further increased when the baby cries which helps to drive lung fluid out of the alveoli and into the pulmonary vascular circulation and helps to establish the resting lung volume.

A rapid labour or a Caesarean section before the onset of labour does not allow the lungs to 'prepare' for their adaptation to extra-uterine life. This partially explains why these babies have a higher incidence of respiratory problems at birth including transient tachypnoea of the newborn (TTN) and Respiratory distress syndrome (RDS) (Madar *et al.* 1999).

Respiratory distress syndrome (RDS)

Respiratory distress syndrome (RDS) is predominantly a pulmonary disorder associated with the immaturity of the neonatal lungs (Donn and Sinha 2006) and is associated with a lack of surfactant. The incidence and severity of RDS are inversely related to gestational age. According to Donn and Sinha (2006), 80 per cent of infants born at 24 weeks' gestational age and 70 per cent born at 28 weeks' gestational age will develop RDS; however, by 32 weeks' gestation, this number has reduced to 25 per cent and only 5 per cent of 36-week gestational-age infants will develop the disease. This reflects the increase in surfactant production the nearer to term an infant is.

RDS presents in the first four hours of life and is characterised by an increase in the respiratory rate >60/ min (tachypnoea) and dyspnoea which is evident by nasal flaring and subcostal and/or sternal recession (from a very compliant ribcage) with a predominantly diaphragmatic breathing pattern. Often there is an expiratory grunt which is caused by the infant forcing air past a partially closed glottis in an effort to retain some air or pressure in the alveoli at the end of each breath to prevent atelectatic collapse (Cameron and Haines 2000). This classic presentation is not often witnessed these days as the most 'at-risk' infants are actively managed at delivery with intubation, exogenous surfactant, mechanical ventilation or continuous positive airways pressure (CPAP).

The surfactant deficient lungs require high-pressure ventilation to maintain their capacity for gas exchange, which leads to inflammatory changes and protein leak on to the alveolar surface which in turn form hyaline membranes. These membranes further inhibit gaseous exchange The name Hyaline Membrane Disease (HMD) was once an accepted term but as it can only truly be diagnosed at post-mortem examination, RDS or surfactant deficient lung disease are now more acceptable terms (Greenough and Milner 2005). The diagnosis of RDS can be suspected by the clinical picture and confirmed by radiological findings. The chest X-ray of an infant presenting with RDS illustrates a typical 'ground glass' or 'reticulogranular' pattern with air bronchograms evident. In severe RDS the X-ray may show near total atelectasis with complete opacification or 'white-out'. In a non-intubated and ventilated infant, the chest X-ray will also show a reduction in the lung volume.

The blood gases of an infant with RDS will present with an acidosis demonstrated by a reduction in the blood pH. This may either be a respiratory acidosis due to the retention of carbon dioxide (hypercarbia) metabolic acidosis from tissue hypoxia or a mixed acidosis having both respiratory and metabolic components. As it may be difficult to differentiate between RDS and congenital pneumonia, it is recommended that antibiotics should be commenced until an infection screen is confirmed as negative.

The loss of protein and impaired renal blood flow during the acute phase of the disease lead to the infant becoming oedematous. As surfactant synthesis commences (approximately 36–48 hours of age), the severity of the disease begins to decline. Characteristically, this period is associated with a spontaneous diuresis and a general improvement in the infant's condition (Kavvadia *et al.* 1998).

The aim of treatment of RDS is to establish adequate gaseous exchange and prevent complications from arising by providing respiratory support until the type II pneumocytes regenerate and begin to produce surfactant. Infants with mild RDS and who have a good respiratory effort and effective ventilation may only require supplemental oxygen to manage their condition. This can be delivered through nasal cannula, via the incubator or a head box or hood. Infants who display an increase in their work of breathing associated with hypercarbia and an increase in oxygen requirements will benefit from increased respiratory support in the form of CPAP. CPAP support can be considered if the infant has a reasonable spontaneous respiratory effort with mild hypercarbia. Infants who present with a decreased respiratory drive or apnoeas with a raised $PaCO_2$ and reduced PaO_2 will need to be intubated and ventilated. Most of these infants will receive surfactant replacement therapy. Exogenous surfactant therapy has been shown to reduce the severity of RDS (Soll 1999; McDonald and Ainsworth 2004) and can be given as a prophylactic medication or as a rescue treatment. Prophylactic surfactant therapy should be given as soon as possible after birth regardless of the respiratory status of the baby. Rescue surfactant therapy is given when signs of respiratory distress are present – usually at approximately 2 hours of age.

Surfactant is delivered to the lungs via the endotracheal tube over a period of a few seconds. The surfactant disseminates homogeneously and works by coating the alveolar surface of the lung which primarily reduces surface tension, improving lung volume, pulmonary perfusion and oxygenation.

Several studies have been undertaken as to which method of treatment provides the best outcome (Yost and Soll 2000; Soll and Morley 2001; Sinha *et al.* 2005). Meta-analysis of these trials demonstrates an improvement in mortality and a reduction in pneumothorax for neonates who are given surfactant as a prophylactic treatment. Infants given surfactant therapy also demonstrated a reduction in oxygen requirement, intensity of ventilation and improvements in blood gases. Research is ongoing for the use of aerosol surfactants which avoids the need for intubation in its delivery.

Initially these infants will require intravenous fluids and Total Parental Nutrition as enteral feeding may compromise respiratory function. Small-volume milk feeds (ideally breast milk) can be introduced once the ventilatory status is more stable. These infants can have their clinical course affected by other problems associated with prematurity, e.g. intraventricular haemorrhage (IVH), infections, and necrotising enterocolitis (NEC).

Pulmonary interstitial emphysema (PIE)

A complication of RDS is pulmonary interstitial emphysema. In PIE, air is trapped outside of the airways, e.g. in the interstitial spaces, rather than the alveoli and is due to terminal bronchiole rupture, usually following high pressure ventilation. PIE alters the pulmonary mechanics by decreasing lung compliance, making the lungs much stiffer. This in turn increases the residual volume within the lungs and increases the dead space impeding pulmonary blood flow which reduces pulmonary perfusion and leads to hypoxemia and hypercarbia. It can be localised but is more commonly widespread throughout both lungs. Clinical signs of PIE include marked respiratory acidosis and hypoxemia. Chest radiography reveals hyperinflation with a characteristic cystic appearance. If PIE is advanced, the X-ray may show large bullae formation within the affected area of the lung. Transillumination of the chest wall with widespread PIE shows an increased transmission of light similar to that seen with a pneumothorax.

Management is focused on preventing further barotrauma to the lungs. In conventional ventilation this involves reducing the peak inspiratory pressure and reducing the positive end-expiratory pressure provided that blood gases can be maintained and it may be that higher than normal $PaCO_2$ levels are tolerated (permissive hypercarbia, see p. 134). PIE is amenable to high frequency oscillatory ventilation (HFOV) as this form of ventilation is effective in treating lung injury (Bunnell 2006). Localised PIE may resolve spontaneously; however, widespread PIE may take several weeks to improve.

Infants with localised PIE should be nursed with the affected side down to compress the lung on that side. Selective intubation of the non-affected side has been suggested to 'deflate' the hyperinflated areas. However, the real treatment for PIE is in its prevention by avoidance of over-distension of the lungs when managing RDS.

Pneumothorax

Spontaneous pneumothorax can occur in up to 1 per cent of infants around the time of birth; however, only 10 per cent of these infants will become symptomatic (Steele *et al.* 1971, cited in Greenough and Milner 2005). This incidence increases with both prematurity and the need for mechanical ventilation, especially where high inspiratory pressures are needed (Greenspan *et al.* 1998). Clinical signs include:

- pallor;
- deterioration in oxygenation;
- bradycardia and hypotension;
- unequal chest movement/air entry which can be rapid and dramatic in tension pneumothorax.

Transillumination of the chest may be helpful, especially in preterm infants and, while a chest X-ray will confirm the presence of free air in the chest, it may not be practicable to wait for this due to the infant's condition. A thoracic drain should be inserted (see p. 356) and attached to an underwater seal drain. This drain should remain in situ until the air is drained, the lung re-expanded and the infant's clinical condition sufficiently stable to allow for its removal.

Pulmonary haemorrhage (PH)

Infants receiving respiratory support may demonstrate some evidence of small amounts of blood in tracheal aspirates following trauma during intubation. The term pulmonary haemorrhage (PH) or haemorrhagic pulmonary oedema is usually reserved for massive bleeding into the lung structure and airways. It is more common in extremely preterm and growth-restricted infants who have been ventilated and treated with exogenous surfactant (van Houten *et al.* 1992). A patent ductus arteriosus is also a significant contributing factor but PH may present in any infant with underlying lung pathology (ADHB 2009). PH is usually detected after an acute deterioration in the baby's condition associated with a degree of tube obstruction. On suctioning the endotracheal tube, a large volume of fresh blood-stained fluid may be present. The treatment is generally supportive. Ventilatory support needs to be increased with a high positive end-expiratory pressure (up to 8cm H_2O) to reduce further alveolar capillary leakage by tamponade, and a higher PIP to re-expand the fluid-filled airways to improve oxygenation and V/Q mismatch. High frequency oscillation ventilation may be beneficial. The rapid loss of blood can lead to shock and resuscitation with volume and blood may be necessary. The administration of plasma and/or platelets may be necessary to correct any clotting disorders as DIC may be an underlying factor (see p. 220). The prognosis is often poor and depends on the degree of respiratory and systemic deterioration following the blood loss (Raju 2006).

Pneumonia

Neonatal pneumonia may be an isolated focal infection but is usually part of a more widespread illness (Itoh *et al.* 1990). As pneumonia can be difficult to distinguish from RDS, all infants with respiratory symptoms at birth should be screened for infection and treated with appropriate antibiotics until proven negative.

Pneumonia in the neonatal period falls into three general categories: congenital or intrauterine pneumonia, early onset or intrapartum pneumonia and late onset pneumonia.

Congenital pneumonia

This form of pneumonia usually occurs as a result of ascending infection and chorioamnionitis following premature rupture of membranes. The mortality rate is high and many affected infants appear asphyxiated at birth. Congenital pneumonia may be viral in origin. Parravicini and Polin (2006) suggest that approximately 20–40 per cent of infants with toxoplasmosis, cytomegalovirus, rubella and herpes simplex viruses present with respiratory symptoms and as a consequence infants should be screened for these viruses as a matter of course.

Early onset pneumonia

Early onset pneumonia presents within the first 48 hours of life. It is commonly due to pathogens acquired from the birth canal with Group B beta-haemolytic streptococcus (GBS) being the most common pathogen accounting for 70 per cent of all cases (Rusin *et al.* 1991; Kinney *et al.* 1993; Roberts 2004). Other pathogens include haemophilus influenza, strep pneumoniae, *Listeria monocytogenes* and *E coli*.

Late onset pneumonia

This pneumonia occurs after 48 hours of life and is usually acquired nosocomially. It is most common in preterm infants who require some form of ventilatory support (Dear 2005). The most common pathogens for late onset pneumonia include gram negative bacilli, enterobacter and *E coli*.

The treatment for all forms of neonatal pneumonia includes the administration of IV antibiotics. There is currently debate as to which antibiotic therapy should be administered. General consensus supports the use of ampicillin or penicillin with an aminoglycoside such as gentamicin. This regime tends to be for congenital and early onset pneumonia. For late onset pneumonia, the treatment is a third-generation cephalosporin plus Vancomycin. Antibiotic therapy should be evaluated when sensitivities to the pathogens have been identified. According to Dear (2005), antibiotic treatment should continue for 10 days for a proven pneumonia unless the pathogen is staphylococcus aureus, in which case a three-week course of antibiotics should be administered. Ventilatory support required during the acute illness will be determined by the degree of respiratory compromise and may vary from supplemental oxygen to full mechanical ventilation.

Meconium aspiration syndrome (MAS)

Meconium stained aminiotic fluid (MSAF) is observed in approximately 13 per cent of all deliveries yet only 4 per cent of infants born through MSAF go on to develop meconium aspiration syndrome (MAS). The overall incidence of MAS may be decreasing with changes in obstetric practice, but despite improvements in maternal and infant care MAS continues to carry the risk of death or significant short- and long-term morbidity (Macfarlane and Heaf 1988; Dargaville *et al.* 2006).

MAS is generally a problem associated with term and post-term infants. Meconium is the sticky black-green material contained within the fetal gastro-intestinal tract. In-utero passage of meconium is often a sign of chronic and/or acute fetal compromise mainly due to hypoxic stress. This hypoxic stress further leads to fetal gasping which causes the meconium stained fluid to be inhaled into the fetal lungs (Rigatto 2004). Postnatal **aspiration** is also possible where the meconium stained amniotic fluid is drawn into the lungs with the first breaths after birth.

The presence of MSAF in the preterm population was thought to be a marker of chorioamnionitis or infection with *Listeria monocytogenes*. This finding is now questioned; however, the presence of meconium at the delivery of preterm infants does appear to detrimentally affect their long-term outcome (Tybulewicz *et al.* 2004).

Meconium within the respiratory tract causes several problems:

- The particulate matter creates a physical obstruction which can be complete leading to ateletatic collapse of the alveoli, or partial, leading to air trapping, over-distension, air leak and pneumothorax.
- Surfactant inactivation by damaging the type II cells which decreases lung compliance.
- Complex inflammatory response leading to chemical pneumonitis and parenchymal lung injury, further inactivating surfactant and increasing pulmonary vascular resistance (PVR).
- Infection by inhibition of the action of alveolar **macrophages**.

These pulmonary effects can lead to ventilation perfusion (V/Q) mismatch which can make oxygenation and ventilation of these infants difficult and hence MAS has a strong association with persistent pulmonary hypertension (PPHN) (see pp. 131 and 170).

Most infants with MAS develop some signs of respiratory distress (e.g. tachypnoea, nasal flaring, sternal recession, cyanosis and grunting) soon after birth (van Ierland *et al.* 2009). In addition, the infant's chest can appear hyper-inflated or barrel-shaped. These signs can be delayed due to the evolving disease process, so any infant delivering through MSAF should have its respiratory status assessed regularly by the attending midwife (see p. 78 for delivery room management).

Up to 50 per cent of infants with MAS develop respiratory failure and can be complex infants to care for. Conventional care focuses on providing respiratory support to correct the hypoxia and hypercarbia. As oxygen is a potent pulmonary vasodilator, high concentrations of inspired oxygen can be used to create a normoxaemic state and although unproven, some clinicians try to maintain a hyperoxaemic state in order to try to reduce the PVR (Wiswell 2006). If CPAP or mechanical ventilation is required, then care must be taken, as the areas of over-distension combined with the parenchymal lung injury put these infants at high risk of air leak with rates of approximately 10 per cent (Dargaville *et al.* 2006). These infants may 'fight' the ventilator, even in synchronised modes, and there is often the need to sedate and administer muscle-relaxing agents for a period of time to achieve compliance and optimal ventilation and oxygenation. Acidosis also increases PVR, so ventilating to achieve a 'normal' pCO_2 (see Table 6.1 on p. 135) will help to keep the pH normal. Exogenous surfactant may have a role in the management of MAS in reducing its severity and reducing the need for ECMO (El Shahed *et al.* 2007).

There may be a role for chest physiotherapy if the X-ray shows areas of collapse or consolidation (Hough *et al.* 2008), although these infants are often sensitive to handling and may not tolerate the procedure.

If there has been a severe acute hypoxic-ischaemic insult, other body systems may require support. This may include the brain, kidneys, liver and heart. Measurement and monitoring of blood pressure, preferably by arterial access, are required to ensure that systemic pressure and organ perfusion are main-tained.

Infants who have suffered chronic intra-uterine stress may have undergone abnormal pulmonary vascular development resulting in them being more at risk of persistent pulmonary hypertension of the newborn (PPHN).

Inotropic therapies may be required (see p. 169). Echocardiography can be helpful in determining which inotrope would be most beneficial by assessing myocardial contractility and cardiac output. It is also useful to confirm a structurally normal heart and determine the degree of PPHN present and whether other drugs such as systemic pulmonary vasodilators or inhaled nitric oxide would be beneficial.

Hypotension and poor tissue perfusion may lead to metabolic acidosis which may need correction by the administration of a base, e.g. sodium bicarbonate (see p. 74).

Renal compromise from ante/intra-partum insult or postnatal hypotension makes the accurate recording of fluid balance an important facet of care in these infants. Fluids are usually restricted to prevent volume overload and as a consequence blood sugar levels should be regularly monitored as hypo-glycaemia can become a problem (see p. 266). As the bladder may not empty spontaneously, expressing or catheterisation may be required (see p. 351). An infection screen should be undertaken to exclude underlying infection, and antibiotics administered proven negative.

If the infant is receiving muscle relaxants, protection of the eyes is necessary to prevent drying and corneal abrasions; additionally, careful supported posi-tioning should be used along with passive limb movements as tolerated.

If this level of conventional support is not sufficient for the infant, further advice needs to be sought regarding the ongoing management which could include transfer to a specialist centre for inhaled nitric oxide (iNO) or extra-corporeal membrane oxygenation (ECMO) (see pp. 133 and 171). Infants with MAS account for approximately 50 per cent of the UK neonatal ECMO workload (Karimova *et al.* 2009).

Persistent pulmonary hypertension of the newborn

Persistent pulmonary hypertension of the newborn (PPHN) is the failure of the normal circulatory transition that occurs after birth (see p. 158). It is charac-terised by increased pulmonary vascular resistance (PVR) which results in a variable degree of right-to-left shunting of blood through the foramen ovale and ductus arteriosis resulting in severe hypoxemia. PPHN is a pathophysiological feature often arising from other disease states affecting the infant and can arise from any of the following (Gomella 2004):

- Primary or idiopathic PPHN +/- presence of mild neonatal lung disease. These babies are profoundly hypoxic with very little evidence of lung disease.
- Secondary to severe intrapartum asphyxia. These babies present with hypoxia and severe acidosis. This combination results in pulmonary artery vasoconstriction preventing the normal postnatal circulatory changes from occurring (Greenough and Milner 2005). The right-to-left shunt may be exacerbated by systemic hypotension secondary to myocardial asphyxial damage.
- Secondary to meconium aspiration syndrome leading to obstruction and inflammation of the airways.
- Secondary to infection, Group B strep being the most prevalent organism.
- Secondary to pulmonary hypoplasia in congenital diaphragmatic hernia or alveolar capillary dysplasia.
- Secondary to congenital heart disease resulting in a right-to-left shunt.

The clinical appearance of a neonate presenting with PPHN is that of respiratory distress with cyanosis.

Infants with primary PPHN present within the first 12 hours of life and very rarely after 24 hours. Where PPHN is secondary to pre-existing lung disease such as infection or MAS, presentation is within the first few hours of life. Infants with PPHN are critically ill and despite mechanical ventilation and 100 per cent oxygen may remain cyanosed with poor perfusion and acidosis.

Simultaneous preductal and postductal oxygen saturation monitoring is useful in diagnosing and managing PPHN. In the presence of right-to-left shunting through the PDA, saturations in preductal blood (right hand) will be higher than those in postductal (left hand or feet). A difference of >5 per cent (Gomella 2004; Kinsella *et al.* 2006) is considered indicative of a right-to-left ductal shunt. If invasive monitoring is used a gradient of 20mmHg (2.7kpa) higher in the preductal PaO_2 than postductal may indicate a right-to-left ductal shunt (Schumacher and Donn 2006).

Oxygenation is often assessed by calculating the oxygen index (OI):

$$OI = \frac{FiO_2 \times MAP \times 100}{PaO_2 \ (mmHg)}$$

OI values of 30–40 are indicative of severe respiratory disease. Mortality often occurs with an OI greater than 80 (Gomella 2004). The higher the OI, the more severe the PPHN. An OI level > 40 is a useful indicator for considering extra-corporeal membrane oxygenation (ECMO) as a management strategy for PPHN.

A full blood count should be undertaken as polycythaemia and hyperviscosity (demonstrated by a high haematocrit) syndrome aggravate PPHN. A white cell count is useful to determine whether an underlying sepsis or pneumonia is present. The platelet count is frequently depressed particularly in newborns with MAS or asphyxia. Blood chemistry should be monitored to ensure hypo-glycaemia and hypocalcaemia do not occur as they tend to worsen PPHN.

Chest radiography is useful in determining whether underlying parenchymal lung disease such as MAS or RDS is present. In newborns with idiopathic PPHN the lung fields are clear with decreased vascular markings. The heart size is typically normal or slightly enlarged. Echocardiography (ECHO) is essential for neonates with PPHN as it will rule out cyanotic congenital heart disease and will give a definitive diagnosis of PPHN (Gomella 2004). ECHO provides information about shunting at the arterial and ductal levels and allows assessment of ventricular output and contractility, both of which may be depressed in neonates with PPHN.

The care of infants with PPHN requires meticulous attention to monitoring, oxygenation, blood pressure and perfusion. Mechanical ventilation is usually required to help maintain adequate oxygenation. Surfactant may need to be administered to reduce alveolar surface tension and decrease the work of breathing. Minimal handling and sedation should be used for these infants to maintain compliance and synchrony with the ventilator. Muscle relaxation, however, is controversial; Walsh-Sukys *et al.* (2000) suggest that the use of paralysing agents in infants with PPHN is associated with an increased risk of death.

Maintenance of systemic arterial blood pressure is achieved through the use of pharmacologic vasopressor support such as dopamine and dobutamine (see

p. 169). These inotropes act by increasing myocardial contractility and systemic blood pressure and reduce the right-to-left shunting of blood.

Pulmonary vasodilatation can be attempted by the administration of drugs known to act on the pulmonary vascular bed, e.g. Tolazoline, Epoprostenol and magnesium sulphate (Neonatal Formulary 2007); however, Steinhorn *et al.* (1997) assert that inhaled nitric oxide (iNO) is the most specific vasodilator modality for neonates with PPHN.

Inhaled nitric oxide (iNO)

Nitric oxide is a colourless gas with a half-life of approximately 2 seconds. It is delivered to the intubated and ventilated infant via the endotracheal tube, where it diffuses from the alveoli to pulmonary vascular smooth muscle causing it to relax, improving oxygenation and decreasing ventilation – perfusion (V/Q) mismatch. Excess iNO diffuses into the bloodstream where it is rapidly inactivated by binding to haemoglobin. This rapid inactivation limits its actions to the pulmonary vasculature and consequently it has no systemic effects.

A Cochrane review (Finer and Barrington 2006) concluded that iNO can improve short-term oxygenation and reduce the need for ECMO in term or near-term infants. Soll (2009) states that iNO has been used to treat both term and preterm infants with respiratory failure and concludes that term infants with PPHN respond to iNO with improvement in oxygenation indices and a decreased need for ECMO. Additional to the reduction in ECMO, Clark *et al.* (2000) noted a reduction in the need for supplemental oxygen at 30 days of age in term infants who received iNO. The use of iNO in preterm infants remains controversial and inconclusive. It is thought to be of little benefit in the prevention of the evolution of chronic lung disease and may contribute to IVH due to its vasodilatory nature (Arul and Konduri 2009; Soll 2009).

Initial research studies reported starting doses of 80 parts per million (ppm). Following review of the studies, the recommended starting dose for iNO is now 20ppm in an infant ≥34 weeks. Increasing the dose to 40ppm does not appear to increase oxygenation in infants who do not respond to 20ppm. Infants who do respond to iNO can be weaned at a fairly rapid rate once the oxygenation levels have fallen to approximately 40 per cent. The basic criterion for weaning iNO is the maintenance of adequate oxygenation and stability of the infant without evidence of rebound pulmonary hypertension (Gomella 2004). Complications associated with iNO include an increase in methaemaglobin (MetHb) which leads to the haemoglobin having a reduced oxygen carrying capacity leading to cyanosis. Levels of MetHb need to be monitored on a regular basis. At levels of 20ppm and less, this is rarely a complication.

ECMO

ECMO is a complex procedure of life support used in severe but potentially reversible respiratory failure in term or near term infants (Mugford *et al.* 2008).

It is generally reserved for when other conventional treatment modalities have failed.

Criteria for ECMO are:

- Birth weight >2.0kg.
- Gestational age >34 weeks.
- No bleeding disorder.
- No congenital anomaly incompatible with quality life.
- OI >40.

(Greenough 1996; Mugford *et al.* 2008)

The latter index is the marker of the severity of the respiratory failure.

ECMO is unsuitable for less mature infants as the amount of anticoagulation required in the circuit makes preterm infants more prone to intra-cranial haemorrhage. Benefits have been shown in terms of both the mortality and morbidity in infants receiving ECMO; however, there are still concerns surrounding the invasive nature of the technique, especially with its disruption to the cerebral circulation. Half of the children who have received ECMO have died or are disabled at 4 years of age. This is thought, however, to be a reflection of the severity of the underlying pathology rather than the technique *per se* (Mugford *et al.* 2008). As ECMO is generally instigated once conventional therapies have failed, earlier referral may result in improved outcomes.

Trends in neonatal respiratory care

It is now widely accepted that positive pressure ventilation in the neonatal period can result in lung injury which increases the risk of respiratory morbidity including air leak and chronic lung disease. Several mechanisms for ventilator induced lung injury (VILI) have been proposed:

- Volutrauma where the alveoli are over-distended by the delivery of too much gas.
- Barotrauma where the alveoli are subjected to high pressures causing alveolar disruption.
- Biotrauma resulting from the injurious effects of inflammation, infection and oxidative stress.
- Atelectotrauma where there is alveolar collapse at the end of expiration requiring re-recruitment with every breath.
- Stretch trauma where the rate of inflation of the alveoli is beyond their normal elastic capability.

(Donn and Sinha 2006)

The modern trend in ventilating preterm newborns is to provide those who need it with the gentlest invasive ventilation possible for the shortest time possible. A strategy for protecting the lungs can be achieved by allowing permissive hypercarbia where the target $PaCO_2$ is higher than the previously accepted norm (usually defined together with a target pH) and permissive hypoxaemia where the oxygen saturation target is lower than in a normal infant (Thorne and Ambalavanan 2009). These strategies may decrease volutrauma and the duration of positive pressure ventilation.

The small group of term infants who require mechanical ventilation have different pathophysiologies and require different targets. Example targets for both groups are shown in Table 6.1.

Acid–base balance, gas transport and monitoring

In well infants, there are homeostatic control mechanisms within in the cardio-respiratory system, brain and kidneys that combine to maintain the acidity (pH) of the blood in the narrow range shown in Table 6.1. Sick infants are vulnerable to disturbances in their homeostasis caused by their disease or treatment (Cifuentes and Carlo 2007).

Nurses caring for ventilated infants need to have an understanding of acid–base balance and blood gases in order to recognise abnormal results and act accordingly (see Table 6.2).

Maintenance of the blood pH within acceptable parameters is necessary since all bodily functions are controlled by enzymes and molecular proteins that are highly sensitive to its changes. A number of factors contribute to the regulation of pH including:

- CO_2 buildup (respiratory acidosis);
- low CO_2 (respiratory alkalosis);
- poor tissue perfusion leading to anaerobic metabolism (metabolic acidosis);
- loss of organic acids from persistent removal of gastric secretions (metabolic alkalosis).

Table 6.1 Acceptable blood gas results for infants requiring respiratory support

Parameter	Normal	Ventilated preterm infants Targets with permissive hypercarbia and permissive hypoxia	Term targets
pH	7.35–7.45	>7.25	7.3–7.4
PaCO$_2$	4.5–6 kPa	6–7.5 kPa	4.5–6 kPa
Arterial PaO$_2$	11–14 kPa	7–12 kPa	>8 kPa
SaO$_2$	100 per cent	90 per cent	>95 per cent

Source: Adapted from Newcastle Neonatal Service, *Ventilation Guideline* (2007).

Table 6.2 Relationships between blood gas parameters and acid–base status

	pH	PaCO$_2$	Bicarbonate	Base excess
Respiratory acidosis	Low	High	Normal	−ve
Compensated respiratory acidosis	Normal	High	High	High +ve
Metabolic acidosis	Low	Normal	Low	High −ve
Respiratory alkalosis	High	Low	Normal	+ve
Metabolic alkalosis	High	Normal or low	High	High +ve
Mixed respiratory/ metabolic acidosis	Low	High	Low	High −ve

The underlying cause for the alteration of the pH needs to be considered. If the pH reflects respiratory acidosis, an increase in ventilation is necessary; however, a low pH in the presence of normal CO$_2$ suggests a metabolic cause that should be treated by eliciting the underlying cause (e.g. hypotension) and treating accordingly, and /or infusion of base (usually sodium bicarbonate).

Sodium bicarbonate therapy needs to be given with caution as it is a hyperosmolar, high sodium solution which can predispose to intraventricular haemorrhage if given too quickly (see p. 187) and it can also lead to an increase in carbon dioxide levels (p. 75). Over-correction can lead to a metabolic alkalosis.

Low CO$_2$ states (hypocapnia) should be avoided as they lead to an increase in cerebro vascular resistance and poor cerebral perfusion which can compound an ischaemic insult (Levene and Evans 2005).

Carbon dioxide is carried in the blood in three ways: (1) dissolved in plasma (10 per cent); (2) bound to haemoglobin (30 per cent); and (3) as bicarbonate (60 per cent). Carbon dioxide dissolved in water produces unstable carbonic acid which in normal states dissociates rapidly to produce a hydrogen and bicarbonate balance (see p. 75). In pulmonary disease states, retention of CO$_2$ leads to a failure of this mechanism and a respiratory acidosis (low pH) results. Hypocarbia may lead to respiratory alkalosis (low levels of CO$_2$ high pH) which can lead to decreased cerebral blood flow and should be avoided or corrected expediently.

Four methods are available to assess an infant's carbon dioxide status:

■ Arterial blood sampling to directly measure the infant's PaCO$_2$ This requires either insertion of an indwelling arterial line or regular arterial puncture (see pp. 337, 339 and 345).

- Heel prick capillary blood sample will directly measure the pCO_2 (see p. 334). A warm, well-perfused foot will give an estimation of the arterial pCO_2 that is accepted by many clinicians.
- Transcutaneous pCO_2 ($TcpCO_2$) monitoring estimates the arterial pCO_2 by the attachment of a probe containing a heated electrode to the skin. The underlying skin is warmed (to 43°C) arterialising the underlying capillary bed; the oxygen level is measured by its diffusion across the electrode's membrane. This method is useful for continuous trending but the electrode needs regular calibration and site changes to avoid burning the skin. The more immature the infant, the greater the risk of skin damage from the heat and from the adhesive fixation rings. The trending is particularly helpful in infants who are changed from conventional ventilation to HFOV, as there can be significant drops in CO_2 during this time.
- End tidal CO_2 monitoring is less commonly used in neonatal care but may be useful for confirming correct ET tube placement (by monitoring the presence of expired CO_2) and is useful for trending (Kugelman *et al.* 2008).

Oxygen crosses the alveolar capillary bed by diffusion and is then carried in the blood predominantly bound to haemoglobin (98 per cent) with a small amount dissolved in the plasma (2 per cent). Oxygen is required by all tissues for efficient cellular metabolism and the production of cellular energy adenosine triphosphate (ATP). Anaerobic metabolism, due to poor tissue perfusion, is less efficient and produces minimal ATP; it also generates the by-product of lactate, which accumulates in the tissues leading to metabolic acidosis. High levels of oxygen (hyperoxia) are injurious to tissues and carry risks of eye, lung and brain injury (Tin and Gupta 2007).

Three methods are available to assess and monitor an infant's oxygenation:

- Arterial blood sampling to directly measure the PaO_2 as above.
- Transcutaneous pO_2 (TcO_2) as above.
- Oxygen saturation (SaO_2) monitoring provides a continuous measure of the haemoglobin that is saturated with oxygen. It is simple to apply, requires no calibration and gives instantaneous readings. Saturation monitoring is, however, prone to being affected by strong ambient light, movement and poor tissue perfusion affecting its accuracy and performance. The probe should have regular position changes (minimum four hourly) to prevent pressure damage from too tight application or in poor perfusion states. SaO_2 has become the commonest method of oxygen monitoring within the NICU despite wide variation between clinicians in recommended safe targeted SaO_2 levels and concerns about its poor ability to detect hyperoxia. The ongoing BOOST-II trial (NPEU 2007) may help to address some of these concerns.

Non-invasive respiratory support

Continuous positive airways pressure (CPAP)

CPAP is a method of delivering a predetermined continuous pressure and supplementary oxygen to the airways of a spontaneously breathing infant (Jones and Deveau 1997). CPAP helps reduce upper airway occlusion and decreases upper airway resistance by mechanically splinting the airways open. This improves ventilation by recruiting collapsed alveoli and increasing the surface area available for gas exchange. It also stabilises the chest wall and reduces the work of breathing.

CPAP can be administered in a variety of ways. It has previously been administered through an ET tube; however, this practice is deemed unsatisfactory, as the resistance from the ET tube makes it difficult for the neonate to breathe effectively for more that a short period of time (Morley 2006). Additionally, the ET tube can get blocked with secretions. CPAP is often used post extubation, particularly for preterm babies who have some degree of RDS. It can also be used as the first line of management for babies with mild RDS or TTN. The starting pressure for CPAP is usually in the range of 6–8cmH$_2$O.

Research has been undertaken comparing preterm infants who commence CPAP initially after birth with those who receive mechanical ventilation. During the COIN trial (Morley *et al.* 2008), infants between 25+0 and 28+6 weeks were randomised to nasal CPAP of 8cmH$_2$O or mechanical ventilation. The outcome demonstrated that in the infants in the CPAP group the use of surfactant was halved and there was a lower incidence of death or chronic lung disease at 28 days. There was, however, an increase in pneumothorax in this group but no other differences in complications due to prematurity were noted.

CPAP delivery

Nasal CPAP (nCPAP) prongs are the most commonly applied means of delivering CPAP (Gomella 2004). As newborn infants are inherent nasal breathers, nCPAP is easily facilitated and usually well tolerated. Binasal (double) prongs are more widely used than single prongs. They need to be carefully sized before insertion into the infant's nares and attaching to the CPAP delivery device. Nasal prongs have been associated with erosion of the nasal septum resulting in facial disfigurement which is generally due to poor overzealous fixation. McCoskey (2008) acknowledges the presence of nares and nasal septum breakdown as a complication of CPAP. This can be primarily overcome by the use of correctly fitting nasal CPAP hats and prongs. Prongs have developed over the intervening years and are now made of more flexible plastic and in a wider variety of sizes. This has reduced the problem somewhat, but the nares should be assessed on a regular basis and if signs of tissue damage are becoming apparent, an nCPAP mask can be used to relieve some of the pressure (McCoskey 2008). A higher flow may be needed for an nCPAP mask to deliver the same pressure as the prongs.

Other problems associated with nCPAP include:

- Obstruction of the nose and prongs from nasal secretions. Regular assessment and nasal suctioning, as necessary, will eliminate this problem.
- Loss of pressure due to an open mouth. Chinstraps can be used with extreme caution as they prevent the infant from clearing its mouth in the event of vomiting or regurgitation and therefore increase the risk of aspiration. Dummies (soothers) can be utilised, with parental permission, although opinions vary as to their use, particularly when contemplating breast feeding in the future.
- Gastric distension increases when a baby is on nCPAP and can be overcome by having a nasal or oral gastric tube *in situ* and either leaving on free drainage or aspirating the tube on a regular basis to decompress the stomach. An oral gastric tube is probably preferable in very small infants to prevent overcrowding of the nostril and potential notching disfigurement.
- Air leak or pneumothorax can be a particular issue in the larger infant with surfactant deficiency syndrome. Any infant suddenly deteriorating or having a significant increase in their oxygen requirements while on CPAP should be immediately investigated for pneumothorax.

Weaning practices from CPAP will vary but once the infant is stable on a CPAP of approximately 4–5cmH$_2$O, a trial off the CPAP for short periods can be attempted. If the infant shows any signs of increased work of breathing or oxygen desaturations, the CPAP can be recommenced. As the infant tolerates time off, the periods can be extended depending on physiological stability and blood gases.

Modes of invasive ventilation

The technology supporting invasive ventilation has improved remarkably in the past 10 years with several strategies now available. The integration of real-time monitoring of inspiratory and expiratory flow (inspired tidal volume VTi and expired tidal volume VTe), processed then to loops and waves (Figures 6.1–6.3), show the interaction between the infant and the ventilator which can assist clinicians and nurses in optimising ventilatory support. These 'new' modes of ventilation potentially allow infant-regulated breath-by breath changes in peak pressures, tidal volumes, inspiration times and rate. The evidence to date to support these new modes of ventilation is sparse (Claure and Bancalari 2007) but they may help reduce the ventilator induced lung injury (VILI) as previously discussed.

As various nomenclatures exist between manufacturers for the modes of ventilation being used, practitioners need to be aware of what is being utilised in their individual clinical settings.

Pressure – Volume loop showing single ventilator cycle
Pressure 20/5cmH$_2$O achieving VT 4mL

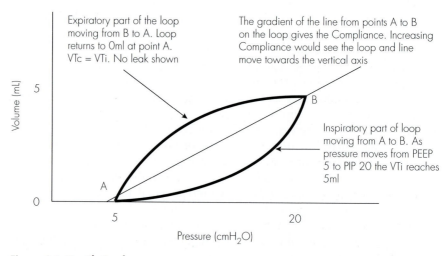

Expiratory part of the loop
moving from B to A. Loop
returns to 0ml at point A.
VTc = VTi. No leak shown

The gradient of the line from points A to B
on the loop gives the Compliance. Increasing
Compliance would see the loop and line
move towards the vertical axis

Inspiratory part of loop
moving from A to B. As
pressure moves from PEEP
5 to PIP 20 the VTi reaches
5ml

Volume (mL)

Pressure (cmH$_2$O)

Figure 6.1 Ventilation loop

Flow – Time wave through two ventilator cycles. The first cycle shows normal flow and the
second shows expiratory flow changes from increasing resistance

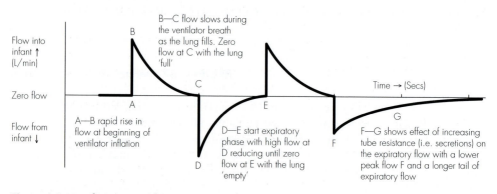

Flow into
infant ↑
(L/min)

Zero flow

Flow from
infant ↓

B—C flow slows during
the ventilator breath
as the lung fills. Zero
flow at C with the lung
'full'

Time → (Secs)

A—B rapid rise in
flow at beginning of
ventilator inflation

D—E start expiratory
phase with high flow at
D reducing until zero
flow at E with the lung
'empty'

F—G shows effect of increasing
tube resistance (i.e. secretions) on
the expiratory flow with a lower
peak flow F and a longer tail of
expiratory flow

Figure 6.2 Ventilation wave form 1

Continuous mandatory ventilation (CMV)

Also known as intermittent mandatory ventilation (IMV) and intermittent
positive pressure ventilation (IPPV). The longest established form of neonatal
ventilation is usually time cycled, pressure limited and with continuous flow.
The clinician sets the inspiratory time (IT), rate, peak inspiratory pressure (PIP)
and prolonged end expiratory pressure (PEEP). These parameters are unchanged

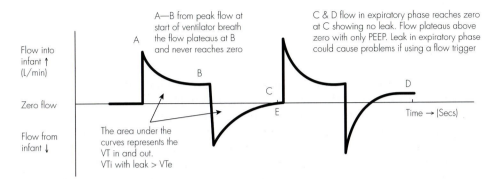

Flow – Time wave through two ventilator cycles. Both cycles show a leak around ETT during the inspiratory phase. The second cycle also shows a leak in expiratory phase

Figure 6.3 **Ventilation wave form 2**

BOX 6.1 Glossary of respiratory function monitoring terms through a ventilator cycle

The pressure in the ventilator circuit rises to PIP. This causes a movement of gas towards the infant from the ventilator circuit through the ET tube – *inspiratory flow*. During the period of the *inspiration time* this gas either collects in the infant's lungs or leaks out around the ET tube up the trachea and is lost. The ventilator calculates the total volume that has gone through the ET tube to give the *inspiratory tidal volume* (VTi).

The *pressure* in the ventilator circuit drops to PEEP which is the pressure maintained in the lung at expiration. The movement of gas from the infant to the ventilator is the *expiratory flow*. During the period of the *expiration time* the gas in the infant's lungs returns to the ventilator circuit and little, if any, is lost around the ET tube. The ventilator calculates the total volume that has gone through the ET tube to give the *expiratory tidal volume* (VTe).

The ventilator will calculate the difference between VTi and VTe giving the amount of *leak*. The VTe is generally accepted as the better measure of the infant's true *tidal volume* (VT) because of the lack of leak.

At the end of expiration, the alveoli and larger airways should still contain gas. The volume left is called the *functional residual capacity* (FRC).

The *minute volume* (MV) is theoretically the sum of all the individual VT measured over one minute (VT × rate per minute).

The behaviour of the lung and chest walls will also affect how much VT is achieved for the pressure delivered by the ventilator. Given the same pressure over the same time, a stiff lung will expand less than a normally functioning lung. This difference is expressed as the *compliance*.

The condition of the airway (ET tube and bronchial tree) can affect the speed of the gas flow and therefore the VT. Increasing length and decreasing diameter of the airway will slow the speed by increasing the *Resistance* to flow.

by any action of the infant and as a consequence are best used in infants who are sedated and muscle-relaxed to prevent any asynchronous breathing from occurring.

Volume control (VC)

This is variously known as volume guarantee, volume assured and volume limited ventilation. The accurate measurement of VT enables alteration of the ventilator breath to deliver a set volume rather than a set PIP. The clinician calculates the required VT (4–6ml/kg in preterm infants) (Greenough and Sharma 2007) and sets the maximum PIP and IT to achieve this. The ventilator will then deliver the predetermined VT but the pressure to deliver it will vary with each infant breath as pulmonary compliance alters. This control can be added to all forms of ventilation (except HFOV). Due to the uncuffed nature of the neonatal ETT and its concomitant variable leak, an accurate volume cannot always be assured.

Assist control ventilation (A/C)

Also known as patient-triggered ventilation (PTV) and synchronised intermittent positive pressure ventilation (SIPPV). A/C uses a signal from the infant to trigger the ventilator breath and hence determine the rate of ventilation. Originally an abdominal capsule was used to detect inspiratory activity; however, there were problems with detection of breath leading to delay in support and asynchrony. The commonest trigger today is the inspiratory flow measured with either pneumotachography or hot wire anemometry. The clinician sets the PIP, PEEP, IT, a back-up rate (in the event of apnoea) and the sensitivity of the trigger level. This sensitivity needs to be at an appropriate level for each infant and the nurse caring for the infant needs to be aware of the signs of trigger thresholds set too high or too low. Artefact from water or secretions in the sensors can cause auto-triggering and affect the infant–ventilator interaction. The IT, PIP and PEEP are unchanged for each breath but every breath the infant initiates crosses the trigger threshold and will be assisted by the ventilator, so the rate is determined by the infant. If the infant stops breathing or if the effort is undetected, the back-up will be activated and ventilation will continue.

Synchronised intermittent mandatory ventilation (SIMV)

Offers less support to the infant than A/C and may be used as a weaning tool. The setting of the trigger, IT, PIP and PEEP are the same as A/C. The rate set is now effectively the maximum number of supported breaths the infant will receive per minute. Any breaths taken in addition to the assisted rate are supported only by PEEP.

Pressure support ventilation (PSV)

A modified version of A/C offering less PIP support to the infant. Each infant breath triggers the ventilator in the usual way but the duration of the assisted breath is variable. The trigger for the termination of the breath is usually when the inspiratory flow has dropped to a clinician-set percentage (e.g. 5 per cent) of the peak flow. PSV can be used in conjunction with SIMV with a higher PIP so that the infant receives a higher level of support for the SIMV breaths.

High frequency oscillation ventilation (HFOV)

High frequency oscillation ventilation is the delivery of small tidal volumes to a neonate at supraphysiological rates (10 Hz = 600/min). It is used to improve gas exchange in patients with severe respiratory failure. As both inspiratory and expiratory phases are active, the likelihood of gas trapping is reduced.

The advantages of HFOV are said to be that it improves ventilation at lower pressure, reduces volutrauma to the lungs and produces a more uniform lung inflation which can reduce air leaks. Studies as yet have not shown any short- or long-term benefits in the use of HFOV over conventional ventilation in either term or preterm populations (Cools *et al.* 2009; Henderson-Smart *et al.* 2009). Disadvantages of the HFOV are rapid reductions in carbon dioxide levels which can lead to alterations in cerebral blood flow and decreased venous return from increased pressure within the thorax which in turn can lead to decreased cardiac output and a fall in blood pressure.

Two volume strategies can be used to deliver HFOV, those of low volume or high volume. A low-volume strategy in which the mean airway pressure (MAP) is limited with the aim of preventing damage due to barotrauma is used for infants with non-homogeneous lung disease, e.g. meconium aspiration syndrome (MAS), air leaks/pneumothorax, diaphragmatic hernia, pulmonary interstitial emphysema and PPHN. High-volume strategy in which MAP is elevated to promote optimum alveolar expansion consequently improving oxygenation is used for infants' more homogeneous disease states, e.g. severe RDS. If a high-volume strategy is used as a rescue support, then the infant should commence HFOV with a MAP $2cmH_2O$ higher than that delivered on conventional ventilation. The MAP is then gradually increased to optimise oxygenation. Infants with severe RDS may need an increase in MAP by as much as $10cmH_2O$. If oxygenation does not improve over the next few hours, additional therapies such as the use of inhaled nitric oxide should be considered.

Carbon dioxide elimination is primarily dependent on the oscillatory amplitude–delta P (Δ P). However, other factors such as frequency and I:E ratio will also effect CO_2 elimination. On commencing HFOV, the oscillatory amplitude is increased until chest wall 'wobbling' or vibration is apparent and then adjusted to manage carbon dioxide level.

Infants receiving HFOV require frequent chest X-rays to check for over- or under-expansion of the lungs. Over-expansion is depicted by the presence of more than nine posterior ribs and a flattened diaphragm and can result in a rapid decrease in carbon dioxide levels and a drop in blood pressure. Under-expansion is demonstrated by fewer than eight posterior ribs and poor aeration of the lung fields. Frequent blood gas analysis is also important for neonates on HFOV as changes in parameters can be rapid. Nursing care of neonates on HFOV is similar to that of any ventilated neonate (see below). However, there are a couple of salient points to consider. There may be increased secretions during HFOV due to the intrapulmonary percussion, so good humidification of the circuit is necessary to prevent blockage of the endotracheal tube (ETT). When undertaking suction an in-line suction procedure should be utilised to avoid reduction in the MAP. If disconnection is necessary, it should be minimised to avoid de-recruitment of the alveoli. Post suction, it may be necessary to temporarily increase the MAP by 1–2cmH$_2$O if the infant's oxygenation has dropped in order to re-recruit the alveoli.

As the infant's condition improves, the MAP and amplitude can be reduced according to blood gas results, and the infant switched to conventional ventilation or CPAP as tolerated.

Weaning from invasive ventilation

The large selection of ventilator modes available and the variation in their use between units mean that there is also wide variation between individual units in weaning methods. As blood gases and respiratory effort improve, gradual reductions in the level of ventilation support are made (i.e. lowering PIP or VT and rate, introducing SIMV and/or PSV). This is commonly followed by extubation to nasal CPAP. There have been several attempts to use some of the measured parameters of infant effort to determine readiness for extubation (Gillespie *et al.* 2003) but most decisions are made following clinical assessment of the individual infant and experience of the clinician.

Nursing care of the ventilated infant

The nursing management of a ventilated infant can be challenging, as the majority of these infants will be initially sick and unstable. Nurses managing these infants need to be vigilant to subtle variations observations, as early recognition of changes may prevent a significant deterioration and collapse. Infants on respiratory support should have constant monitoring of their heart rate, blood pressure and oxygen saturation as a minimum. End tidal CO$_2$ and transcutaneous monitoring can also help manage infants more effectively (see p. 259). As the nurse is probably the infant's best monitor, no ventilated baby should ever be left unattended.

Maintenance of patency and security of the ETT is a prime consideration. The ETT may be introduced either nasally or orally (Spence and Barr 1999) with the size appropriate to the weight of the infant (see p. 259). The largest appropriate tube should be used as the smaller its diameter, the greater the resistance to flow and increased risk of leak around the tube resulting in suboptimal ventilation. However, when using a larger diameter tube, there is a greater risk of complications from pressure damage to the nose, larynx and tracheal walls. The correct tip position for an ETT is below the larynx and above the carina (approximately T2). This distance is small in VLBW infants and increases their risk of tube displacement. The tube size and position should be clearly documented in the infant's notes. The ETT can be secured in many ways (Lai *et al.* 2009), each having their advantages and disadvantages, but failure of secure tube fixation is the commonest reason for accidental extubation (Veldman *et al.* 2006) and means the infant is subjected to emergency re-intubation which may cause trauma and destabilisation.

When an ETT is *in situ*, the normal mucocilliary action is suppressed and removal of secretions will be necessary if tube patency and optimal ventilation are to be maintained. Good humidification is necessary in order to liquefy secretions and prevent drying and damage to the mucosa (Williams *et al.* 1996). Inspired gases should be delivered at 37°C and as close to 100 per cent relative humidity as possible (Rankin 1998). Tarnow-Mordi *et al.* (1989) reported that the incidence of pneumothorax and chronic lung disease is reduced in infants <1500g when appropriate humidity is used.

ET suctioning should not be performed as routine but rather according to the needs of the baby (LaMar 2006). Indications for suction include:

- secretions visible in ETT;
- reduced or coarse breathe sounds;
- a decrease in oxygen saturation;
- deterioration in blood gases;
- change in pulmonary graphics.

Complications of ET suctioning include:

- hypoxemia;
- **bradycardia;**
- raised intra-cranial pressure;
- atelectasis;
- trauma;
- sepsis;
- dislodgement of the ET tube.

Deep suctioning where the catheter goes beyond the end of the ET tube can cause mucosal damage and perforation of the carina. To avoid this, the length of insertion of the suction catheter should be carefully measured (e.g. the length of the ETT plus the connector prior to the procedure) and the depth adhered to. If resistance is met following insertion, the catheter should be withdrawn slightly before suction is applied. The suction pressure should not exceed 10kpa, and suction only applied during withdrawal of the catheter. The duration of the procedure should be less than 20 seconds.

The use of saline as a lavage during the procedure is contentious. The instillation of saline was thought to loosen secretions and aid their removal. According to Puchalski (2007), this practice does not thin secretions or improve pulmonary function, and can further reduce oxygen saturation and increase the risk of bacterial colonisation of the lower airways.

Suctioning can be performed using open method (infant disconnected from the ventilator circuit) or closed (suction catheter is integrated into the ventilator circuit). In a 2001 review of available literature, Woodgate and Flenady reported that there was insufficient evidence at that time to ascertain the best approach; they conclude though that the procedure should only be undertaken by practitioners proficient in the technique. Recording of the nature, colour and volume of the secretions should be undertaken, as this is useful clinical information that may lead to a review or change in current management.

Infants requiring respiratory support should be nursed in a thermal neutral environment (see p. 92), as hypothermia can result in a decrease in surfactant production, and an increase in oxygen consumption (Bailey and Rose 2000). The environment should also be conducive to rest, enabling the baby's condition to improve. Minimal handling should be observed with the baby in a quiet environment away from bright lights and noise (see pp. 26 and 27). Additional to this, a pain assessment scoring chart may be useful in gauging the level of sedation the baby may need (see p. 237) in order to maintain safety and comfort.

Conclusion

Respiratory failure from prematurity or underlying disease processes are the most common reasons for admission to NICU. With decreasing gestational age, clinicians need to correlate therapies to the stage of development of the infant in order to optimise efficacy and prevent further VILI. While there have been significant technological advancements in the provision of respiratory support it is clear from review of the literature that more research is necessary to define the best way to ventilate this vulnerable population.

Case study: ventilatory management

Ralph is 27+3 weeks' gestation and weighs 810g. He was delivered by lower segment Caesarean section for maternal pregnancy-induced hypertension. His mother is a primigravid and received a full course of antenatal steroids prior to delivery.

At birth, Ralph had a good heart rate but had a weak respiratory effort. His cord blood gas was pH 7.15, $PaCO_2$ 7.6kpa PaO_2 2.3kpa. He was intubated and given a dose of surfactant. He remained ventilated and was transferred to NICU for further management.

On arrival at NICU, Ralph was put on to cycle pressure-limited ventilation with pressures 24/5, rate of 40 to maintain adequate tidal volumes he required 43 per cent oxygen. Umbilical lines were sited and a chest X-ray was performed which showed a white-out. Ralph's arterial blood gas at 5 hours of age was pH 7.20, $PaCO_2$ 8.8kpa, PaO_2 6.1kpa.

Q.1. What would you do next and why?

At 12 hours of age, Ralph was given a second dose of surfactant. His arterial blood gas a few hours later was pH 7.39, $PaCO_2$ 5.1kpa, PaO_2 7.5kpa.

Q.2. What would you do next and why?

The following day, Ralph has had his cares performed. The nurse notices he is not ventilating adequately and that his tidal volumes have reduced. There is no chest wall movement and Ralph develops a bradycardia with a decrease in his oxygen saturations.

Q.3. What do you think has happened?

Q.4. What would you do next and why?

Over the next few days Ralph's condition improves. His ventilation is weaned to pressures of 14/5, rate 40 and FiO2 is now between 21-25 per cent. He is given a loading dose of caffeine and is successfully extubated to nasal CPAP 6cmH$_2$O.

Q.5. What condition do you think Ralph presented with?

Q.6. What other aspects of Ralph's care need to be addressed?

References

ADHB (Auckland District Health Board) (2009) 'Newborn teaching resources', available at: http://www.adhb.govt.nz/newborn/TeachingResources/radiology/LungParenchyma. htm#PulmonaryHaemorrhage (accessed June 2009).

Arul, N. and Konduri, G.G. (2009) 'Inhaled nitric oxide for preterm neonates', *Clinics in Perinatology* 36(1): 43–61.

Bailey, J. and Rose, P. (2000) 'Temperature measurement in the preterm infant: a literature review', *Journal of Neonatal Nursing* 6(1): 35–8.

Bhutani, V.K. (2006) 'Development of the respiratory system', in S.M. Donn and S.K. Sinha (eds) *Manual of Neonatal Respiratory Care*, 2nd edn, Philadelphia, PA: Mosby Elsevier.

Bland, R.D. (1988) 'Lung liquid clearance before and after birth', *Seminar Perinatology* 12: 124–33.

Bland, R.D. (1998) 'Formation of fetal lung liquid and its removal near birth', in R. Polin and W.W. Fox (eds) *Fetal and Neonatal Physiology*, 2nd edn, Philadelphia, PA: W.B. Saunders, pp. 1947–2054.

Bunnell, J.B. (2006) cited in S.M. Donn and S.K. Sinha (eds) *Manual of Neonatal Respiratory Care*, 2nd edn, Philadelphia, PA: Mosby-Elsevier.

Cameron, J. and Haines, J. (2000) 'Management of respiratory disorders', in G. Boxwell (ed.) *Neonatal Intensive Care Nursing*, London: Routlledge.

Cifuentes, J. and Carlo, W. (2007) 'Respiratory system', in C. Kenner and J.. Lott (eds) *Comprehensive Neonatal Care*, 4th edn, Missouri: Saunders Elsevier, pp. 1–4.

Clark, R.H., Kueser, T.J., Walker, M.W. *et al.* (2000) 'Low dose nitric oxide therapy for persistent pulmonary hypertension of the newborn', *The New England Journal of Medicine* 342(7): 469–74.

Claure, N. and Bancalari, E. (2007) 'New modes of ventilation in the preterm newborn: evidence of benefit', *Archives of Disease in Childhood: Fetal and Neonatal Edition* 92: 508–12.

Cools, F., Henderson-Smart, D.J., Offringa, M. and Askic, L.M. (2009) 'Elective high frequency oscillatory ventilation versus conventional ventilation for acute pulmonary dysfunction in preterm infants', *Cochrane Database of Systematic Reviews 2009*, Issue 3, Art. No. CD000104, pub 3.

Crowley, P. (1999) 'Prophylactic corticosteroids for preterm delivery (Cochrane Revi), in *The Cochrane Library*, Issue 3, Oxford: Update Software.

Dargaville, P.A., Copnell, B. and the Australian and New Zealand Neonatal Network (2006) 'The epidemiology of meconium aspiration syndrome: incidence, risk factors, therapies, and outcome', *Pediatrics* 117: 1712–21.

Dear, P. (2005) 'Infection in the newborn', in J.M. Rennie (ed.) *Roberton's Textbook of Neonatology*, 4th edn, Philadelphia, PA: Elsevier Churchill Livingstone.

Donn, S. and Sinha, S.K. (2006) 'Minimising ventilator induced lung injury in preterm infants', *Archives of Disease in Childhood: Fetal and Neonatal Edition* 91: 226–30.

El Shahed, A.I., Dargaville, P.A., Ohlsson, A. and Soll, R. (2007) 'Surfactant for meconium aspiration syndrome in full term/near term infants', *Cochrane Database of Systematic Reviews*, Issue 3, Art. No. CD002054. DOI: 10.1002/14651858. CD002054, pub 2.

Ellis, J. (2005) 'Neonatal hypothermia', *Journal of Neonatal Nursing* 11: 76–82.

Finer, N. and Barrington, K. (2006) 'Nitric oxide for respiratory failure in infants born at or near term', *The Cochrane Database of Systematic Reviews 2006*, Issue 4, Art No. CD000399.

Gillespie, L.M., White, S.D., Sinha, S.K. and Donn, S.M. (2003) 'Usefulness of the minute ventilation test in predicting successful extubation in newborn infants: a randomized controlled trial', *Journal of Perinatology* 23: 205–7.

Gomella, T.L. (2004) 'Neonatology, management procedures', in *Call Problems: Diseases and Drugs*, 5th edn, New York: McGraw-Hill.

Greenough, A. (1996) 'Respiratory support', in A. Greenough, N.R.C. Roberton and A.D. Milner (eds) *Neonatal Respiratory Disorders*, London: Arnold.

Greenough, A. and Milner, A.D. (2005) 'Pulmonary disease of the newborn', in J.M. Rennie (ed.) *Roberton's Textbook of Neonatology*, 4th edn, Philadelphia, PA: Elsevier Churchill Livingstone.

Greenough, A. and Sharma, A. (2007) 'What is new in ventilation strategies for the neonate?' *European Journal of Pediatrics* 166(10): 991–6.

Greenspan, J., Schaffer, T., Fox, W. and Spitzer, A. (1998) 'Assisted ventilation: physiologic implications and complications', in R. Polin and W. Fox (eds) *Fetal and Neonatal Physiology*, 2nd edn, Philadelphia, PA: W.B. Saunders.

Henderson-Smart, D.J., De Paoli, A.G., Clark, H. and Tushar, B. (2009) 'High frequency ventilation versus conventional ventilation for infants with severe pulmonary dysfunction born near or at term', *Cochrane Database of Systematic Reviews 2009*, Issue 3, Art. No. CD002974, pub 2.

Hough, J.L., Flenady, V., Johnston, L. and Woodgate, P.G. (2008) 'Chest physiotherapy for reducing respiratory morbidity in infants requiring ventilatory support', *Cochrane Database of Systematic Reviews*, Issue 3, Art. No. CD006445, DOI: 10.1002/14651858.CD006445, pub. 2.

Itoh, K., Aihara, H., Takada, S. *et al.* (1990) 'Clinicopathological differences between early-onset and late-onset sepsis and pneumonia in very low birth weight infants', *Pediatric Pathology* 10: 757–68.

Jones, D. and Deveau, D. (1997) 'Continuous positive airway pressure for neonates', in D. Askin (ed.) *Acute Respiratory Care of the Neonate*, 2nd edn, California: NICU Ink, pp. 281–98.

Karimova, A., Brown, K., Ridout, D., Beierlein, W., Cassidy, J., Smith, J., Pandya, H., Firmin, R., Liddell, M., Davis, C. and Goldman, A. (2009) 'Neonatal extracorporeal membrane oxygenation: practice patterns and predictors of outcome in the UK', *Archives of Disease in Childhood: Fetal and Neonatal Edition* 94: 129–32.

Kavvadia, V., Greenough, A., Dimitriou, G. and Forsling, M. (1998) 'Comparison of respiratory function and fluid balance in very low birthweight infants given artificial or natural surfactant or no surfactant', *Journal of Perinatal Medicine* 26: 469–74.

Kinney, J.S., Johnson, K., Papasian, C. *et al.* (1993) 'Early onset Haemophilus influenzae sepsis in the newborn infant', *Pediatric Infectious Disease Journal* 12: 739–43.

Kinsella, J.P., Cutter, G.R., Walsh, F.W., Gerstmann, D.R., Bose, C.L. *et al.* (2006) 'Early inhaled nitric oxide therapy in premature newborns with respiratory failure', *New England Journal of Medicine* 355: 354–64.

Kugelman, A., Zeiger-Aginsky, D., Bader, D., Shoris, I. and Riskin, A. (2008) 'A novel method of distal end-tidal CO_2 capnography in intubated infants: comparison with arterial CO_2 and with proximal mainstream end-tidal CO_2', *Pediatrics* 122: e1219–e1224.

Lai, M., Inglis, G.D.T., Hose, K., Jardine, L.A. and Davies, M.W. (2009) 'Methods for securing endotracheal tubes in newborn infants', *Cochrane Database of Systematic Reviews*, Issue 2, Art. No. CD007805, DOI: 10.1002/14651858.CD007805.

LaMar, K. (2006) 'Nursing care of the ventilated neonate', in S.M. Donn and S.K. Sinha (eds) *Manual of Neonatal Respiratory Care*, 2nd edn, Philadelphia, PA: Mosby Elsevier.

Levene, M. and Evans, D.J. (2005) 'Hypoxic-ischaemic brain injury', in J.M. Rennie (ed.) *Roberton's Textbook of Neonatology*, 4th edn, Philadelphia, PA: Elsevier Churchill Livingstone.

Madar, J., Richmond, S. and Hey, E. (1999) 'Surfactant-deficient respiratory distress after elective delivery at "term"', *Acta Paediatrics* 88: 1244–8.

McCoskey, L. (2008) 'Nursing care guidelines for prevention of nasal breakdown in neonates receiving nasal CPAP', *Journal of Advanced Neonatal Care* 8(2): 116–24.

McDonald, C.L. and Ainsworth, S.B. (2004) 'An update on the use of surfactant in neonates', *Current Paediatrics* 4: 284–9.

Macfarlane, P.I. and Heaf, D.P. (1988) 'Pulmonary function in children after neonatal meconium aspiration syndrome', *Archives of Disease in Childhood* 63: 368–72.

Morley, C. (2006) 'Continuous positive airway pressure', in S.M. Donn and S.K. Sinha *Manual of Neonatal Respiratory Care*, 2nd edn, Philadelphia, PA: Mosby Elsevier, pp. 183–90.

Morley, C.J., Davis, P.G., Doyle, L.W. *et al.* (2008) 'Nasal CPAP or intubation at birth for very preterm infants', *New England Journal of Medicine* 358: 700–8.

Mugford, M., Elbourne, D. and Field, D. (2008) 'Extra corporeal membrane oxygenation for severe respiratory failure in newborn infants', *Cochrane Database of Systematic Reviews* 2008, Issue 3, Art. No. CD001340, pub. 2.

Neonatal Formulary (2007) *Neonatal Formulary Drug Use in Pregnancy and the First Year of Life*, 5th edn, Oxford: Blackwell Publishing Limited and BMJ Books.

NPEU (National Perinatal Epidemiology Unit, Oxford, UK) (2007) *Benefits of Oxygen Saturation Targeting Trial (BOOST-II UK)*, available at: http://www.npeu.ox.ac.uk/boost.

Parravicini, E. and Polin, R.A. (2006) 'Pneumonia in the newborn infant', in S.M. Donn and S.K. Sinha (eds) *Manual of Neonatal Respiratory Care*, 2nd edn, Philadelphia, PA: Mosby Elsevier, pp. 183–90.

Puchalski, M.L. (2007) 'Should normal saline be used when suctioning the endotracheal tube of the neonate?' Available at: http//www.medscape.com/viewarticle/552862.

Raju, T.N.K. (2006) 'Neonatal pulmonary hemorrhage', in S.M. Donn and S.K. Sinha (eds) *Manual of Neonatal Respiratory Care*, 2nd edn, Philadelphia, PA: Mosby Elsevier.

Rankin, N. (1998) 'What is optimum humidity?', *Respiratory Care Clinics of North America* 4(2): 321–8.

Resuscitation Council (UK) (2006) *Newborn Life Support: Resuscitation at Birth*, 2nd edn, London: Resuscitation Council (UK).

Rigato, H. (2004) 'Control of breathing in fetal life and onset and control of breathing in the newborn', in R.A. Polin, W.W. Fox and S.H. Abman (eds) *Fetal and Neonatal Physiology*, 3rd edn, Philadelphia, PA: W.B. Saunders.

Roberts, R. (2004) 'Prevention of sepsis at birth', in J. Wyllie (ed.) *Postnatal Care of the Newborn Baby: Guidelines for NICU and Postnatal Ward, March 2008–March 2009*, Newcastle: South Tees Hospital NHS Trust.

Rooney, S.A. (1998) 'Regulation of surfactant assisted phospholipids syntheses and secretion', in R. Polin and W. Fox (eds) *Fetal and Neonatal Physiology*, 2nd edn, Philadelphia, PA: W.B. Saunders, pp. 1283–99.

Rusin, P., Adam, R.D., Peterson, E.A. *et al.* (1991) 'Haemophilus influenzae: an important cause of maternal and neonatal infections', *Obstetrics and Gynaecology* 77: 92–6.

Schumacher, R.E. and Donn, S.M. (2006) 'Persistent hypertension of the newborn', in S.M. Donn and S.K. Sinha (eds) *Manual of Neonatal Respiratory Care*, 2nd edn, Philadelphia, PA: Mosby Elsevier, pp. 183–90.

Sherer, D., Davis, J. and Woods, J. (1990) 'Pulmonary hypoplasia: a review', *Obstetrical and Gynaecological Survey* 45(11): 792–803.

Sinha, S.K., Lacaze-Masmonteil, T., Valls I., Soler, A. *et al.* (2005) 'A randomized, controlled trial of lucinactant versus poractant alfa among very premature infants at high risk for respiratory distress syndrome', *Journal of Paediatrics* 115: 1030–8.

Soll, R.F. (1999) 'Natural surfactant extract versus synthetic surfactant for neonatal respiratory distress syndrome (Cochrane Review)', in *The Cochrane Library*, Issue 3, Oxford: Update Software.

Soll, R.F. (2009) 'Inhaled nitric oxide in the neonate', *Journal of Perinatology* 29(S2): S63–S65.

Soll, R.F. and Morley, C.J. (2001) 'Prophylactic versus selective use of surfactant in preventing morbidity and mortality in preterm infants', *Cochrane Database Systematic Review*, 2: CD000510.

Spence, K. and Barr, P. (1999) 'Nasal versus oral intubation for mechanical ventilation of newborn infants', *Cochrane Database of Systematic Reviews*, Issue 2, Art. No. CD000948, DOI: 10.1002/14651858.CD000948.

Steinhorn, R.H., Cox, P.N., Finemanm, R., Finer, N., Rosenberg, E.M. *et al.* (1997) 'Inhaled nitric oxide enhances oxygenation but not survival in infants with alveolar capillary dysplasia', *Journal of Pediatrics* 130: 417–22.

Strang, L.B. (1991) 'Fetal lung fluid secretion and reabsorption', *Physiology Review* 71: 991–1016.

Subhedar, N. and Shaw, N.J. (1997) 'Changes in oxygenation and pulmonary haemodynamics in preterm infants treated with inhaled nitric oxide', *Archives of Disease in Childhood: Fetal and Neonatal Edition* 77(3): F191–F197.

Tarnow-Mordi, W.O., Reid, E., Griffiths, P. and Wilkinson, A.R. (1989) 'Low inspired gas temperature and respiratory complications in very low birthweight infants', *Journal of Pediatrics* 114: 438–42.

Thome, U.H. and Ambalavanan, N. (2009) 'Permissive hypercapnia to decrease lung injury in ventilated preterm neonates', *Seminars in Fetal and Neonatal Medicine* 14(1): 21–7.

Tin, W. and Gupta, S. (2007) 'Optimum oxygen therapy in preterm babies', *Archives of Disease in Childhood: Fetal and Neonatal Edition* 93: F143–F147.

Tybulewicz, A.T., Clegg, S.K., Fonfé, G.J. and Stenson, B.J. (2004) 'Preterm meconium staining of the amniotic fluid: associated findings and risk of adverse clinical outcome', *Archives of Disease in Childhood: Fetal and Neonatal Edition* 89: F328–F330.

Van Houten, J., Long, W. and Mullet, M. (1992) 'Pulmonary haemorrhage in premature infants after treatment with synthetic surfactant; an autopsy evaluation', *Journal of Pediatrics*, suppl. 120: S40.

van Ierland, Y., de Boer, M. and de Beaufort, A.J. (2009) 'Meconium-stained amniotic fluid: discharge vigorous newborns', *Archives of Disease in Childhood: Fetal and Neonatal Edition*, published online 23 April 2009; doi:10.1136/adc.2008.150425,

Veldman, A., Trautschold, T., Weiss, K., Fischer, D. and Bauer, K. (2006) 'Characteristics and outcome of unplanned extubation in ventilated preterm and term newborns on a neonatal intensive care unit', *Paediatric Anaesthesia* 16: 968–73.

Walsh-Sukys, M.C., Tyson, J.E., Wright, L.L., Bauer, C.R., Korones, S.B., Stevenson, D.K. *et al.* (2000) 'Persistent pulmonary hypertension of the newborn in the era before nitric oxide: practice variation and outcomes', *Pediatrics* 105: 14–20.

Webber, S., Wilkinson, A.R., Lindsell, D. *et al.* (1990) 'Neonatal pneumonia', *Archives of Disease in Childhood* 65: 207–11.

Williams, R., Rankin, N., Smith, T., Galler, D. and Seakins, P. (1996) 'Relationship between the humidity and temperature of inspired gas and the function of the airway mucosa', *Critical Care Medicine* 24(11): 1920–9.

Wiswell, T.E. (2006) 'Meconium aspiration syndrome', in S.M. Donn and S.K. Sinha (eds) *Manual of Neonatal Respiratory Care*, 2nd edn, Philadelphia, PA: Mosby Elsevier.

Woodgate, P.G. and Flenady, V. (2001) 'Tracheal suctioning without disconnection in intubated ventilated neonates', available at http://www.nichd.nih.gov/cochrane/Woodgate2/Woodgate.htm.

Yost, C.C. and Soll, R.F. (2000) 'Early versus delayed selective surfactant treatment for neonatal respiratory distress syndrome', *Cochrane Database Systematic Review* (2): CD001456.

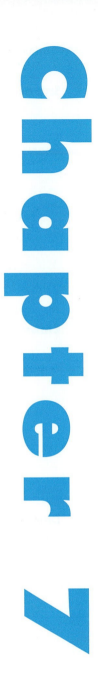

Chapter 7

Management of Cardiovascular Disorders

Rosarie Lombard

Contents

Introduction

Cardiovascular anomalies, congenital or acquired, are common problems in neonatal care. It is therefore inevitable that every neonatal nurse will encounter an infant with cardiac compromise within their practice. Recognising and treating cardiovascular anomalies are challenging and require good observational skills. To understand the complexities of the cardiac anomalies, it is imperative to have an understanding of fetal, transitional and neonatal circulations and the common associated problems in order to gain a greater understanding of the medical and nursing management required for each baby.

The aim of this chapter is to give an overview of the embryonic and neonatal cardiovascular system and to discuss the common conditions that are encountered in neonates.

Embryology of the cardiovascular system

The cardiovascular system refers to the heart and its supporting blood vessels. It is one of the first systems to function in the embryo (Blackburn 2007). Each system develops independently and simultaneously in utero, evolving into a closed functional cardiac system (Moore and Persaud 2003). The embryonic heart maintains the blood flow throughout the embryo, facilitating the exchange of fetal wastes for oxygen and nutrients in the placenta (Carlson 2004). A brief overview of this process will be discussed in four sections: development of the primitive heart, septation of the heart, blood vessels, and cardiac conduction.

Development of the primitive heart

The heart begins to form from the third week of gestation and it is fully developed by the eighth week (Moore and Persaud 2003). A heartbeat is present at 21 to 23 days (Carlson 2004). Initially, two endothelial tubes are formed from mesodermal cells. These tubes fuse together as the embryo undergoes lateral folding and become a single primitive heart tube. This primitive structure eventually becomes the endocardium. Mesenchymal tissue surrounding this endocardial tube thickens, cardiac jelly forms between the tissue and tube, and this gradually separates the layers that will eventually form the myocardium and the pericardium (Moore and Persaud 2003).

Five distinct areas are formed within the heart tube by day 20: sinus venous, atrium, ventricle, bulbus cordis and truncus arteriosus (Carlson 2004). Over the next few days, the structure assumes an S-shape due to the rapid expansion of the ventricle and bulbus cordis areas. The atrium expands laterally and ventrally and, in addition with the sinus venous, assumes a superior position to the ventricle, bulbus cordis and truncus arteriosus. This further divides into two atria. Simultaneously, the ventricle is moved upward and becomes the left ventricle. The right ventricle evolves from the bulbus cordis. The rudimentary layout of the heart

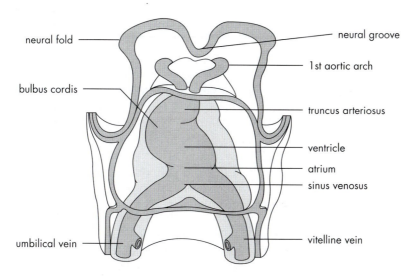

Figure 7.1 **The heart tubes fuse to form a single heart tube**
Source: After Moore and Persaud (1998, p. 356), with permission.

is now evolving. By day 22, the heart begins to beat, pumping blood from the sinus venosus (lower section) through the tubular-structured heart (Figure 7.1).

Septation of the heart

Late in the fourth week the endocardial cushions appear. These cushions contain mesenchymal cells and grow, expanding towards each other. During this process, the atrioventricular canals are formed (Moore and Persaud 2003). In addition, the septum primum develops downward from the top of the atrium. This results in a large opening which enables oxygenated blood to flow from the right atrium into the left atrium. This opening is gradually obliterated when fusion occurs between the cushions and the septum primum. The atrial septum secundum evolves beside the septum primum. The septum primum recesses on the upper atrial aspect; however, the lower atrial aspect remains and acts as a flap for the foramen ovale (Carlson 2004). This opening is one of the key factors of fetal circulation, facilitating the free flow of oxygenated blood from the right atrium to the left atrium and hence, into systemic circulation.

The ventricles continue to evolve from active proliferation of the septal tissue. Fusion of the bulbar ridges and the atrioventricular cushions occurs, resulting in closure of the intraventricular foramen. By week six, the semilunar valves, the papillary muscles and the atrioventricular valves are present and the heart

155

assumes a *normal* appearance. The membranous section of the interventricular septum continues to develop and is completed by week eight (Moore and Persaud 2003).

Blood vessels

By week three, the rudimentary aortic arch develops from the truncus arteriosus and it continues to develop over the next few weeks (Carlson 2004). The carotid and subclavian arteries, aortic arch, pulmonary artery and ductus arteriosus form. The formation of the aorta and pulmonary artery is facilitated by the presence of the aorticopulmonary septum. This septum is a longitudinal spiral structure which separates the aorta and pulmonary trunk and supports the normal intertwining of the aorta and pulmonary artery (Moore and Persaud 2003). By week five, the aorta and pulmonary artery are clearly identifiable (see Figures 7.2a and 7.2b).

In addition, by week five, the sinus venosus integrates into the right atrium and eventually becomes the inferior and superior vena cava blood vessels (Moore and Persaud 2003). The pulmonary veins are now recognisable in the left atrium. By week six, the coronary circulation is forming.

Cardiac valves form in the aorta, pulmonary artery and between the atrioventricular structures. The valves' function is to prevent the backward

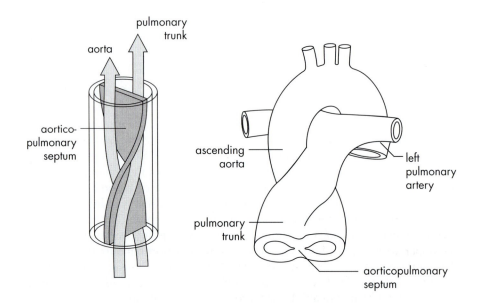

Figure 7.2 (a) Diagram illustrating the spiral form of the aorticopulmonary septum. (b) The spiral effect allows the vessel to twist upon itself as it divides to form the aorta and pulmonary artery

Source: After Moore and Persaud (1998, p. 373), with permission.

reflux of blood. The aortic and pulmonary artery valves are formed from subendothelial tissue, resulting in three-cusp valves. The atrioventricular valves, mitral and tricuspid, are formed from subendothelial and connective tissue and are connected to the ventricular wall by papillary muscle and cordae tendineae (Carlson 2004).

Cardiac conduction

The primitive heart is controlled by a temporary pacemaker in the cardiac tube. Once the sinus venous develops in the atrium, the sinoatrial node can be identified in the right atrium adjacent to the superior vena cava. The atrioventricular node on the atrial septal wall and the Purkinje fibres are then formed, resulting in a conductive system for the developing embryonic heart (Moore and Persaud 2003).

During this rapid development of the heart, defects can occur at several stages. Contributory environmental factors can also influence this process (see Table 7.1 for further details). Some of the common abnormalities will be discussed later in this chapter.

Table 7.1 Most common environmental triggers and specific defects associated with each

Potential trigger	% of disease	Most common malformations
DRUGS		
Alcohol	25–30	VSD, PDA, ASD
Amphetamines	5–10	VSD, PDA, ASD, TGA
Anticonvulsants	2–3	Pulmonary stenosis, aortic stenosis
		Coarctation of aorta, PDA
Lithium	10	Ebstein's anomaly, tricuspid atresia, ASD
Sex hormones	2–4	VSD, TGA, tetralogy of Fallot
INFECTIONS		
Rubella	35	Pulmonary artery stenosis, VSD, PDA, ASD
		MATERNAL
Diabetes	3–5	TGA, VSD, coarctation of aorta
	30–50	Cardiomegaly, myopathy
Lupus erythematosus		Heart block

Notes: VSD = ventricular septal defect; PDA = patent ductus arteriosus; ASD = atrial septal defect; TGA = transposition of great arteries

Source: Modified from Knight and Washington (2006), with permission.

157

Fetal circulation

The fetal circulation facilitates the delivery of oxygen and nutrients from the placenta to the growing fetus (Carlson 2004). There are three main structures associated with fetal circulation: (1) the ductus venosus; (2) the foramen ovale; and (3) the ductus arteriosus. In addition, the fetal circulation has a high-resistance pulmonary vascular system due to the collapsed lungs, thickened medial smooth muscle layer, and a low-resistance systemic circuit (Lakshminrushimba and Steinharn 1999).

In utero, blood enters under pressure from the placenta into the umbilical vein (Carlson 2004). Approximately 50 per cent of the blood travels via the ductus venosus, bypassing the smaller liver blood vessels, into the inferior vena cava (IVC). The remainder of the blood enters the liver sinusoids and enters the IVC via the hepatic veins (Moore and Persaud 2003). Blood from the IVC flows into the right atrium and flows across the foramen ovale and foramen secundum into the left atrium. In the left atrium, this blood mixes with the low-oxygenated blood from the lungs (via the pulmonary veins). The blood flows into the left ventricle and into the aorta. Approximately 65 per cent of this blood is returned to the placenta via the umbilical arteries – the remainder of the blood perfuses the viscera and the inferior part of the body.

The opening of the inferior vena cava is larger than the inter-atrial opening and, consequently, some of the highly oxygenated blood enters into the right ventricle and exits the heart via the pulmonary artery (Carlson 2004). In addition, low-oxygenated blood is returned from the head to the right atrium by the superior vena cava. This blood enters the right ventricle and also exits by the pulmonary artery. This blood flows towards the lungs; however, the fetal lungs are collapsed and are unable to denature the blood. Due to the high pulmonary vascular resistance (PVR), only 12 per cent of blood passes to the lungs, providing oxygen and nutrients for lung development. The remainder of the blood is shunted via the ductus arteriosus into the aorta whereby the majority of the blood will be returned to the placenta via the umbilical arteries. The patency of the ductus arteriosus is maintained by circulating prostaglandin E_2 and low circulating oxygen concentration (Figure 7.3).

Transitional neonatal circulation

At birth, profound haemodynamic changes occur in the transition from fetal to ex-utero circulation (Moore and Persaud 2003). The two major initial changes are the clamping of the placental blood flow and the expansion of the lung fields (Carlson 2004).

As the baby is delivered, ideally it cries and the lungs open up. Residual lung fluid is reabsorbed by the pulmonary epithelial cells, a process stimulated by increased levels of arginine vasopressin and adrenaline (Carlson 2004). The cessation of the placental blood flow results in decreased blood pressure in the IVC and right atrium (Moore and Persaud 2003). Consequently, the pressure in the left atrium supersedes the right atrium due to the increased pulmonary

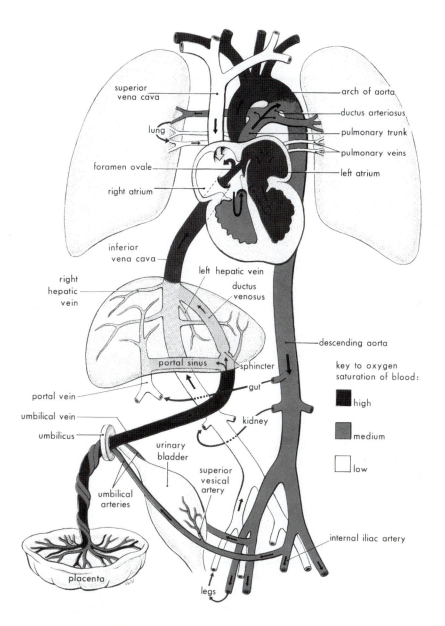

Figure 7.3 Schematic illustration of the fetal circulation. The shading indicates the oxygen saturation of the blood, and the arrows show the course of the blood from the placenta to the heart. The organs are not drawn to scale. Observe that three shunts permit most of the blood to bypass the liver and lungs: the ductus venosus, the foramen ovale and the ductus arteriosus. The poorly oxygenated blood returns to the placenta for oxygen and nutrients through the umbilical arteries

Source: After Moore and Persaud (1998, p. 392), with permission.

blood flow and the pressure closes the valve of the foramen ovale against the septum secundum (Carlson 2004). The blood flow from the right ventricle is now directed to the pulmonary circulation increasing the pulmonary blood flow. At this point, the PVR is lower than the systemic vascular resistance (Archer 2005). This is influenced by lung aeration, increased oxygen levels, prostaglandins (vasodilators), nitric oxide and endothelium-derived relaxing factor (EDRF) (Blackburn 2007). The lowered PVR results in reversed ductus arteriosus flow from the aorta to the pulmonary trunk.

Normal physiology

In *normal* physiology, the ductus arteriosus continues to constrict and gradually closes, aided by the presence of a higher circulatory oxygen concentration. The action of cytochrome P-450 is also understood to contribute to this process; however, the exact mechanism is not fully understood (Carlson 2004). The ductus venosus gradually closes over weeks and eventually becomes the ligamentum venosum. The umbilical vein becomes the ligamentum teres and the umbilical arteries become the lateral umbilical ligaments and the superior vesical arteries (ibid.).

The function of the heart is to pump blood throughout the body (Tortora and Derrickson 2009). There are many factors contributing to cardiac function and output.

Cardiac cycle

The cardiac cycle is composed of contraction of the atria (atrial systole), contraction of the ventricles (ventricular systole), and complete cardiac **diastole** (relaxation of the atria and ventricle) (ibid.).

Blood fills the right and left atria simultaneously from the inferior and superior vena cava and the pulmonary veins respectively. The sinuatrial node, located in the right atrium, is stimulated and emits an impulse of contraction across the atria, causing blood to be ejected from the atria into the ventricles through the atrioventricular valves. The atrioventricular node is stimulated by this contraction and it generates an impulse of contraction down the Purkinje fibres, resulting in contraction of the ventricles and expulsion of the blood into the pulmonary artery and the aorta. The heart relaxes, completing the cardiac cycle before the process restarts (ibid.).

Cardiac output

Cardiac output (CO) refers to the total amount of blood ejected from both ventricles each minute and is dependent on stroke volume (SV) and heart rate (HR) (ibid.):

$$CO = SV \times HR$$

Changes to adrenoreceptors, namely alpha (α), beta$_1$ (β_1), beta$_2$ (β_2) and dopaminergic, can also induce altered states of cardiac function and output (Rang *et al.* 2007). **Stroke volume** refers to the volume of ventricular blood ejected with each heartbeat. It is comprised of three phases: preload, afterload and contractility (Tortora and Derrickson 2009).

Preload is the amount of blood distending the ventricle. The filled ventricular blood volume reflects end-diastolic flow volume. The relationship between the lengthening of the myocardial fibres during this filling process is known as the Frank-Starling Law. The greater the lengthening of the fibres, the greater the ventricular contraction and hence, increased SV and CO (Blackburn 2007). However, as the neonatal heart has fewer myocardial fibres, the efficiency of the cardiac contractions is influenced by underfilling or overfilling during the preload period. Both processes can lead to reduced contractility and ultimately, reduced CO (Levene *et al.* 2008).

Afterload refers to the high pressure required by the ventricles to overcome the high pressures of the pulmonary trunk and the aorta. It is the resistance the heart must pump against (Tortora and Derrickson 2009). This is influenced by pulmonary vascular resistance and the viscosity of the blood (Levene *et al.* 2008). Afterload reflects arterial blood pressure measurements (Bell 1998).

Contractility relates to the myocardial intrinsic pumping mechanism and it is controlled by intrinsic and extrinsic factors (Rang *et al.* 2007) and is mainly dominated by intracellular calcium (Tortora and Derrickson 2009). The main factors that control the calcium entry into the cell membrane are the voltage-gated calcium channels, and the intracellular sodium levels which affect the calcium–sodium exchange (Rang *et al.* 2007). In addition, **catecholamines,** cardiac glycosides, drugs and other mediators can alter this process.

Regulation of neonatal circulation

Blood pressure (BP) reflects blood flow and peripheral resistance. The regulation of neonatal circulation is controlled by hormonal and neural regulation (Tortora and Derrickson 2009). The cardiovascular centre is located in the medulla oblongata in the brain:

Blood pressure = blood flow $\times$ peripheral resistance

Neural regulation

Baroreceptors, located in the aortic arch, the right atrium and the carotid sinuses, are sensitive to fluctuations in BP (Tortora and Derrickson 2009). Negative feedback mechanisms relay systemic BP fluctuations to the cardio-vascular centre in the medulla oblongata. For example, raised pressure increases the parasympathetic impulses and decreases the sympathetic impulses resulting in reduced HR and force of contraction and, ultimately, reduced CO. Conversely, reduced pressure increases the sympathetic impulses, decreases the parasympathetic impulses, and increases the secretion of adrenaline and nor-adrenaline from the adrenal medulla, and thus increases the blood pressure.

Chemoreceptors are located in the carotid sinus (carotid bodies) and the arch of the aorta (aortic bodies) and are sensitive to oxygen, carbon dioxide and hydrogen ion concentrations (ibid.). Hypoxia, hypercapnia or high hydrogen ion concentrations (acidosis) stimulate the chemoreceptors and send feedback to the cardiovascular centre. The sympathetic supply is stimulated resulting in vasoconstriction of the arterioles and veins and thus raises the BP.

Hormonal regulation

Hormones, produced in differing systems and circumstances, influence BP and blood flow (ibid.). The following is an overview of the major hormonal influences on BP:

- Adrenaline and noradrenaline, produced by the adrenal medulla, increase the CO by raising the rate and force of the heart.
- Antidiuretic hormone (ADH) is produced by the hypothalamus, released by the posterior pituitary gland and induces vasoconstriction in blood loss situations.
- Renin is produced by the afferent arterioles in the kidneys in response to a fall in BP. Combined with circulatory globulin, angiotension is produced which results in the adrenal cortex releasing aldosterone. Aldosterone increases the reabsorption of sodium and water resulting in raised BP.
- Atrial natriuretic peptide is released in the atria of the heart. It causes vasodilatation, promotes sodium and water loss, with the result in lowered BP.

History and clinical examination

Nurses need to have a good understanding of normal cardiac physiology, cardiac adaptations post delivery, and common cardiac anomalies to aid diagnosis and management of each presenting baby. Although detailed antenatal screening has improved the detection of primary congenital heart defects (CHD), 25 per cent of undiagnosed CHD present from home (Brown *et al.* 2006). This heightens the need for good nursing and medical clinical and observational skills. In addition, a sick preterm or term baby may develop secondary cardiac complications as a result of underlying altered pathophysiology (Archer 2005; Abman 2007).

History

A detailed medical history is essential for diagnosis and management of the baby (Archer 2005). This includes family history risk (2–5 per cent if other sibling has CHD; 5–10 per cent chance of an affected person passing to the next generation), social history, antenatal history (including scans' results, complications of pregnancy, medications, labour, delivery, and resuscitation if required), and presenting signs and symptoms in primary or secondary heart abnormalities. Heart disease can present in four different ways: cyanosis, respiratory distress, collapse or asymptomatic (Archer 2005).

Physical examination

Colour

Cyanosis is characterised by blue-grey mucus membranes, nail beds and skin and presents when deoxygenated haemoglobin is >3g/dl in arterial blood (Wechsler and Wernovsky 2008). Cardiac abnormalities (primary and secondary) can be associated with cyanosis or acyanosis (Archer 2005). At birth, peripheral cyanosis (acrocyanosis) is a common normal finding. Any condition where there is reduced haemoglobin may manifest as a greyish hue which can be mistaken for actual cyanosis. This includes facial **petechiae**, polycythaemia, anaemia, methemoglobinemia or other haemoglobinopathies. If a baby's pallor improves with oxygen and/or crying, the cause is likely to be pulmonary. If there is persistent central cyanosis, it is usually cardiac or respiratory (Levene *et al.* 2008).

Respiratory effort

Signs of respiratory distress include tachypnoea, wheeze, retractions and cardiopulmonary collapse (Wechsler and Wernovsky 2008). The presence of rales (coarse crackles) is associated with severe congestive heart failure (CHF), indicating fluid present in the alveolar and interstitial spaces (Furdon 1997). With some CHD, there are no obvious signs of respiratory distress, so vigilance is essential in detecting early signs and symptoms.

Peripheral perfusion

Before **auscultation**, the capillary refill time (CRT) should be assessed. Delayed CRT (≥3 seconds) indicates poor peripheral perfusion due to redistribution (Knight and Washington 2006). There may be a discrepancy between the peripheral and central temperature. Babies may also appear mottled.

Hepatamegaly

In congestive heart failure, blood outflow from the right ventricle is less compliant. This causes venous congestion and results in a palpable liver (≥3 cm below the costal margin) (Knight and Washington 2006).

Auscultation

Heart rate should be assessed for rate, rhythm, regularity and any abnormal finding(s). As the cardiac output decreases, the heart rate increases in an attempt to compensate (Knight and Washington 2006). Heart sounds are divided into four distinctive sounds: S1, S2, S3 and S4 (Lott 1993). In neonates, the 'lub-dub' sound is usually heard and represents the S1 and S2 sounds – 'lub' is produced by mitral and tricuspid valve closure; 'dub' is produced by pulmonary and aortic valve closure. The presence of a gallop rhythm (third heart sound) indicates abnormal filling due to dilation of the ventricles (Knight and Washington 2006). This is associated with impaired myocardial performance (Furdon 1997).

The presence of a murmur, systolic or diastolic, helps in the diagnosis of an underlying cardiac defect (Wechsler and Wernovsky 2008). Cardiac murmurs are classified according to their location, intensity, timing (systolic or diastolic) and quality (high-pitched or rough) and are graded 1–6. A murmur at less than 24 hours of age has a 1:12 risk of being CHD related (Burton and Cabalka 1994); however, it may also be a normal physiological finding (Arlettaz *et al.* 1998). If the murmur is present after 24 hours, oxygen saturations, four-limb BP measurements and an echocardiogram should be performed to rule out CHD.

Pulses

Distal pulses should be assessed. Decreased cardiac output causes redistribution of the peripheral blood supply to vital organs (Knight and Washington 2006). Reduced or absent pulses are indicative of obstruction of the aorta. The precordium should be palpated. The presence of a precordial thrill suggests reduced pulmonary or aortic outflow or, in some cases, a ventricular septal defect (Wechsler and Wernovsky 2008).

Diaphoresis

Babies with cardiac abnormalities, especially with congestive heart failure, can appear sweaty (Knight and Washington 2006). **Diaphoresis** is sweating. The increase in sweat production results from the raised metabolic rate as the body tries to cope with the extra demands on it.

Feeding

Frequently, there is a history of poor feeding with an underlying cardiac defect. This is multifactorial: tachypnoea, tachycardia, and increased energy consumption due to increased metabolic rate. In relation to weight, the baby may have poor weight gain overall; however, there may also be inappropriate weight gain due to oedema as a consequence of heart failure.

Investigations

Radiological

A chest X-ray is essential as part of cardiac investigations. Information such as the heart size and lung calibre is useful for diagnostic purposes. Dark or poorly perfused lung fields are indicative of reduced pulmonary blood flow; whereas opaque lung fields are indicative of increased pulmonary blood flow (Wechsler and Wernovsky 2008).

Blood pressure (BP)

A four-limb BP should be performed if cardiac abnormalities are suspected. A systolic difference of 20mmHg between the upper limbs and one of the lower limbs is indicative of a coartation (Archer 2005).

Electrocardiogram (ECG)

A 12-lead ECG may be performed as part of the assessment of the heart rate, and atrial and ventricular function/abnormalities (Archer 2005). Interpreting the ECG requires a skilled clinician. The age of the baby is important for analysis as there are many differences between the preterm, term and adult ECG.

Echocardiogram (ECHO)

An ECHO is a non-invasive investigation that provides information on cardiac structures, assessment of pressures, measurement of gradients, and overall function of the heart (Archer 2005). The incidence of cardiac catherisation has dramatically reduced since the evolution of detailed ECHO. It is also used as a guide for interventions such as balloon atrial septostomy.

Magnetic resonance imaging (MRI)

MRI provides a three-dimensional image of the heart and blood vessels. It is becoming increasingly prominent in planning treatment and management of babies with cardiac abnormalities. Cardiac catherisation has reduced as a consequence.

Hyperoxic test (nitrogen washout)

This test rules out or confirms CHD. To perform the test, oxygen saturations are recorded in air (pre- and post-ductal), 100 per cent oxygen is administered for 10 minutes. If the problem is respiratory in origin, the oxygen saturations will increase; if it is CHD, the saturations will not improve. Similarly, a PaO_2 >20kPa is indicative of respiratory; a PaO_2 <20kPa is indicative of CHD (Archer 2005). This test should be undertaken with caution as high oxygen concentrations can cause the ductus to close and bring about significant clinical deterioration in infants with duct-dependent cardiac lesions. If a duct-dependent lesion is suspected, a prostaglandin infusion should be commenced to maintain the patency of the duct.

Cardiac catherisation

This is an invasive procedure that can be used as a diagnostic or therapeutic strategy. Nowadays, it is mainly used for data collection and therapeutic interventions such as balloon septostomy.

Pathophysiology of common and relevant neonatal conditions

Cardiac abnormalities can be primary (congenital), maladaptive at birth or acquired (secondary). The following is an overview of the more common cardiac conditions.

PDA

In normal circumstances, the PDA is functionally closed at 10–15 hours post delivery and is completely closed within 5–7 days through a process of muscular and endothelial changes (Moore and Persaud 2003). Its structural closure does not occur until 4–6 weeks of age. Failure in closure compromises circulation, resulting in blood shunting from the aorta into the pulmonary artery. The increased pulmonary circulation results in decreased perfusion throughout the body, compromising major organs such as the brain, kidneys and gut and, consequently, increasing the risk of mortality and morbidity (e.g. necrotising enterocolitis (NEC), chronic lung disease (CLD), intraventricular haemorrhage (IVH)) (Herrera *et al.* 2007). In persistent PDA, prematurity and respiratory distress syndrome (RDS) are two of the main contributory factors (Archer 2005).

Symptoms of a symptomatic PDA include bounding pulses, active pre-cordium, murmur (not always audible on examination), apnoea (non-ventilated babies), desaturations, ventilator dependency, NEC, progressive cardiomegaly, and worsening lung shadowing on X-ray (Archer 2005; Levene *et al.* 2008). Confirmation of the PDA is by chest X-ray and an ECHO.

PDA treatment choices are pharmaceutical intervention with prostaglandin synthetase inhibitors (e.g. indomethacin, ibuprofen) or surgical ligation. The drugs act by inhibiting prostaglandin production by blocking the cyclo-oxygenase (COX) action on arachidonic acid, and thus facilitating closure of the PDA (Bell 1998). Successful pharmaceutical intervention is optimised if treatment is within the first two weeks of life and gestational age is between 30–34 weeks (Levene *et al.* 2008). There is also evidence that prophylactic indomethacin in <1000-gram babies can significantly reduce the presence of PDA and IVH (Schmidt *et al.* 2001). Fluid restriction in symptomatic babies can also benefit management.

In relation to drug choice, duration and dosage, PDA treatment varies considerably between neonatal units due to a paucity of definitive data (Cooke *et al.* 2003; Aranda and Thomas 2006; Herrera *et al.* 2007). Traditionally, indomethacin was used for treatment; however, ibuprofen is now regularly used as an alternative. Comparative studies have shown equivalence for PDA closure; however, ibuprofen appears to reduce renal dysfunction (Thomas *et al.* 2005; Ohlsson *et al.* 2008). Although Ibuprofen is renal sparing, there are some concerns that it increases the risk of pulmonary complications, for example, chronic lung disease (Ohlsson *et al.* 2008). Data are warranted from long-term follow-up studies to support clinical decision-making in relation to drug choice.

Vigilance for NEC detection is essential. It can result from an untreated PDA as well as pharmaceutical treatment (Archer 2005). NEC is a contraindication to starting treatment and if it presents during treatment, the drug should be stopped immediately (see p. 413). Treatment should be stopped or delayed if creatinine is >200μmol/L, platelet count is <100,000mm-3, unconjugated jaundice >200μmol/L or oliguria (Archer 2005; Levene *et al.* 2008).

Two options need to be considered if there is an unsuccessful primary treatment – a second drug course or surgical referral. A second indomethacin course has a low success rate (Hafeez and Watkinson 2007). Older infants have only a 50 per cent chance of closure. Persistent Doppler flow on ECHO post-primary indomethacin treatment in <28 weeks' gestation babies is indicative of surgical referral for ligation (Keller and Clyman 2003). Surgical ligation involves clipping the duct through a lateral thoracotomy incision. Minimally invasive endovascular techniques are also an option whereby a device is fed into the duct via a large vein, guided by radiological imaging (see www.nice.org.uk).

Hypotension

Hypotension is the blood pressure that results when **autoregulation** of blood flow to vital organs is lost (Seri 2006a). The definition of a normal BP varies considerably and factors such as gestational age, weight, cuff size and alert state need to be considered. Sick, premature babies are particularly vulnerable. These babies are more prone to cerebral blood flow fluctuations due to poor autoregulation (Tsuji *et al.* 2000) and are, consequently more at risk of IVH. Hypotension can predispose babies to increased risk of mortality and morbidity (Seri 2006a).

The gestation and age of the baby influence the blood pressure and, consequently, the management required for each baby (Levene *et al.* 2008). Preterm babies with low apgar scores, birth asphyxia or ventilated babies have lower systolic and diastolic BP measurements while those born to hypertensive mothers have higher BP measurements (Hegyi *et al.* 1994, 1996). A 'rule of thumb' for mean arterial pressure is the corrected gestational age up to 4 days of age (Levene *et al.* 2008).

Invasive BP measurement is essential in ill babies for accuracy (Archer 2005). Although current management is based on physical examination and mean blood pressure readings, there is increasing evidence to support the use of non-invasive Doppler ECHO measurements of superior vena cava (SVC) flow as a means of assessing blood pressure (Kluckow and Evans 2000; Groves *et al.* 2008). As 80 per cent of blood returning via the SVC is from the brain, the Doppler readings are reflective of cerebral blood flow and consequently can reflect hypo- or hyperperfusion of the brain.

Up to 50 per cent of babies become hypotensive in the first 24 hours in NNU (Patwardhan 2009). In the absence of primary pathophysiological factors (e.g. hypovolaemia, shock), delayed circulatory adaptation and/or myocardial dysfunction should be considered as causative factors in the first 24 hours of life (Seri 2006a). From day 2 onward, other causes such as NEC, sepsis, PDA, adrenal insufficiency and/or vasopressor/inotrope resistance should be considered. Treatment options include volume expansion, inotropes, hydrocortisone, noradrenaline and adrenaline (BAPM 1998; Seri 2006a).

Volume

Volume loss can relate to blood or transepidermal water losses (Patwardhan 2009). The average newborn blood volume is 80ml/kg (Wechsler and Wernovsky 2008). Volume replacement, isotonic saline (10–20ml/kg), should be considered as an initial treatment for hypovolaemaia (BAPM 1998; Kourembanas 2008). Saline is proven to be as effective as human albumin and it reduces the infection risks associated with albumin (So *et al.* 1997).

Inotropes

An inotrope is a sympathomimetic amine that improves myocardial performance (Rang *et al.* 2007). Dopamine, dobutamine and adrenaline are the most commonly used inotropes in hypotension in neonates.

Dopamine is a dose-dependent inotrope which acts on dopaminergic, α, and β adrenergic receptors (Rang *et al.* 2007). Low doses (1–5 micrograms/kg/min) induce dopaminergic action, increasing urinary output, slightly increasing the HR and cardiac contractility; medium doses (6–10 micrograms/kg/min) induce β_1 actions, increasing HR, contractility and BP; and high doses (11–20 micrograms/kg/min) are α-adrenergic, increasing HR, contractility, BP and SVR (Levene *et al.* 2008; Wechsler and Wernovsky 2008). Caution is required at higher doses as reduced renal blood flow can result due to increased PVR (Levene *et al.* 2008). Decreased CO can also manifest from myocardial dysfunction secondary to increased systemic vascular resistance (Seri 2006a).

Dobutamine has β_1, β_2 and minor α adrenergic actions (Rang *et al.* 2007). Dosage is 5–20 micrograms/kg/min and it acts by decreasing the SVR, increasing contractility and CO (Levene *et al.* 2008). If myocardial dysfunction or poor CO is suspected, dobutamine should be the first drug choice (Seri 2006a). If ineffective, then dopamine should be used as an adjunct therapy.

Adrenaline is an endogenous catecholamine (Rang *et al.* 2007). At low doses, it acts on the beta receptors, resulting in pulmonary and systemic vasodilatation. There is an increase in cardiac contractility, stroke volume and heart rate. At higher doses, it acts on alpha receptors inducing increased SVR.

Hydrocortisone

Hydrocortisone can be used if volume expansion and inotropic interventions are unsuccessful and vasopressor resistance is suspected (Seri 2006b). Vasopressor resistance can be defined as a dopamine requirement ≥ 15 micrograms/kg/min with or without other inotropes and/or vasoactive amines support to maintain normal BP. The exact mechanisms of hydrocortisone treatment are not fully understood; however, there is evidence that premature babies have adrenocortical insufficiency (Ng *et al.* 2001). In addition, cardiac adrenergic receptors are regulated by glucocorticoids. Reduced glucocorticoid production in sick neonates causes downregulation of the cardiovascular receptors and, consequently, vasopressor resistance results. Hydrocortisone improves BP without compromising cardiac function and organ blood flow (dose range: 1mg/kg every eight hours) (Ng *et al.* 2006).

Nursing babies on hydrocortisone therapy requires vigilance for complications. These include hyperglycaemia, system infections, osteoporosis, growth suppression and muscle wasting. Concurrent use of indomethacin and hydrocortisone should be avoided due to the increased incidence of intestinal perforations (Seri 2006b).

Persistent pulmonary hypertension of the newborn (PPHN)

The transitional circulatory changes at birth were described earlier in this chapter. Failure of the lungs to decrease PVR leads to severe respiratory distress and hypoxaemia, resulting in PPHN (see p. 131) (Abman 2007). It affects 1–2 per 1000 live births, predominantly term or post-term babies (Van Marter 2008). The causes of PPHN are:

- Idiopathic (20 per cent).
- Pulmonary parenchymal disease, e.g. surfactant deficiency, pneumonias, meconium aspiration syndrome. Less commonly, RDS, TTN and CLD.
- Abnormal pulmonary development, e.g. congenital diaphragmatic hernia, alveolor capillary dysplasia.
- Maladaption at birth, hypoxia with metabolic acidosis, metabolic (e.g. hypoglycaemia, hypocalcaemia), polycythaemia.
- Sepsis – bacterial or viral.
- In-utero exposure to prostaglandin synthetase inhibitor, e.g. aspirin, indomethacin.

(Levene *et al.* 2008; Van Marter 2008)

Generally, the onset of PPHN is at delivery or within hours of delivery. Presentation includes respiratory distress (grunting, tachypnoea, intercostal and sternal recession) and cyanosis. Hypoxaemia and acidaemia are evident on arterial blood gas. Pre- (right upper extremity) and post- (lower extremity) ductal oxygen saturation gradient difference of >10 per cent in the absence of congenital cardiac disease are indicative of PPHN (Van Marter 2008). A chest X-ray and an ECHO are essential to help rule out congenital cardiac disease and confirm PPHN (Levene *et al.* 2008; Van Marter 2008).

General principles of treatment include maximising oxygenation, reducing pulmonary vasoconstriction, normalising systemic blood pressure, correcting metabolic problems (hypocalcaemia, hypoglycaemia, hypomagnesium), and treating polycythaemia (Levene *et al.* 2008). The following is an overview of management.

Ventilation

- Give up to 100 per cent oxygen in term babies to maintain oxygen saturations >95 per cent and keep arterial blood oxygen level 9–13 kPa.
- Intubate and ventilate if progressively worsening respiratory distress and arterial oxygen level <7 kPa in 100 per cent oxygen. Consider high-frequency oscillation ventilation (HFOV).
- Aim to ventilate in mild alkalotic state (pH 7.40; pCO_2 4.5–5.0 kPa). Alkalosis helps reduce PVR. Sodium bicarbonate may be used to achieve desired blood gas levels (Van Marter 2008).
- Use paralysing agent to optimise ventilation.

Systematic haemodynamic

- Inotropes – see hypotension.
- Volume expansion – see hypotension. Packed red blood cells transfusion may also benefit.

Increased blood pressure will improve oxygenation and help reduce right-to-left shunting (Kinsella and Abman 2000).

Vasodilation

- Nitric oxide (NO) therapy. NO is a natural-occurring vasodilator (Rang *et al*. 2007). Inhaled NO (iNO) acts as a pulmonary vasodilator in the reduced/absence of endogenous NO. It is very effective for treating PPHN and reducing the need for extra-corporeal membrane oxygenation (ECMO) in term or near-term infants (Finer and Barrington 2006; Field *et al*. 2007); however, its use in preterm babies is unclear (Barrington and Finer 2007; Huddy *et al*. 2008). Therapeutic dose is 5–40ppm (parts per million).
- Prostacyclin. This is a vasodilator produced in the lungs in response to vasoconstriction (Rang *et al*. 2007). Some evidence suggests that it also enhances endogenous NO release (Levene *et al*. 2008). Hypotension can manifest during this treatment, thereby increasing the need for inotropes. Therapeutic dose is 2–20 nanograms/kg/min as an infusion (*BNF for Children* 2008).
- Magnesium sulphate is also a non-specific vasodilator and may be considered as an adjunct to treatment (Levene *et al*. 2008). Although improved oxygenation occurs, there are insufficient data to support safe usage in PPHN (Ho and Rasa 2007).
- Sildenafil is a cGMP-specific phosphodiesterase inhibitor which has inotropic and vasodilatation properties (Patwardhan 2009) and thus can improve oxygenation. Limited studies in neonates restrict its use in PPHN (Shah and Ohlsson 2007).

Extracorporeal membrane oxygenation (ECMO)

ECMO is a temporary life support technique that acts as a bypass for the heart and lungs, allowing the PPHN to subside (see p. 133). It should be considered if there are persistent problems with cardiac and respiratory function once other treatment measures have been maximised. Increased oxygen index (OI) >40 is indicative of severe respiratory distress and is used as a referral indication for ECMO (UK Collaborative Trial Group 1996). In addition, babies need to have a reversible condition, be >1.5 kilograms, >34 weeks, and lack severe IVH for eligibility (Wolf and Arnold 2008). Each ECMO centre has a referral criterion and this should be consulted for appropriate referrals at local level.

$$OI = \frac{FiO2 \times MAP \times 100}{PaO2 \ (mmHg)}$$

Note:
MAP = Mean Airway Pressure
mmHg = kPa × 7.5

Arrhythmias

Arrhythmias can include heart block (first-degree to third-degree) or tach-yarrhythmias. They can be associated with CHD, intracardiac tumours or structurally normal hearts (Penny and Skekerdemian 2001). Connective tissues disease, for example, systemic lupus erythema, can also cause heart block. A 12-lead electrocardiography (ECG) provides essential information in the diagnosis. Both conditions can present with signs of shock.

Treatment for ventricular tachycardia (VT) is dictated by the cause and severity of presentation (Archer 2005). Hyperkalaemia is a common cause of VT. Treatment is warranted when the potassium level exceeds 7.5mmol/L (Levene *et al.* 2008). Treatment includes correcting electrolyte imbalance (see p. 259). Other treatment measures include lignocaine in mildly symptomatic babies. Pulseless VT requires full resuscitation and cardioversion (1–2 Joules/kg). Amiodarone should be considered if there is unsuccessful cardioversion. Propranolol (beta-blocker) may be used as a preventative measure. See *BNF for Children* (BNF 2008) for drug doses.

Complete heart block (third-degree) with low cardiac output requires prompt intervention. Isoprenaline may be considered to increase the heart rate (Levene *et al.* 2008). Management may also include inotropes and diuretics (Archer 2005). Temporary and/or permanent pacemaker insertion may be necessary if pharmaceutical measures are unsuccessful.

Congestive heart failure (CHF)

CHF can be insidious and early signs can be missed due to their subtleness (Furdon 1997). It is clinically diagnosed through presenting signs and symptoms and supported by radiological findings (Wechsler and Wernovsky 2008). The signs and symptoms are caused by the inability of the heart to meet the metabolic demands of the tissues. There are many contributing underlying causes – hypoxia, haematological abnormalities (anaemia, hydrops fetalis, fetomaternal haemorrhage, polycythaemia), impaired myocardial contractility (metabolic, arrhythmias), structural abnormalities (congenital heart defects), pulmonary disorders (PPHN), renal disorders (renal failure, hypertension) and endocrine (hyperthyroidism, adrenal insufficiency).

Management of CHF includes supportive measures such as minimising respiratory distress (consider intubation if symptomatic), strict fluid balance of intake and output, and correcting any underlying metabolic derangement. Anaemia should be treated with a blood transfusion. Fluid restriction and diuretics may also be helpful. Digitalisation is an option; however, the newborn's myocardium has minimal inotropic reserve and it is, therefore, not as effective as when used in older children (Levene *et al.* 2008).

Congenital heart defects (CHD)

The incidence of CHD is estimated at 8 per 1000 live births (Ainsworth *et al.* 1999). To date, at least 35 CHD defects (cyanotic and acyanotic) have been identified. Acyanotic lesions relate to volume load (atrial septal defect (ASD), Ventricular septal defect (VSD), Atrioventricular (AV) canal, PDA) or pressure load (pulmonary valve disease, aortic stenosis, coarctation of aorta). Cyanotic lesions relate to increased pulmonary flow (transposition of the great arteries (TGA), single ventricle, truncus arteriosus) or decreased pulmonary flow (tetralogy of Fallot, pulmonary atresia, tricuspid atresia) (Levene *et al.* 2008).

Acyanotic defects include PDA and coarctation of the aorta. Cyanotic defects include transposition of the great arteries, tetralogy of Fallot, pulmonary stenosis or atresia, hypoplastic left heart, Ebstein's anomaly, truncus arteriosus and tricuspid atresia.

PDA

See p. 166.

Coarctation of the aorta

Incidence: 1:2500. Coarctation of the aorta is a narrowing of the descending aorta, usually distal to the left subclavian artery. It may exist in isolation or co-exist with other cardiac lesions. Although this is more commonly found in males, there is also a strong association with Turner's syndrome ($\geq$15 per cent) (Archer 2005). While some lesions are detected on antenatal scans, there are some lesions that are difficult to diagnose and may present with a collapsed baby. Specific management options include prostaglandin infusion, diuretics, and inotropic support. Surgical repair is a priority in the sick, collapsed baby once the baby is stabilised. The main surgical option is excision of the coarctation and end-to-end anastomosis or a subclavian flap (Waldhaussen) repair. Balloon angio-plasty under cardiac catherisation, with or without a stent insertion, is a less invasive procedure for some cases (see www.nice.org.uk).

Transposition of the great arteries (TGA)

Incidence: 1:3500 live births. More common in males (3:1). In TGA, the aorta and pulmonary artery are reversed. This results in deoxygenated blood from the right ventricle flowing into the aorta and hence is pumped around the body. Oxygenated blood from the left ventricle flows into the pulmonary artery and returns to the lungs. Other anomalies such as ASD, VSD, PDA, pulmonary stenosis, or aortic coarctation may also be present. Approximately 50 per cent will have a VSD (Wechsler and Wernovsky 2008).

Presentation is usually within hours of delivery if undiagnosed antenatally. The aim of management is to reduce oxygen consumption and maximise oxygen delivery (Wechsler and Wernovsky 2008). Mechanical ventilation, sedation, paralysis, blood transfusion and inotropes should be considered. A prostaglandin infusion will maintain the patency of the PDA to improve oxygenation. A balloon septostomy, performed by cardiac catherisation, enlarges the foramen ovale to promote mixing of oxygenated and deoxygenated blood. Traditionally, Mustard or Senning's operations were performed as a primary surgical intervention; however, in view of the incidence of arrhythmias and right ventricular failure associated with these procedures, early neonatal (2–3 weeks) corrective surgery is now the preferred surgical management. An uncomplicated TGA has a <5 per cent mortality rate (Archer 2005).

Tetralogy of Fallot

Incidence: 1:3500. Tetralogy of Fallot consists of four anomalies: right ventricular outflow obstruction (pulmonary stenosis), a VSD, an overriding aorta over the ventricular septum, and hypertrophy of the right ventricle (Archer 2005). Polycythaemia can manifest over time due to the persistent hypoxia. Hypoxia stimulates the red cell production in the bone marrow.

Presentation of cyanosis can be at birth (20 per cent) while other babies have mild cyanosis that worsens progressively in the first year of life (Archer 2005). A chest X-ray shows a boot-shaped cardiac outline and an ECHO confirms diagnosis. A prostaglandin infusion should be given during the diagnostic and stabilisation period to ensure patency of the ductal lesions. Babies can experience episodes of hypoxemia and cyanosis while awaiting surgery, known as hyper-cyanotic episodes. The management of these episodes includes knee-to-chest position to increase systemic resistance, oxygen therapy and morphine. Propranolol should also be considered. Surgical repair for an asymptomatic baby is recommended within the first six months of life; a symptomatic baby will need more urgent intervention (Archer 2005; Wechsler and Wernovsky 2008).

Pulmonary stenosis or atresia

Incidence: 1:5000. Pulmonary stenosis is the narrowing at the artery entrance. This predisposes to right ventricular hypertrophy, shunting of blood right-to-left through the foramen ovale, and congestive heart failure (Spilman and Furdon 1998). Pulmonary atresia is more severe than stenosis. Fusion of the commissures (valve leaflets) causes occlusion of blood flow from the right ventricle; hence systemic circulation becomes duct-dependent. The right lung tends to be hypoplastic and the more severe it is, the poorer the prognosis (Levene *et al.* 2008). Approximately 30 per cent of babies with TGA have pulmonary atresia.

Both conditions can present similarly to Fallot's tetralogy; however, cyanosis presentation is sooner. A chest X-ray may show a mildly enlarged heart. A prostaglandin infusion is essential in the initial management as this is a duct-dependent lesion. Cardiac catherisation provides information that will assist decision-making for surgical intervention. Open surgery pulmonary valvotomy is one treatment option that creates an outflow from the right ventricle (Wechsler and Wernovsky 2008). Alternatively, balloon dilatation of the valve is a minimally invasive procedure via cardiac catherisation (see www.nice. org.uk).

Hypoplastic left heart

Incidence: 1:5500. In this condition, the left ventricle and atrium fail to develop and the mitral and aortic valves are usually atretic (Wechsler and Wernovsky 2008). In addition to the pulmonary circulation, the right ventricle shunts blood via the ductus arteriosus to maintain the systemic circulation. As the PVR falls, the pulmonary circulation increases, the systemic circulation flow reduces, and this further compromises the systemic circulation. As this progresses, the baby will deteriorate (gradual or sudden). Signs include tachypnoea, respiratory distress, hepatomegaly, weak or absent peripheral pulses, poor CRT, and increased cyanosis. A chest X-ray shows a large heart and plethoric lung fields (Levene *et al.* 2008).

Management includes a prostaglandin infusion to maintain duct patency; however, if the foramen ovale is small or absent, the drug will have little effect (Wechsler and Wernovsky 2008). Balloon dilation via cardiac catherisation is an urgent requirement at this stage. Inotropes may be needed to treat hypotension. The standard treatment is staged surgical interventions (Norwood procedure followed by a Fontan operation) or heart transplantation. In recent years, the hybrid procedure is being considered as an option as it reduces the incidence of open heart surgery for the individual baby. This involves banding of the pulmonary artery and endovascular techniques to insert a stent in the PDA and perform an atrial balloon septostomy (see www.nice.org.uk).

Ebstein's anomaly

Incidence: 1:25,000. Although an uncommon anomaly, there is a high mortality associated with Ebstein's anomaly. It can be associated with Wolff-Parkinson-White syndrome (30 per cent) and SVT (Levene *et al.* 2008). The tricuspid valve, between the right atrium and ventricle, has a 'downward displacement' presentation. The non-compliant valve increases regurgitation from the right ventricle back into the right atrium, resulting in an enlarged right atrium. There is a large right-to-left shunting of blood at atrial level. In addition, there is reduced blood outflow into the pulmonary circulation. A chest X-ray shows cardiomegaly with diminished vascular markings (Wechsler and Wernovsky 2008).

Management includes prostaglandin infusion and measures to reduce the high PVR – oxygenation, mild respiratory acidosis and nitric oxide. Pulmonary hypoplasia as a result of an enlarged right heart in utero contributes to the difficult management of these babies, and hence it carries a high mortality rate (Levene *et al.* 2008).

Truncus arteriosus

Incidence: 5–15:100,000. This is a rare complex malformation that is characterised by a single artery arising from the heart that forms the pulmonary artery and aorta. A single similunar valve (truncal valve) is present between the ventricles and the single artery. The valve is often abnormal – stenotic, thickened, and/or regurgitant (Wechsler and Wernovsky 2008). A large ventricular septal defect is present in >98 per cent. In a third of cases, the aortic arch is on the right side of the heart instead of the left side. Over a third of babies have a deletion of chromosome 22 at 22q11.

Undiagnosed truncus arteriosus presents with cyanosis and signs of CHF in the first week of life. Pulmonary hypertension is often present due to the increased pulmonary blood flow. If untreated, 15–30 per cent of babies survive the first year of life. Complete surgical repair in neonatal or early infancy is recommended.

Tricuspid atresia

Incidence: 1:5500. In this abnormality, the tricuspid valve is absent and there is no communication between the right atrium and the right ventricle. The right ventricle is severely hypoplastic or absent in some cases. The majority of babies have a ventricular septal defect that allows left-to-right ventricular blood flow and pulmonary stenosis. Atrial communication (right-to-left blood flow) is essential to survival. Thirty per cent of babies have associated TGA (Wechsler and Wernovsky 2008).

These babies are cyanosed due to mixing of the blood supplies at atrial and ventricular levels. Prostaglandin infusion is vital to maintain the patency of the duct. Surgical correction in early neonatal period is vital. A Blalock–Taussig shunt or a Fontan procedure are options for surgical intervention. Other palliative measures may also be considered.

Nursing considerations

The management of a cardiac baby will be individualised to their specific cardiac abnormality and associated complications. The overall aims of management include the following instructions.

Maximise oxygenation

- Careful monitoring of physiological status – heart rate, respiratory rate, blood pressure, oxygen saturations, transcutaneous oxygen and carbon dioxide levels.
- Ongoing assessment of the baby's clinical condition and nursing and medical requirements.
- Blood gas analysis for respiratory and metabolic status.
- Supplementary oxygen if required to maintain oxygen saturations at acceptable parameters. Consider ambient, funnel or mechanical ventilation (CPAP or intubation) with oxygen supplementation.
- Blood transfusion if anaemic or hypovolaemic.
- Pharmaceutical intervention, for example, diuretics, inotropes, propanolol, prostaglandin.
- Vigilance for complications that can reduce systemic oxygen delivery, for example, IVH, severe infection.

Reduce oxygen requirements

- Nurse in a thermoneutral environment.
- Reduce stress by nursing the baby in a developmentally supportive environment, adhering to the principles of developmental care (see p. 16).

Maximise comfort

- Good positioning – elevate head of cot; use positioning aids for support.
- Give analgesia as appropriate – mechanical ventilation; hypercyanotic events; post-operative; painful procedures.
- Consider sucrose for pain relief for minor painful procedures.
- May need to paralyse, for example, part of management for severe PPHN.

Maximise nutritional status

- Close monitoring and recording of intake and output.
- Feeding – if oral feeding, monitor feeding closely for any signs of distress with feeding (increased signs of respiratory distress, tachycardia, diaphoresis, mottled, prolonged feeding). If distressed feeding, consider nasogastric tube feeding, partial or all of the feed depending on the baby's status; support breastfeeding and if unable to fully breastfeed, provide assistance and support for expressing and storage of breast milk. If the baby is unable to have enteral feeds, nutrition should be maximised by administering total parental nutrition via longline access or Hickman line.
- Liaise with dietician to maximise calorific intake.
- Careful monitoring of weight and growth (head and body) on the percentile growth chart.
- Monitor urea, electrolytes, blood sugars, jaundice levels. Correct any metabolic imbalance.
- Some babies will need fluid intake restriction (e.g. PDA, CHF).

Minimise infection risk

- Good handwashing.
- Adherence to local policies for infection control measures.
- Be aware of side effects of drugs that increase the risk of infection, for example, inotropes and NEC.
- Babies and children who have undergone palliative or corrective heart surgery are more at risk of subacute bacterial endocarditis. As the incidence is rare, prophylactic antibiotics are no longer routinely indicated (www.nice.org.uk). Parents need to be educated regarding the recommendations and need to be aware of the signs, symptoms and actions required for management of an unwell baby with heart problems.

Safe administration of drugs

- Ensure that drug information and resources are readily available for reference.
- Nurses have a good knowledge of each drug that the baby is on – dose, administration, actions, interactions, compatibilities, side effects.
- Good documentation of drug administration.
- Abide by hospital and professional governing body guidelines and professional standards for drug administration (NMC 2008).

Provide family support

- Ensure parents are kept updated regularly with regard to the baby's management and care.
- Have information readily available – leaflets relating to conditions, website addresses, general information of the NNU services and contact details.
- Provide support – counselling services, family support group (e.g. CAF directory), social worker, cardiac specialist nurse (if applicable), interpreters (if applicable), pastoral care team (if required or requested).
- Financial support – assistance may be available to support travel expenses, etc.
- Discharge planning (as appropriate). Educate parent(s) in resuscitation, medication administration, signs and symptoms of unwell child, when to seek further assistance.

Innovative strategies and ongoing research

Advances in prenatal and postnatal diagnosis of CHD have improved considerably in the past 20 years; however, undiagnosed or delayed diagnosis of CHD is still a concerning issue. Global medical research and technical advances strive for greater detection of CHD and improved treatment strategies for both congenital and acquired cardiac abnormalities.

Imaging has improved detection of cardiac problems in both antenatal and postnatal periods. MRI is increasingly informative in the detection of cardiac abnormalities. Software has been improved over the years to enhance 3-D imaging (MRI and ECHO) and interpretation of the results. Clinical studies using imaging are ongoing. Other developments include a new stethoscope that provides a wider range of heart sounds on auscultation. This is currently undergoing clinical trials.

Geneticists endeavour to identify new causative genes. High resolution chromosome analysis, fluorescence in situ hybridisation (FISH) and gene mutation analysis provide valuable information for specific CHD. Currently, new heart valves, generated from stem cells from the umbilical cord blood, are being trialled in laboratory conditions and these may prove to be clinically viable in the future. Some of the current medical and surgical treatments mentioned in this chapter are relatively new and will need ongoing research (short- and long-term) to ensure that treatment is evolving safely.

Case study: cardiovascular management

Jane was delivered by spontaneous vaginal delivery at 30 weeks' gestation following premature rupture of membranes. The pregnancy was, otherwise, uneventful. Apgars 8 at 1 minute; 9 at 5 minutes. She was transferred to NNU. A partial septic screen was performed for prolonged rupture of membranes and grunting at 10 minutes of age. She was placed on to nasal continuous positive airway pressure (CPAP) in 28 per cent oxygen and commenced on intravenous (IV) benzylpenicillin and gentamicin. IV maintenance fluids were commenced and on day 1 nasogastric feeding of expressed breast milk was commenced.

Jane appeared relatively stable until day 3 when her oxygen requirement increased to 45 per cent and she started having profound desaturations and apnoeas. She had increased work of breathing. On examination, a loud murmur was audible, loudest at the left upper costal margin.

Q.1. What is the possible diagnosis?

Q.2. What is the differential diagnosis?

Jane was intubated and ventilated due to a profound apnoea. Her feeding was stopped and IV fluids were given at 120ml/kg/day. A chest X-ray was done and this showed bilateral hazy lung fields with cardiomegaly. An ECHO was performed and this showed a large patent ductus arteriosus.
Q.3. What treatment options are available for treatment of the PDA?
A decision was made to treat the PDA with ibuprofen.

Q.4. What specific nursing observations are required for caring for Jane during treatment?

Q.5. What physiological and/or clinical measures would halt treatment?

Jane completed her course of ibuprofen but still continued to have a PDA. An ECHO showed that it was still patent.

Q.6. What treatment options would you consider next?

References

Abman, S.H. (2007) 'Recent advances in the pathogenesis and treatment of persistent pulmonary hypertension of the newborn', *Neonatology* 91: 283–90.

Ainsworth, S.B., Wylie, J.P. and Wren, C. (1999) 'Prevalence and clinical significance of cardiac murmurs in neonates', *Archives of Disease in Childhood* 80: F43–F45.

Aranda, J.V. and Thomas, R. (2006) 'Systematic review: intravenous Ibuprofen in preterm newborns', *Seminars in Perinatology* 30(3): 114–20.

Archer, N. (2005) 'Cardiovascular disease', in J.M. Rennie (ed.) *Roberton's Textbook of Neonatology*, 4th edn, Philadelphia, PA: Elsevier Churchill Livingston.

Arlettaz, R., Archer, N. and Wilkinson, A.R. (1998) 'Natural history of innocent heart murmurs in newborn babies: controlled echocardiographic study', *Archives of Disease in Childhood: Fetal and Neonatal Edition* 78: F166–F170.

BAPM (1998) *Report of the Second Working Group of the British Association of Perinatal Medicine: Guidelines for Good Practice in the Management of Neonatal Respiratory Distress Syndrome*, London: British Association of Perinatal Medicine.

Barrington, K.J. and Finer, N.N. (2007) 'Inhaled nitric oxide for preterm infants: a systematic review', *Pediatrics* 120: 5, 1008.

Bell, S.G. (1998) 'Neonatal cardiovascular pharmacology', *Neonatal Nursing* 17(20): 7–15.

Blackburn, S.T. (2007) *Maternal Fetal, and Neonatal Physiology: A Clinical Perspective*, 3rd edn, St Louis, MO: W.B. Saunders.

BNF (2008) *BNF for Children*, London: BMJ Publishing Group (www.bnfc.org).

Brown, K.L., Ridout, D.A., Hoskote, A., Verhulst, L., Ricci, M. and Bull, C. (2006) 'Delayed diagnosis of congenital heart disease worsens preoperative condition and outcome of surgery in neonates', *Heart* 92: 1298–302.

Burton, D.A. and Cabalka, A.K. (1994) 'Cardiac evaluation of infants in the first year of life', *Pediatric Clinics of North America* 41(5): 991–1015.

Carlson, B.M. (2004) *Human Embryology and Developmental Biology*, 3rd edn, Philadelphia, PA: Mosby.

Cooke, L., Steer, P.A. and Woodgate, P.G. (2003) 'Indomethacin for asymptomatic patent ductus arteriosus in preterm infants', *Cochrane Database of Systematic Reviews*, Issue 1, Art. No. CD003745. DOI: 10. 1002/14651858.CD003745.

Field, D., Elbourne, D., Hardy, P., Fenton, A.C., Ahluwalia, J., Halliday, H.L., Subhedar, N., Heinonen, K., Aikio, O., Grieve, R., Truesdale, A., Tomlin, K., Normand, C. and Stocks, J. (2007) 'Neonatal ventilation with inhaled nitric oxide vs. ventilatory support without nitric oxide for infants with severe respiratory failure born at or near term: the INNOVA multicentre randomised controlled trial', *Neonatology* 91: 73–82.

Finer, N.N. and Barrington, K.J. (2006) 'Nitric oxide for respiratory failure in infants born at or near term', *Cochrane Database of Systematic Reviews*, Issue 4, Art. No. CD000399. DOI: 10.1002/14651858.CD000399. pub 2.

Furdon, S.A. (1997) 'Recognizing congestive heart failure in the neonatal period', *Neonatal Network* 16(7): 5–13.

Groves, A.M., Kuschel, C.A., Knight, D.B. and Skinner, J.R. (2008) 'Relationship between blood pressure and blood flow in newborn preterm infants', *Archives of Disease in Childhood: Fetal and Neonatal Edition* 93: F29–F32.

Hafeez, U. and Watkinson, M. (2007) 'When is a second course of indomethacin effective in ventilated neonates with patent ductus arteriosus?' *Infant* 3(4): 140–3.

Hegyi, T., Carbone, M.T., Anwar, M., Ostfeld, B., Hiatt, M., Koons, A., Pinto-Martin, J. and Paneth, N. (1994) 'Blood pressure ranges in premature infants. I. The first hours of life', *Journal of Pediatrics* 124(4): 627–33.

Hegyi, T., Anwar, M., Carbone, M.T., Ostfeld, B., Hiatt, M., Koons, A., Pinto-Martin, J. and Paneth, N. (1996) 'Blood pressure ranges in premature infants. II. The first hours of life', *Journal of Pediatrics* 97(3): 336–42.

Herrera, C., Holberton, J. and Davis, P. (2007) 'Prolonged versus short course of indomethacin for the treatment of patent ductus arteriosus in preterm infants', *Cochrane Database of Systematic Reviews*, Issue 2, Art. No. CD003480, DOI: 10.1002/14651858.CD003480. pub 3.

Ho, J.J. and Rasa, G. (2007) 'Magnesium sulphate for persistent pulmonary hypertension of the newborn (Review)', *Cochrane Database of Systematic Reviews*, Issue 3, Art. No. CDOO5588. DOI.10.1002/14651858.CDOO5588. pub 2.

Huddy, C.L., Bennett, C.C., Hardy, P., Field, D., Elbourne, D., Grieve, R., Truesdale, A. and Diallo, K. (2008) 'The INNOVA multicentre randomised controlled trial: neonatal ventilation with inhaled nitric oxide versus ventilatory support without nitric oxide for severe respiratory failure in preterm infants: follow up at 4–5 years', *Archives of Disease in Childhood: Fetal and Neonatal Edition* 93: F430–F435.

Keller, R.L. and Clyman, R.I. (2003) 'Persistent Doppler flow predicts lack of response to multiple courses of indomethacin in premature infants with recurrent patent ductus arteriosus', *Paediatrics* 112: 583–7.

Kinsella, J.P. and Abman, S.H. (2000) 'Clinical approach to inhaled NO therapy in the newborn', *Journal of Pediatrics* 136: 717–26.

Kluckow, M. and Evans, N. (2000) 'Superior vena cava flow in newborn infants: a novel marker of systemic blood flow', *Archives of Disease in Childhood: Fetal and Neonatal Edition* 82: F182–F187.

Knight, S.E. and Washington, R.L. (2006) 'Cardiovascular diseases and surgical interventions', in G.B. Merenstein and S.L. Gardner (eds) *Handbook of Neonatal Intensive Care*, 6th edn, St. Louis, MO: Mosby.

Kourembanas, S. (2008) 'Shock', in J.P. Cloherty, , E.C. Eichenwald and A.R. Stark (eds) *Manual of Neonatal Care*, 6th edn, Philadelphia, PA: Lippincott.

Lakshminrushimba, S. and Steinharn, R.H. (1999) 'Pulmonary vascular biology during neonatal transition', *Clinics in Perinatology* 26(3): 601–19.

Levene, M.I., Tudehope, D.I. and Sinha, S. (2008) *Essential Neonatal Medicine*, 4th edn, Oxford: Blackwell.

Lott, J.W. (1993) 'Assessment and management of cardiovascular dysfunction', in C. Kenner, A. Brueggemeyer and L.P. Gunderson (eds) *Comprehensive Neonatal Nursing: A Physiological Perspective*, Philadelphia, PA: W.B. Saunders.

Moore, K. and Persaud, T.V.N. (1998) *The Developing Human – Clinically Oriented Embryology*, 6th edn, Philadelphia, PA: W.B. Saunders.

Moore, K.L. and Persaud, T.V.N. (2003) *Before We Are Born: Essentials of Embryology and Birth Defects*, 6th edn, Philadelphia, PA: W.B. Saunders.

Ng, P.C., Lam, C.W., Fok, T.F., Lee, C.H., Ma, K.C. and Chan, I.H.S. (2001) 'Refractory hypotension in preterm infants with adrenocorticol insufficiency', *Archives of Disease in Childhood: Fetal and Neonatal Edition* 84: F122–F124.

Ng, P.C., Cheuk, L.H., Bnur, F.L., Chan, I.H.S., Anthony, L.W.Y., Wong, E., Chan, H.B., Lam, C.W.K., Lee, B.S.C. and Fok, T.F. (2006) 'A double-blind, randomised, controlled study of a "stress dose" of hydrocortisone for rescue treatment of refractory hypotension in preterm infants', *Pediatrics* 117: 367–75.

Nursing and Midwifery Council (2008) *Standards for Medicines Management*, London: NMC.

Ohlsson, A., Walia, R. and Shah, S.S. (2008) 'Ibuprofen for the treatment of patent ductus arteriosus in preterm and/or low birth weight infants', *Cochrane Database of Systematic Reviews*, Issue 1, Art. No. CD003481.DOI: 10.1002/14651858.CD003481. pub 3.

Patwardhan, K. (2009) 'Inotropes in term neonates', *Infant* 5(1): 32–47.

Penny, D.J. and Skekerdemian, L.S. (2001) 'Management of the neonate with symptomatic congenital heart disease', *Archives of Disease in Childhood: Fetal and Neonatal Edition* 84: F141–F145.

Rang, H.P., Dale, M.M., Ritter, J.M. and Flower, R.J. (2007) *Rang and Dale's Pharmacology*, 6th edn, Philadelphia, PA: Churchill Livingstone Elsevier.

Schmidt, B., Davis, P., Moddemann, D., Ohlsson, A., Roberts, R.S., Saigal, S., Solimano, A., Vincer, M. and Wright, L.L. (2001) 'Long-term effects of Indomethacin prophylaxis in extremely low birth weight infants', *North England Journal of Medicine* 344: 1966–72.

Seri, I. (2006a) 'Management of hypotension and low systemic blood flow in the very low birth weight neonate during the first postnatal week', *Journal of Perinatology* 26: S8–S13.

Seri, I. (2006b) 'Hydrocortisone and vasopressor-resistant shock in preterm neonates', *Pediatrics* 117: 516–18.

Shah, S. and Ohlsson, A. (2007) 'Sildenafil for pulmonary hypertension in neonates', *Cochrane Database of Systematic Reviews*, Issue 3, Art. No. CD005494. DOI: 10.1002/14651858.CD005494. pub 2.

So, K.W., Fok, T.F., Ng, P.C., Wong, W.W. and Cheung, K.L. (1997) 'Randomised controlled trial of colloid or crystalloid in hypotensive preterm infants', *Archives of Disease in Childhood: Fetal and Neonatal Edition* 76: F43–F46.

Spilman, L.J. and Furdon, S.A. (1998) 'Recognition, understanding, and current management of cardiac lesions with decreased pulmonary blood flow', *Neonatal Network* 17(4): 7–18.

Thomas, R.L., Parker, G.C., Van Overmeire, B. and Aranda, J.V. (2005) 'A meta-analysis of Ibuprofen versus Indomethacin for closure of patent ductus arteriosus', *European Journal of Pediatrics* 164(3): 135–40.

Tortora, G.J. and Derrickson, B.H. (2009) *Principles of Anatomy and Physiology*, Vol. 2, 12th edn, Chichester: Wiley.

Tsuji, M., Saul, J.P., du Plessis, A., Eichenwald, E., Sobh, J., Crocker, R. and Volpe, J.J. (2000) 'Cerebral intravascular oxygenation correlates with mean arterial pressure in critically ill premature infants', *Pediatrics* 106: 625–32.

UK Collaborative Trial Group (1996) 'UK collaborative randomised trial of neonatal extracorporeal membrane oxygenation', *Lancet* 348: 75–82.

Van Marter, L.J. (2008) 'Persistent pulmonary hypertension of the newborn', in J.P. Cloherty, E.C. Eichenwald and A.R. Stark (eds) *Manual of Neonatal Care*, 6th edn, Philadelphia, PA: Lippincott.

Wechsler, S.B. and Wernovsky, G. (2008) 'Cardiac disorders', in J.P. Cloherty, E.C. Eichenwald and A.R. Stark (eds) *Manual of Neonatal Care*, 6th edn, Philadelphia, PA: Lippincott.

Wolf, G.K. and Arnold, J.H. (2008) 'Extracorporeal membrane oxygenation', in J.P. Cloherty, E.C. Eichenwald and A.R. Stark (eds) *Manual of Neonatal Care*, 6th edn, Philadelphia, PA: Lippincott.

Further reading

American Heart Association http://americanheart.com
British Heart Foundation http://www.bhf.org.uk
Children's Heart Federation http://www.childrens-heart-fed.org.uk
NICE guidelines www.nice.org.uk

Chapter 8

Neonatal Brain Injury

Anja Hale

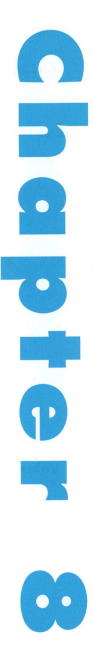

Contents

Introduction

Despite great advances in the understanding of the contributing mechanisms of injury to the developing brain and the many attempts at prevention, perinatal cerebral brain injury still remains a major cause of neonatal morbidity and mortality. Current data suggest that approximately 2–5 infants per 1000 live births experience a brain injury as a result of events that occur before, during or after birth. However, this may be more in developing countries although no strong data exist (Bhutta *et al.* 2005).

There are many potential mechanisms of injury such as: hypoxic-ischaemic insults, haemorrhage, perinatal infection or inflammation, metabolic disturbances and potentially the stressful neonatal intensive care environment itself. Such insults can affect the infant's ability to survive the perinatal and neonatal periods with approximately 30–40 per cent of infants with brain injury dying; for those surviving there are significant implications for later development and cognitive outcome, with 20–30 per cent developing some degree of neurological impairment. This has ramifications for the infant, their family, and indeed society. Today, although the overall rates of neurological disability remain the same, increased survival of more high-risk infants through improved neonatal care and management has seen the number of infants discharged from NICU with neurologic deficits increase. This is of concern to all involved in the care of newborns and presents a formidable challenge to health care professionals.

Vulnerability of the neonatal brain

In order to better understand neonatal brain injury, it is important to recognise that there are specific vulnerabilities that distinguish the response of the immature or neonatal brain, from that of the mature adult brain. Brain development begins in the embryonic period of fetal development from four to eight weeks of gestation, and continues well into childhood. Development is in an organised, stepwise fashion involving the unfolding of discrete, sequential processes including the division, migration, differentiation and maturation of neurons. This protracted course of development makes the brain particularly vulnerable to a variety of insults. In particular, the neonatal brain is susceptible to damage to the developing oligodendrocytes in the presence of oxygen-free radicals, the release of which is a well-established consequence of hypoxia, ischaemia and reperfusion. This can lead to **apoptosis** or programmed cell death, loss of oligodendrocytes and impaired myelinisation (Ferriero 2004).

The preterm brain has more vulnerability to brain injury than that of the term infant as it is more vascular with a prominent germinal matrix, has proportionally higher water content, a relatively lower amount of myelin, and a poorly developed cortex. Most importantly though is the premature infant's limited capacity to induce **autoregulation** or maintain a constant cerebral blood flow by arterial vasodilation or constriction in the event of systemic hyper- or hypotension. The ability to autoregulate is further impaired in the presence of hypoxia, hypercapnia or hypocarbia, all too frequent occurrences in NICU (Fritz and Delivoria-Papadopoulos 2006). When exposed to fluctuations in systemic blood pressure, a pressure-passive cerebral circulation results. Rupture of the fragile germinal matrix blood vessels may occur in the presence of raised cerebral blood pressure whereas low cerebral blood pressure damages the vessels leaving them prone to rupture when the blood pressure returns to normal.

Germinal matrix and intraventricular haemorrhage

Aetiology

The subependymal germinal matrix is an embryonic structure which is richly vascularised and located adjacent to the lateral ventricles. It contains immature neurological cells prior to their migration to cortical and subcortical areas to form the cerebral cortex. It is most prominent at 24–26 weeks' gestation and gradually reduces in size as the brain matures, with complete involution by 40 weeks' gestation. Germinal matrix haemorrhage (GMH) and intraventricular haemorrhage (IVH) are the most common types of intracranial haemorrhage seen in the neonatal period. These are seen almost exclusively in preterm infants, and in particular those weighing less than 1500g. Indeed, the incidence of GMH/IVH is inversely related to the gestational age with incidence around 30 per cent for infants <750g and 1 per cent for infants weighing more than 1500g. It is therefore uncommon to see a GMH beyond 32 weeks' gestation.

The immature capillary bed of the germinal matrix is embedded in gelatinous material, with the vessels large and thin walled with little supportive elements surrounding them. This increases the germinal matrix's vulnerability to rupture. In many preterm infants the haemorrhage begins as a small rupture of the capillaries or a micro-vascular event that may clot off and remain isolated to the subependymal area. However, the original haemorrhage may rupture into the lateral ventricles and then into the third and fourth ventricles. The blood eventually collects in the subarachnoid space of the posterior fossa and may extend into the basal cistern. It is thought that the rupture of the haemorrhage from the germinal matrix into the ventricles may serve as a protective function, decompressing the haemorrhagic area and reducing further tissue destruction. Following a severe haemorrhage, blood may also be found in the periventricular white matter. This usually is not due to extravasation of blood from the ventricles but to an associated insult in the white matter. As a result of blood clots obstructing the flow of cerebral spinal fluid (CSF) at the aqueduct of sylvius or the foremen of monro, or an obliterative arachnoiditis, progressive ventricular dilation may occur (Volpe 2001a).

GMH/IVH is usually detected within the first week of life with diagnosis at the bedside. In the newborn infant the anterior fontanelle provides an ideal window, through which cranial or head ultrasound scanning (HUSS) may be performed. HUSS is especially helpful in identifying brain injury in newborn infants and allows grading of the injury according to the location and severity of the haemorrhage, of which a well-defined system has been established:

Grade I Isolated germinal matrix haemorrhage

Grade II Intraventicular haemorrhage filling up to 50 per cent of the ventricles

Grade III Intraventricular haemorrhage filling greater than 50 per cent of the ventricles, with evidence of ventricular dilation

Grade IV Periventricular haemorrhagic venous infarct
(Adapted from Volpe 2001a)

For more than 90 per cent of newborn infants with GMH/IVH, bleeding occurs within the first 72 hours after birth, with 50 per cent of the bleeding occurring in the first 24 hours. For approximately 10–20 per cent of infants, there is a progressive increase in the size of haemorrhage over a 24–48-hour period. Late haemorrhages may be seen after a few days or weeks in a small number of infants, that is, around 10 per cent; however, these are seen primarily in those preterm infants with a more complicated history, such as a severe, prolonged respiratory problem.

The clinical manifestations of a GMH/IVH are non-specific. Volpe (2001a) describes three classic syndromes: catastrophic, salutary, or silent. The catastrophic syndrome occurs most infrequently but is one of sudden dramatic deterioration with a decrease in blood pressure and haematocrit, a full fontanelle and seizure activity. Catastrophic deterioration usually involves major haemorrhages that evolve rapidly over several minutes or hours. Some infants exhibit a more protracted or saltatory course where symptoms 'wax and wane' over a period of time. Findings include changes in alertness and tone, abnormal eye position and movement, an abnormally tight popliteal angle, with respiratory distress progressing to apnoea. These signs evolve over many hours and may cease, only to begin again. They may also be so subtle they are missed. Infants with a clinically silent syndrome, the most common of the three, fail to show any neurological signs but may have an unexplained fall in haematocrit or failure of haematocrit to raise following red blood cell transfusion. Diagnosis of silent haemorrhages is usually by cranial ultrasound.

As previously described, the immature vasculature and probable passive-pressure circulation leave the preterm brain vulnerable to injury. Therefore hypoxia and/or fluctuations in the infant's systemic blood pressure and cerebral blood flow are mechanisms of injury strongly linked to the pathogenesis of GMH/IVH. Many perinatal factors may be linked to hypoxia. Antenatal events include antepartum haemorrhage, fetal distress, asphyxia, prolonged labour and malpresentation. Following birth, hypoxic events such as respiratory distress, apnoea and hypotension are associated with an increased risk.

Postnatally episodes of high systemic blood pressure are linked to an increased cerebral blood flow. Causes of systemic hypertension include the following: noxious stimulation, spontaneous activity or handling, crying, tracheal suctioning, excessive light and noise. Pneumothorax, rapid volume expansion, decreased haematocrit and blood glucose levels may also increase cerebral blood flow. Marked hypercarbia leads to vasodilation of the cerebral arteries and a subsequent increase in cerebral perfusion. This has led to the more cautious use of sodium bicarbonate as a buffer due to its effect of causing an abrupt rise in arterial carbon dioxide following administration. Systemic hypotension significantly decreases cerebral blood flow. Postnatal events such as severe apnoea, myocardial failure and sepsis lead to hypotension. There is a strong correlation between a patent ductus arteriosus and fluctuations in cerebral blood flow (Gressens *et al.* 2002).

Prevention or risk reduction begins in the perinatal period with the prevention of preterm birth, the single most important method of preventing IVH. It is desirable for high-risk pregnancies to be managed in a tertiary centre able to provide optimal delivery, resuscitation and neonatal intensive care, as a consequence, in-utero transfer may be required. Prenatal administration of antenatal steroids is associated with a decreased risk and incidence of GMH/IVH as they aid maturation of the infant's lungs decreasing the incidence or respiratory distress syndrome with its concomitant acid–base balance disturbances. Additionally, antenatal steroids may also decrease IVH by promoting cardiovascular stability postnatally and may contribute to maturation of the germinal matrix itself. Numerous prophylactic regimes including the administration of phenobarbital and vitamin K have been evaluated as prenatal and postnatal interventions; however, neither has proved to be an effective enough therapy to warrant its use (Crowther *et al.* 2001, 2003).

Although the administration of indomethacin has been shown to reduce the incidence of severe IVH and the need for surgical ligation of PDA, its administration has not resulted in the improvements in long-term neurocognitive improvements as hoped. Many practitioners feel the potential unwanted side effects of indomethacin, such as reduced organ perfusion, particularly to the renal and gastrointestinal tracts, outweigh the clinical benefit (Fowlie and Davis 2002). Recently delayed cord clamping of the umbilical cord for 30–45 seconds and lowering the infant below the perineum or Caesarean section incision site has been shown to be associated with a lower incidence of IVH (Mercer *et al.* 2006).

Acute management of the infant once IVH has occurred is supportive in nature with control of ventilation, fluid, metabolic and nutritional states, temperature, and if a catastrophic bleed, management of seizures. The outcome for an infant suffering an IVH is largely determined by the severity and extent of the haemorrhage. The presence of associated problems such as respiratory distress syndrome, perinatal hypoxic ischaemic injury and sepsis all increase morbidity and mortality. However, generally for infants with small or mild haemorrhages the outcome is good. Nearly all survive and there is a low incidence of post-haemorrhagic ventricular dilation or major neurological sequelae. For those with moderate haemorrhage there is a 5–20 per cent mortality rate and ventricular dilation occurs in 15–25 per cent of survivors. Following severe haemorrhages, mortality averages 50 per cent with progressive ventricular dilation in 55–88 per cent of survivors. Although significant motor and cognitive deficits are seen commonly in those infants with severe haemorrhages, some do seem to escape long-term sequelae (Volpe 2001a).

Post-haemorrhagic hydrocephalus (PHH)

Post-haemorrhagic **hydrocephalus** is seen in 15-80 per cent of GMH/IVH infants. The term hydrocephalus refers to a progressive dilation of the cerebral ventricular system due to a production of CSF that exceeds the absorption rate. In the infant suffering an IVH, a particulate blood clot may occlude or obliterate the microscopic arachnoid villi rendering them non-functional, resulting in insufficient absorption of CSF. In many infants ventricular dilation occurs slowly. Increased intracranial pressure does not usually occur due to the neonate's soft malleable skull, open sutures and fontanelles which for a period of time allow head size to increase without an appreciable raise in pressure. In approximately half of the infants ventricular dilation spontaneously arrests within about 30 days. However, for the remaining infants, dilation continues with accompanying signs of raising intracranial pressure such as bulging fontanelles, setting sun eye sign, dilated scalp veins and widely spaced sutures. Progressive ventricular dilation may be managed with a ventricular peritoneal shunt or temporary ventricular drainage via needle aspiration if the infant is too small or ill for surgery.

Periventricular haemorrhagic infarction (PVHI)

About 15 per cent of newborn infants with IVH also exhibit a characteristic parenchymal lesion, known as a periventricular haemorrhagic infarction (PVHI). This is a relatively large area of haemorrhagic necrosis in the periventricular white matter, situated dorsal and lateral to the external angle of the lateral ventricle. It is seen in approximately 80 per cent of those with large intraventricular haemorrhages; however, these lesions are usually unilateral. It is thought that the GMH or its associated IVH leads to obstruction of the terminal veins and thus impairs the blood flow in the medullary veins leading to a haemorrhagic infarction and necrosis. This necrotic area may eventually form a porencephalic cyst and communicate with the ventricle. Although PVHI is distinguishable from PVL, distinction may be difficult as the pathogenesis of PVHI and PVL overlap. Destruction of the periventricular white matter may result in neurological deficits associated with learning, speech, behaviour, personality, intelligence, muscle strength and control.

Pereventricular leukomalcia (PVL)

Pereventricular leukomalcia (PVL) is a less common but more severe form of brain injury seen primarily in preterm infants with the incidence ranging from 4–26 per cent. Again, the greatest period of risk is less than 32 weeks' gestation;

however, it may be diagnosed in term infants especially those suffering hypoxic-iscaemic insults. PVL refers to injury of periventicular white matter most commonly seen in areas at the interface of two arterial distributions sometimes called the watershed area where the long penetrating arteries terminate. These are the frontal-parietal white matter (between the arterial supply of the anterior cerebral and the middle cerebral arteries) and the parietal-occipital white matter (between the posterior cerebral and the middle cerebral arteries (Volpe 2001c). The cystic lesions may be located in the frontal, parietal and less commonly the occipital regions of the brain.

PVL often accompanies IVH, but is not caused by the haemorrhage itself. PVL can be caused by ischaemia secondary to hypotension from previously discussed mechanisms, but recent evidence suggests a strong correlation between maternal chorioamnionitis, cytokine release and PVL (Volpe 2001c). Over a period of days or weeks, the periventricular areas of injury often develop multiple small bilateral white matter cysts not communicating with the lateral ventricle. These may initially be seen on HUSS as 'brightness' or 'flares' at the lateral angle of the lateral ventricle. The lesions may be focal with small areas of cyst formation, or diffuse with more of the white matter destroyed. Over a period of weeks, these echo densities may no longer be visible on HUSS as the cavities constrict, or they may become more prominent. These cysts disturb subsequent cortical organisation and neuronal connections.

The outcome of infants with PVL depends upon the size of the initial lesion and the time of the acute insult. Between 60–100 per cent of infants with PVL develop cerebral palsy, most typically spastic diplegia which usually correlates with the more focal form of PVL. Diffuse PVL is more often associated with quadriplegia along with cognitive and behavioural deficits (Deguchi and Millar 2007).

Hypoxic-ischaemic brain injury in the term infant

Despite advances in obstetric and neonatal care, hypoxic-ischaemic (HI) brain injury continues to have an incidence of approximately 3–5 out of 1000 full term infants. It is a significant problem worldwide as 10–75 per cent of infants affected die, and of those surviving 25 per cent have neurological complications which result in chronic handicapping conditions. The previously used term 'birth asphyxia' has now been discarded with neonatal hypoxic-ischaemic encephalopathy (HIE) now being the preferred terminology. Birth asphyxia was thought to be imprecise and implied that the infant's condition was a consequence of the birthing process; however, as the understanding of the mechanisms of hypoxic-ischaemic brain injury has increased it is now known that this injury may occur before, during or after labour and delivery. Volpe (2001b) lists the relative proportions of the timing of hypoxic-ischaemic insults as 20 per cent before labour, 35 per cent during labour and delivery, 35 per cent during delivery alone and 10 per cent after delivery.

Neonatal HI brain injury occurs because of hypoxia – diminished oxygen in the blood supply or from ischaemia – decreased blood perfusion to a tissue bed.

Table 8.1 Mechanisms of injury

Failure of gas exchange across the placenta
  Prolonged or excessive uterine contractions
  Placental abruption
  Ruptured uterus

Interruption of umbilical blood flow
  Cord compression (including tight nuchal cord, shoulder dystocia, cord prolapse, true knots)

Inadequate placental perfusion
  Maternal hypo-/hypertension

Impaired maternal oxygenation
  Asthma
  Pulmonary embolism
  Pneumonia

Compromised fetus
  IUGR
  Anaemia

Failure of cardiorespiratory adaptation at birth

Hypoxia can occur in utero because of placental insufficiency or after birth from respiratory or cardiac failure (Table 8.1). Both hypoxia and ischaemia lead to asphyxia or impaired gas exchange, resulting in acidosis affecting the brain as well as other organs. Although once thought to be a simple relationship between energy failure and tissue necrosis, it is now known that a complex biochemical cascade results in neuronal cell death (Grow and Barks 2002).

Cerebral ischaemia results in reduced delivery of the energy substrates oxygen and glucose to brain tissue. This causes a switch to anaerobic metabolism which rapidly depletes the neonate's brain stores of glucose and high energy phosphates (ATP and phosphocreatine) resulting in an accumulation of lactate and inorganic phosphate. If the insult is severe enough, there may be immediate primary neuronal death. Following resuscitation and subsequent reperfusion there is some recovery of high energy phosphates; however, this is followed by a delayed or 'secondary' energy failure occurring after a latent phase of at least six hours and up to 24–48 hours later. At this time encephalopathy and increased seizure activity are usually evident. Mechanisms involved in neuronal death during this delayed stage include accumulation of excitatory neurotransmitters, generation of reactive oxygen radicals, intracellular calcium accumulation and mitochondrial dysfunction. Apoptosis or programmed cell death occurs. Even after a severe insult with primary cell death, the delayed phase contributes to a significant proportion of the final cell loss (Volpe 2001c).

HI brain injury is reflected by a constellation of signs seen at or shortly after birth which form the clinical entity of HIE. The newborn infant who is encephalopathic may have difficulty initiating and maintaining respirations at birth, an altered state of consciousness, seizures, tone and reflex abnormalities, and feeding difficulties. Although definitions vary, the degree of HIE is commonly defined as follows:

Mild: hyperalert, hyperexcitable, normal or increased muscle tone, no seizures

Moderate: hypotonia, decreased movements, often seizures

Severe: stuporous, flaccid, absent primitive reflexes, usually with seizures
(Adapted from Lissauer and Fanaroff 2006)

Utilising the definitions above, for those term infants with mild neonatal encephalopathy in the first few days of life there is a high likelihood of being completely normal at follow-up. For those with moderate encephalopathy there is a 20–35 per cent risk of neurological sequelae, although those with normal neurological examinations and feeding well within two weeks of birth are likely to have normal outcomes. Infants with severe encephalopathy have a 75 per cent risk of dying with coma persisting, or progressing to brain death by 72 hours of life. If the infant survives for longer than 72 hours without losing all cerebral function, a variable amount of improvement may be seen; however, there is an almost universal risk of poor neurological outcome in survivors (Wu 2008). The patterns of injury predominantly found in term infants following a HI insult are selective neuronal necrosis, status marmoratus or hypermylinated lesions, focal and multifocal ischaemic injury, and most commonly parasagittal cerebral injury. Permanent sequelae may be mild such as learning difficulties or attention deficit disorder or may be severe and disabling including cerebral palsy, epilepsy, visual impairment and severe cognitive and developmental disorders.

The most effective intervention against HI brain injury remains prevention with vigilant intrapartum monitoring to help detect those fetuses at risk. The hallmarks of intrapartum asphyxia are the occurrence of fetal heart rate abnormalities and the passage of meconium in utero. Robust intrapartum assessment allows appropriate obstetric management and effective resuscitation following delivery.

A better understanding of the biological processes contributing to the secondary phase of neuronal cell death have led to investigation of several pharmacological treatments such as calcium channel blockers, free-radical scavengers, glutamate receptor blockers, anti-inflammatory agents and growth factors to advance repair. However, it is the 'window of opportunity' or latent phase that exists following resuscitation of the asphyxiated newborn before the secondary phase of impaired energy metabolism and injury that has been of particular interest, with modest reductions in brain temperature, in the order of 2–4° Celsius appearing to be the most promising of the specific neuro protective therapies to emerge over the past 10–15 years (Azzopardi and Edwards 2007).

Hypothermia for neuroprotection

Between 1959 and 1972, numerous reports exist where newborn infants were subjected to hypothermia as an additional treatment to standard resuscitative measures. However, hypothermia as an intervention essentially stopped around 1970 as new evidence showed the benefit of thermal regulation in preterm infants. Although for many decades hypothermia has been found valuable for neuroprotection during cardiac bypass surgery, it is only over the past 20 years, with the recognition that temperature of the brain has an important influence on the extent of brain injury following hypoxia-ischemia, that interest in modest/moderate hypothermia or cooling as a therapeutic measure has resumed.

There are a number of postulated mechanisms by which hypothermia is thought to be neuroprotective. It may protect neurons by reducing cerebral metabolic rate, attenuating the release of excitatory amino acids, ameliorating the ischaemia-impaired uptake of glutamate and lowering production of toxic nitric oxide and free radicals. Hypothermia may also modify cells programmed for apoptosis, leading to their survival. Cooling needs to be initiated within six hours of birth; that is, within the latent phase before the secondary phase of injury occurs. This has been based on animal data, which suggest the effectiveness of cooling diminishes as the time increases from the hypoxic-ischaemic insult to initiation of cooling. The aim of intervention with hypothermia is to lower the core body temperature to 33–34° Celsius for 72 hours (Azzopardi and Edwards 2007).

Currently there are three potential ways to reduce brain temperature: (1) cool the head alone; (2) cool the body alone; or (3) cool the head and body. The aim of selective head cooling is to adequately cool the brain, with only a small reduction in body temperature, therefore minimising potentially harmful side-effects. This is achieved using a cooling cap; however, the drawback to this method is the difficulty in establishing the actual brain temperature as a true measurement is not possible. Whole body cooling, in contrast, assumes that the core temperature approximates brain temperature. This is measured by rectal or oesophageal probe as standard bedside digital thermometers are unlikely to record temperatures in the target range required. Cooling is achieved through the use of cold packs around the infant or a cooling mattress or fan.

Hypothermia appears to be well tolerated. Adverse effects such as sinus bradycardia, increased blood pressure and increased oxygen requirement are generally transient and reversible with re-warming. Severe hypotension, however, may be problematic, but generally only occurs with too rapid re-warming (Thoresen 2008).

A Cochrane Review by Jacobs *et al.* (2007) concluded that cooling decreases mortality, without increasing major neurodevelopmental disability in survivors. For parents, this means they could expect that cooling would decrease their baby's chance of dying, and that if their baby did survive, the chance of major disability would decrease if he or she had been cooled. However, the potential for rescue hypothermia was demonstrated to be greatest following moderate, rather than severe hypoxic-ischaemic insults. It is hoped by all that these early promising results, which are based on neurodevelopmental assessment at 12–24 months, will translate into improved long-term outcomes. Some aspects of cooling remain controversial such as how soon after the insult or birth does cooling need to be started, what length and depth of hypothermia is required, and what method should be used, although given the paucity of other therapies for HIE, this is unlikely to deter implementation of cooling (Barks 2007). Additionally, it is hoped that cooling may provide a further window of opportunity for adjunctive therapy with pharmacologic agents as previously described.

The selection of infants for cooling remains challenging. Other causes of encephalopathy which may mimic HIE such as maternal drug administration, sepsis and metabolic conditions need to be ruled out so that these infants are not subjected to an unnecessary intervention. This must be accomplished within six hours of birth. Generally if two of the following are present, the infant is considered for cooling:

- Umbilical cord blood gas or arterial blood gas within one hour of delivery showing a pH <7.
- Base deficit >12mEq/L.
- Apgar score of <5 at 5 minutes.
- Need for respiratory support at 5 minutes of age.

Traditionally normothermia has been a crucial aspect of neonatal care and nursing an infant undergoing an emergent therapy such as cooling may precipitate feelings of uncertainty and discomfort. Maintaining physiological stability in a critically ill, hypothermic infant is challenging requiring labour-intensive and skilful care. Pulmonary secretions are stickier during hypothermia; therefore infants benefit from frequent turning, suctioning and instillation of saline as needed. Enteral feeds are generally withheld to relieve the burden on a gastrointestinal tract made vulnerable by hypoxic-ischaemia and the additional risk for hypothermia. Perceptions of patient discomfort during cooling, with anecdotal experiences of restlessness and shivering, have arisen in those caring for these infants. Clinicians have acknowledged this as a major barrier for nursing staff and provision for providing comfort with sedation is standard in protocols. Support of the family, especially following the often traumatic events of a hypoxic-ischemic insult, is paramount.

Neonatal seizures

Seizures are the most common neurologic sign during the neonatal period resulting from abnormal electrical impulses generated by the brain. Excessive synchronous electrical discharge or depolarisation in the brain produces stereotypic, repetitive behaviours which may be the first, and at times only, sign of central nervous system (CNS) dysfunction. Although the precise mechanism that causes neonatal seizures is unknown, they are thought to result from one or more of these mechanisms: disturbances in the Na+/K+ energy production pump, altered neuronal permeability to sodium, or imbalance in excitatory (glutamate) and inhibitory (GABA) neurotransmitters (Volpe 2001d). Seizures are important as they indicate a potentially serious underlying disease process, and may have a detrimental effect on the developing brain. They also interfere with supportive care and result in an increase in glucose metabolism and alter cerebral blood flow. Repetitive seizures may eventually alter brain lipid, protein and energy metabolism or result in damage from asphyxia or oedema.

Seizures occur more often in the newborn infant than at any other period of life, with the incidence in term infants being 0.7 to 2.8 per 1000 live births and more commonly than this in the preterm population. The clinical manifestations of neonatal seizures differ from those of older children with five major varieties described: subtle, generalised tonic, multifocal clonic, focal clonic and myoclonic (see Table 8.2).

Seizures generally indicate an underlying, potentially treatable, aetiology. Therefore determining and treating the cause of the seizures are the priority in preventing further seizures and neurological injury. The timing of the onset of seizures may provide insight into possible aetiology.

Causes of seizures by time of onset

Day 1   Perinatal asphyxia, Birth injury, hypoglycaemia, congenital infection, subarachnoid hemorrhage.

Day 2   Intracerebral bleed, HIE, hypoglycaemia.

Day 3   Hypoglycaemia, inborn errors of metabolism (as milk intake increases and placental dialysis ends).

Day 4–7   Hypocalaemia, meningitis, drug withdrawal, 'fifth day fits' (cause unknown).

The time of onset of seizures following a hypoxic-ischaemic event may add some clarity to the timing of the insult. With a prelabour insult the first seizures generally occur before 12 hours of age, whereas in infants with a peripartum insult the onset of seizures is generally after 18–20 hours of age (Filan 2004).

The issue of when to treat with anticonvulsant drugs and for how long, however, remains controversial. Generally if a seizure is longer than three minutes' duration or number more than three per hour, treatment is required. The first line anticonvulsant remains phenobarbital despite the known long-term effects on brain growth. Other drugs often used include phenytoin, and benzodiazepines such as midazolam. Newer agents such as levetiracetam look promising with no evidence of neurotoxicity in the developing brain at anticonvulsant concentrations in experimental studies (Rennie and Boylan 2007). As anticonvulsants can be respiratory, myocardial and CNS depressants, the infant's respiratory effort and heart rate must be assessed to maintain adequate ventilation and perfusion. The neurological status is monitored in addition to drug effectiveness. As anticonvulsants also compete with

Table 8.2 Neonatal seizures (in order of decreasing frequency)

Type of seizure	Manifestations	Comments
Subtle seizures	Horizontal deviation of the eyes or repetitive blinking/fluttering of eyelids	Most common seizure in newborns especially preterm infants
	Drooling, sucking and/or tongue thrusting, lip smacking, yawning	Difficult to distinguish from normal movements; therefore may be missed
	Swimming or rowing movements of limbs or cycling movements of legs	
Tonic seizures	Tonic extension or flexion (less common) of all extremities or may be limited to one	Generalised tonic seizures may be mistaken for decerebrate (extension of arms and legs) or decorticate posturing (extension of legs, flexion of arms) where there are no EEG changes
	May be accompanied by eye deviations, apnoea, occasional clonic movements	Seizure most frequently seen in preterm infant especially following IVH and asphyxia
Clonic seizures	Rhythmic jerky movements	More frequent in term infants
	Multifocal – migration in non-ordered fashion	May be confused with jitteriness
	Focal – usually focal injury	Often associated with: ■ CNS injury ■ Severe acidosis ■ Asphyxia
Myoclonic seizures	Sudden single or multiple jerks with flexion of upper (more common) or lower extremities	Uncommon in term infants
		Rarely seen in preterm infants
		Often associated with: ■ inborn errors of metabolism ■ other metabolic problems
Benign myoclonic seizure	Brief, intermittent jerk (no EEG changes)	Seen during sleep only

bilirubin for albumin binding sites, the infant must be monitored for signs of jaundice.

Neonatal seizures must be differentiated from non-seizure behaviours of the newborn which can at times be problematic. Normal behaviour such as stretching, yawning, jitteriness, startling and clonus may raise suspicions of seizure activity. Traditionally diagnosis in the NICU has been based upon clinical observation; however, in recent years, continuous brain function monitoring has become increasingly acknowledged as a method for continuous evaluation of brain function in neonates, and is now a daily part of clinical surveillance of sick newborn infants (Hellström-Westas and Rosén 2006).

Continuous brain function monitoring

Amplitude-integrated electroencephalography (aEEG) is increasingly being used in the NICU today. The aEEG records single channel EEG from biparietal electrodes and the signal is filtered, rectified, smoothed and amplitude integrated. Both thin subdermal needles and gel electrodes are available. The aEEG display is time-compressed to allow an overview of long-term trends in cerebral activity with interpretation based primarily on pattern recognition (see Table 8.3). The monitor can be used at the bedside without interruption of daily care and does not require extensive formal training. Primarily the aEEG is used to detect seizure activity, gauge response to anticonvulsant therapy and as part of routine clinical monitoring, especially for those infants pharmacologically paralysed.

Studies have shown that the aEEG is very accurate in outcome prediction of term infants with HIE between 3 and 48 hours' postnatal age, especially when the early aEEG is combined with clinical evaluation. A poor background pattern (BS, CLV, and FT) persisting beyond the first 12–24 hours after birth is known to carry a poor prognosis (Spitzmiller *et al.* 2007; Toet and deVries 2008).

Table 8.3 Classification of aEEG traces in full-term infants

Continuous normal voltage pattern (CNV): continuous activity with lower margin of amplitude around (5) to 7 to 10µV and maximum amplitude around 10 to 25µV (to 50). Sleep–wake cycling (SWC) should be present.

Discontinuous normal voltage pattern (DNV): discontinuous background, with variable minimal amplitude, but < 5µV and maximum amplitude greater than 10µV

Burst suppression (BS): discontinuous background with minimum amplitude without variability at 0 to 1 (2)µV

Continuous low voltage (CLV): continuous background pattern of extremely low voltage (less than or around 5µV)

Inactive flat trace (FT): mainly inactive (isoelectric tracing) background less than 5µV

It must be remembered, however, that due to the limited number of electrodes, epileptic seizure activity may be missed and the standard EEG remains the gold standard. Although not as extensively evaluated in preterm infants, research studies are beginning to demonstrate the utility of the aEEG in this population.

Other mechanisms of brain injury

Chorioamnionitis and brain injury

Strong epidemiologic data link maternal infection with neonatal brain injury. Although chorioamnionitis is itself associated with premature delivery and low gestational age, cytokines may contribute further to brain injury. Cytokines are produced by, or act on, the immune system mediating responses associated with infection, inflammation and tissue injury. Recent work links increased amniotic fluid or blood concentrations of cytokines with perinatal brain injury. It is thought that maternally or fetally derived circulating inflammatory mediators may cross the immature blood–brain barrier either directly injuring neurons or increasing their vulnerability to subsequent hypoxic-ischaemic insults. Alternatively intra-uterine infection could initiate injury by producing in-utero septic shock with its resultant decreased cerebral perfusion. The neurologic outcome linked most commonly with chorioamnionitis is cerebral palsy (Willoughby and Nelson 2002; Rocha *et al*. 2007).

Hypoglycaemic injury to the brain

Hypoglycaemia (see p. 267) remains a common preventable cause of neurological injury in the newborn infant. Like oxygen, glucose is essential for brain function. The major source of cerebral glucose is the blood supply; therefore it is easy to understand how encephalopathy and brain injury may occur when the glucose content in the blood is deficient (Volpe 2001e).

Conclusion

Newborn infants at risk of, or suffering from, a brain injury present a significant challenge to neonatal nurses. A knowledge of the nature and implications of types of brain injury aids optimal care of these infants. Nursing management involves recognition of factors that increase the risk of further hypoxia, interventions to restore oxygenation and supportive care of infants and their families. Fluctuations in systemic blood pressure with increased intracranial pressure may result from care-giving or environmental stress; therefore interventions to avoid rapid alterations in cerebral blood flow, and developmental care to reduce stress is essential. Owens (2005) has devised a useful table of potentially better practices for preventing intracranial haemorrhage and PVL which is recommended as further reading.

For parents, ongoing support is needed in understanding and dealing with their infant's serious illness, the changes in infant responsiveness or irritability, the possibility of death, or possible implications for future poor neurological outcome.

Case study: infant at risk of IVH

Luke is a 26-week gestation infant born by precipitous vaginal delivery, weighing 890g. The pregnancy had been complicated with intermittent vaginal bleeding from 12 weeks' gestation. Following the premature rupture of membranes, his mother was transferred to a tertiary perinatal centre four days prior to his delivery. His mother received erythromycin and betamethasone. Several hours prior to delivery his mother began to feel unwell with an increased temperature and uterine tenderness. Luke delivered following a further APH. He required resuscitation at birth including intubation and positive pressure ventilation. Following a dose of surfactant, he was transferred to the neonatal intensive care unit.

Q.1. What antenatal factors place Luke at risk for GMH/IVH and/or PVL brain injury?

On admission to NICU, Luke was commenced on synchronised inter-mittent positive pressure ventilation. Umbilical venous and arterial catheters were inserted. Findings consistent with respiratory distress syndrome were evident on his chest X-ray. He went on to receive a further two treatment doses of surfactant. In the first 24 hours of life Luke's blood pressure was problematic and he required two doses of volume expansion which was followed by inotropic support. On day three Luke became more unstable and hypotensive. There was a murmur present on auscultation and a patent ductus arteriosus was confirmed on cardiac echo. On the routine day 7 head ultrasound scan there was evidence of intraventricular haemorrhage with blood present in normal-sized ventricles.

Q.2. During Luke's initial care and management what potential mechan-isms for injury were present and how could the presentation of his IVH be described? Identify potential care-giving practices that may aid in the prevention and management of IVH.

Follow-up head ultrasound scan at 14 days of age revealed further bleeding had occurred and the ventricles were now slightly dilated. Despite this, Luke's condition had allowed him to be extubated to continuous positive airways pressure (CPAP). Further regular ultrasounds were planned as although it was unlikely that further bleeding would occur, there was risk of post-haemorrhagic hydrocephalus. Successive scans showed mild progressive dilation which stopped at around 30 days. During this period Luke appeared well and his head circumference remained unchanged.

Q.3. What is Luke's likely long-term outcome?

Case study: infant with HIE

Emily is a 39-week gestation female infant born by emergency Caesarian section subsequent to her mother presenting in the delivery suite following a large antepartum haemorrhage. A fetal bradycardia was present. Emily was born pale, floppy, with no respiratory effort, and a heart rate of less than 60. She required inflation breaths followed by bag and mask ventilation, chest compressions, intubation and adrenaline. A fluid bolus of 10ml/kg/dose of normal saline was given for poor perfusion. Her first spontaneous respiration was noted at 10 minutes of age. Apgar scores were 1, 1, 5 and 7 at 1, 5, 10 and 15 minutes respectively. On admission to NICU her breathing pattern was stabilising but she was irritable with abnormal posturing. On the first arterial gas obtained, her pH was 6.9 with a base deficit of 16mEq/L.

Q.1. Describe potential mechanisms of HIE. Would cooling be likely to be beneficial to Emily?

The aEEG initially showed a discontinuous pattern without sleep–wake cycling; however, at 18 hours of age she was noted to have repetitive jerky movements of her upper extremities with eye flickering lasting 45 seconds. She was given a loading dose of phenobarbital for recurrent episodes of jerking movements correlating to seizure activity on aEEG.

Q.2. Describe the significance of the timing of onset of seizures. Identify potential care-giving practices required while Emily is being cooled.

Over the next 12 hours her seizures stopped. She was re-warmed after 72 hours of cooling and was extubated to room air. Over the course of the next 10 days Emily established breast feeding well.

Q.3. What is Emily's long-term outcome likely to be?

References

Azzopardi, D. and Edwards, A.D. (2007) 'Hypothermia', *Seminars in Fetal and Neonatal Medicine* 12(4): 303–10.

Barks, J.D.E. (2008) 'Current controversies in hypothermic neuroprotection', *Seminars in Fetal and Neonatal Medicine* 13(1): 30–4.

Bhutta, Z.A., Darmstadt, G.L., Hasan, B.S. and Haws, R.A. (2005) 'Community-based interventions for improving perinatal and neonatal outcomes in developing countries: a review of the evidence', *Pediatrics* 115(2): 519–617.

Crowther, C., Crosby, D.D. and Henderson-Smart, D.J. (2001) 'Vitamin K prior to preterm birth for preventing neonatal periventricular haemorrhage', *Cochrane Database of Systematic Reviews*, Issue 1, Art. No. CD000229. DOI:10.1002/14651858.CD000229.

Crowther, C., Crosby, D.D. and Henderson-Smart, D.J. (2003) 'Phenobarbital prior to preterm birth for preventing neonatal periventricular haemorrhage', *Cochrane Database of Systematic Reviews*, Issue 3, Art No. CD000164.DOI:10.1002/14651858.CD000164.

Deguchi, K. and Millar, G. (2007) *Periventricular leukomalacia* [Online]. Available at: http://www.utdol.com/utd/content/topic.do?topicKey=ped_neur/22941 (accessed 9 February 2008).

Ferriero, D.M. (2004) 'Neonatal brain injury', *The New England Journal of Medicine* 351(19): 1985–96.

Filan, P., Boylan, G.B., Chorley, G., *et al.* (2004) 'The relationship between the onset of electrographic seizure activity after birth and time of cerebral injury in utero', *British Journal of Obstetrics* 111: 1–4.

Fowlie, P.W. and Davis, P.G. (2002) 'Prophylactic intravenous indomethacin for preventing mortality and morbidity in preterm infants', *Cochrane Database of Systematic Reviews*, Issue 3, Art. No. CD000174. DOI: 10.1002/14651858.CD000174.

Fritz, K.I. and Delivoria-Papadopoulos, M. (2006) 'Mechanisms of injury to the newborn brain', *Clinics in Perinatology* 33: 573–91.

Gressens, P., Rogido, M., Paindaveine, B. and Sola, A. (2002) 'The impact of neonatal intensive care practices on the developing brain', *Journal of Pediatrics* 140(6): 646–53.

Grow, J. and Barks, J.D.E. (2002) 'Pathogenesis of hypoxic-ischemic cerebral injury in the term infant: current concepts', *Clinics in Perinatology* 29: 585–602.

Hellström-Westas, L. and Rosén, I. (2006) 'Continuous brain-function monitoring: state of the art in clinical practice', *Seminars in Fetal and Neonatal Medicine* 11(6): 503–11.

Jacobs, S., Hunt, R., Tarnow-Mordi, W., Inder, T. and Davis, P. (2007) 'Cooling for newborns with hypoxic ischaemic encephalopathy (review)', *Cochrane Database of Systematic Reviews*, Issue 4, Art. No. CD003311. DOI: 10-1002/14651858.CD003311. pub 2.

Lissauer, T. and Fanaroff, A. (2006) *Neonatology at a Glance*, Malden, MA: Blackwell Publishing.

Mercer, J.S., Vohr, B.R., McGrath, M.M., Padbury, J.F., Wallach, M. and Oh, W. (2006) 'Delayed cord clamping in very preterm infants reduces the incidence of intraventricular hemorrhage and late-onset sepsis: a randomized, controlled trial', *Pediatrics* 117(4): 1235–42.

Owens, R. (2005) 'Intraventricular hemorrhage in the premature neonate', *Neonatal Network* 24(3): 55–71.

Rennie, J. and Boylan, G. (2007) 'Treatment of neonatal seizures', *Archives of Disease in Childhood: Fetal and Neonatal Edition* 92: F148–F150.

Rocha, G., Proença, E., Quintas, C., Rodrigues, T. and Guimarães, H. (2007) 'Chorioamnionitis and brain damage in the preterm newborn', *The Journal of Maternal-Fetal and Neonatal Medicine* 20(10): 745–9.

Spitzmillar, R.E., Phillips, T., Meinzen-Derr, J. and Hoath, S.B. (2007) 'Amplitude – integrated EEG is useful in predicting neurodevelopmental outcome in full-term infants with hypoxic-ischemic encephalopathy: a meta-analysis', *Journal of Child Neurology* 22(9): 1069–78.

Thoresen, M. (2008) 'Supportive care during neuroprotective hypothermia in the term newborn: adverse effects and their prevention', *Clinics in Perinatology* 35: 749–63.

Toet, M.C. and de Vries, L.S. (2008) 'The use of amplitude integrated electroencephalography for assessing neonatal neurologic injury', *Clinics in Perinatology* 35: 665–78.

Volpe, J.J. (2001a) 'Intracranial hemorrhage: germinal matrix-intraventricular hemorrhage of the premature infant', in J.J. Volpe (ed.) *Neurology of the Newborn*, 4th edn, Philadelphia, PA: W.B. Saunders Company, pp. 428–93.

Volpe, J.J. (2001b) 'Hypoxic-ischaemic encephalopathy: clinical aspects', in J.J. Volpe (ed.) *Neurology of the Newborn*, 4th edn, Philadelphia, PA: W.B. Saunders Company, pp. 331–94.

Volpe, J.J. (2001c) 'Hypoxic-ischaemic encephalopathy: neuropathology and pathogenesis', in J.J. Volpe (ed.) *Neurology of the Newborn*, 4th edn, Philadelphia, PA: W.B. Saunders Company, pp. 296–330.

Volpe, J.J. (2001d) 'Neonatal seizures', in J.J. Volpe (ed.) *Neurology of the Newborn*, 4th edn, Philadelphia, PA: W.B. Saunders Company, pp. 178–214.

Volpe, J.J. (2001e) 'Hypoglycaemia and brain injury', in J.J. Volpe (ed.) *Neurology of the Newborn*, 4th edn, Philadelphia, PA: W.B. Saunders Company, pp. 497–520.

Willoughby, R.E. and Nelson, K.B. (2002) 'Chorioamnionitis and brain injury', *Clinics in Perinatology* 29: 603–21.

Wu, Y. (2008) 'Clinical features, diagnosis and treatment of neonatal encephalopathy' [Online]. Available at: http://www.uptodate.com/online/content/topic.do?topicKey=ped_neur/4411 (accessed 9 February 2008).

Chapter 9

Management of Haematological Disorders

Jackie Dent and Katie McKenna

Contents

Introduction

Caring for infants with haematological disorders presents the neonatal nurse with many challenges. In order to correctly interpret clinical signs, monitor changes and provide information to support parents, a background knowledge of the haematological system is necessary. This chapter will review four of the more common haematological disorders in the newborn: jaundice, haemorrhagic disease of the newborn (Vitamin K deficient bleeding), disseminated intravascular coagulopathy and anaemia. The pathophysiology and treatment modalities of each condition will be presented to enable the nurse to anticipate problems, assess the effectiveness of treatment and limit complications that may impact on the infant.

Jaundice

It is estimated that 60 per cent of term and 80 per cent of preterm infants develop neonatal jaundice, which usually appears 2–4 days after birth and resolves spontaneously after 1–2 weeks (Evans 2007). Jaundice, a yellow coloration of the skin and sclera, is a sign of hyperbilirubinemia, which is a result of elevated unconjugated bilirubin. Hyperbilirubinaemia occurs as a result of excessive production of bilirubin and decreased bilirubin elimination. Elevated levels of serum bilirubin (SBR) are common in the newborn and generally benign unless occurring in the first 24 hours; prolonged for more than two weeks; or are excessive. Unconjugated bilirubin levels that rise above the threshold of albumin binding and clearance are taken up by the central nuclei in the brain and are toxic. This leads to bilirubin encephalopathy and **kernicterus**, which are irreversible and lead to choreoathetoid cerebral palsy and if untreated lead to death (American Academy of Pediatrics Subcommittee on Hyperbilirubinemia 2004). Non-immune 'physiological' jaundice starts to rise after the first 24 hours, peaks at 72 hours and then reduces by day 7. This condition reflects the immaturity of the liver and the breakdown of fetal haemoglobin, resolution of bruising from birth and often the establishment of the breast milk supply and enterohepatic circulation.

Bilirubin encephalopathy and kernicterus

Elevated levels of SBR may cross the blood–brain barrier and deposit in the basal ganglia and cerebellum. Acute bilirubin encephalopathy describes the neurological effects evident in the first few weeks while kernicterus describes the longer-term neurological sequelae and refers to the yellowish staining in the central nuclei within the basal ganglia (ibid.). Acute effects of bilirubin enecephalopathy include lethargy, hypotonia and a diminished suck. Symptoms will then progress to hypertonia, arching, seizures and high-pitched cry (Juretschke 2005). Longer-term effects can include cerebral palsy, sensorineural hearing loss, mental retardation and death (ibid.).

Physiology of bilirubin production

In utero, the placenta is responsible for the excretion of unconjugated bilirubin. Following delivery, the neonatal liver assumes responsibility for bilirubin metabolism. The predominant source of bilirubin is the breakdown of haem containing proteins, in particular haemoglobin (Hb), a major constituent of red blood cells. Haemoglobin accounts for 70–80 per cent of bilirubin production (Blackburn 2003). One gram of haemoglobin produces approximately 600μmol of bilirubin that is unconjugated and fat-soluble. This means that it is unable to be excreted via the gut or kidney and can easily pass through the lipid membranes of cells such as fatty tissue and the brain.

Infants produce higher rates of bilirubin than adults as a result of the shortened lifespan of fetal red blood cells (40–70 days compared with 120 days in adults), and an increased circulating red cell mass. Newborns produce 6mg/kg/day of bilirubin, which is double the level produced by an adult (Maisels and McDonagh 2008). Bilirubin production is a two-stage process. During the first stage, haem is degraded by the enzyme haem oxygenase, which causes the release of iron and the formation of biliverdin and carbon monoxide. Biliverdin is then broken down by biliverdin reductase to form bilirubin.

Bilirubin metabolism and excretion

Conjugation occurs in the liver. The transport of free bilirubin into hepatocytes is facilitated by binding with albumin. Once bound, the bilirubin enters the smooth endoplastic reticulum of the hepatocyte in a carrier-mediated process, with the help of carrier proteins Y (ligandin) and Z. In the liver a series of reactions occur, catalysed by the enzyme uridine diphosphate glucuronyl transferase (UGT) resulting in the joining of bilirubin with two molecules of glucuronic acid to produce bilirubin diglucuronide or conjugated bilirubin (Figure 9.1). Conjugated bilirubin, in bile, enters the small intestine via the common bile duct, and during its passage through the intestinal tract, bacterial enzymes convert bilirubin into urobilinogen and stercobilinogen. As these compounds are now water-soluble, they can be excreted in the urine and stools.

Physiological jaundice

Neonatal jaundice may be classified as either physiological or pathological. Several factors contribute to the neonate's predisposition to developing physiological jaundice including increased bilirubin production, decreased bilirubin clearance and increased enterohepatic circulation of bilirubin (Wong et al. 2007). Physiological jaundice may be exacerbated by prematurity, administration of albumin-bound medications, bruising, polycythaemia, short life span of fetal red blood cells, inadequate oral intake, delayed passage of stool and breastfeeding (Truman 2006).

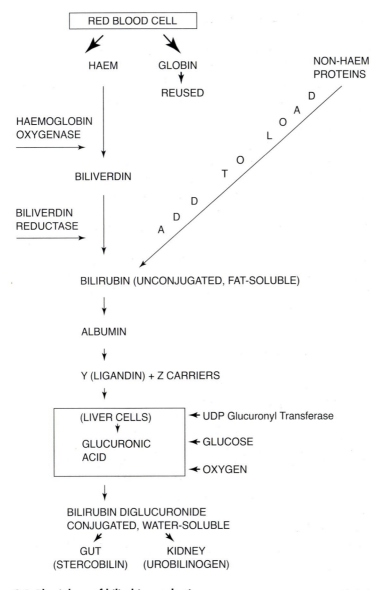

Figure 9.1 **Physiology of bilirubin production**

Other causes of jaundice

While physiological jaundice is a naturally occurring phenomenon, jaundice may occur for other reasons, and is often the result of various disease processes. Table 9.1 summarises these, and some of the more common causes are discussed in more detail.

Table 9.1 Causes of jaundice

Example	Mechanism
G6PD deficiency ABO/Rhesus incompatibility Haemoglobinopathies	Increased red cell breakdown
Trauma	Sequestered blood
Physiological	Temporary reduction in efficiency of normal process
Breast milk	? Pregnanediol ? Free fatty acids Low fluid intake
Hypothyroidism Galactosaemia	Interfere with metabolism and excretion
Drugs	Need albumin binding sites
Infection	May affect liver +/− increase haemolysis
Biliary atresia Cystic fibrosis Tumours	Impair ability to excrete the conjugated bilirubin

Rhesus incompatibility

Haemolytic disease of the newborn (HDN) with resultant red cell haemolysis and overproduction of bilirubin may occur with blood group incompatibilities such as Rhesus (Rh or Anti D), ABO or when the mother carries more rare antibodies such as Anti E Anti C, Kell or Duffy. The fetal and maternal circulations, although intimately positioned in the placenta, are essentially separate from one another. Small tears in the placental capillaries or placental separation during delivery may facilitate the passage of fetal cells into the normally separate maternal circulation. Passage of Rh-positive fetal cells into the Rh-negative maternal circulation generates an immune response and the production of anti-Rh-antibodies. During this Rh-isoimmunisation, **antibodies** from an Rh-negative mother cause destruction of the Rh-positive fetal red blood cells. A number of scenarios exist in which an Rh-negative mother carrying an Rh-positive fetus may become sensitised to Rh antigens, including fetal-maternal blood transfusion during pregnancy, delivery, miscarriage, termination or **amniocentesis**. The immune response in the Rh-negative mother following exposure to Rh-positive cells is not usually significant during the first pregnancy; however, during subsequent pregnancies the risk of fetal red cell haemolysis increases secondary to an elevated level of maternal anti-Rh antibodies.

Severe haemolysis in the fetus from Rh incompatibility can result in the condition erythroblastosis fetalis (EBF) where the resultant anaemia of the fetus promotes red cell production from unusual sites such as the liver. The most severe form of EBF causes fetal hypoxia, cardiac failure and this leads to hydrops fetalis with generalised oedema and pleural, pericardial and/or peritoneal effusions (Bagwell 2007). This is now a rare condition due to the production of therapeutic Anti D immunoglobulin. Anti D gamma globulin is donor-pooled immunoglobulin that binds to fetal cells and promotes their destruction prior to the initiation of a maternal immune response. Administration of Anti D immunoglobulin provides passive protection from further sensitisation. The routine administration of Anti D gamma globulin to Rh-negative mothers during the second trimester (26–28 weeks) and following any high-risk event during pregnancy is now accepted obstetric practice.

ABO incompatibility

The decline of Rhesus Disease has meant that ABO blood group incompatibility is now the most frequent cause of haemolytic disease of the newborn. ABO incompatibility occurs in the following situations:

- Maternal blood type is O and infant's blood type A (most common type) or B (most severe type).
- Maternal blood type is B and infant's blood type is A or AB.
- Maternal blood type is A and infant's blood type is B or AB.

(Mundy 2005)

Naturally occurring maternal antibodies attach to the antigens on the incompatible fetal red cells, causing haemolysis and the production of bilirubin. The infant presents with anaemia and jaundice. The direct antiglobulin test (Coombs) is positive.

G6PD deficiency

Glucose-6 phosphate dehydrogenase is an enzyme, which is responsible for maintaining the integrity of the red cell membrane. A deficiency of this enzyme renders the cell liable to haemolyse. In affected individuals, this can occur during ingestion or exposure to oxidants such as naphthalene (moth balls), sulphonamide medications, Fava beans (broad beans), or during periods of infection. Newborns are usually symptom-free until exposed to an oxidant, which triggers haemolysis. It can be very difficult to identify the oxidant stress in some situations; however, a thorough history and/or home investigation will usually be able to identify the oxidant. This condition has a sex-linked recessive inheritance pattern, which means that heterozygous females are carriers and males are affected. Once diagnosis is established, the family need advice on how to avoid the oxidants. G6PD is usually only clinically significant in infancy where there is a risk of developing kernicterus and is not a clinical problem in adults.

Jaundice associated with breastfeeding

There appear to be two aetiologies surrounding breastfeeding and jaundice:

- *Breastfeeding jaundice* – Breastfeeding mothers require support and education if they are to be successful. Newborns who are breastfed have a lower fluid intake compared with formula-fed infants in the first few days and as a consequence relatively higher levels of serum bilirubin. Newborns also have slower intestinal transit times which increases exposure to beta-glucuronidase and increases the unconjugation process via the enterohepatic circulation. Infants who lose weight early in the establishment of breastfeeding are more likely to become more jaundiced (Frank and Frank 2006) and are also at increased risk of hypernatraemia (Oddie *et al.* 2001).
- *Breast milk jaundice* – this is a benign condition of prolonged jaundice occurring in a small percentage of breastfed infants. A factor in human milk increases the enterohepatic circulation of bilirubin resulting in prolonged jaundice (Gartner 2001). Breast milk jaundice is a diagnosis of exclusion and can be confirmed by the (brief) cessation of breastfeeding leading to a fall in bilirubin levels. This practice is not necessary as it may lead to a complete cessation of breastfeeding as the mother feels she has 'caused' the jaundice. The potential harms of stopping breastfeeding outweigh any risks of a mild or moderate hyperbilirubinaemia.

Measurement of jaundice

Jaundice becomes clinically evident when serum levels of bilirubin reach 86μmol/L (5mg/dl) (Dennery *et al.* 2001) and progress **cephalocaudally**, e.g. commencing with the head and moving towards the plantar and palmar surfaces (Kramer 1969). This visual progression of jaundice may indicate the level of bilirubin, however; it should not replace actual serum bilirubin measurement. Transcutaneous bilirubinometers (TcB) are an accurate and non-invasive screening method for clinically significant jaundice in the well term infant (Maisels and McDonagh 2004; Sanpavat and Nuchprayoon 2005). TcB measures have a linear correlation with SBR in the lower range and their use as a screening device to detect clinically significant jaundice decreases the need for frequent blood sampling in the well term infant. Reduction in invasive blood tests will have an ensuing reduction in pain and discomfort for the newborn and a reduction in health care costs (Bredemeyer *et al.* 2007).

Measurement of end-tidal carbon monoxide (CO) levels in breath corrected for inhaled CO is also under investigation as a potential screening tool for jaundice. Haem degradation produces equal amounts of biliverdin, CO and iron (Stevenson and Vreman 2001). While biliverdin further reduces and forms bilirubin, CO binds to haemoglobin and is eliminated via the lungs during exhalation. Consequently, CO measurements give an approximation of bilirubin production.

Despite these advances, serum measurement of total bilirubin remains the gold standard for diagnosing and treating hyperbilirunaemia.

Jaundice should be treated according to the infant's gestational and postnatal age. Figure 9.2 shows suggested treatment levels and Table 9.2 outlines investigations for jaundice related to time of onset.

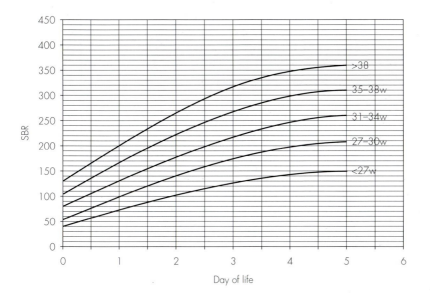

Summary of healthy term infants

Day of life	1	2	3	4	5
SBR	200	260	320	350	360

Figure 9.2 **Suggested treatment levels of jaundice**
Source: Reproduced with permission Beeby (2009).

Management of jaundice

As with many conditions in the neonate, the management of jaundice depends upon the underlying pathophysiology and the severity of the hyperbiliru-binaemia. The aim of any treatment is to prevent serum bilirubin levels

Table 9.2 Investigations of jaundice related to timing of onset

Jaundice in the first 24 hours	Jaundice appearing at 2–5 days	Prolonged jaundice (longer than 14 days)
Serum bilirubin levels including the conjugated fraction	As per jaundice in the first 24 hours plus the following	As per jaundice in the first 24 hours plus the following
Full blood count with haematocrit/packed cell volume	Blood cultures	Liver function tests
Blood group and direct antiglobulin test	Urine metabolic screening looking for metabolic disorders	Thyroid function tests
Maternal blood group	Total serum bilirubin including the conjugated fraction < 20μmol/l excludes obstruction in the biliary tree	
G6PD screening (be aware that this can be false during acute haemolysis)		
Galactose-1-PO$_4$ uridyl transferase (to detect galactosaemia)		
TORCH screen for evidence of congenital infection (to detect Toxoplasmosis, other including hepatitis/HIV/parvovirus Rubella, Cytomegalovirus and Herpes)		

from rising to such a degree that they will cause bilirubin encephalopathy or kernicterus. A number of therapies are available for mild/moderate cases o f hyperbilirubinaemia.

Phenobarbital

Since the mid-1960s, phenobarbital has been used to increase the conjugation and excretion of bilirubin, by increasing uptake and enhancing bile flow. Phenobarbital's onset of action is not immediate and is even slower in the preterm infant and as a result, it has not been widely accepted as a standard treatment for hyperbilirubinaemia. It may be used to augment other therapies and in conjugated jaundice to accentuate excretion prior to diagnostic scanning.

Intravenous immunoglobulin (IVIG)

Administration of IVIG combined with phototherapy has been shown, in randomised controlled trials, to significantly reduce the maximum serum bilirubin and need for exchange transfusion in babies with isoimmune haemolytic jaundice (Alcock and Liley 2003). It works by binding the antibodies in the newborn's blood and halts the immune mediated haemolysis. The Cochrane review (ibid.) suggested that in circumstances where there is a strong need to avoid transfusion, it is justifiable to use IVIG.

Metalloporphyrin

Metalloporphyrins, specifically tin-mesoporphyrin (SnMP) or tin proto-porphyrin (SnPP), are potent inhibitors of haem oxygenase (HO), an important enzyme involved in bilirubin production. Tin-mesoporphyrin, administered as a single intramuscular injection, competitively inhibits the production of haem oxygenase. Limiting haem oxygenase prevents the breakdown of haem and thus reduces the production of bilirubin. The Cochrane Review in 2003 (Alcock and Liley 2003) concluded that its use was not justified based on the evidence at the time (Suresh et al. 2003). However, two further randomised controlled trials have demonstrated that intramuscular administration of tin-mesoporphyrin (SnMP) to jaundiced term and near term infants within the first few days of life greatly reduced the need for phototherapy (Evans 2007). At present, tin-mesoporphyrin is not licensed for routine clinical use in the United Kingdom or the USA and further studies are required to support its use in clinical practice.

Phototherapy

Phototherapy has been demonstrated to rapidly reduce the serum bilirubin concentration and has been the standard of care for treatment of neonatal jaundice for the past four decades. The use of phototherapy to prevent SBR levels associated with bilirubin encephalopathy and kernicterus is now universal. Phototherapy works on the skin, due to the processes of photo-oxidation and photoisomerisation which convert unconjugated bilirubin into an excretable form (Vreman *et al.* 2004):

- *Photo-oxidation* involves the oxidation of bilirubin pigment deposited in the skin and its conversion into colourless products that are water-soluble and able to be excreted in the urine (Bagwell 2007). Only a small fraction of the bilirubin load is excreted in this way.
- *Photoisomerisation* involves the conversion of bilirubin polymers present in the skin into excretable isomers. Photoisomerisation occurs when bilirubin is exposed to light at 450 nanometers (nm), which is light at the blue end of the spectrum. This causes bilirubin to change from a lipid-soluble substance into five water-soluble isomers. Four of these isomers are excreted in bile without undergoing conjugation. The fifth isomer, lumibilirubin (also known as photobilirubin), is a stable water-soluble form of bilirubin and is excreted in bile and urine (Robertson 1993). The isomerisation process is possibly the most important in terms of bilirubin elimination.

Phototherapy lamps/units emitting visible blue light in the wavelength of 420–460nm are the most effective in reducing serum bilirubin. There are several methods available for delivering phototherapy, all of which deliver varying dosages of light intensity (spectral irradiance) to the infant. The higher the level of irradiance, the higher the rate of bilirubin decline.

Methods of administration of phototherapy

Fluorescent tubes

Fluorescent tubes incorporate different colours of light including cool white, blue, turquoise or green using either straight or U-shaped tubes. The most effective light for reducing bilirubin is blue light and many units use two blue and two white fluorescent tubes which in combination deliver an irradiance of $12\mu W/cm^2/nm$ (Tan 1994). Irradiance decreases exponentially the further the distance of the infant from the phototherapy source, thus the fluorescent tubes should be positioned to achieve irradiance of $12\mu W/cm^2/nm$, measured at the infant's skin.

Halogen spotlights

Halogen spotlight systems, positioned directly above the infant, use either single or multiple metal halide lamps and provide irradiance from $10\mu–30\mu W/cm^2/nm$. These units are capable of generating considerable heat with the potential for causing thermal injury to both infants and clinicians. Manufacturers recommend not positioning the lights any closer than 52cm from the infant. Ad hoc positioning for the convenience of care-givers is a potential benefit of spotlight systems. However, the ability to vary the position of the light source, affecting the angle of application and distance to infant, may lead to unreliable dosing and unpredictable clinical responses (Vremen *et al*. 2004).

Fibreoptic systems (Bili blanket)

Fibreoptic systems utilise plastic filaments, which carry a high-intensity halogen light source, woven into a pad which is placed in direct contact with the infant's skin. These devices may deliver up to $35\mu W/cm^2/nm$ and may be used as a sole phototherapy source or as an adjunct to spotlights or fluorescent tubes. Combination of fibreoptic systems with other systems is often referred to as 'double' phototherapy and increases the surface area exposed to the light source with a resultant increase in irradiance dose. The main advantages of fibreoptic systems are that the infant may be held and it eliminates the need to shield the eyes (Vremen *et al*. 2004).

Intermittent vs. continuous phototherapy

Clinical studies comparing intermittent with continuous phototherapy have produced conflicting results (Maurer *et al*. 1973). Because all light exposure increases bilirubin excretion (compared with darkness), no plausible scientific rationale exists for using intermittent phototherapy (American Academy of Pediatrics Subcommittee on Hyperbilirubinemia 2004). Individual judgement should be exercised to permit phototherapy to be interrupted during feeding, care-giving episodes and briefly during parental visits.

Nursing care with phototherapy

Early animal studies suggested that retinal damage may occur following exposure to phototherapy lights (Noell *et al*. 1966; Messner *et al*. 1975). Although these studies were conducted over 40 years ago, it has never been conclusively established that this may or may not occur in humans and thus it remains important to shield the infant's eyes during phototherapy. Eyes can be shielded by opaque 'goggles' which should be removed at regular intervals to check for abrasions or infection. These shields need to be tight enough to prevent slipping and potential airway obstruction, but not too tight as to restrict blood flow or cause tissue damage. Orange Perspex shields can be used to obliterate the light but these minimise the amount of skin exposed compared to goggles. To facilitate infants' visual stimulation and to promote parental interaction, stopping the lights and removing eye shields for short periods each day, such as during feeding and parental visits, should be considered if clinically appropriate.

Skin care with phototherapy

Controlled trials have demonstrated that increased skin surface area exposure, achieved by nursing infants naked under the phototherapy lights, will cause a greater reduction in serum bilirubin levels (Tan 1994). Regular position changes permit maximum skin exposure to light. A potential side-effect of lumirubin excretion is diarrhoea/loose stools. As a result, some form of nappy is desirable while still maximising skin exposure to the lights. Nappies comprising UV light-permeable material are now available in Australia and the USA. The use of lotions, creams and oils is not recommended since the action of the light upon them may cause burns. A further side-effect of phototherapy is skin rashes due to **histamine** release (Blackburn 2003); this is a temporary rash which resolves when therapy is discontinued.

Fluid balance during phototherapy

There is a lack of consensus regarding increasing the free water intake, either parenterally or enterally during phototherapy treatment to account for insensible water losses. In the absence of a consensus or supporting evidence for this practice, it would seem prudent that attention to fluid balance, infant weight, serum electrolyte results, urine output and specific gravity would determine the need for administration of increased fluids rather than an indiscriminate increase alone.

Thermoregulation

To maximise skin surface area exposed to phototherapy light, the infant should be nursed naked. Consequently, the infant's temperature should be closely monitored. The action of the light on the perspex incubator or cot lid may increase environmental temperature, while small babies may need a heat shield to prevent heat loss.

Parental support during phototherapy

Support, explanations and reassurance for the need for phototherapy are vital for parents of infants undergoing treatment. Encouraging parents to continue feeding, caring for and visiting their infant may be necessary.

Exchange transfusion

Exchange transfusion may be required to reduce the SBR levels if they are dangerously high to prevent neurodevelopment sequelae. Twice the infant's blood volume should be exchanged (2×85ml/kg) and is best performed by slow removal of aliquots of blood (e.g. 10ml) from an artery (usually peripheral) and simultaneous infusion of a similar volume of blood into a vein (usually peripheral). This is the preferred method as it causes less fluctuations of blood volume and pressure. However, umbilical artery and venous lines can be used.

The rate of exchange is usually 2–4ml/min. The bilirubin level should decrease by around 45 per cent of the immediate pre-exchange level (Frank and Frank 2007). The actual serum bilirubin level at which an exchange transfusion should be performed will vary from unit to unit as consideration is given not only to the actual SBR level but also to the rate of rise of the concentration, the expected peak and the infant's age and condition.

Vitamin K deficient bleeding (VKDB)

Vitamin K deficiency (formerly haemorrhagic disease of the newborn) is the most important bleeding disorder in the otherwise stable neonate. The most obvious predisposing factor is the omission of postnatal administration of prophylactic Vitamin K. Other factors include hepatic dysfunction, perinatal asphyxia and maternal ingestion of anticonvulsant or anticoagulant therapy.

To understand the processes involved in VKDB, it is important to understand the physiology of blood clotting.

Coagulation

When blood vessel injury occurs, platelets adhere to the damaged area and release adenosine diphosphate (ADP) which activates the process of clotting. The platelets are pulled together because they have an affinity for the blood protein fibrinogen and together they form a mesh over the tear. In order to prevent the mesh from being torn away the platelet prostaglandin pathway releases thromboxane, which encourages vasoconstriction and decreased blood flow in the damaged area. A process known as the clotting cascade is then initiated (see Table 9.3), in which a series of proteins and enzymes are activated sequentially and, through a variety of complex biochemical reactions, will produce a blood clot. Other proteins work to regulate the process and ensure that clotting does not occur in the systemic circulation with potentially disastrous results. A number of the proteins/enzymes – 'clotting factors' – are vitamin K dependent and need the vitamin to become functional. The dependent factors are Factor II, VII, IX and X. The vitamin K promotes carboxylation and following this process, the calcium-binding proteins in the clotting process can be activated.

Sources of vitamin K

In the newborn, levels of the vitamin K dependent clotting factors are significantly lower compared to older infants and these levels increase. Vitamin K is obtained naturally from plants (vitamin K1 – phylloquinone) and bacteria

Table 9.3 Blood clotting factors

Factor I	Fibrinogen
Factor II	Prothrombin*
Factor III	Thromboplastin
Factor IV	Calcium ions
Factor V	Pro-accelerin
Factor VI	Is no longer recognised in the clotting pathway
Factor VII	Pro-convertin* (Serum prothrombin conversion accelerator)
Factor VIII	Antihaemophilic factor
Factor IX	Plasma thromboplastin component* (Christmas factor)
Factor X	Thrombokinase* (Stuart–Power factor)
Factor XI	Plasma thromboplastin antecedent
Factor XII	Hageman factor
Factor XIII	Fibrin stabilising factor

* Vitamin K dependent

(vitamin K2 – menaquinone). The main source of vitamin K1 is the most important in newborns. The absorption of bacterial vitamin K2 is reported by some writers (Kelnar *et al*. 1995) but disputed by others (Passmore and McNinch 1995). Unfortunately, the placental transfer of K1 is low, with a maternal:fetal ratio of 4:1 so the infant is dependent on dietary sources. Infant formulas contain on average 50µg/l of vitamin K. Breast milk, on the other hand, has about 2µg/l (Passmore and McNinch 1995). Equally, if the bacterially produced K2 is actually absorbed as some suggest, the breastfed baby is also at a further disadvantage. This relates to the fact that due to the different types of colonisation in breastfed infants, this process of absorption may take longer than in the formulae fed infant. This difficulty in acquiring vitamin K coupled with a normal postnatal drop in the levels of Factor II, VII, IX and X means that the newborn, especially the breastfeeding newborn, is at risk from vitamin K deficient bleeding (Blackburn 2003).

Characteristics of vitamin K deficient bleeding

VKDB is classified into early, classical and late, based on the age of presentation (Sutor *et al*. 1999):

- Early onset – the least common form, presents within the first 24 hours and is associated with maternal intake of medications which interfere with vitamin K metabolism. These medications include anticonvulsants such as phenytoin or carbemazepam and vitamin K antagonists such as warfarin. Postnatal administration of vitamin K cannot prevent early neonatal bleeding. In pregnant women receiving anticonvulsant therapy, oral vitamin K (10mg) for 10 days prior to delivery may be of benefit to the infant (Bagwell 2007).

- Classical onset – usually presents between 2–7 days of life and is more common in infants who are unwell at delivery or with delayed onset of feeding. Classical VKDB manifests as generalised and dramatic haemorrhage from such sites as the gastrointestinal tract, umbilical cord stump and skin punctures. Inadequate breast milk intake in infants who have not received prophylactic vitamin K is thought to be the cause of classical onset VKDB. When breast milk is consumed in sufficient quantities, it provides adequate vitamin K to prevent this disorder.

- Late onset – occurs from 1 week to 6 months after delivery, with the most common presentation at 3 months of age. It is associated with a higher incidence of intracranial haemorrhage and permanent neurological sequelae. Chronic disease states that interfere with fat absorption such as cystic fibrosis or biliary atresia are often associated with this form of VKDB.

Vitamin K prophylaxis

Since the 1950s, the use of artificial vitamin K, Konakion 1mg/0.5ml to prevent VKDB has been common practice. Intramuscular (IM) administration continued until the 1980s when it became more prevalent to give the IM preparation via the oral route. During the 1990s, administration of IM vitamin K to all newborn infants became routine. In 1992, Golding *et al.* reported an association between IM (not oral) vitamin K and childhood cancer which caused controversy at the time, resulting in many parents not wishing their infants to receive the drug. Golding's studies were criticised methodologically and subsequent large-scale international studies have not supported the association of vitamin K to malignancy. The current recommendations are that healthy newborn infants should receive an intramuscular injection of 1mg of vitamin K at birth or three 2mg oral doses administered at birth, at 3–5 days of age and in the fourth week of life. Infants receiving the oral regime need to be closely observed at the time of dosing to ensure ingestion. It is recommended that infants with a birth weight of less than 1.5kg receive a smaller IM dose of 0.5mg (0.25ml). Many units require informed parental consent prior to any administration of vitamin K (NHMRC 2006).

Disseminated intravascular coagulation (DIC)

DIC is a complex serious thrombohaemorrhagic disorder which affects infants who are already critically ill and, as such, is a secondary coagulation disorder. Disease processes that may predispose the development of DIC are severe hypoxia/acidosis sepsis and necrotising enterocolitis (NEC). The underlying pathology, while poorly understood, appears to be an inappropriate triggering of the clotting mechanisms leading to increased consumption of platelets and plasma clotting factors causing haemorrhage to occur (Emery 1992). Clot formation also results in the activation of thrombin, leading to fibrinolysis and the production of fibrin degradation products. These products lead to release of anticoagulants leading to further haemorrhage and prolongation of the cycle of DIC (Kuehl 1997) (Figure 9.3). The incidence of DIC is difficult to establish since it is a secondary disease process, but mortality rates are reported as 60–80 per cent in infants with severe DIC who experience severe bleeding (Bagwell 2007). Physical manifestations of DIC include prolonged oozing from puncture sites, bruising and petechiae.

Management of DIC

Correction of the underlying disease process triggering the condition is the key to successfully treating the infant with DIC. Concurrent treatments to control the haemorrhage/clotting cycle include the administration of cryoprecipitate, fresh frozen plasma (FFP), platelet and blood transfusion. Exchange transfusions may be used to 'wash out' any toxins in the infant's blood and to replace clotting factors. Cryoprecipitate increases Factor VIII and fibrinogen levels. FFP can increase coagulation factors by 15–20 per cent and a platelet infusion of 10ml/kg can increase the platelet count by up to 100000/mm^3 (Emery 1992; Kenner *et al.* 1993; Kuehl 1997). Vitamin K may also be given.

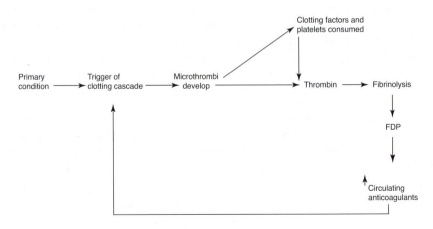

Figure 9.3 **Disseminated intravascular coagulation**

Anaemia

Anaemia is a deficiency in the concentration of red cells and haemoglobin (Hb) in the blood and results in tissue hypoxia and acidosis (Manco-Johnson *et al.* 2006) An infant may be considered anaemic if the haemoglobin or haematocrit value is more than two standard deviations below normal for their gestational age group (Luchtman-Jones *et al.* 2002). All term and preterm infants experience a degree of physiological anaemia due to the conversion of fetal haemoglobin to adult haemoglobin during the first few weeks of postnatal life. Certain conditions may exacerbate this and lead to acute and chronic anaemia. These include acute or chronic blood loss or venesection and acute or chronic red blood cell haemolysis.

Physiological anaemia

During the first weeks of life all infants will experience a decrease in the number of circulating red blood cells from that of the in-utero level. It is universally acknowledged that healthy term infants will experience a drop in haemoglobin to 11–12g/dL at 10–12 weeks of age, which is well tolerated, and the Hb will then remain low for most of the first year of life. This postnatal decrease in Hb is commonly referred to as physiological anaemia (Strauss 2008).

Anaemia of prematurity

The majority of ELBW infants develop a normocytic, normochromic, hypopro-liferative anaemia characterised by inadequate production of erythropoietin (EPO).This is in addition to venesection losses causing low haematocrits (Bishara and Ohls 2009).

The mechanisms responsible for diminished EPO plasma levels in preterm infants have not been completely defined; however, one well-documented mechanism is that the liver is the primary site of EPO production in preterm infants, rather than the kidneys (Dame *et al.* 1998). This results in a less than optimal trigger for RBC production in this population as the hepatic response to hypoxia is less efficient than the renal response (Downey 1997).

Causes of pathological anaemia

Feto-maternal transfusion, twin-to-twin transfusion, obstetric difficulties and internal haemorrhage are causes of acute neonatal blood loss or haemorrhage (Bagwell 2007). Chronic anaemia may be associated with red cell destruction and haemolysis secondary to maternal–fetal blood group incompatibilities, acquired or congenital defects of red blood cells.

Feto-maternal transfusion is a common cause of occult fetal blood loss. Cohen and Manno (1996) suggest that some form of feto-maternal haemorrhage occurs in 50 per cent of pregnancies, though the blood loss is not usually significant. Confirmation of the presence of fetal cells in the maternal circulation is performed using the Kleihauer-Betke acid elution test.

Twin-to-twin transfusion is another cause of occult blood loss and occurs in 15–33 per cent of all monochorionic twins (Bagwell 2007). Weight differences greater than 20 per cent indicate that the smaller twin is the donor twin, though for weight differences less than 20 per cent either twin may be the donor and haematocrit values are used to determine donor and recipient. The donor twin is often anaemic with elevated reticulocytes. Conversely, the recipient twin is polycythaemic and may exhibit signs of congestive cardiac failure. The degree of anaemia will depend upon the duration and extent of the transfusion.

There are a number of obstetric complications that may occur during labour and delivery resulting in acute or chronic blood loss. Anaemia, secondary to chronic blood loss, results from conditions such as placental abruption and placenta praevia, while acute blood loss occurring at the time of delivery is seen in cases of severe placental abruption, umbilical cord rupture or incision/severing of the placenta during Caesarean section.

Anaemia may occur as a result of 'hidden' haemorrhages, for example, following intraventricular haemorrhage (see p. 187) associated with prematurity or other intracranial bleeds such as subdural, subarachnoid or subapnoneurotic haemorrhages, which can occur at any gestation. Massive cephalhaematoma, peritoneal, adrenal, renal and hepato-splenic haemorrhage secondary to traumatic or breech delivery may also result in anaemia.

Iatrogenic anaemia due to repeated blood sampling is an important consideration in the neonatal unit. Measures which may reduce blood volume depletion and the incidence of iatrogenic anaemia include: diagnostic testing based on individual infant condition rather than routine testing, micro sample laboratory techniques, non-invasive monitoring methods and documentation of blood sample volumes collected. This may in turn reduce the need for replacement blood transfusion therapy.

Red blood cell haemolysis

Neonatal haemolysis is now most commonly caused by G6PD deficiency and less commonly with isoimmunisation, as seen in ABO and Rh incompatibilities. Haemolysis of red blood cells may occur as a result of bacterial sepsis and viral infections, drug ingestion, either maternal or direct administration of the drug to the newborn. Other rare causes of red blood cell haemolysis are thalassemia and hereditary spherocytosis (Bagwell 2007).

Signs and symptoms of anaemia

In acute haemorrhage the infant will exhibit signs of acute cardiorespiratory compromise including **tachycardia**, hypovolaemia, hypotension, tachypnoea, pallor and poor peripheral perfusion. Infants with chronic anaemia will exhibit less obvious signs and symptoms and will have developed some tolerance to the condition. Although treatment is less urgent, the cause of chronic anaemia must be actively sought. Infants with chronic anaemia may present with lethargy, pallor, poor growth and a persistent or elevated oxygen requirement. Hepatosplenomegaly is not an uncommon finding on physical examination in infants with chronic anaemia because of extramedullary haematopoiesis.

Identification of the cause of anaemia through maternal and perinatal history review, laboratory data analysis and signs and symptoms will guide management and treatment options.

Management of anaemia

Iron supplementation

Without an exogenous source of iron, the preterm infant's iron stores are depleted by about 8 weeks and prophylactic oral iron supplementation from 2 months of age is an accepted practice across neonatal units (Rao and Georgieff 2002). Although formula milk has a greater iron content than that of breast milk, the iron in breast milk has a greater bioavailability. The recommended oral dosage of supplemental iron is 2mg/kg/day (Klein 2002). Concurrent administration of calcium and phosphorus supplements should be avoided as together with iron they form insoluble compounds, which reduce the bio-availability of each mineral (Jones and King 2005).

Transfusion therapy

RBC transfusion therapy has long been the standard of care for neonatal anaemia and ELBW infants are among the most highly transfused group of patients. Despite its widespread use, many aspects of RBC transfusion therapy are controversial and transfusion practices vary between neonatal units. Much of the controversy surrounding RBC transfusion therapy originates with the lack of consensus regarding criterion for transfusion. Diagnostic accuracy of clinical signs and correlation with laboratory findings of anaemia are yet to be defined, and at present local policies should guide practice.

Disease transmission and multiple donor exposure are two of the more significant risks associated with red blood cell transfusion; however, several methods of screening and blood preparation have been identified to minimise these risks. Bacterial/viral contamination should be a rare event since blood is screened for many of the known organisms including Hepatitis B and C, Human

Immunodeficiency Virus (HIV) and cytomegalovirus (CMV). Irradiation of blood products prevents Transfusion Associated Graft versus Host Disease (TA-GVHD), which is a potentially fatal incompatibility between recipient and donor cells. This rare condition is said to be more likely when the recipient receives blood from multiple donors (McCormack 1998) and the use of smaller packs of irradiated blood produced from one donor, stored for as long as possible, may help to prevent this (Strauss 2008).

First identified in 1996, Variant CJD (vCJD) is a transmissible spongiform encephalopathy (TSE) that is thought to be caused by the same agent as bovine spongiform encephalopathy (BSE). During the late 1990s and early 2000s, a number of successful vCJD precautionary measures were undertaken by the UK blood and tissue services to minimise potential transmission.

Recombinant Human Erythropoietin Therapy (r-HuEPO)

Erythropoietin is the glycoprotein that regulates the production rate of red blood cells. Studies in the USA and the UK have demonstrated that r-HuEPO is equally effective in raising haemoglobin levels and maintaining haematocrit levels during the normal phase of anaemia in the preterm infant (Bagwell 2007). Treatment with r-HuEPO is usually commenced when infants are stable, receiving enteral feeds and can tolerate iron supplementation. The recommended dose is 200–250 units/kg r-HuEPO given intravenously or via subcutaneous injection three times per week. Concurrent oral iron supplementation of 3mg/kg/day increasing to 6mg/kg/day is also recommended. Treatment is administered for 6 weeks or until 36 weeks' post-conceptual age is reached (Manco-Johnson *et al.* 2006).

Conclusion

Many questions remain unanswered about the optimum treatment for hae-matological disorders. As primary care-givers, neonatal nurses have a duty to keep abreast of clinical developments which lead to the introduction of new therapies and to be ready to incorporate these therapies when planning appropriate nursing care.

Case study: infant with jaundice

Steven is a 34-week gestation baby who is now 54 hours old. He is being breastfed and is reported to be sucking well. During a feed his mother asks you if he 'looks yellow'.

Q.1. What is the most likely cause of Steven's jaundice?

Q.2. Give your rationale for excluding the other causes.

Q.3. What are the physiological processes happening to cause it?

Q.4. Outline the investigations that will need to be undertaken.

Case study: infant with vitamin K deficient bleeding

Rose has just been admitted to your neonatal unit. She is 38 weeks' gestation and is 20 minutes old. Rose was diagnosed antenatally with congenital heart disease. Her condition is stable. Her mother intends to breastfeed.

Q.1. Prior to administering vitamin K, what information should you give the parents?

Q.2. What is the underlying pathophysiology in vitamin K deficient bleeding?

Q.3. What are the implications of the mother's choice to breastfeed?

Acknowledgements

Jackie Dent was the author of this chapter in the first edition.

References

Alcock, G.S. and Liley, H. (2003) 'Immunoglobulin infusion for isoimmune haemolytic jaundice in neonates', *Cochrane Database of Systematic Reviews*, Issue 3, Art. No. CD003313. DOI: 10.1002/14651858.CD003313.

American Academy of Pediatrics Subcommittee on Hyperbilirubinemia (2004) 'Clinical Practice Guideline management of hyperbilirubinemia in the newborn infant 35 or more weeks of gestation', *Pediatrics* 114(1): 297–316.

Ansell, P., Bull, D. and Roman, E. (1996) 'Childhood leukaemia and intramuscular vitamin K: findings from a case control study', *British Medical Journal* 313: 204–5.

Bagwell, G. (2007) 'A hematologic system', in C. Kenner and J.W. Lott (eds) *Comprehensive Neonatal Care: An Interdisciplinary Approach*, 4th edn, Philadelphia, PA: W.B. Saunders, pp. 249–50.

Beachy, J.M. (2007) 'Investigating jaundice in the newborn', *Neonatal Network* 26(5): 327–33.

Beeby, P. (2009) Department of Newborn Care, Royal Prince Alfred Hospital, Camperdown, New South Wales (personal communication).

Bishara, N. and Ohls, R.K. (2009) 'Current controversies in the management of the anemia of prematurity', *Seminars in Perinatology* 33(1): 29–34.

Blackburn, S.T. (1995) 'Hyperbilirubinaemia and neonatal jaundice', *Neonatal Network* 14(7): 15–25.

Blackburn, S.T. (2003) 'Bilirubin metabolism', in *Maternal, Fetal and Neonatal Physiology: A Clinical Perspective*, St Louis, MO: W.B. Saunders.

Bredemeyer, S., Polverino, J. and Beeby, P. (2007) 'Assessment of jaundice in the term infant: accuracy of transcutaneous bilirubinometers compared with serum bilirubin levels', *Neonatal, Paediatric and Child Health Nursing* April, 10: 1.

Cloherty, J. (1991) 'Neonatal hyperbilirubinaemia', in J. Cloherty and A. Stark (eds) *Manual of Neonatal Care*, 3rd edn, Boston, MA: Little, Brown.

Cohen, A. and Manno, C. (1996) 'Anemia: intensive care of the fetus and neonate', in A.R. Spitzer (ed.) *Intensive Care of the Fetus and Neonate*, St Louis, MO: Mosby.

Cremer, R., Perryman, P. and Richards, D. (1958) 'Influence of light on the hyper-bilirubinaemia of infants', *Lancet* i: 1094–7.

Dame, C., Fahnenstich, H., Freitag, P, Hofmann, D., Abdul-Nour, T., Bartmann, P. and Fandrey, J. (1998) 'Erythropoietin mRNA expression in human fetal and neonatal tissue', *Blood* 92: 3218–25.

Dennery, P.A., Seidman, D.S. and Stevenson, D.K. (2001) *New England Journal of Medicine* 344(8): 581–90.

Dodd, K. (1993) 'Neonatal jaundice, a lighter touch', *Archives of Disease in Childhood: Fetal and Neonatal Edition* 68: F529–F533.

Downey, P. (1997) 'Recombinant human erythropoietin as a treatment for anaemia of prematurity', *Journal of Perinatal and Neonatal Nursing* 11(3): 57–68.

Edwards, S. (1995) 'Phototherapy and the neonate: providing safe and effective nursing care for jaundiced infants', *Journal of Neonatal Nursing* Oct: 9–12.

Ehrenkranz, R. (1994) 'Iron requirements of preterm infants', *Nutrition* 10(1): 77–8.

Emery, M. (1992) 'Disseminated intravascular coagulation in the neonate', *Neonatal Network* 11: 5–14.

Evans, D. (2007) 'Neonatal jaundice', *BMJ Clinical Evidence* 12: 319.

Fleming, P., Speidel, B., Marlow, N. and Dunn, P. (1991) *A Neonatal Vade Mecum*, 2nd edn, London: Edward Arnold.

Frank, C.G. and Frank, P.H. (2006) 'Jaundice', in G.B. Merenstein and S.L. Gardner (eds) *Handbook of Neonatal Intensive Care*, 6th edn, St Louis, MO: Mosby, pp. 548–68.

Gartner, LM. (2001) *Journal of Perinatology* 21 Suppl. 1: S25–9; discussion S35–9.

Golding, J., Greenwood, R. and Birmingham, K. (1992) 'Childhood cancer, intramuscular vitamin K and pethidine given during labour', *British Medical Journal* 305: 341–6.

Golding, J., Paterson, M. and Kinlen, L. (1990) 'Factors associated with childhood cancer in a national cohort study', *British Journal of Cancer* 62: 304–8.

Hey, E. (1995) 'Neonatal jaundice: how much do we really know?', *MIDIRS Midwifery Digest* 5(1): 4–8.

Hey, E. (1998) 'Vitamin K: the debate continues', *MIDIRS Midwifery Digest* 8(2): 234–6.

Johnson, M., Rodden, D. and Collins, S. (1998) 'Newborn haematology', in G. Merenstein and S. Gardner (eds) *Handbook of Neonatal Care*, 4th edn, St Louis, MO: Mosby.

Jones, E. and. King, C. (eds) (2005) *Feeding and Nutrition in the Preterm Infant*, Oxford: Elsevier.

Juretschke, L.J.(2005) ' Kernicterus: still a concern', *Neonatal Network* 24: 7–19.

Kelnar, C., Harvey, D. and Simpson, C. (1995) *Care of the Newborn*, 3rd edn, London: Baillière Tindall.

Kemper, K., Forsyth, B. and McCarthy, P. (1989) 'Jaundice terminating breastfeeding and the vulnerable child', *Paediatrics* 84(5): 773–8.

Kenner, C., Brueggemeyer, A. and Gunderson, L. (1993) *Comprehensive Neonatal Nursing: A Physiologic Perspective*, Philadelphia, PA: W.B. Saunders.

Klebanoff, M., Read, J. and Mills, J. (1993) 'The risk of childhood cancer after neonatal exposure to vitamin K', *New England Journal of Medicine* 329(13): 905–8.

Klein, C.J. (2002) 'Nutrient requirements for preterm infant formulas', *Journal of Nutrition* 1232 (suppl. 1): 1395S–577S.

Kramer, L.I. (1996) 'Advancement of dermal icterus in the jaundiced newborn', *American Journal of Diseases of Children* 118: 454–8.

Kuehl, J. (1997) 'Neonatal disseminated intravascular coagulation', *Journal of Perinatal and Neonatal Nursing* 11(3): 69–77.

Letsky, E. and de Silva, M. (1994) 'Preventing Rh immunisation', *British Medical Journal* 30: 213–14.

Luchtman-Jones, L., Schwartz, A.L. and Wilson, D.B. (2002) 'Hematologic problems in the fetus and neonate', in A.A. Fanaroff and R.J. Martin (eds) *Neonatal-Perinatal Medicine*, 7th edn, St Louis, MO: Mosby.

Maisels, M.J. and McDonagh, A.F. (2008) 'Phototherapy for neonatal naundice', *New England Journal of Medicine* 8(358): 920–8.

Manco-Johnson, M., Rodden, D. and Collins, S. (2006) 'Newborn haematology', in G. Merenstein and S. Gardner (eds) *Handbook of Neonatal Intensive Care*, 4th edn, St Louis, MO: Mosby.

Mayne, S., Parker, J. and Harden, T. (1997) 'Rate of RhD sensitisation before and after implementation of a community based ante natal prophylaxis programme', *British Medical Journal* 3: 1588.

McClelland, D.B.L. (ed.) (2007) *Handbook of Transfusion Medicine*, 4th edn, London: The Stationery Office.

McCormack, K. (1998) 'Neonatal blood transfusions: a case for guidelines', *Journal of Neonatal Nursing* 4(5): 12–17.

MacDonald, M.G. (1995) 'Hidden risks: early discharge and bilirubin toxicity due to glucose-6 phosphate dehydrogenase deficiency', *Paediatrics* 96: 734–8.

Merenstein, G. and Gardner, S. (eds) (2006) *Handbook of Neonatal Intensive Care*, 6th edn, St Louis, MO: Mosby.

Messner, K., Leure-Dupree, A. and Maisels, M. (1975) 'The effect of continuous prolonged illumination on newborn retina', *Paediatric Research* 9: 368.

Modi, N. (1991) *A Guide to Phototherapy for Neonatal Hyperbilirubinaemia*, London: S. and W. Vickers.

Mundy, C.A. (2005) 'Intravenous immunoglobulin in the management of hemolytic disease of the newborn', *Neonatal Network* 24: 17–24.

Neonatal Formulary (2007) *Neonatal Formulary*, 5th edn, Oxford: Blackwell Publishing.

NHMRC (2006) *Joint Statement and Recommendations on Vitamin K Administration to Newborn Infants to Prevent Vitamin K Deficiency Bleeding in Infancy*, Canberra: National Health and Medical Research Council.

Noell, W.K., Walker, V., Kang, B.S. and Berman, S. (1966) 'Retinal damage by light in rats', *Investigative Ophthalmology* 5: 450–73.

Oddie S., Richmond, S. and Coulthard, M. (2001) 'Hypernatraemic dehydration and breast feeding: a population study', *Archives of Disease in Childhood* 85: 318–20.

Passmore, S. and McNinch, A. (1995) 'Vitamin K in infancy', *Current Paediatrics* 5: 36–8.

Raafat, A. and Urbaniak, S. (1996) 'Economic appraisal of prophylactic antepartum Rh programme', *Transfusion Medicine* 6 (Suppl.).

Rao, R. and Georgieff, M.K. (2002) ' Perinatal aspects of iron metabolism', *Acta Paediatrica* (Suppl.) 91: 124–9.

Roberton, N.R.C. (1992) *Textbook of Neonatology*, 2nd edn, London: Churchill Livingstone.

Robertson, K. (1993) 'Neonatal jaundice: a management update', *Modern Midwife* Nov/Dec: 24–7.

Rosenfield, W. (1990) 'A new device for phototherapy treatment of jaundiced infants', *Journal of Perinatology* 10: 243.

Royal College of Physicians (Edinburgh)/Royal College of Obstetricians and Gynecologists (1997) *Final Consensus Statement Relating to Anti D Prophylaxis in the UK: From the Consensus Panel: Consensus Conference on Anti D Prophylaxis*, London: author.

Ruchala, P.L., Seibold, L. and Stremsterfer, K. (1996) 'Validating assessment of neonatal jaundice with transcutaneous bilirubin measurement', *Neonatal Network* 15(4): 33–7.

Sanpavat, S. and Nuchprayoon, I. (2005) *Southeast Asian Journal of Tropical Medicine and Public Health* 36(6): 1533–7.

Schwoebel, A. and Sakraida, S. (1997) 'Hyperbilirubinaemia – new approaches to an old problem', *Journal of Perinatal and Neonatal Nursing* Dec: 78–97.

Seidman, D., Gale, R. and Stevenson, D. (1997) 'What should we do about jaundice?', in T. Hansen and N. McIntosh (eds) *Current Topics in Neonatology (2)*, London: W.B. Saunders.

Shannon, K., Keith, J. and Mentzer, W. (1995) 'Recombinant human erythropoietin stimulates erythropoiesis and reduces erythrocyte transfusions in very low birthweight preterm infants', *Paediatrics* 95: 1–8.

Steffensrud, S. (1998) 'Tin-metalloporphyrins: an answer to neonatal jaundice', *Neonatal Network* 17(5): 11–17.

Stevenson, D.K. and Vreman, H.J. (1997) 'Carbon monoxide and bilirubin production in neonates', *Pediatrics* 100(2): 252–9.

Strauss, R.G. (2008) 'How I transfuse red blood cells and platelets to infants with the anemia and thrombocytopenia of prematurity', *Transfusion* 48: 209–17.

Suresh, G.K., Martin, C.L. and Soll, R.F. (2003) 'Metalloporphyrins for treatment of unconjugated hyperbilirubinemia in neonates', *Cochrane Database of Systematic Reviews* 2003, Issue 1, Art. No. CD004207. DOI: 10.1002/14651858.CD004207.

Sutor, A.H., Von Kries, R., Cornelissen, E.A.M., McNinch, A.W. and Andrew, M. (1999) 'Vitamin K deficiency bleeding (VKDB) in infancy', *Journal of Thrombosis and Haemostasis* 81: 456–61.

Swanwick, T. (1989) 'The causes of neonatal jaundice', *Nursing* 3(39): 3–5.

Tan, K.L. (1994) 'Comparison of the efficacy of fiberoptic and conventional phototherapy for neonatal hyperbilirubinemia', *Journal of Pediatrics* 125: 607–12.

Todd, N. (1995) 'Isovolaemic exchange transfusion of the neonate', *Neonatal Network* 14(6): 75–7.

Truman, P. (2006) 'Jaundice in the preterm infant', *Paediatric Nursing* 18(5): 20–2.

Vreman, H.J., Wong, R.J. and Stephenson, D.K. (2004) 'Phototherapy: current methods and future directions', *Seminars in Perinatology* 28: 326–33.

Wong, R.J., Stevenson, D.K., Ahlfors, C.E. and Vreman, H.J. (2007) 'Neonatal jaundice: bilirubin physiology and clinical chemistry', *NeoReviews* 8: e58–e67.

Yeo, H. (1998) *Nursing the Neonate*, Oxford: Blackwell Science.

Chapter 10

Pain and Its Management in NICU

Kaye Spence

Contents

Introduction

In the past three decades there have been major changes in the attitudes and practices of clinicians in recognising and managing pain in neonates. Prior to this, pain was not seen as a priority and was often unrecognised or treated. Today, ground-breaking research has impacted on how pain is managed and the understanding of short-term and long-term consequences of pain. Unfortunately pain still remains an emotive issue for clinicians and the infant's inability to express pain can still result in under- or over-treatment of pain. More research needs to be undertaken on the treatment of pain in both the fetal and neonatal periods (American Academy of Pediatrics 2000; Anand *et al.* 2006).

Pain assessment and management remain controversial. There are many assessment tools available for acute pain; however, the assessment of pain remains underused in the neonatal intensive care and special care units. Choosing a suitable tool has been a challenge for many nurses and guideline statements now recommend that procedural pain is covered with some analgesia.

This chapter aims to provide the evidence for best practice in terms of assessment and management of pain in neonates. Nurses remain on the front line in ensuring that neonates and their families receive the best care for managing painful interventions. Despite an overwhelming volume of evidence, there still remains an evidence–practice gap for the assessment and management of pain in neonates (Gray *et al.* 2006; Harrison *et al.* 2006; Gharavi *et al.* 2007; Heaton *et al.* 2007).

Development of the pain pathways

Pain pathways consist of a network that communicates unpleasant sensations of noxious stimuli throughout the body. At birth, neonates have a developing and incomplete myelinated nervous system; however, all the components of the nociceptive (pain) pathways are present. Thus a newborn infant's nervous system is fully capable of transmitting, perceiving, responding to and remembering noxious stimuli even though it is not yet fully developed (Fitzgerald 1998).

Nociception occurs when harmful stimuli are signalled to the spinal cord through thinly myelinated and unmyelinated nerve fibres. These neuronal connections to the cortex are essential for the experience of pain and these occur late in gestation (ibid.). Physiological and behavioural response to noxious stimulation may occur early in development as the connections to the cortex where pain perception is mediated are immature (Slater *et al.* 2007) (Figure 10.1). Responses to noxious stimuli, such as limb withdrawal and increased heart rate, do not require the involvement of higher (cortical) brain structures; they are reflexes mediated at the level of the brainstem or spinal cord. As a result, these responses are measures of nociception (the detection of noxious stimuli) rather than the perception of pain (ibid.).

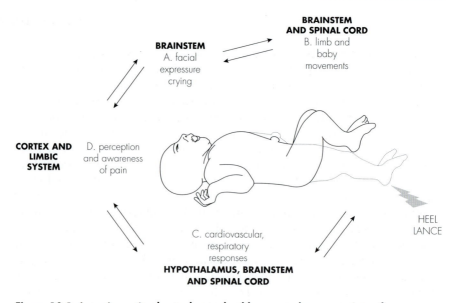

Figure 10.1 **A noxious stimulus such as a heel lance produces a variety of measurable responses in infants resulting from activation of neural circuits at different levels of the nervous system. Individual responses may be linked by the common stimulus or by interconnections. However, the presence of one of these responses does not necessarily mean that the others have occurred. Importantly, the presence or absence of A, B, and/or C does not predict D.**
Source: Slater *et al.* (2007), with permission from Elsevier.

There are three key aspects of sensory processing in the spinal cord which underlie responses to pain in the neonate. First, an infant's spinal sensory nerve cells are more excitable than an adult's. This makes their spinal reflex response to a harmful stimulus much greater and more prolonged. Second, individual sensory nerve cells in neonates have a much larger area of skin – or receptive fields than in adults. This means reflex responses can be triggered from a larger body area. Receptive fields combine to form a 'map' or image of our body surface in our brain and enable us to locate a stimulus in a particular part of our body. In neonates, the larger receptive fields result in a less precise or 'smeared' body map where the newborn responds less selectively and produces the same reflex to a light touch (Fitzgerald 2005; Bartocci *et al.* 2006).

Outcomes of pain

There are several consequences of untreated and unmanaged pain in the newborn period. Untreated pain which results in the release of stress hormones may exacerbate injury, delay wound healing, increase risk of infection and prolong hospitalisation (Anand *et al.* 2006).

Early pain experiences

The plasticity of the developing brain contributes to its vulnerability to the stressors that cause long-term developmental changes, ultimately leading to adverse neurological outcomes (Lowery *et al.* 2007). Observational studies have highlighted the impact of early pain experience upon later pain behaviour (Grunau *et al.* 1994; Taddio *et al.* 1997; Peters *et al.* 2005).

NICU environmental influences

Preterm infants often experience lengthy hospital stays that entail repeated painful procedures (Simons *et al.* 2003; Carbajal *et al.* 2008). Infants who are sicker and have been exposed to more painful procedures were found to have lower pain scores (Evans *et al.* 2005), and preterm infants who were subjected to painful procedures had a greater response to endo-tracheal tube suctioning (Grunau *et al.* 2000). Other procedures commonly carried out in the NICU have been found to be painful such as suprapubic aspiration (Kozer *et al.* 2006), eye examination (Mitchell *et al.* 2004), nappy change (Holsti *et al.* 2005) and central line placement (Taddio *et al.* 2006). Developmental care practices were found to decrease the pain response to a routine nursing procedure in medically stable preterm infants (Sizun *et al.* 2002). It is important to consider these influences and the context of the infant experiencing painful procedures during care.

Surgery

Taddio *et al.* (1997) found that male infants who had been circumcised at birth without analgesia responded with increased distress to vaccinations at 4 and 6 months of age compared with male infants who had not been circumcised. Term infants have learnt to anticipate pain following repeated skin-breaking procedures (Taddio *et al.* 2002), and hypersensitivity has been found in the same region as the surgery occurred (Andrews and Fitzgerald 2002) which may last for up to three years after the initial surgical tissue injury (Peters *et al.* 2005). These results suggest that pain responses may be mediated by factors such as experience in the neonatal intensive care unit, stress of the surgery and the emotion of separation.

Chronic pain

Chronic pain has been defined as a pathological pain state without apparent biological value that persists beyond normal tissue healing time. The assessment of neonates who are ventilated in terms of their need for analgesia is inadequate because of the limited ability to assess chronic pain in this group (Stevens *et al.* 2007; Whit Hall *et al.* 2007). Opioids are not recommended for routine use in ventilated babies (Bellù *et al.* 2008); however, this does not deny the presence of pain (Whit Hall *et al.* 2007). Nurses who are providing direct care for these neonates have an obligation to ensure that pain relief is given for stress indicators.

The message for the clinical nurse is that being aware of the consequences of pain, no matter how harmless it may appear, is to know that it has the potential to cause harm. Modifications of practice to meet the individualised needs of each infant should be part of each nurse's practice.

Expression of pain

Pain can be classified as physiologic, inflammatory, neuropathic or visceral and each of these classifications can have degrees of severity. None of these responses can be used in isolation; however, they may be used in conjunction to assess the degree of pain in neonates. The infant pain response is not merely immature compared to the adult's, but rather stems from a quite different underlying clinical and functional significance within developmental neurobiology (Fitzgerald and Beggs 2001).

Physiological response to pain

There are several parameters that may be measured to assess physiological responses to pain, including heart rate, blood pressure, respiratory rate, oxygenation, palm sweating, vagal tone and intracranial pressure. However, changes in these parameters may occur for other reasons and it is important to determine this when assessing whether the neonate is in pain (Anand *et al.* 2007). The systems that control cardiovascular function are closely associated with systems that modulate the perception of pain (ibid.). Heart rate can be bi-directional; that is, it increases first before decreasing; however, in the extremely **low birth weight** or fragile infant **bradycardia** alone may be the initial response.

Behavioural responses to pain

Pain expression in newborns has been described as a function of ongoing behavioural state, rather than solely reflecting tissue damage (Grunau and Craig 1987). Infants as young as 28 weeks' gestation have been observed to have a behavioural response to painful procedures (Johnston *et al.* 1996), therefore gestational age should not be used as a reason for excluding this component of an assessment of pain.

Cry is the most important method available to the infant to signal emotional and painful distress (Stevens *et al.* 2007). Analysis of pain cries has shown specific features such as sudden onset, high-pitched and prolonged cry followed by a protracted episode of inspiration and then a transition to further cycles of cry (Grunau *et al.* 1994).

Behavioural and physiologic responses to pain are different as the physiological signs such as heart rate can return to baseline soon after a procedure, whereas behavioural responses can remain elevated (Holsti *et al.* 2008). An emerging component of behavioural responses is taking into consideration the behavioural states of the infant.

Endocrine/metabolic manifestations of pain

Most of the early research concerning the endocrine response to pain has been undertaken on neonates undergoing surgery with minimal anaesthesia. Anand *et al.* (2007) demonstrated that the term infant appears to respond similarly to adults where **catcholamines**, glucagon, growth hormone, cortisol, aldosterone and other corticosteroids are released, resulting in a stress response of insulin suppression, increased metabolism of fat stores and carbohydrates and hyperglycaemia.. Frank *et al.* (2000) found that critically ill premature neonates have catecholamine concentrations equal to or greater than those of full-term neonates. The stress response may last for a longer period of time in the preterm infant because of their limited carbohydrate, protein and fat stores (Sparshott 1996).

The use of biochemical responses such as cortisol to assess pain in neonates in clinical practice is not readily available due to the requirement of blood collection, which in itself is a painful and distressing procedure (Harrison *et al.* 2005). Skin conductance is a potential measure for a metabolic response to pain (Harrison *et al.* 2006; Eriksson *et al.* 2008). Slater *et al.*'s (2007) research group has begun measuring cortical responses to noxious stimulation using near-infrared spectroscopy (NIRS). These advances in haemodynamic and electrical brain imaging have enabled a more precise assessment of the cortical activity required for the true experience of pain in the neonate. This cutting-edge research will allow examination of the behavioural correlates of cortical pain processing using haemodynamic and electrical brain imaging. The research will enable the development of a validated behavioural pain scale, combining the accuracy of cortical measurements with the ease of behavioural observations. We wait for the results of this research to enable assessment of pain to be more accurate.

Assessment of pain

The assessment of pain is an essential role for the clinical nurse and this should form part of the routine assessment procedure for infants assigned to the nurse. The difficulty in accurate measurement of pain in infants is a major impediment in providing effective analgesia for infants undergoing neonatal intensive care (Slater *et al.* 2008). There are over 40 tools for the assessment of acute neonatal pain and these have been reviewed by several authors (Duhn and Medves 2004;

Burton and MacKinnon 2007; Crellin *et al.* 2007). There has been a call for the validation of existing tools rather than developing even more (Franck 2002; Anand *et al.* 2006). Even though there are many pain assessment tools available, no single tool is seen as superior for use across the varied painful conditions or clinical situations and under-recognition and under-treatment of pain in infants still persist (Ranger *et al.* 2007).

When choosing a pain assessment tool, the infant population and setting, and the type of pain experienced must be taken into consideration (Boyle *et al.* 2006). The choice of a tool to use should be made after carefully considering the existing published options. Confidence that the tool will assess pain in a reproducible way is essential, and must be demonstrated with validity and reliability testing. Using an untested tool or combining tools is not recommended, and should only occur within a research protocol, with appropriate ethics and parental approval.

Pain tools have their limitations and can only be used as a guide for practice and decisions. By undertaking a pain assessment using a chosen tool, it opens up the dialogue between clinicians and often leads to joint decisions in relation to the management of an infant's pain and discomfort. For example, a painful stimulation generally evokes parallel cortical and behavioural responses in infants and pain may be processed at the cortical level without producing detectable behavioural changes. As a result, an infant with a low pain score based on behavioural assessment tools alone may not be pain-free (Slater *et al.* 2008). Table 10.1 describes a few of the tools in current use. There are many, and clinicians need to have a consensus based on the published literature and their specific context in deciding which tool they will use in clinical practice.

Behavioural states

In addition to using a multimodal pain assessment tool, consideration needs to be given to the behavioural state of the infant when the assessment is being undertaken. Behavioural states have been described by Als and Gilkerson (1995) and accommodate both term and preterm infants. State behaviours refer to sleeping and waking cycles. The link between behavioural states and pain responses in premature infants was observed during a study by Ahn (2006). In this study it was found that relatively healthy, premature infants who were in a state of quiet or active sleep could adequately express pain-related responses to NICU procedures. Ahn found that clinicians paid little attention to the infant's state before performing procedures, regardless of their invasive and stimulatory nature. In an attempt to consider the infant's behavioural states, Holsti *et al.* (2008) developed the Behavioural Indicators of Infant Pain (BIIP) scale which combines changes in sleep/wake states, five facial actions and two hand actions into a single score. This score has potential for measuring prolonged and chronic pain. However, nurses need to be familiar with the behavioural states as these should be included in their routine assessment of the infant (see p. 20).

Table 10.1 Some frequently used pain assessment tools

Tool	Variables	Type of pain	Clinical use	Resources available
BIIP (Behavioural Indicators of Infant Pain) (Holsti et al. 2008)	Sleep/wake states, five facial actions and two hand actions	Procedural Preterm	Reliability, moderate concurrent validity with a multidimensional pain scale (NIPS)	
COMFORT Scale (Van Dijk et al. 2005)	Movement, calmness, facial tension, alertness, respiration rate, muscle tone, heart rate, blood pressure	Post-operative pain in 0- to 3-year-old infant Ventilated and non-ventilated	Reliability, validity, clinical utility	CD available from author
NIPS (Neonatal Infant Pain Score) (Lawrence et al. 1993)	Facial expression, crying, breathing patterns, arm and leg movements, arousal	Procedural Preterm and full term	Reliability, validity	
NFCS (Neonatal Facial Coding System) (Peters et al. 2003)	Facial actions	Procedural	Reliability, validity, clinical utility, high degree of sensitivity to analgesia	
N-PASS (Neonatal Pain, Agitation, and Sedation Scale)	Crying, irritability, behavioural state, facial expression, extremity tone, vital signs	Post-operative, procedural, ventilated	Reliability, validity, includes sedation end of scale, does not distinguish pain from agitation	
PAT (Pain Assessment Tool) (Spence et al. 2005)	Physiological, behavioural, nurse's, perception	Post-operative, ventilated Term and preterm	Reliability and validity Comfort measures part of use Clinical utility	
PIPP (Premature Infant Pain Profile) (Stevens et al. 1996)	Heart rate, oxygen saturation, facial actions; takes state and gestational age into account	Procedural, post-operative (minor) Preterm, GA variable	Reliability, validity, clinical utility well established	Training CD

Guidelines for a pain assessment

Before undertaking a pain assessment, a guideline should be followed to ensure consistency and reliability in the assessment so that when handing over the patient at the end of a shift, the criteria used is similar and the context is the same:

- Familiarise yourself with the components of the assessment tool and the recommended actions from the score obtained.
- Stand where you can clearly see the baby's face and all of the body.
- Note the gestational age of the neonate.
- Observe the neonate's behavioural state for 30 seconds and take into consideration during your assessment.
- At conclusion of the observation, gently touch neonate's limb to determine muscle tone/tension.
- Complete the physiological and behavioural parameters.

During the score consider:

- Physiological conditions that may influence the score. For example, neonates with cyanotic heart disease would score their colour as normal unless there is a change in the intensity of the cyanosis or duskiness in response to pain.
- Medications the neonate is receiving or has recently received that may affect behaviour or physiological responses.
- Other environmental issues that may contribute to an elicited response from the neonate. For example, sudden bright lights, noise, activity around the bedspace.
- Document these potential distracters on the chart or in the notes at the time of the score.

When to do the assessment and score:

- At the commencement of your shift – think of pain assessment as a vital sign and a priority in assessment.
- Prior to and at the completion of a painful intervention.
- At least once per nursing shift (every four to six hours) and continue as long as analgesia is being used for pain relief.
- When analgesia is being weaned continue to score when the analgesia has been completed for a further 48 hours.

Action to be taken on the results of the pain assessment score:

- Depending on the assessment tool being used and the recommended thresholds, institute comfort measures or analgesia when the score is above baseline.
- Reassess one to two hours after administering analgesia or comfort measures.
- If the score continues to rise, then consider increasing dose of analgesia.

■ Reassess after one to two hours.
■ If score constantly at 0 and analgesia maintained, consider reducing the analgesia according to the guidelines.

Ensuring the reliability of staff in using a pain assessment score

Each clinician needs to be able to demonstrate their reliability in their assessment of a neonate's pain using a pain score. To assess the reliability of all staff and to teach new staff the following criteria for pain assessment skill is recommended:

■ Clinicians in groups of two or three observe the neonate as described above and each clinician scores the neonate's pain separately.
■ Compare scores and see where differences occur.
■ Reobserve neonate or a different neonate until consensus is reached for each parameter of the assessment tool.
■ This test and retest should occur on a regular basis for all staff.

Management of pain

A multidisciplinary approach to management of pain is required in the neonatal intensive care unit (Dunbar *et al.* 2006). This involves initially identifying stress and pain triggers and communicating these between the clinical teams. Stressors may include: a noisy, crowded environment, frequent handling followed at intervals by painful procedures, lack of soothing touch, poor use of analgesia during painful procedures, and frequent uncontrolled weaning of pain medications. A multidisciplinary approach involves identifying these triggers and, if possible, removing or justifying the noxious stimuli (Anand *et al.* 2001).

Comfort

The first line of care is to ensure basic comfort measures are instituted. Comfort measures include positioning the infant in a non-stressful way and ensuring there are boundaries to assist in self-regulation as a method of relieving stress. In addition, the use of a pacifier to encourage non-nutritive sucking, ensuring the nappy is dry and comfortable, and environmental modification to ensure the lights are dimmed and the noise and activity kept to a minimum. Handling infants has been found to increase the pain response after procedures (Cameron *et al.* 2007).

To protect the neurodevelopment of preterm and sick term infants and to provide best practice in neonatal intensive care, emphasis has been put on humane neonatal care, individualised developmentally supportive care, and family-centred care (Simons *et al.* 2001).

Non-pharmalogical interventions

A number of non-pharmacological therapies have been used for managing pain in neonates (Golianu *et al.* 2007). A systematic literature review undertaken by Cignacco *et al.* (2007) provides evidence of the pain-relieving effects of non-pharmacological interventions among preterm and term neonates. Non-pharmacological interventions include: non-nutritive sucking, swaddling, **facilitated tucking** as well as the use of breastfeeding and sucrose for procedural pain. It needs to be emphasised, however, that non-pharmacological interventions cannot replace pharmacological treatment in cases of severe and chronic pain.

Sucrose

The use of oral sucrose solution with and without non-nutritive sucking (NNS) (pacifier use) has been shown to reduce the physiological and behavioural responses to procedural pain in neonates. Its administration has been the most frequently studied non-pharmacologic intervention for relief of procedural pain in neonates (Stevens *et al.* 2004).

Sucrose is considered an ideal analgesia for use prior to a painful procedure because it is commercially available, inexpensive, easily administered, non-invasive, short-acting and non-sedating. The administration of sucrose does not require additional training for administration or monitoring of the infant and does not expose the infant to risks greater than those associated with breast or bottle-feeding. The rapid onset and the absence of long-term effects of the analgesia support the utilisation of sucrose during many procedures in hospital settings (Hatfield *et al.* 2008).

Sucrose is administered orally where it is absorbed through the buccal mucosa. As it is not ingested, it can be given to infants who are not yet enterally fed. It is ineffective if given via a gastric tube. The recommended dose is 0.5ml of 24 per cent sucrose (Stevens *et al.* 2004). This dose is administered by one drop on the tongue two minutes prior to the procedure and further drops repeated during the procedure if necessary. It is contra-indicated to give the complete dose in one go. The action is triggered by the sweet taste of the sucrose.

There are several myths surrounding the use of sucrose as an analgesia for procedural pain in neonates and these can be a barrier to the use of sucrose (Harrison 2008). The concerns about sucrose causing unwanted complications such as an increased risk of necrotising enterocolitis, hyperglycaemia, adverse neurodevelopmental outcomes, or a tolerance to sucrose analgesia are unfounded.

Breastfeeding

If available, breastfeeding or breast milk can be used to alleviate procedural pain in neonates undergoing a single painful procedure (Shah *et al.* 2006). The analgesic effects of breastfeeding or breast milk include the presence of a comforting person (mother) (Blass and Shide 1995), physical sensation (skin-to-skin contact with comforting person) (ibid.), diversion of attention (Gunnar 1984) and sweetness of breast milk (presence of lactose or other ingredients present in the breast milk) (Blass 1997). Breast milk contains a higher concentration of tryptophan (Heine 1999), a precursor of melatonin which has been shown to increase the concentration of beta endorphins (Barrett *et al.* 2000) and could possibly be one of the mechanisms for the nociceptive-relieving effects of breast milk.

The effectiveness of breast milk for repeated painful procedures is not established and further research is needed (Shah *et al.* 2006). However, breastfeeding should be encouraged as a first line analgesia for procedural pain. For this to occur there needs to be a substantial effort made to inform the families of this strategy and support them in their efforts to help manage their infant's pain.

Non-nutritive sucking (NNS)

'Non-nutritive sucking' refers to the use of a pacifier in an infant's mouth to promote sucking behaviour without breast or formula milk to provide nutrition. Non-nutritive sucking achieves a moderate effect on the behaviour of preterm and term neonates, regardless of neonatal complications. NNS was found to have no effect on respiratory rate or transcutaneous oxygen tension; however, it reduced the time of crying and increased heart rate during a heel lance (Corbo *et al.* 2000). NNS can be recommended to reduce distress in newborns undergoing invasive routine procedures.

Skin-to-skin care (also known as Kangaroo Mother Care)

Skin-to-skin care can lead to a decrease in stressful neurobehavioural signs after blood-taking procedures in premature infants. The analgesic effects of skin-to-skin care occur due to endogenous mechanisms which are elicited through the continuous tactile stimulation during the interaction which may serve as a pain inhibitory system by activating endogenous pain-modulating systems (Johnston *et al.* 2008; Kostandy *et al.* 2008). Painful procedures such as the heel lance in premature infants can be performed while the infant is being held in the skin-to-skin position (Ferber and Makhou 2008). Skin-to-skin care before and during a heelstick has been found to be effective in reducing the crying response in medically stable premature infants (Ludington-Hoe *et al.* 2005; Kostandy *et al.* 2008).

As skin-to-skin care can lead to lessening of painful reactions after heelstick and venepuncture in premature infants, consideration needs to be given (where practical) for infants to be held skin-to-skin during these painful procedures. This practice will require organisation and preparation to enable the intervention to be successful.

Odour

The use of a familiar odour, such as the mother's milk or smell, has been used to help settle and soothe infants (Rattaz *et al.* 2005). During short-term procedural pain, such as venepuncture, infants exposed to a familiar odour demonstrated little to no crying (Goubet *et al.* 2003). These findings are supported by evidence on early memory and olfactory competence in foetuses and newborns. Goubet's (2003) study showed that a familiar odour prevented crying, and therefore limited the energy spent during blood collection.

Some of the non-pharmacological interventions have an evident favourable effect on pulse rate, respiration and oxygen saturation, on the reduction of motor activity, and on the excitation states after invasive measures (Figure 10.2). It is recommended that further research should emphasise the use of validated pain assessment instruments for the evaluation of the pain-alleviating effect of non-pharmacological interventions (Cignacco *et al.* 2006).

Pharmacological interventions

Pharmacological agents may be required to alleviate pain in neonates in intensive care who are subjected to numerous invasive procedures or in the post-operative period. There is considerable clinical and experimental evidence to support the practice of providing adequate analgesia for newborns undergoing invasive procedures, medical, surgical, diagnostic or therapeutic or who develop condi-

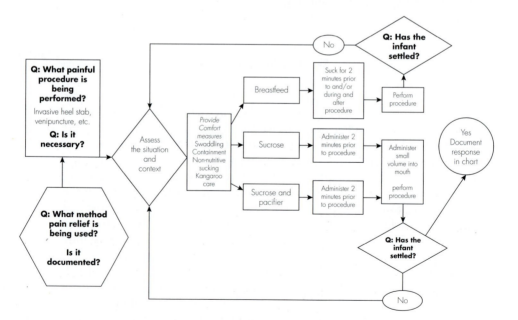

Figure 10.2 Algorithm for the management of procedural pain

tions associated with considerable pain such as necrotising enterocolitis. Despite an overwhelming volume of evidence, analgesia still remains underutilised (Carbajal *et al.* 2008). A neonatal pain control group was established to further address issues related to pain management and they identified three main themes: (1) procedural pain; (2) sedation and analgesia during mechanical ventilation; and (3) pain and stress following surgery (Anand *et al.* 2006).

Opioids

Opioids remain the gold standard for relief of moderate to severe pain in neonates. However, there is scant data on morphine or fentanyl dosing regimens that uniformly relieves pain in non-intubated neonates (Anand *et al.* 2006). A systematic review found that there is insufficient evidence to recommend routine use of opioids in mechanically ventilated newborns (Bellù *et al.* 2008); therefore opioids should be used selectively, when indicated by clinical judgement and through the evaluation of pain indicators.

Potential adverse effects of opioids include the slowing of gastric and intestinal motility, feeding intolerance, dependence and tolerance and adverse neurological effects (Taddio *et al.* 2002). Concerns have been raised about the potential inhibition of the respiratory drive, leading to difficulties in weaning from mechanical ventilation. Although it is well known that the prolonged use of opioid analgesics results in opioid tolerance, even the use of a single dose or a few doses of opioids during critical periods of early development may lead to opioid tolerance in neonates (Suresh and Anand 2001).

Morphine

Morphine is the most widely used and studied opioid in critically ill infants and those undergoing post-operative pain management. Although it is commonly used in the NICU as a continuous infusion, its use for pain relief for acute procedural pain is less effective (Carbajal *et al.* 2005). When used in combination with a local application of tetracaine, it was found to be effective for the procedure of insertion of a percutaneous central venous catheter (Taddio *et al.* 2006).

There are several effects of morphine that need to be considered. Morphine is commonly used for ventilated infants; however, these infants have a slower morphine metabolism than spontaneously breathing neonates (Bouwmeester *et al.* 2003). Side effects include marked respiratory depression, bradycardia and hypotension. Some authors suggest the clinical importance of this hypotension may be minimal, as the measures of overall blood pressures together with the use of volume expanders and vasopressor drugs showed no significant difference between infants treated with morphine or a placebo (Simons *et al.* 2006).

Morphine has a long half life (6 to 14 hours in preterm, 2 to 11 hours in term babies) and provides greater sedation than other opioids (see p. 448). Tolerance may develop after prolonged use and it is recommended that it is weaned slowly (Young and Magnum 2008). Behavioural observation can be used as indication for tapering off the morphine infusion, thus preventing overdosing with its associated risks (Bouwmeester *et al.* 2003).

Fentanyl

Fentanyl is synthetic opioid that is 50 to 100 times more potent than morphine on a weight basis (see p. 448). It penetrates the CNS rapidly and the serum half life is 1 to 15 hours and is prolonged in infants with liver failure (Young and Magnum 2008). Infants receiving a fentanyl infusion should be observed closely for chest wall rigidity, urine retention and laryngospasm. Infants who have been on a continuous infusion of fentanyl for more that five days have shown significant withdrawal symptoms.

Opioid withdrawal

Clinical and experimental data suggest that the duration of opioid receptor occupancy is an important factor in the development of tolerance and dependence and that continuous administration of opioids may produce tolerance more rapidly than intermittent therapy (Suresh and Anand 2001). Indirect clinical evidence suggests a more rapid development of tolerance occurs in preterm neonates than in term neonates.

Withdrawal symptoms can appear from one hour to three days after a decrease in analgesia or sedation dose. Symptom onset appears to be related to increment or speed of weaning. In one study, the withdrawal symptoms occurred as late as six days after commencement of weaning greater than 10 per cent (Franck *et al.* 2004).

The clinical features specific to opioid withdrawal primarily include neurological, gastrointestinal, as well as autonomic signs and symptoms (Suresh and Anand 2001). The four most common signs of withdrawal are: sleeplessness, diarrhoea, mydriasis and tremors (Franck *et al.* 2004).

Regular assessment for iatrogenic narcotic withdrawal includes both physiological and behavioural parameters during the weaning of the analgesia to enable a diagnosis of opioid withdrawal to be made and appropriate management instituted. There are multiple validated assessment scales available, although many have come from assessment of infants of drug-dependent women. However, instead of nominating an ideal scale, it is more important to use a consistent scoring system using a familiar scale (Suresh and Anand 2001).

Oral and parenteral opioids have been used successfully for the management of tolerance. Various preparations of morphine are frequently used to treat withdrawal. The dosage is adjusted to offset the signs and symptoms of withdrawal. There are different views of weaning from opioids. There have been reports of rapid decrease in opioid dosing over a period of two to three days with success; however, it is preferable for a gradual decrease (approximately 10 per cent of the current dose) of opioids over a period of time (Suresh and Anand 2001).

Post-operative pain management

Neonates who undergo a surgical operation in the neonatal period are vulnerable to pain in the post-operative period. Infants experience pain during the post-operative period as a result of the surgical procedure as well as from continuing post-operative interventions which can be many and repeated.

The ideal medicines and doses that provide sufficient analgesia after major surgery in neonates remain largely unknown. Morphine given as a continuous infusion is more feasible and might be regarded as safer in neonates (Bouwmeester *et al.* 2003).

Neonates who are younger than 7 days old require significantly less morphine post-operatively than older neonates (Fitzgerald and Beggs 2001; Bouwmeester *et al.* 2003) and maintain higher plasma morphine levels. For neonates older than 7 days a morphine dose of 10µg/kg per hour was found to be sufficient for post-operative analgesia after noncardiac major surgery (Bouwmeester *et al.* 2003). The dose may need to be adjusted if there are hepatic and renal disturbances. For neonates aged 7 days or younger, a morphine infusion of 5–10µg/kg per hour is recommended (ibid.). However, these doses are recommendations and each infant needs to be assessed and their pain management regime altered based on their individual responses.

Epidural

Epidural anaesthesia can be accomplished at various sites along the epidural space (see p. 376). Caudal catheters were found to account for 50 per cent of neonatal epidural catheters (Llewellyn and Moriarty 2007; Sethna and Suresh 2007). This may be a reflection of the relative ease of access and catheter placement in this group. The commonest drugs are: bupivavaine, lidocaine and ropivacaine. All staff caring for a neonate with an epidural infusion need to ensure that thorough prescribing, checking and administration guidelines are in place (Llewellyn and Moriarty 2007).

Topical agents

Topical anaesthetics are now available as creams, gels and a heat-activated patch system. Lidocaine injection continues to be widely used for pain associated with circumcision, lumbar puncture, or placement of central venous lines. Local anesthetics reduce pain during common medical procedures performed in neonates with the exception of heel lances. Topical treatments include liposomal lidocaine, lidocaine–prilocaine mixture and tetracaine, in addition to lidocaine injections, and can be effective analgesic options for neonates (Lehr and Taddio 2007).

Professional issues

Clinical guidelines and practice

Position statement and clinical practice recommendations for pain assessment in the nonverbal patient have been developed and issued in many countries (American Academy of Pediatrics 2000; Royal Australian College of Physicians 2006). Guidelines are a useful way of putting the evidence for pain assessment and management into practice. However, it is the responsibility of practising clinicians to be aware of the guidelines supporting their own practice and to adhere to these recommendations.

Caregiver knowledge and response to newborn pain

Gaps in knowledge can be attributed to the lack of basic knowledge about pain behaviour, overreliance on an invasive short-term pain model, pain measurement issues, and lack of knowledge about contributing factors to the painful experience (Warnock and Lander 2004). How nurses respond to the infant's pain is often influenced by their personal perception of pain and their work with others in the care team.

Studies (Pillai Riddell and Craig 2007) have shown that similar ratings on a pain scale may have different meanings for various caregiver groups which can result in different management strategies. Nurses were found to appropriately identify pain display indicators such as crying, vital sign changes and body movement; however, having this specific pain assessment knowledge did not translate to their care practices (Campbell-Yeo 2008). When caring for a neonate in pain, nurses can have emotional reactions (Nagy 1998) or an empathetic response (Campbell-Yeo 2008), both of which have a central role in the recognition and treatment of pain.

Part of the nurse's role is as an advocate for best practice by ensuring there are guidelines available; these are used to inform practice. Practice is measured by way of clinical audits to ensure pain management is individualised and best practice based on evidence.

Ethical aspects of neonatal pain

Pain assessment and management can raise ethical issues for neonatal staff with the infant's best interests being of primary concern. When neonates are subjected to painful procedures, it can be argued that it is not in the infant's best interest (see p. 478) to withhold pain relief (Spence 2000). If pain relief is withheld on the assumption that the medicine may be harmful to the infant, then this raises the issue of the boundaries of preserving life and health. The ethical issues associated with the treatment for neonatal pain are complex. All the long-term consequences of continued exposure to pain experienced by neonates are unknown. Therefore, the focus for this dilemma is to try to reduce the exposure to pain. Consideration of each potentially painful procedure needs to be a priority for each caregiver. The number of painful procedures carried out in the NICU needs to be reduced and the indiscriminate use of routines without a clear rationale reviewed by the multidisciplinary team.

Families

Parents of infants in the neonatal intensive care unit may worry that their infant may experience pain, and this concern may contribute to increased parental stress. Franck *et al.* (2005) identified six conceptual categories which parents found distressing about their infant's pain. These were: (1) causes of infant pain; (2) parent concerns about infant pain and pain management; (3) parent information needs; (4) parent involvement; (5) differing views among parents and health care professionals about the care of infant pain; and (6) parent views on how health care professionals can improve infant pain care. Nurses can assist parents by being aware of these issues and address them as they talk about the baby's pain or potential pain.

Nurses cannot care for neonates without considering the parents and their involvement in their infant's care. Communication regarding neonatal pain is a challenge and may be difficult between parents and nurses, leading to frustration for both (Simons *et al.* 2001) and an undercurrent of anxiety (Table 10.2). Parents may be apprehensive about actively participating in their infant's

Table 10.2 Suggested wording for parents' information brochure to support their infants during a painful procedure

Identifying your baby's responses. You can assist the nurses and doctors by describing your baby's responses to them. The nurses may assess your baby's signals by using a standard chart.

How to comfort your baby. If a procedure is required that is likely to cause your baby pain, you can comfort the baby by holding or supporting them during the procedure. If you are breastfeeding, it can be helpful to give your baby a breastfeed a couple of minutes before the procedure. If you are not breastfeeding, then ask the nurses to provide some sucrose for your baby prior to the procedure.

Being present during procedures. Holding your baby during a procedure may comfort your baby; however, you may decide that this is too uncomfortable for you to do.

pain care in case they are labelled as 'demanding'. There needs to be good communication and support for the parents as witnessing their baby's pain can be very distressing.

Conclusion

Neonatal pain is an emotive issue and nurses can help alleviate pain and suffering through careful assessment and ensuring appropriate interventions are provided. By having an understanding of the mechanisms of neonatal pain pathways, nurses should be able to demonstrate effective assessment skills which in turn contribute to best practice. Despite a large amount of evidence regarding painful procedures and effective management, there remains a gap in what actually occurs in practice.

It is envisaged that nurses who learn about pain in the newborn will be empowered to provide interventions to ensure that neonates in NICU and SCN will receive adequate relief not only from procedural pain but also from chronic pain associated with ventilation and surgery.

Case study: pain management

George is a 26-week gestation infant weighing 875 grams. He delivered by emergency Caesarean section following maternal antepartum haemorrhage. His mother did not receive antenatal steroids. He was born in fair condition and was intubated and given surfactant immediately after delivery. Following stabilisation, he is transferred to the neonatal intensive care unit, where he continues to require mechanical ventilation. Umbilical arterial and venous lines are sited for monitoring and intravenous therapy and medication.

Q.1. Does George need any pain relief given that he is so premature? Please qualify your answer.

Q.2. How would you assess George's need for pain relief?

Q.3. What drugs could be used in this situation?

Q.4. Are there any non-pharmacological strategies you could employ to keep George comfortable?

Q.5. How would you assess whether the pain-relieving strategies were effective?

On day two of life it is decided to site a percutaneous long line to administer total parenteral nutrition.

Q.6.   What would you consider prior to this procedure being undertaken?

George establishes full enteral feeding over the subsequent week and is also extubated to CPAP. By day 21 of life he is self-ventilating in air and is being cared for in the special care nursery.

Q.7.   George will still require regular blood tests and naso-gastric tube changes during his stay in the nursery; what strategies could you use to ensure his safety and comfort during these procedures?

Q.8.   Are there any long-term sequela for George following his admission to NICU with regard to painful procedures and noxious stimulation?

References

Ahn, Y. (2006) 'The relationship between behavioral states and pain responses to various NICU procedures in premature infants', *Journal of Tropical Pediatrics* 52(3): 201–5.

Als, H. and Gilkerson, L. (1995) 'Developmentally supportive care in the neonatal intensive care unit', *Zero to Three* 16(6): 1–10.

American Academy of Pediatrics (Committee on Fetus and Newborn. Committee on Drugs. Section on Anesthesiology. Section on Surgery. Canadian Paediatric Society. Fetus and Newborn Committee) (2000) 'Prevention and management of pain and stress in the neonate', *Pediatrics* 105(2): 454–61.

Anand, K.J.S. and International Evidence-based Group for Neonatal Pain (2001) 'Consensus statement for the prevention and management of pain in the newborn', *Archives of Pediatric and Adolescent Medicine* 155(2): 173–80.

Anand, K.J.S., Stevens, B. and McGrath, P.J. (2007) *Pain in Neonates and Infants*, Philadelphia, PA: Elsevier.

Anand, K.J.S., Aranda, J., Berde, C., Buckman, S., Capparelli, E., Carlo, W. *et al.* (2006) 'Summary proceedings from the neonatal pain-control group', *Pediatrics* 117(3): S9–S22.

Andrews, K. and Fitzgerald, M. (2002) 'Wound sensitivity as a measure of analgesic effects following surgery in human neonates', *Pain* 99: 185–95.

Barrett, T., Kent, S. and Voudoris, N. (2000) 'Does melatonin modulate beta-endorphin, corticosterone, and pain threshold?', *Life Sciences* 66: 467–76.

Bartocci, M., Bergqvist, L., Lagercrantz, H. and Anand, K.J.S. (20006) 'Pain activates cortical areas in the preterm newborn brain', *Pain* 122: 109–17.

Bellù, R., de Waal, K.A. and Zanini, R. (2008) 'Opioids for neonates receiving mechanical ventilation', *Cochrane Database of Systematic Reviews*, Issue 1, Art. No. CD004212. DOI: 10.1002/14651858.CD004212. pub 3.

Blass, E.M. (1997) 'Milk-induced hypoalgesia in human newborns', *Pediatrics* 99: 825–9.

Blass, E.M. and Shide, D.J. (1995) 'Mother as a shield: differential effects of contact and nursing on pain responsivity in infant rats: evidence for nonopioid mediation', *Behavioral Neuroscience* 109: 342–53.

Bouwmeester, N., Hop, W., van Dijk, M., Anand, K.J.S., van den Anker, J. and Tibboel, D. (2003) 'Postoperative pain in the neonate: age-related differences in morphine requirements and metabolism', *Intensive Care Med* 29: 2009–15.

Boyle, E.M., Freer, Y., Wong, C.M., McIntosh, N. and Anand, K.J.S. (2006) 'Assessment of persistent pain or distress and adequacy of analgesia in preterm ventilated infants', *Pain* 124: 87–91.

Burton, J. and MacKinnon, R. (2007) 'Selection of a tool to measure post-operative pain on a neonatal surgical unit', *Infant* 3(5): 188–96.

Cameron, E.C., Raingangar, V. and Khoor (2007) 'Handling procedures on pain responses of very low birth weight infants', *Pediatric Physical Therapy* 19: 40–7.

Campbell-Yeo, M., Latimer, M. and Johnston, C.M. (2008) 'The empathetic response in nurses who treat pain: concept analysis', *Journal of Advanced Nursing* 61(6): 711–19.

Carbajal, R., Lenclen, R., Jugie, M., Paupe, A., Barton, B. and Anand, K. (2005) 'Morphine does not provide adequate analgesia for acute procedural pain among preterm infants', *Pediatrics* 115(6): 1494–500.

Carbajal, R., Rousset, A., Danan, C., Coquery, S., Nolent, P. *et al.* (2008) 'Epidemiology and treatment of painful procedures in neonates in intensive care units', *JAMA* 300(1): 60–70.

Cignacco, E., Hamers, J.P.H., Stoffel, L., van Lingen, R.A., Gessler, P., McDougall, J. and Nelle, M. (2007) 'The efficacy of non-pharmacological interventions in the management of procedural pain in preterm and term neonates: a systematic literature review', *European Journal of Pain* 11(2): 139–52.

Corbo, M.G., Mansi, G., Stagni, A., Romano, A., Van den Heuvel, J., Capasso, L., Raffio, T., Zoccali, S. and Paludetto, R. (2000) 'Nonnutritive sucking during heelstick procedures decreases behavioral distress in the newborn infant', *Biol Neonate* 77: 162–7.

Crellin, D., Sullivan, P., Babel, F., O'Sullivan, R. and Hutchinson, A. (2007) 'Analysis of the validation of existing behavioral pain and distress scales for use in the procedural setting', *Pediatric Anesthesia* 17: 720–33.

Duhn, L. and Medves, J. (2004) 'A systematic integrative review of infant pain assessment tools', *Advances in Neonatal Care* 4(3): 126–40.

Dunbar, A.E., Sharek, P.J., Mickas, N.A., Coker, K.L., Duncan, J., McLendonf, D., Pagano, C., Puthoff, T., Reynolds, N.L., Powers, R.J. and Johnston, C.C. (2006) 'Implementation and case-study results of potentially better practices to improve pain management of neonates', *Pediatrics* 118, Suppl. 2: 87–94.

Eriksson, M., Storm, H., Fremming, A. and Schollin, J. (2008) 'Skin conductance compared to a combined behavioural and physiological pain measure in newborn infants', *Acta Pædiatrica* 97: 27–30.

Evans, J., McCartney, E., Lawhon, G. and Galloway, J. (2005) 'Longitudinal comparison of preterm pain responses to repeated heelsticks', *Pediatric Nursing* 31(3): 216–21.

Ferber, S.G. and Makhou, I.R. (2008) 'Neurobehavioural assessment of skin-to-skin effects on reaction to pain in preterm infants: a randomized, controlled within-subject trial', *Acta Paediatrica* 97: 171–6.

Fitzgerald, M. (1998) 'The birth of pain', *MRC News*: 20–3.

Fitzgerald, M. (2005) 'The development of nociceptive circuits', *Nature Reviews: Neuroscience* 6: 507–20.

Fitzgerald, M. and Beggs, S. (2001) 'The neurobiology of pain: developmental aspects', *The Neuroscientists* 7: 246–57.

Franck, L (2002) 'Some pain, some gain: reflections on the past two decades of neonatal pain research and treatment', *Neonatal Network: The Journal of Neonatal Nursing* 21(5): 37–41.

Franck, L., Naughton, I. and Winter, I. (2004) 'Opioid and benzodiazepine withdrawal symptoms in paediatric intensive care patients', *Intensive and Critical Care Nursing* 20: 344–51.

Franck, L., Allen, A., Cox, S. and Winter, I. (2005) 'Parents' views about infant pain in neonatal intensive care', *Clinical Journal of Pain* 21(2): 133–9.

Franck, L., Boyce, W., Gregory, G., Jemerin, J., Levine, J. and Miaskowski, C. (2000) 'Plasma norepinephrine levels, vagal tone index, and flexor reflex threshold in premature neonates receiving intravenous morphine during the postoperative period: a pilot study', *Clinical Journal of Pain* 16(2): 95–104.

Gharavi, B., Schott, C., Nelle, M., Reiter, G. and Linderkamp, O. (2007) 'Pain management and the effect of guidelines in neonatal units in Austria, Germany and Switzerland', *Pediatrics International* 49: 652–8.

Golianu, B., Krane, E., Seybold, J., Almgren, C. and Anand, K.J.S. (2007) 'Non-pharmacological techniques for pain management in neonates', *Seminars in Perinatology* 31: 318–22.

Goubet, N., Rattaz, C., Pierrat, V., Bullinger, A. and Lequien, P. (2003) 'Olfactory experience mediates response to pain in preterm newborns', *Developmental Psychobiology* 42: 171–80.

Gray, P.H., Trotter, J.A., Langbridge, P. and Doherty, C.V. (2006) 'Pain relief for neonates in Australian hospitals: a need to improve evidence-based practice', *Journal of Paediatric Child Health* 42: 10–13.

Grunau, R.V. and Craig, K.D. (1987) 'Pain expression in neonates: facial action and cry', *Pain* 28: 395–410.

Grunau, R.V., Holsti, L. and Whitfield, M. (2000) 'Are twitches, startles, and body movements pain indicators in extremely low birth weight infants?', *Clinical Journal of Pain* 16: 37–45.

Grunau, R.V., Whitfield, M.F. and Petrie, J.H. (1994) 'Early pain experience, child and family factors, as precursors of somatization: a prospective study of extremely premature and full-term children', *Pain* 56: 353–9.

Gunnar, M. (1984) 'The effects of a pacifying stimulus on behavioral and adrenocortical responses to circumcision in the newborn', *Journal of the American Academy of Child and Adolescent Psychiatry* 23: 34–8.

Harrison, D. (2008) 'Oral sucrose for pain management in infants: myths and misconceptions', *Journal of Neonatal Nursing* 14: 39–46.

Harrison, D., Johnston, L. and Loughnan, P. (2006) 'Pain assessment and pain management practices in Australian neonatal units', *Journal of Paediatric Child Health* 42: 6–9.

Harrison, D., Spence, K., Gillis, D., Johnston, L. and Nagy, S. (2005) 'Salivary cortisol measurements in sick infants: a feasible and objective method of measuring stress', *Journal of Neonatal Nursing* 11: 10–17.

Harrison, D., Boyce, S., Loughnan, P., Dargaville, P., Storm, H. and Johnston, L. (2006) 'Skin conductance as a measure of pain and stress in hospitalised infants', *Early Human Development* 82(9): 603–8.

Hatfield, L.A., Gusic, M.E., Dyer, M.A. and Polomano, R.C. (2008) 'Analgesic properties of oral sucrose during routine immunizations at 2 and 4 months of age', *Pediatrics* 121(2): e327–e334.

Heaton, P., Herd, D. and Fernando, A. (2007) 'Pain relief for simple procedures in New Zealand neonatal units: practice change over six years', *Journal of Paediatrics and Child Health* 43: 394–7.

Heine, W.E. (1999) 'The significance of tryptophan in infant nutrition', *Advances in Experimental Medicine and Biology* 467: 705–10.

Holsti, L., Grunau, R., Oberlander, T. and Osiovich, H. (2008) 'Is it painful or not? Discriminant validity of the behavioral indicators of infant pain (BIIP) scale', *Clinical Journal of Pain* 24: 83–8.

Holsti, L., Grunau, R., Oberlander, T. and Whitfield, M. (2005) 'Prior pain induces heightened motor responses during clustered care in preterm infants in the NICU', *Early Human Development* 81: 293–302.

Johnston, C.C., Filion, F. Campbell-Yeo, M., Goulet, C., Bell, L., McNaughton, K., Byron, J., Aita, M., Finley, G.A. and Walker, C.D. (2008) 'Kangaroo mother care diminishes pain from heel lance in very preterm neonates: a crossover trial', *BMC Pediatrics* 8: 13.

Johnston, C.C., Stevens, B., Yang, F. *et al.* (1996) 'Developmental changes in response to heel stick in preterm infants: a prospective cohort study', *Developmental Medicine and Child Neurology* 38: 438–45.

Kostandy, R.R., Ludington-Hoe, S.M., Cong, X., Abouelfettoh, A., Bronson, C., Stankus, A. and Jarrell, J.R. (2008) 'Kangaroo care (skin contact) reduces crying response to pain in preterm neonates: pilot results', *Pain Management Nursing* 9(2): 55–65.

Kozer, E., Rosenbloom, E., Goldman, D., Lavy, G., Rosenfeld, N. and Goldman, M. (2006) 'Pain in infants who are younger than 2 months during suprapubic aspiration and transurethral bladder catheterization: a randomized, controlled study', *Pediatrics* 118: e51–e56.

Lawrence, J., Alcock, D., McGrath, P., Kay, J., MacMurray, S.B. *et al.* (1993). 'The development of a tool to assess neonatal pain', *Neonatal Network* 12(6): 59–66.

Lehr, V.T. and Taddio, A. (2007) 'Topical anesthesia in neonates: clinical practices and practical considerations', *Seminars in Perinatology* l(31): 323–9.

Llewellyn, N. and Moriarty, A. (2007) 'The National Pediatric Epidural Audit', *Pediatric Anesthesia* 17: 520–33.

Lowery, C., Hardman, M., Manning, N., Whit Hall, R. and Anand, K.J.S. (2007) 'Neurodevelopmental changes of fetal pain', *Seminars in Perinatology* 31: 275–82.

Ludington-Hoe, S., Hosseini, R. and Torowicz, D.L. (2005) 'Skin-to-skin contact (kangaroo care) analgesia for preterm infant heel stick', *AACN Clinical Issues* 16(3): 373–87.

Mitchell, A., Stevens, B., Mungan, N., Johnson, W., Lobert, S. and Boss, B. (2004) 'Analgesic effects of oral sucrose and pacifier during eye examinations for retinopathy of prematurity', *Pain Management Nursing* 5(4): 160–8.

Nagy, S. (2006) 'A comparison of the effects of patients' pain on nurses working in burns and neonatal intensive care units', *Journal of Advanced Nursing* 27(2): 335–40.

Paediatrics and Child Health Division, the Royal Australasian College of Physicians (2006) 'Guideline statement: management of procedure-related pain in neonates', *Journal of Paediatrics and Child Health* 42: S31–S39.

Peters, J., Koot, H., de Boer, J. *et al.* (2003) 'Major surgery within the first three months of life and subsequent biobehavioral pain responses to immunisation at a later age: a case comparison study', *Pediatrics* 111: 129–35.

Peters, J., Schouw, R., Anand, K., van Dijk, M., Duivenvoorden, H. and Tibboel, D. (2005) 'Does neonatal surgery lead to increased pain sensitivity in later childhood?', *Pain* 114: 444–54.

Pillai Riddell, R. and Craig, K. (2007) 'Judgments of infant pain: the impact of caregiver identity and infant age', *Journal of Pediatric Psychology* 32(5): 501–11.

Ranger, M., Johnston, C. and Anand, K.J.S. (2007) 'Controversies regarding pain assessment in neonates', *Seminars in Perinatology* 31: 283–8.

Rattaz, C., Goubet, N. and Bullinger, A. (2005) 'The calming effect of a familiar odour on full-term newborns', *Developmental and Behavioral Pediatrics* 26(2): 86–92.

Sethna, N. and Suresh, S. (2007) 'Central and peripheral regional analgesia and anaesthesia', in K.J.S. Anand, B. Stevens and P.J. McGrath (eds) *Pain in Neonates and Infants*, 3rd edn, Philadelphia, PA: Elsevier.

Shah, P.S., Aliwalas, L.L. and Shah, V. (2006) 'Breastfeeding or breast milk for procedural pain in neonates', *Cochrane Database of Systematic Reviews*, Issue 3, Art. No. CD004950.DOI: 10.1002/14651858. CD004950.pub 2.

Simons, J., Franck, L. and Roberson, E. (2001) 'Parent involvement in children's pain care: views of parents and nurses', *Journal of Advanced Nursing* 36(4): 591–9.

Simons, S., van Dijk, M., Anand, K.S., Roofthooft, D., van Lingen, R.A. and Tibboel, D. (2003) 'Do we still hurt newborn babies? A prospective study of procedural pain and analgesia in neonates', *Archives of Pediatric and Adolescent Medicine* 157(11): 1058–64.

Simons, S., Roofthooft, D., van Dijk, M., van Lingen, R., Duivenvoorden, J., van den Anker, J. and Tibboel, D. (2006) 'Morphine in ventilated neonates: its effects on arterial blood pressure', *Archives of Disease in Childhood: Fetal and Neonatal Edition* 91: F46–F51.

Sizun, J., Ansquer, H., Browne, J., Tordjman, S. and Morin, J. (2002) 'Developmental care decreases physiologic and behavioral pain expression in preterm neonates', *The Journal of Pain* 3(6): 446–50.

Slater, R., Cantarella, A., Franck, L., Meek, J. and Fitzgerald, M. (2008) 'How well do clinical pain assessment tools reflect pain in infants?', *PLoS Medicine* www. plosmedicine.org 5(6): 928–33.

Slater, R., Fitzgerald, M. and Meek, J. (2007) 'Can cortical responses following noxious stimulation inform us about pain processing in neonates?', *Seminars in Perinatology* 31: 298–302.

Sparshott, M.M. (1996) 'The development of a clinical distress scale for ventilated newborn infants: identification of pain and distress based on validated behavioural scores', *Journal of Neonatal Nursing* 2: 5–11.

Spence, K. (2000) 'The best interest principle as a standard for decision making in the care of neonates', *Journal of Advanced Nursing* 31(6): 1286–92.

Spence, K., Gillies, D., Harrison, D., Johnston, L. and Nagy, S. (2005) 'A reliable pain assessment tool for clinical assessment in the neonatal intensive care unit', *Journal of Obstetric, Gynecologic, and Neonatal Nursing* 34(1): 80–6.

Stevens, B., Yamada, J. and Ohlsson, A. (2004) 'Sucrose for analgesia in newborn infants undergoing painful procedures', *Cochrane Database of Systematic Reviews*, Issue 3, Art. No. CD001069.DOI: 10.1002/14651858.CD001069.pub 2.

Stevens, B., Johnston, C., Petryshen, P. and Taddio, A. (1996) 'Premature infant pain profile: development and initial validation', *Clinical Journal of Pain* 12: 13–22.

Stevens, B., McGrath, P., Gibbins, S., Beyene, J., Breau, L., Camfield, C., Finley, A., Franck, L., Howlett, A., Johnston, C., McKeever, P., O'Brien, K., Ohlsson, A. and Yamada, J. (2007) 'Determining behavioural and physiological responses to pain in infants at risk of neurological impairment', *Pain* 127: 94–102.

Suresh, S. and Anand, K. (2001) 'Opioid tolerance in neonates: a state-of-the-art review', *Paediatric Anaesthesia* 11: 511–21.

Taddio, A., Katz, J., Ilersich, A.L. and Koren, G. (1997) 'Effect of neonatal circumcision on pain response during subsequent routine vaccination', *Lancet* 345: 291–2.

Taddio, A., Lee, C., Yip, A., Parvez, B., McNamara, P. and Shah, V. (2006) 'Intravenous morphine and topical tetracaine for treatment of pain in preterm neonates undergoing central line placement', *JAMA* 295: 793–800.

Taddio, A., Shah, V., Gilbert-Macleod, C. *et al.* (2002) 'Conditioning and hyperalgesia in newborns exposed to repeated heel lances', *JAMA* 288: 857–61.

van Dijk, M., Peters, J., van Deventer, P. and Tibboel, D.(2005) 'The COMFORT behaviour scale: a tool for assessing pain and sedation in infants', *American Journal of Nursing* 105(1): 33–6.

Warnock, F. and Lander, J. (2004) 'Foundations of knowledge about neonatal pain', *Journal of Pain and Symptom Management* 27(2): 170–9.

Whit Hall, R., Boyle, E. and Young, T. (2007) 'Do ventilated neonates require pain management?' *Seminars in Perinatology* 31: 289–97.

Young, T. and Magnum, B. (2008) *Neofax(r): A Manual of Drugs Used in Neonatal Care*, Raleigh, NC: ed 21.

Chapter 11

Fluid and Electrolyte Balance

Dee Beresford and Glenys Connolly

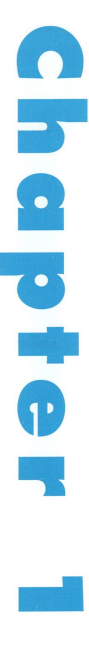

Contents

Introduction

Water and electrolytes are vital components of physiological stability at any point in life. In the newborn infant this stability is often impaired due to immaturity or lack of function, in the term infant, by an underlying disease process such as hypoxia or sepsis. These problems can be further compounded by the administration of **nephrotoxic** drugs. Fluid and electrolytes imbalances in the newborn period can lead to significant morbidity if not detected early enough. As it is the role of the neonatal nurse to administer fluid therapy and monitor fluid balance, meticulous attention to detail should highlight imbalances early to avoid serious complications.

The aim of this chapter is to highlight the pertinent aspects of fluid and electrolyte balance in order to enable the nurse to anticipate problems, to assess the adequacy of renal function, and subsequently to plan the management of infants in intensive care.

Embryological development

The development of the kidneys is along a continuum that begins in the fifth week of gestation and continues until 34–36 weeks' postconceptual age. Formation of the nephrons – nephrogenesis – occurs from week seven, with glomerular filtration and urine formation occurring two weeks later. The urine produced is excreted into the amniotic cavity, contributing to a major part of the amniotic fluid volume (Moore and Persaud 2003). Initially, the kidneys develop in the pelvis and lie close together. Slowly their position changes, following a path along the dorsal aorta to the lumbar region and then rotating medially (Bissinger 1995). By nine weeks of gestation, they are separated and have taken up the adult, retroperitoneal, position in the abdomen.

At term, each kidney contains the adult complement of 800,000–1,000,000 nephrons. In the preterm infant, nephrogenesis continues at the same rate as it would in utero (Bonilla-Felix *et al.* 1998). Therefore, an infant born at 24 weeks' gestation will not complete this process for 10–12 weeks. At 24 weeks, the kidney measures 2.5cm and has grown to 4.5cm at term. The adult size of 6cm is achieved postnatally by the elongation of the proximal renal tubules and the loops of Henle (Moore and Persaud 2003).

Physiology of urine production

Urine production begins with the process of glomerular filtration. As the blood flows through the afferent arteriole into the glomerulus, non-selective filtration occurs in which fluid and solutes pass through the capillary membrane into Bowman's capsule. The rate of filtration is affected by several factors, but the most important is the hydrostatic pressure. **Glomerular filtration rate** (GFR) is low in newborns, 20ml/min/1.73m^2 at term compared with the adult rate of

80ml/min. This decreases to 10ml/min/1.73m^2 at 28 weeks and further to 2ml/min/1.73m^2 at 25 weeks (Blackburn 2003; N.B. 1.73m^2 is a correction factor for difference in surface area between persons of different sizes). The GFR rises after birth due to a progressive rise in systemic blood pressure, fall in renal vascular resistance and an increase in renal blood flow from 4 per cent of the cardiac output to 10 per cent. This will further rise to the adult level of 25 per cent in the first few days of life. The GFR appears to increase in a programmed way at least from 26 weeks' gestation and from the second postnatal day unaffected by the gestation at birth (Wilkins 1992a). The preterm infant should produce a minimum of 25–60ml of urine per kilogram per 24 hours, which can rise maximally to 300ml/kg per 24 hours with acute increases in fluid intake. The minimum value (1ml/kg/hr) represents the lowest acceptable volume, as below this level **solute** accumulation will occur. Infants producing such a low volume warrant further investigation as a matter of urgency.

The majority of infants (95 per cent) will pass urine in the first 24 hours of life. Approximately 21 per cent will pass urine at delivery and as this may be missed or not recorded, anxieties may be raised unnecessarily that an infant has not passed urine since birth.

Sodium balance

Sodium is the major **cation** in extracellular fluid, and is vital for the regulation of circulating blood volume as well as weight gain and tissue growth.

The newborn term kidney can filter and reabsorb sodium reasonably efficiently. Utilising approximately 9 per cent of the infant's oxygen consumption for energy, sodium and water are reabsorbed from the nephron back into the circulation. Due to the high concentration gradient of sodium, it is the first ion to move from the filtrate in the tubular lumen to tubular epithelial cell. A normal physiological negative balance of sodium and water has been found to occur in healthy newborn infants during the first few days of life.

The preterm infant is less efficient at both filtering a delivered sodium load and reabsorbing filtered sodium, and is thus at risk of both hypernatraemia and hyponatraemia. Studies have demonstrated a high sodium excretion rate of 5–15 per cent, with infants becoming hyponatraemic before or after the first postnatal week (Wilkins 1992b). The very preterm infant is also at risk of high transepidermal water losses (see p. 95), increasing the propensity of hypernatraemia.

Modi (2004) suggests that in sick preterm infants an early intake of sodium is unnecessary and possibly harmful, and should be avoided until the physiological postnatal diuresis, or a weight loss of 6 per cent of the birth weight has occurred. Thereafter, normal maintenance requirements are 2–3mmol/kg per day.

Sick infants' requirements, however, will vary according to a number of factors, and this requires careful clinical assessment prior to supplementation. The serum sodium level should be measured once or twice a day in the acutely sick infant. Reasons for sodium imbalances are shown in Table 11.1.

Table 11.1 Reasons for sodium imbalances

Hyponatraemia	Hypernatraemia
Excess renal loss (particularly very preterm)	Excess transepidermal losses (particularly very preterm)

Insufficient replacement:
    Sodium-poor intravenous therapy
    Expressed breast milk with low sodium
    fortifiers
	Insufficient fluid replacements:
	    While under phototherapy or radiant
	    heaters
	Glycosuria causing osmotic diuresis

Diuretics and xanthines (i.e. caffeine)	Drugs or parenteral nutrition fluids containing excessive sodium supplementation
Inappropriate ADH secretion	
Adrenocortical failure	
Barrter's syndrome (associated with hypokalaemia)	
Salt-losing congenital adrenal hyperplasia	

Hyponatraemia

Hyponatraemia is often evident at birth, reflecting the maternal value (Modi 2005). Hyponatraemia occurring during the first week of life may be due to water retention or sodium wastage, although opinion is mixed as to which is the most likely (Haycock and Aperia 1991). Inappropriate antidiuretic hormone (IADH) syndrome is frequently implicated as the factor responsible for the hyponatraemia (Rees *et al.* 1984). Elevated ADH levels are often seen along with hyponatraemia; this may be due to infant conservation of water to maintain circulating volume, at the expense of the plasma osmolality. It is likely that in these situations, secretion of ADH syndrome is physiologically appropriate. This differentiation is important, as a true case of IADH requires restriction of fluids, whereas in physiological adaptation due to low circulating volume an increase of fluid volume and sodium may be what is really necessary (Wilkins 1992b).

Irrespective of the cause of the hyponatraemia, an appropriate positive sodium balance is vital, since a chronic deficiency is associated with poor skeletal and tissue growth with adverse neurodevelopmental outcome (Haycock 1993).

BOX 11.1 How to calculate an infant's sodium deficit

To calculate an infant's sodium deficit the following formula is used:

Sodium deficit = $0.7 \times$ body weight (kg) $\times$ (140 − actual sodium)

To correct the deficit, aim to replace two-thirds of the deficit within 24 hours, with monitoring of plasma and urine electrolytes at least daily to determine subsequent replacement.

Where the sodium deficit is due to inappropriate ADH secretion, fluids are restricted along with sodium replacement.

Hypernatraemia

Hypernatraemia usually presents in the very preterm infant secondary to TEWL, or without regard being given to 'hidden' sodium supplementation from saline infusions for arterial lines, flushes following drugs or sodium bicarbonate infusions. In moderate hypernatraemia (serum level of up to 155mmol/L), sodium supplements are best avoided and appropriate fluid replacement should correct the imbalance.

At higher levels (serum level >155mmol/l) care must be taken not to lower the plasma concentration faster than 10mmol/day. Rapid falls in sodium concentration can precipitate cerebral oedema and convulsions. Judicious additional sodium may be required, while the fall in plasma sodium is carefully monitored.

Potassium balance

Potassium is the principal intracellular **cation** and is required for maintenance of the intracellular fluid volume. Potassium reabsorption, which occurs mainly in the distal tubule, is mediated by aldosterone which regulates the sodium potassium pump to maintain cellular electroneutrality. Renal regulation of potassium is linked to the arterial pH. In a metabolic alkalotic state, the kidney will excrete potassium in exchange for sequestering bicarbonate within the cells, resulting in hypokalaemia. In a metabolic acidotic state, potassium is exchanged for hydrogen ion in the proximal tubule, increasing the plasma concentration.

In infants requiring parenteral fluids, potassium supplementation should commence when urine output is adequate, providing that the plasma level is not elevated. The daily requirement is 2mmol/kg per 24 hours. Serum potassium levels should be measured once or twice daily in the acutely sick infant. Reasons for potassium imbalances are shown in Table 11.2.

Hypokalaemia

It has been found that extreme variations in the plasma concentration of potassium can occur in neonates, both above and below the normal range of 3.8–5.0mmol/l, indicating rapid changes between the intracellular and extracellular compartments (Rogan 1998). A deficiency invariably involves an excessive loss

Table 11.2 Reasons for potassium imbalances

Hypokalaemia	Hyperkalaemia
Insufficient replacement	Tissue damage
	Excessive bruising
Excess losses:	Nephrotoxic drugs
Renal – polyuric states	
– Diuretics and other drugs	Renal failure:
– Hyperaldosteronism	Acute tubular necrosis
– Bartter's syndrome (with	Urethral valves
hyponatraemia)	Renal vein thrombosis
– Renal tubular acidosis	Congenital chronic renal failure
Gastrointestinal	
– Gastric aspiration	
– Vomiting	
– Ileostomy losses	
– Diarrhoea	

via either the intestinal or renal routes, or both, or a lack of appropriate supplementation.

Potassium supplements should be commenced on the third postnatal day at a rate of 1–2mmol/kg per day, provided an adequate urine output (over 1ml/kg/hr) has been observed and the plasma level is not elevated. To correct hypokalaemia, it is recommended administering appropriate replacements as indicated by normal maintenance requirements and to estimate ongoing losses with careful monitoring of serum levels.

Hyperkalaemia

Hyperkalemia (level >6.5mmol/l) is usually associated with a failure of the renal excretory mechanisms or secondary to an overwhelming situation from acidosis or severe infection. Elevated levels can also occur if there has been extensive bruising or ischaemic insult. Hyperkalaemia can also be reported following haemolysis of blood cells during sampling. True hyperkalaemia is extremely serious and potentially a lethal condition; the management must be prompt. All potassium supplementation or drugs containing potassium must be stopped and increased ECG surveillance commenced, closely observing for arrhythmias. Calcium gluconate may be infused slowly to counteract the toxic effects of potassium on the myocardium. As calcium gluconate extravasation injury causes severe and permanent tissue damage, it is best infused via a central line. If it is infused peripherally, the infusion site should be clearly visible and carefully observed. Other management strategies involve removing potassium from the body by the use of ion exchange agents such as rectal calcium resonium, or reducing the serum potassium level by altering the cell membrane threshold to 'push' potassium back into the cell. This can be achieved by the intravenous infusion of sodium bicarbonate (4mmol/kg 4.2 per cent solution over 5–10 minutes), glucose and insulin solution (0.3 units of insulin per kilogram per hour), monitoring blood glucose levels carefully, or salbutamol (4μcg/kg over 10 minutes; Neonatal Formulary 2007). Intravenous sodium bicarbonate (1mmol/kg) is said to be effective in reducing serum potassium levels even if the patient is not acidotic (Haycock 2003).

Chloride balance

Chloride is the abundant **anion** in extracellular fluid. Hypochloraemia may result from increased losses from gastric aspiration due to obstruction or surgery leading to metabolic alkalosis. Hyperchloraemia can occur in infants who are hypernatraemic or on parenteral nutrition and results in metabolic acidosis.

Calcium and phosphate balance

Calcium and phosphate are essential minerals required for normal growth and development and, in particular, bone mineralisation. There is active transport of calcium and phosphate via the placenta to the fetus with a gradient of 1:1.4, consequently the fetus is relatively hypocalcaemic in relation to the mother (Cheetham 2005). Perinatal asphyxia can also lead to a fall in calcium levels due to altered cell metabolism and phosphorus release, with alkalosis either from alkali therapy or over-ventilation reducing the ionised serum calcium levels further (Cruz and Tsang 1992).

Calcium and phosphate absorption is regulated by calcitonin, parathormone and the active metabolites of vitamin D, namely 1,25 dihydroxyvitamin D.

Term infants are able to convert vitamin D in the liver and kidneys, but this process is limited in the preterm infant, and does not occur at significant rates until 36 weeks' gestation (Specker and Tsang 1986). Calcium maintenance requirements are 1.5–2.0 mmol/kg per 24 hours (Cairns 2005).

In infants presenting with signs of hypocalcaemia, for example, tremors, twitching, irritability, laryngospasm, high-pitched cry, apnoea or seizures, an intravenous dose of 2ml/kg of 10 per cent calcium gluconate over 10 minutes (Cheetham 2005) may be warranted, but should be given with extreme caution under strict ECG control as bradycardia and asystole can occur if given too rapidly. Ideally this should be via a central line as calcium is notorious for severe extravasation injury and scarring; if it is given via peripheral line, close observation of the cannula site is mandatory.

Water management

Water management has to include not only water being administered, but also endogenously produced water. Approximately 10 per cent of body water is produced by oxidative cellular metabolism (Blackburn 2003). This has to be balanced with all that is lost via the differing routes.

Term infants' urinary losses are in the region of 5–10ml/kg per 24 hours. Stool water losses are minimal in the first few days but are subsequently estimated at 5–10ml/kg per 24 hours. Basal insensible water losses in the term newborn are approximately 20ml/kg per 24 hours, with 70 per cent being lost through the skin and 30 per cent via the respiratory tract. Water losses via the skin are primarily influenced by gestational age and postnatal age. There is an exponential relationship between TEWL and gestational age, with a 15-fold increase in water losses in infants born at 25 weeks to those born at term. The losses are markedly different (steeper) between those born at 25 weeks and those born at 28 weeks of gestation (see p. 96). Increasing the ambient humidity of the infant's environment to 50–90 per cent substantially reduces these losses to approximately 40ml/kg/day (see p. 105). Care of the skin and reduction in epidermal stripping are major nursing priorities. The use of skin-protecting films (e.g. cavilon™ or duoderm™) prior to application of fixation tapes for ET tubes or urine bags is useful. The use of water-impermeable creams has been suggested to maintain skin integrity but as they appear to increase the incidence of CONS infection (Conner *et al.* 2003) should only be used with this borne in mind.

Fluid requirements

Fluid intake is usually calculated on the infant's birth weight, until that weight is exceeded, unless weight gain is thought to be due to fluid retention and/or oedema.

The fluid requirement for growth in a preterm infant is thought to be 120–150ml/kg per 24 hours, but until the postnatal diuresis begins much less is required and usual starting figures are 60ml/kg in a well-humidified environment. Bell and Acarregui (2008) suggest that careful restriction of fluid intake so that physiological requirements are met, without creating dehydration, is beneficial in reducing the incidence of necrotising enterocolitis, patent ductus arteriosus and intraventricular haemorrhage.

Some infants may require a more rapid increase in fluid intake, for example, very preterm infants with high insensible losses that are not minimised, while term infants, following asphyxial injury, require a more cautious approach and may undergo fluid restriction.

When calculating an infant's fluid requirement, the weight, disease state, general condition, urine output, fluid losses and blood biochemistry need to be taken into consideration.

Monitoring fluid balance

Recording and monitoring the fluid balance of infants in intensive care is principally the role of the nurse caring for the infant. This aspect of care is as important as any other type of physiological monitoring, as imbalances and inaccuracies in fluid balance can cause serious deterioration or impair the infant's recovery. It is for these reasons that fluid balance recording should become second nature to neonatal nurses and observation and recording of the fluid status be meticulous.

Accurate measurement of body weight

Monitoring of fluid balance includes accurate measurement of body weight. Weight correlates very well with total body water content during the first few days of life (Shaffer *et al.* 1986). While infants in NICU are physiologically unstable and warrant minimal handling, weighing is an important marker for fluid balance and should be undertaken daily in most instances. The risks of the procedure, for example, accidental extubation, temperature instability and brief disconnection from IPPV, have to be balanced against the infant's condition and the benefits from the information gained. The procedure should be well planned and executed by skilled personnel, to lessen the occurrence of potential problems. Many intensive care incubators now have integral scales so that the infant does not need to be taken out for weighing. While this weight may not be as accurate as taking the infant out it does allow for trending of weight if it is undertaken around the same time each day with the same amount of equipment attached.

Weight loss is normally in the region of 1–3 per cent of the body weight per day, reaching a maximum of 10–15 per cent by day 5 in the preterm, with weight gain commencing by 7–10 days.

Measurement of urine volume

Urine output must be accurately measured as it is a marker for not only water balance but also renal perfusion. The volume voided can be estimated in several ways. Weighed nappies provide the simplest method, but evaporation of the urine into the environment or further damping of the nappy by incubator humidity may create spurious results. Commercially available adhesive bags may be used but the fixation and retention without leakage can be a problem. Additionally, when the bag is removed, significant epidermal stripping can occur. The use of the finger of a polythene glove fixed to the skin with a smear of soft paraffin is sometimes successful in small inactive males, and some success can be achieved in female infants by using the thumb of a glove applied in the same way. Urine output should be in the region of 1ml/kg per hour on day 1 rising to >2–3ml/kg per hour subsequently.

Urinalysis

Urinalysis is a procedure nurses undertake from very early in their clinical practice experience and yet it is often overlooked in its importance in renal compromise. Catching volumes of the urine can be difficult in the newborn (see above), but as only a small amount is needed for urinalysis, simply placing cotton wool balls into the infant's nappy, and then aspirating the absorbed urine with a syringe, is sufficient for the task and avoids skin damage from the application of adhesive urine bags.

Specific gravity (SG)

SG reflects the ability to concentrate and dilute urine. As the ability to concentrate urine is limited, the maximum specific gravity is usually 1.015 to 1.020, but the minimum may be as low as 1.001 to 1.005. As other factors such as glucose and protein can alter SG, osmolality measurement of both blood and urine should be undertaken and compared if concentrating ability is being questioned. A preterm infant has a limited capacity to concentrate its urine beyond 500mOsmlos/kg. (NB: SG of 1020–1030 is equivalent to 400mOsmol/l (Modi 2005).)

Urine pH

The pH reflects the kidneys' ability to acidify urine, but it is usually relatively alkalotic at 6.0. Many neonates can acidify the urine to 5.0 by one to two weeks of age. In extreme prematurity' urinary bicarbonate losses may be high increasing the pH to 7.0 or above.

Glycosuria

This estimation reflects the kidneys' ability to handle glucose and is usually associated with a high blood glucose level. High blood glucose levels associated with renal losses can contribute to osmotic diuresis and dehydration.

Proteinuria

Proteinuria is frequently seen in small amounts and is related to gestational age. If proteinuria persists, 12–24-hour urine collection should be undertaken as it may indicate renal injury, congestive heart failure, sepsis or elevated venous pressure (Boineau and Levy 1992).

Haematuria

Haematuria is not a normal finding and may be associated with renal damage following asphyxia, embolisation in the renal artery from umbilical arterial catheterisation, renal vein thrombosis, coagulopathies or congenital abnormality, for example, cystic disease or obstruction.

Glucose homeostasis

Monitoring of blood glucose levels of infants, both on admission and subsequently, is a primary responsibility of the nurse and should be undertaken if the adverse event of glucose instability is to be avoided. It is important therefore that neonatal nurses have an understanding of the factors surrounding maintenance of blood glucose levels.

During intra-uterine life the fetus is dependent upon a constant supply of transplacental glucose to provide energy for metabolic functions and substrate for growth. Fetal glucose utilisation, at 6mg/kg per minute, is greater than the neonatal requirement of 3.5–5.5mg/kg per minute, which is approximately twice the adult requirement.

Fetal blood glucose levels are approximately 70–80 per cent of the maternal level which allows the process of facilitated diffusion across the placenta to occur.

While the stored form of glucose, glycogen, is laid down from as early as 9 weeks, the rate of deposition accelerates during the third trimester. Thus, the more preterm the infant is, the smaller the reserves are, increasing susceptibility to hypoglycaemia. The timing of the increased deposition of stored substrate is probably related to the fetal energy needs during the process of labour and delivery in order to maintain blood glucose levels during the anaerobic conditions. Should the labour become difficult or prolonged, substrate utilisation increases during anaerobic metabolism, depleting hepatic and cardiac stores rapidly, making the term asphyxiated infant susceptible to hypoglycaemia (see p. 67).

At birth, the fetus undergoes a shift from an intra-uterine anabolic-dominant state to a neonatal catabolic state (Blackburn 2003), as separation from the maternal supply occurs. All newborns, therefore, have a potential for glucose instability but the susceptibility increases in certain situations (see Table 11.3), and is probably greatest in infants requiring admission to NICU.

Glucose is the main substance required by the body to create adenosine triphosphate, referred to as the energy 'currency' (Karp *et al.* 1995). After birth, the neonate has to regulate its own glucose metabolism. To survive, the newborn infant utilises the processes of **glycogenolysis**, the breakdown of stored **glycogen** to glucose, and **gluconeogenesis**, which is glucose produced from non-carbohydrate sources, such as alanine from skeletal muscle. Additionally it is also recognised that ketone bodies and lactate may also be metabolised by the fetal and neonatal brain as an energy source. This pathway is impaired in most of the infants admitted to NICU, e.g. preterm or growth-restricted infants and those following hypoxic insults.

Renal handling of glucose

The ability of the tubules to reabsorb glucose is decreased in the preterm infant and increases towards term. The preterm infant has a low renal threshold for glucose conservation, and varying degrees of glycosuria are not uncommon. Glycosuria in conjunction with hyperglycaemia may cause an osmotic diuresis whereby water is lost due to the high urinary solute concentration; this is unlikely to occur unless blood glucose levels exceed 12mmol/l (Coulthard and Hey 1999).

Hypoglycaemia

The healthy well-grown term infant will have a low blood glucose level (if measured) following birth; however, due to its compensatory mechanisms at this time its brain has the ability to utilise other metabolic fuels such as ketone bodies. Infants who require admission to NICU do not fall into this category and as a consequence hypoglycaemia must be identified and actively managed.

The definition of neonatal hypoglycaemia has long courted controversy, with definitive values ranging from below 1mmol/l to below 4mmol/l (Koh and Aynsley-Green 1988). While the academics continue to debate this issue, practitioners need guidance on what is a 'safe' level. Cornblath et al. (2000) suggest that an infant with a blood glucose level <2.0mmol/l should be closely observed and that intervention is required if the level does not increase after a feed or if clinical signs develop. Babies experiencing perinatal complications as in those admitted to NICU should have their levels maintained at >2.6mmol/L (Hawdon 2007). It is recommended that in infants with profound, recurrent or persistent hyperinsulinaemic hypoglycaemia, a higher level of 3.3mmol/L should be maintained (Cornblath et al. 2000; Hawdon 2007).

Management of hypoglycaemia

Close surveillance, early identification and the instigation of prophylactic measures for the prevention of hypoglycaemia in the high-risk population constitute by far the best management strategy. Commencement of early feeding, either enterally or intravenously with 10 per cent glucose at 3ml/kg/hour (5mg/kg/min) should be sufficient for most infants (Hawdon 2005).

If hypoglycaemia occurs despite this, a bolus of 10 per cent glucose at 3–5ml/kg should be given slowly followed by an infusion (Digiacomo and Hay 1992; Hawdon 2005). Higher concentration should be avoided due to the risk

Table 11.3 Infants at risk of hypoglycaemia

Infant group	Mechanism	Expected duration
Decreased stores 　Preterm	Decreased stores of glycogen and fat Enteral feed intolerance Fluid (caloric) restriction Impaired hormonal responses	Transient
Intra-uterine growth retardation	Decreased stores of glycogen and fat Impaired hormonal responses	Transient
Inborn errors of metabolism	Glycogen storage disease Enzyme deficiencies impairing glycogenolysis and gluconeogenesis	Prolonged
Increased utilisation 　Perinatal hypoxia	Anaerobic cellular metabolism exhausting stores	Transient
Sepsis	Increased metabolic rate	Transient
Hypothermia	Increased metabolic rate and brown fat metabolism	
Infant of diabetic mother	Hyperinsulinaemia	Transient
Beckwith–Wiedeman syndrome	Hyperinsulinaemia from islet hyperplasia	Prolonged
Erythroblastosis fetalis	Hyperinsulinaemia from islet hyperplasia	Transient
Exchange transfusion	Excess insulin secretion due to glucose level in stored blood	Transient
Islet cell dysplasias	Hyperinsulinism	Prolonged
Other causes 　Iatrogenic	'Tissued' IVs abruptly reducing supply	Transient
	Glucose infusion via UAC if tip is close to the coeliac access	Transient
Maternal drugs	Beta-agonist tocolytics	Transient

of tissue injury and rebound hypoglycaemia. If higher concentrations are required to maintain blood glucose levels, the infusion must be administered via a central venous line in order to prevent vessel damage, extravasation injury and scarring due to the sclerosing effects of the solution (Hawdon and Aynsley-Green 1999). Vigilant observation of the infusion site and infusion pump pressures must be undertaken. Hypoglycaemia resistant to high glucose infusions are usually secondary to hyperinsulinism. In these situations other therapies can be instigated such as diazoxide, glucagon, somatostatin and hydrocortisone. These agents should only be used following referral and advice from a specialist centre as their use can precipitate serious complications (Hawdon 2005).

While the consequences of asymptomatic hypoglycaemia are not well established (Cornblath et al. 2000), Lucas et al. (1988) did report lower motor and mental development scores following five episodes of blood glucose levels below 2.6mmol/l in the very low birth weight population. Any baby with a low blood sugar who is demonstrating seizure activity warrants urgent intravenous treatment.

Hyperglycaemia

Neonatal hyperglycaemia is defined as a blood glucose level >7mmol/l in term infants and >8mmol/l in the preterm (Hawden 2005), and is a much less common condition in the newborn than hypoglycaemia. Neonatal diabetes mellitus occurs in 1 in 400,000 livebirths (Shield et al. 1997), but the incidence of 'transient diabetes' (see Table 11.4) appears to be increasing as more extremely low birth weight infants are actively managed within NICU. This is probably reflective of an immaturity of the usual regulatory mechanisms, including decreased insulin response, and the provision of a high glucose load (King et al. 1986; Hawdon et al. 1993).

The consequences of hyperglycaemia are not well defined. There may be an increased risk of intracranial haemorrhage if serum osmolality is increased due to the high serum glucose level, but this remains largely speculation (Digiacomo and Hay 1992). It has to be remembered though that hyperglycaemia without a significant change in infused glucose concentration may be an indicator of sepsis and should be investigated.

Glycosuria in conjunction with hyperglycaemia may cause an osmotic diuresis whereby water is lost due to the high urinary solute concentration. This situation can result in other electrolyte instabilities, such as hypernatraemia. Osmotic diuresis, however, is unlikely to occur in blood glucose levels below 12mmol/l (Coulthard and Hey 1999).

Reducing the concentration of infused glucose to a level that will reduce the blood glucose level is often all that is required. Infants not responding to this measure may be prescribed intravenous insulin therapy. While this practice appears to occur relatively frequently, there have been no controlled studies to validate it and it must therefore be undertaken with caution (McGowan et al. 1998; Hawdon and Aynsley-Green 1999; Hawdon 2005). A recent study on the early use of insulin in the VLBW infants to avoid hyperglycaemia conferred no benefit and increased the incidence of hypoglycaemia in the treatment group (Beardsall *et al.* 2008).

Table 11.4 Infants at risk of hyperglycaemia

infant group	Mechanism	Expected duration
Extremely low birth weight infants	High intravenous glucose concentralion Immalure insulin and regulatory mechanisms	Transient
Infants receiving methyl xanthines		Transient
Infants undergoing surgery	Release of stress-related hormones Infusion of high glucose-containing solutions Transfusion of blood with high glucose levels	Transient
Neonatal diabetes mellitus	Decreased insulin production	Prolonged

Acute renal failure

Acute renal failure (ARF) is characterised by a deterioration of renal function over a period of hours or days resulting in failure to excrete nitrogenous waste and maintain fluid and electrolyte balance (Moghal and Shenoy 2008). It is said to occur in up to 8 per cent of neonates admitted to the NICU (Stapleton *et al.* 1987).

Renal failure is classified into three main categories, those of: pre-renal, intrinsic and post-renal or obstructive failure (see Table 11.5). Pre-renal failure often precedes established renal failure and is reversible if prompt attention is paid to correcting renal perfusion. As the first clinical sign of pre-renal failure is the onset of **oliguria**, careful monitoring of urine output is mandatory for an infant requiring intensive care.

The commonest reasons for ARF are asphyxia, sepsis, necrotising enterocolitis and major surgery, but it should be considered in any neonate whose urine output falls abruptly or drops below 1ml/kg /hr in the first few days of life (Modi 2005).

If readily available. a renal ultrasound is useful as it may clearly identify any anatomical abnormality, obstructive problem, congenital malformations such as polycystic disease or aplasia, or renal vascular thrombosis.

Table 11.5 Causes of renal failure in infants

Pre-renal	Intrinsic	Obstructive

Due to systemic hypovolaemia
  Haemorrhage
  Septic shock
  Necrotising enterocolitis
  Dehydration
	Acute tubular necrosis
	
	Congenital malformations
	  Agenesis
	  Polycystic kidneys
		Congenital malformations
		  Strictures
		  Obstructive lesions
		
		Renal calculi

Due to hypoperfusion
  Asphyxia
  Heart failure
  Respiratory distress
  syndrome
	Infection
	
	Renal vascular thrombosis
	
	Nephrotoxic drugs
		Fungal balls
		
		Neurogenic bladder
		
		Compression
		  Teratomas

Adapted from Karlowicz and Adelman (1996).

Investigations

When oliguria is first recognised, the bladder should be palpated to eliminate acute urine retention, which is not uncommon after asphyxial insults or in infants on morphine infusions. Assessment of the circulation, blood pressure, capillary refill time and core–periphery gap must also be undertaken to assess the adequacy of renal perfusion.

Paired blood and urine analysis may assist in establishing the diagnosis of renal failure. Measurement of fractional excretion of sodium (Fe_{Na}) is said to be the best indicator to distinguish between pre-renal and established renal failure. It is calculated from the sodium and creatinine concentrations of serum and spot urine samples. For example:

$$\frac{\text{Urine sodium}}{\text{Serum sodium}} \times \frac{\text{Serum creatinine}}{\text{Urine creatinine}} \times 100$$

In low perfusion states sodium and water will be conserved and the Fe_{Na} will be less than 2.5 per cent; however, if tubular damage is causing the oliguria, the Fe_{Na} will be greater than 2.5 per cent.

These values are only pertinent to the term population as in the VLBW population the Fe_{Na} can be up to 15 per cent, due to kidney immaturity, so the test in this population is unreliable. Other indices are listed in Table 11.6.

Provided there is no evidence of circulatory overload the response to a fluid challenge may be helpful. This consists of administering 10–20ml/kg of 0.9 per cent saline over 1–2 hours, followed by a single dose of furosemide on completion of the infusion. If the infant responds with an increase in urine output, a diagnosis of pre-renal failure is likely and further management should be directed towards maintaining adequacy of renal perfusion. Furosemide may be given as a single dose of up to 5mg/kg (Modi 2005). If the fluid challenge does

Table 11.6 Indices of renal failure in infants

	Pre-renal failure	Established renal failure
Urine sodium	Low (<10mmol/L)	High (>20mmol/l)
Urine urea	High	Low
Urine creatinine	High	Low
Urine specific gravity	High (>1025)	Low (approx. 1010)
Urine osmolality	High (> 500mosmol/kg)	Low (approx. 300mosmol/kg)
Fractional excretion Na	Low (<1%)	High (>2.5–3.0%)
Urea : plasma creatinine	High (>40)	Low

not elicit a diuresis fluid intake should be reduced as outlined below. As the half-life of furosemide is up to 8 hours in term infants and 24 hours in preterm (Neonatal Formulary 2007), repeated high doses cannot be advocated due to its potential ototoxic and nephrotoxic effects.

Management of ARF

Management of ARF should be directed to correcting the underlying cause, for example, correcting poor perfusion, hypotensive states and sepsis. Successful management of these infants is pivotal upon meticulous measuring and accurate recording of urine output, in conjunction with a fastidious account of *all* fluids administered.

All nephrotoxic drugs should be stopped where possible. The adjusting of dose schedules of all renally excreted drugs also needs consideration, with drug assays guiding the adjustments. Fluids should be calculated as insensible losses plus urine output, and any gastrointestinal losses. Furosemide may be given in doses up to 5mg/kg. Low-dose dopamine 2μg/kg per minute may aid renal perfusion. In hypotensive infants, inotropic support may be required, but as high-dose dopamine causes vasoconstriction decreasing renal blood flow, dobutamine 5–10μcg/kg per minute should probably be used. Acidosis may require treatment with sodium bicarbonate 4.2 per cent. Hyperphosphataemia and hypocalcaemia, if persistent, may require oral calcium carbonate 2–3ml t.d.s. to bind intestinal phosphate. Symptomatic hypocalcaemia with serum Ca <1.7mmol or ionised Ca <0.7mmol/l may be treated with infusion of calcium gluconate 10 per cent at 0.5–1mmol/kg per 24 hours. Treatment of hyperkalaemia (see p. 260) may also be instigated. While these are very sick and often unstable infants, regular weighing 12–24 hourly is essential in order to gauge fluid gains and losses. The same weighing scales should always be used.

If the condition is not improving with conservative management and there is severe fluid overload, metabolic acidosis, hyperkalaemia, electrolyte disturbances with uraemic central nervous system depression, dialysis should be considered (Haycock 2003).

Dialysis

Dialysis is the process of removing solute molecules by means of diffusion down their concentration gradients, via a semi-permeable membrane. While dialysis as a treatment of infants in renal failure is a rare occurrence in NICU, it can be implemented by three methods:

- Haemodialysis: this is not really an option for most infants due to lack of suitably sized machines and their availability outside highly specialised centres.
- Peritoneal dialysis (PD): this is the commonest and most easily available technique.
- Continuous arteriovenous haemofiltration (CAVH).

PD and CAVH will be further described.

Peritoneal dialysis (PD)

PD is useful in management of renal failure and is probably the technique most commonly available in most NICUs. PD works by the process of diffusion and ultrafiltration across the semi-permeable peritoneal membrane (see Figure 11.1).

A soft catheter is inserted into the peritoneal space, following systemic and local analgesia, and securely fixed in position with sutures and carefully applied tape to reduce potential skin damage. The site of insertion should be visible at all times and observed for fluid leakage, which can affect skin integrity, inflammation and signs of infection. Once the catheter is deemed patent, the fluid cycles can commence. Cycle frequency, dwelling time and volume are dependent on the infant's toleration of the procedure.

A typical dialysis prescription is 10–30ml/kg volume of fluid infused over 10 minutes, dwelling for 35 minutes and draining for 10 minutes (Modi 1999).

Nursing management of an infant undergoing PD is focused upon prevention of complications of the procedure. These are peritonitis, fluid overload or dehydration, thermal instability and respiratory compromise during dwelling time. To prevent these from occurring, a sterile technique should be adopted whenever changing fluids or PD circuitry. The drained PD fluid should be observed for turbidity, and additionally sampled daily and sent for culture and sensitivity. Fastidious attention must be paid to fluid balance recording of cycle volumes both in and out to establish whether the infant is in a positive or negative balance state. The circuitry should be well secured and supported, and not subject to kinking, which may impede flow either in or out.

PD fluid should be warmed by the use of a blood warmer set at 37°C, so that dramatic cooling does not occur from cold dialysate being instilled.

Impairment of the infant's respiratory status can occur during cycles, due to increased intra-abdominal pressure causing diaphragmatic embarrassment. This

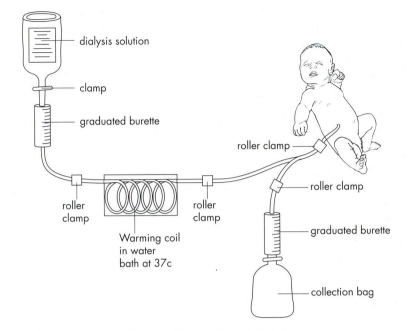

Figure 11.1 **Diagram of an infant receiving peritoneal dialysis**

can be lessened by reducing the cycle volume, and nursing the infant in a pronounced head-up tilt position to reduce the infra-diaphragmatic pressure.

Continuous arteriovenous haemofiltration (CAVH)

Unlike PD, this requires vascular access in order to be commenced, via either the umbilical venous and arterial routes or a double lumen central venous catheter. CAVH is a convection-based extracorporeal therapy, which involves a haemofilter constructed of semi-permeable membranes within a circuit of tubing (see Figure 11.2). Because the extracorporeal blood volume will be in most cases 10–20 per cent of the infant's blood volume, priming of the lines with heparinised saline (5000IUI/l), followed by whole blood, will help the infant tolerate the connection process more readily. It is also prudent to have fluid for volume replacement immediately accessible in order to correct any precipitate falls in blood pressure during the process.

As blood flows through the haemofilter, ultrafiltrate moves across the semi-permeable membranes, mimicking the process of glomerular filtration (Dudley and Sherbotie 1992). CAVH provides slow, continuous and gradual removal fluid and electrolytes without adverse effects on the haemodynamic status (Dudley and Sherbotie 1992; Bonilla-Felix *et al.* 1998). It is driven by the infant's blood pressure, which needs to be in the region of 45mmHg systolic to be adequate to sustain the flow. Infants may well require inotropic therapy (see p. 169) to achieve this.

273

While the nursing management from fluid balance, infection and temperature perspectives is not that dissimilar to the infant undergoing PD, the risk of bleeding is a major consideration in these infants. Due to the extracorporeal nature of the circuit, significant heparinisation is usually required to prevent clotting within the circuit and filter. Careful observation of the skin for **petechiae** and for oozing needs to be undertaken. Procedures that can create trauma to tissue, for example, oral or endotracheal suction and removal of sticking tape, should be carefully undertaken and kept to a minimum. Infants should not have intramuscular injections and blood sampling should be undertaken via the circuit rather than venepuncture. Clotting studies should be undertaken regularly to ascertain how much heparinisation is required.

The filter needs to be observed constantly for the flow through it. Flow ceasing abruptly suggests that the filter is blocked and needs to be changed.

While in 1995 Coulthard claimed that many clinicians agreed that PD was the preferable technique, Bonilla-Felix and colleagues (1998) state that CAVH is now their first choice for dialysis of infants. Irrespective of which technique is chosen, the prognosis for these infants remains poor, usually due to the severity of the underlying disease processes. It is for this reason that the decision to undertake dialysis should only be taken following careful deliberations with the family regarding the infant's probable outcome, prior to commencement of either of these techniques (Coulthard and Sharp 1995; Coulthard and Vernon 1995; Modi 1999).

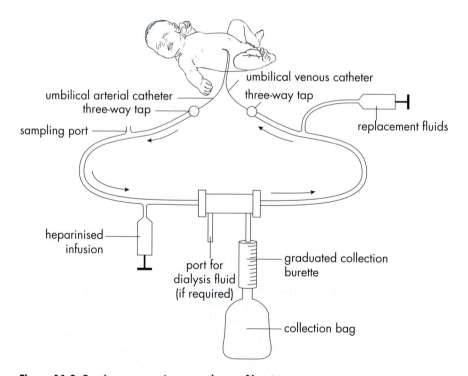

Figure 11.2 **Continuous arteriovenous haemofiltration**

Conclusion

While fluid and electrolyte balance may not appear as exciting or demanding as some of the newer technologies present within NICU, maintenance of the fluid and electrolyte homeostasis has a significant role in the progress and subsequent outcome of infants. This has never been more apparent than in recent times with the management of increasingly preterm infants who, with their exquisitely fragile skin coupled with organ immaturity, make fluid and electrolyte therapy a great challenge.

Maintaining stability and detection of potential (and real) problems is a pivotal role of the nurse and should not be underestimated.

Case study: fluid and electrolyte disturbances in a preterm infant

Stephanie was born at 25 weeks' gestation weighing 680g. She is now 36 hours of age. Stephanie has been ventilated since birth for respiratory distress syndrome and has required both 0.9 per cent saline and bicarbonate infusions to correct hypotension and acidaemia. She is also receiving phototherapy.

Her current fluid intake is 100ml/kg of IV 10 per cent dextrose and arterial line fluids. Her most recent serum electrolyte result is:

Sodium	156mmol/l
Potassium	4.8mmol/l
Urea	7.2mmol/l
Creatinine	90µmol/l

Q.1. What does this result suggest?

Q.2. What are the factors that may have contributed to this state?

Q.3. What nursing actions need to be considered?

Q.3. What other parameters should be considered in conjunction with the above result?

Q.4. What should the plan of action include for Stephanie?

Case study: fluid and electrolyte disturbances in a term infant

Edward is a 3kg male infant delivered by emergency Caesarean section at 38 weeks for fetal distress. He had respiratory depression at birth and required resuscitation by intubation and positive-pressure ventilation.

Following admission to NICU, he developed persistent seizures which required ventilatory support and anticonvulsant therapy. He is currently prescribed 60ml/kg of IV 10 per cent dextrose.

A diagnosis has been made of grade three hypoxic-ischaemic encephalopathy. The following results are obtained:

Sodium	122mmol/l	Urea	2.0mmol/l
Potassium	3.9mmol/l	Creatinine	55µmol/l
Calcium	2.0mmol/l	Plasma osmolality	275mosmol/l
Magnesium	0.7mmol/l	Urine osmolality	320mosmol/l
Phosphate	1.6mmol/l	Glucose	2.0mmol/l

Q.1. What are the areas of concern within this result?

Q.2. What are the contributing factors to this situation?

Q.3. What plan of action is necessary to correct this situation?

Q.4. What observations does Edward require?

Acknowledgements

Dee Beresford was the co-author of this chapter in the first edition.

References

Beardsall, K., Vanhaesebrouck, S., Ogilvy-Stuart, A.L., Vanhole, C. and van Weissenbruch, M. *et al.* (2008) 'The use of early continuous insulin infusion in very low birth weight infants: effects on glucose control, mortality and morbidity', *Archives of Disease in Childhood* 193: 82.

Bell, E.F. and Acarregui, M.J. (2008) 'Restricted versus liberal water intake for preventing morbidity and mortality in preterm infants', *Cochrane Database of Systematic Reviews*, Issue 1: CD00503.

Bissinger, R.L. (1995) 'Renal physiology part I: structure and function', *Neonatal Network* 14(4): 9–20.

Blackburn, S.T. (2003) 'Renal system and fluid and electrolyte homeostasis', in *Maternal Fetal and Neonatal Physiology: A Clinical Perspective*, Philadelphia, PA: W.B. Saunders.

Boineau, F.G. and Levy, J.E. (1992) 'Nephrological problems in the newborn', in N.R.C. Roberton (ed.) *Textbook of Neonatology*, 2nd edn, London: Churchill Livingstone, pp. 839–51.

Bonilla-Felix, M., Brannan, P. and Portman, R.J. (1998) 'Neonatal nephrology', in G.B. Merenstein and S.L. Gardner (eds) *Handbook of Neonatal Intensive Care*, 4th edn, St Louis, MO: Mosby.

Cairns, P. (2005) 'Parenteral nutrition', in J.M. Rennie (ed.) *Roberton's Textbook of Neonatalogy*, 4th edn, London: Churchill Livingstone.

Cheetham, T. (2005) 'Endocrine disorders', in J.M. Rennie (ed.) *Roberton's Textbook of Neonatalogy*, 4th edn, London: Churchill Livingstone.

Conner, J.M., Soll, R.F. and Edwards, W.H. (2003) 'Topical ointment for preventing infection in preterm infants', *Cochrane Database of Systemic Reviews*, Issue 4: CD001971.

Cornblath, M., Hawdon, J.M., Williams, A.F. *et al.* (2000) 'Controversies regarding definition of neonatal hypoglycaemia: suggested operational thresholds', *Pediatrics* 105: 1141–5.

Coulthard, M.G. and Hey, E.N. (1999) 'Renal processing of glucose in well and sick neonates', *Archives of Disease in Childhood: Fetal and Neonatal Edition* 81: F92–F98.

Coulthard, M.G. and Sharp, J. (1995) 'Haemodialysis and ultrafiltration in babies weighing under 1000 g', *Archives of Disease in Childhood: Fetal and Neonatal Edition* 73: F162–F165.

Coulthard, M.G. and Vernon, B. (1995) 'Managing acute renal failure in very low birthweight infants', *Archives of Disease in Childhood: Fetal and Neonatal Edition* 73: F187–F192.

Cruz, M.L. and Tsang, R.C. (1992) 'Disorders of calcium and magnesium homeostasis', in T.F. Yeh (ed.) *Neonatal Therapeutics*, 2nd edn, St Louis, MO: Mosby.

Digiacomo, J.E. and Hay, W.W. (1992) 'Abnormal glucose homeostasis', in J.C. Sinclair and M.B. Bracken (eds) *Effective Care of the Newborn*, Oxford: Oxford University Press.

Dudley, T.E. and Sherbotie, J.E. (1992) 'Continuous hemofiltration in neonates', in R.A. Polin and W.W. Fox (eds) *Fetal and Neonatal Physiology*, Philadelphia, PA: W.B. Saunders.

Hawdon, J. (2005) 'Disorders of blood glucose homeostasis in the neonate', in J.M. Rennie (ed.) *Roberton's Textbook of Neonatalogy*, 4th edn, London: Churchill Livingstone.

Hawdon, J. (2007) 'The medicolegal implications of hypoglycaemia in the newborn', *Clinical Risk* 13(4): 135–7.

Hawdon, J.M. and Aynsley-Green, A. (1999) 'Metabolic disease', in J. Rennie and N.R.C. Roberton (eds) *Textbook of Neonatology*, 3rd edn, London: Churchill Livingstone.

Hawdon, J.M., Aynsley-Green, A., Bartlett, K. and Ward Platt, M.P. (1993) 'The role of pancreatic insulin secretion in neonatal glucoregulation: infants with disordered blood glucose homeostasis', *Archives of Disease in Childhood* 68: 280–5.

Haycock, G.B. (1993) 'The influence of sodium on growth in infancy', *Pediatric Nephrology* 7: 871–5.

Haycock, G.B. (2003) 'Management of acute and chronic renal failure in the newborn', *Seminars in Neonatology* 8: 325–34.

Haycock, G.B. and Aperia, A. (1991) 'Salt and the newborn kidney', *Pediatric Nephrology* 5: 65–70.

Karp, T.B., Seardino, C. and Butler, L.A. (1995) 'Glucose metabolism in the neonate: the short and sweet of it', *Neonatal Network* 14(8): 17–22.

King, R.A., Smith, R.M. and Dahlenburg, G.W. (1986) 'Long term postnatal development of insulin secretion in newborn dogs', *Early Human Development* 13: 285–7.

Koh, T.H.H.G. and Aynsley-Green, A. (1988) 'Neonatal hypoglycaemia – the controversy regarding definition', *Archives of Disease in Childhood: Fetal and Neonatal Edition* 63: F1386–F1389.

Lucas, A., Morley, R. and Cole, T.F. (1988) 'Adverse neurodevelopmental outcome of moderate neonatal hypoglycaemia', *British Medical Journal* 297: 1304–8.

McGowan, J.E., Enzman Hagedorn, M.I. and Hey, W.W. (1998) 'Glucose homeostasis', in G.B. Merenestein and S.L. Gardner (eds) *Handbook of Neonatal Intensive Care*, 4th edn, St Louis, MO: Mosby.

Modi, N. (1999) 'Renal function, fluid and electrolyte balance and neonatal renal disease', in J. Rennie and N.R.C. Roberton (eds) *Textbook of Neonatology*, 3rd edn, London: Churchill Livingstone.

Modi, N. (2004) 'Management of fluid balance in the very immature neonate', *Archives of Disease in Childhood: Fetal and Neonatal Edition* 89: F108–F111.

Modi, N. (2005) 'Fluid and electrolyte balance', in J.M. Rennie (ed.) *Roberton's Textbook of Neonatalogy*, 4th edn, London: Churchill Livingstone.

Moghai, N.E. and Shenoy, M. (2008) 'Furosemide and acute kidney injury in neonates', *Archives of Disease in Childhood: Fetal and Neonatal Edition* 93: F313–F316.

Moore, K.L. and Persaud, T.V.N. (2003) 'The urogenital system', in *The Developing Human: Clinically Oriented Embryology*, 7th edn, Philadelphia, PA: W.B. Saunders.

Neonatal Formulary (2007) *Neonatal Formulary*, Oxford: Blackwell Publishing.

Rees, I., Brook, C.G., Shaw, J.L. and Forsling, M.L. (1984) 'Hyponatraemia in the first week of life in preterm infants: Part I: Arginine vasopressin secretion', *Archives of Disease in Childhood* 59: 414–22.

Rogan, R.W. (1998) 'Fluid, electrolyte and acid base disturbances', in A.G.M. Campbell and N. McIntosh (eds) *Textbook of Pediatrics*, 4th edn, New York: Churchill Livingstone.

Shaffer, S.G., Bradt, S.K. and Hall, R.T. (1986) 'Post natal changes in total body water and extracellular volume in the preterm infant with respiratory distress syndrome', *Journal of Pediatrics* 109: 1028–33.

Shield, J.P.H., Gardener, R.J., Wadsworth, E.J.K., Whiteford, M.L., James, R.S., Robinson, D.O., Baum, J.D. and Temple, I.K. (1997) 'Aetiopathology and genetic basis of neonatal diabetes', *Archives of Disease in Childhood: Fetal and Neonatal Edition* 76: F39–F42.

Specker, B.L. and Tsang, R.C. (1986) 'Vitamin D in infancy and childhood: factors determining vitamin D status', *Advanced Pediatrics* 33: 1–18.

Stapleton, F.B., Jones, D.P. and Freen, R.S. (1987) 'Acute renal failure in neonates: incidence, etiology and outcome', *Pediatric Nephrology* 1: 314–17.

Wilkins, B.H. (1992a) 'Renal function in sick very low birthweight infants. 1: Glomerular filtration rate', *Archives of Disease in Childhood* 67: 1140–5.

Wilkins, B.H. (1992b) 'Renal function in sick very low birthweight infants. 2: Sodium, potassium and water excretion', *Archives of Disease in Childhood* 67: 1154–61.

Chapter 12

Nutritional Management of the Infant in NICU

Kaye Spence

Contents

Introduction

Nutritional management of the preterm or sick term infant is essential for survival and an optimal outcome. Nutritional needs of the preterm infant differ from the term infant, but they also differ for each infant according to the infant's gestation, degree of growth restriction, postnatal age and accompanying disease (Steer *et al.* 1992). Nurses are faced with many challenges as they aim to meet the nutritional goals of the infant in their care and at the same time decide on the most appropriate method of feeding according to the individual infant's stage of development. In the past ten years there have been changes in the approach for neonatal nutrition and there is a growing body of evidence to support these changes, i.e. the Cochrane Collaboration.

This chapter provides an individualised approach to feeding neonates in intensive care and supporting families in their choice for feeding. It is beyond the scope of this chapter to provide an in-depth coverage of nutritional requirements and breastfeeding practices. These topics are readily available in a range of reference material.

An overview of the development and function of the gastrointestinal tract is provided to enable the reader to make an informed choice for initiating enteral feeds. The outcomes of nutrition are explored, with particular emphasis on the assessment of adequate nutrition evidenced by optimal growth and development and clinical outcomes.

Challenges of feeding sick infants with reference to appropriate nutritional requirements, feeding methods and parental choices are examined based on current research. The chapter concludes by considering the important role of families in meeting the nutritional goals of their infant.

The gastrointestinal system

The gastrointestinal tract's role in ingestion, digestion and elimination is important for long-term growth and survival in infants. Development occurs in utero and the tract is structurally prepared for oral feeding by 20 weeks' gestation; however, many of the functions required for successful feeding are not fully developed. Functional maturity occurs after anatomical maturity with many functions still immature at birth and continues to develop for up to four years (Berseth 2005). After birth, the newborn's gastrointestinal tract takes over from the placenta in the task of assimilation of nutrients. In healthy full-term infants this transition proceeds smoothly. When the function is impaired, however, due to disease such as infection, shock or hypoxia, or extreme prematurity, the results may be a delay in gastric emptying and intestinal peristalsis, resulting in impaired digestion and absorption.

The most critical period of embryonic development of the gastrointestinal tract is from around 15 days to 60 days. During this time there is a period when the development may be affected by teratogens. Birth represents a challenge and demands several responses from the gastrointestinal tract, including coordinated sucking and swallowing, efficient gastric emptying and intestinal motility, regulated salivary, gastric, and pancreatic and hepatobiliary secretion, effective absorption, secretion and mucosal protection. The major functions of the gastrointestinal tract are digestion, absorption of nutrients and water, and as a protective barrier against infection (Berseth 2005).

Successful transition to extrauterine nutrition requires the gut to be able to function rapidly and efficiently. Two factors are important in this transition: first, the gestational age of the neonate, and second, the composition of the food the neonate receives after birth.

Studies have shown that there is a gestational dependent pattern of development of small intestinal motility. Increasing gestational age results in an increase of the migrating motor complex which is responsible for the forward movements of nutrients (Berseth 2005). There are different types of motor activity during feeding and fasting. During fasting, few infants display a migrating motor complex. Instead, episodes of non-migrating phasic activity of clusters of contractions followed by an absence are seen. Normal motor activity following feeding, despite an immature small intestine, suggests that infants can respond to enteral nutrition before complete maturation of their gastrointestinal motility, thereby accelerating motor development of the preterm gut (Berseth 2005).

Gastric emptying is delayed in preterm infants as compared with term infants; this may also reflect immaturity of motor function and a lack of coordination between the antrum, fundus, pylorus and duodenum. Intestinal transit is also slower in preterm infants with a range of 8–96 hours compared with 4–12 hours seen in adults (Berseth 2005). The varying times for the transit through the gastrointestinal tract can be an important factor in deciding an appropriate feeding regime for the neonate with special needs.

In the first 3–6 months of life the gastrointestinal function is immature, which places the infant at risk for a variety of infectious and non-infectious diseases. Within a few hours of birth, the neonate is faced with antigens from both the diet and microbial sources. Following birth, mucosal protection can be divided into non-immune, which includes the luminal and mucosal defence mechanisms, and immune defence mechanisms, which include both humoral and cellular immune responses which are activated in response to specific antigens that are present in the lumen or surface of the gastrointestinal tract (Berseth 2005). Non-immune defence mechanisms include gastric acid, motility, pancreatic secretions, breast milk, mucus and a microvillus membrane. Immune defence mechanisms include secretory IgA, **macrophages, lymphocytes** and leucocytes.

Despite the immaturity of many of the digestive mechanisms, the well neonate is able to compensate to achieve adequate digestion of nutrients (Hamosh 1996). Sugars present in human milk and formula are assimilated by both small intestinal digestion and, especially in the case of lactose, colonic bacterial fermentation (Kien 1996). Diarrhoea may be caused by the malabsorption of sugars in the small bowel. Carbohydrate absorption is limited due to a deficiency of lactase that is reduced in the preterm infant to less than 30 per cent of that in the term infant. Gradual introduction of enteral feeds may enhance lactase production, so avoiding the osmotic diarrhoea of sugar malabsorption (Schanler

2005). Therapy to reduce diarrhoea may involve slowing of motility, by using a prokinetic agent to facilitate fermentative activity. However, there have been studies which have shown that there is no benefit for some agents given intravenously (Stenson *et al.* 1998). Immaturity of other organs poses additional problems for nutrition. For example, reduced renal sodium conservation may necessitate large sodium supplements. The preterm infant is also at risk for deficiencies of some amino acids that may be achieved through supplementation.

The nutritional requirements, calories, vitamins and minerals and water are supplied by the breakdown of food through digestion and absorption. Digestion and absorption involve complex mechanisms that may differ from the adult and between the preterm and term infants. These include both inefficient protein and fat absorption. Infants who have had intestinal damage following necrotising enterocolitis or who have a prolonged ileus with a resulting atrophy may have disaccharide intolerance and yet absorb glucose polymers. These variations between the term and preterm infant require caution to be used when commencing enteral feeds in very small and preterm infants.

Illness and some diseases can inhibit the function of the gastrointestinal tract thereby making it difficult for nutritional goals to be achieved. The administration of nutrients using the vascular system has been in clinical practice for more than 30 years. Total Parental Nutrition (TPN) is recommended for all extremely preterm infants and those unable to receive enteral nutrition within a few days of birth if the gastrointestinal tract is unsuitable for normal nutritional function due to illness or disease (Kilbride *et al.* 2006).

Functional problems of the gastrointestinal tract may occur which can limit the ability to achieve nutritional requirements by the enteral route. One of the more common problems is gastro-oesophageal reflux (GOR), which has been described in 50 per cent of healthy infants at the age of 2 months (Novak 1996). The contributing pathogenesis has been identified as a decrease in lower oesophageal sphincter tone, transient sphincter relaxation, increases in intra-abdominal pressure, and delayed gastric emptying. Other functional problems, although rare, may be due to congenital anomalies of the gastrointestinal tract such as oesophageal atresia or stenosis, pyloric stenosis, extrahepatic biliary atresia and malformation of the small and large intestines.

Outcomes of nutrition

The most effective method of determining whether nutritional goals have been achieved in the short term is growth. This may be assessed by measurement of weight, length, head circumference and skin fold thickness. The pattern of growth rate may influence the management of the infant and their length of stay in the NICU or step-down nursery. For graduates of intensive care it is important to ensure that their dietary management is appropriate as it may influence long-term growth, neurological development and subsequent illnesses such as allergies (Steer *et al.* 1992). Lucas *et al.* (1998) propose that suboptimal nutrition during sensitive stages in early brain development may have long-term effects on cognitive function and they recommend that avoidance of under-nutrition in sick preterm infants is important to optimise neurodevelopmental outcomes.

Human milk and colostrum contain all the nutrients for healthy growth and development, including neurodevelopment of the newborn term infant (Lucas 1993), and is the preferred milk. However, additives to formula or mother's expressed milk have been used to promote optimal growth and prevent morbidities associated with feeding preterm infants. The addition of lactase to feeds has shown no significant benefit (Cry *et al.* 2005). There are no beneficial effects of long chain polyunsaturated fatty acid (LCPUFA) supplementation of formula milk on the physical, visual and neurodevelopmental outcomes of term or preterm infants (Simmer *et al.* 2008a, 2008b). Similarly there is no difference between medium chain triglycerides (MCT) and long chain triglycerides (LCT) on short-term growth, gastrointestinal intolerance, or necrotising enterocolitis (Nehra *et al.* 2002). All of these systematic reviews recommend that further research is undertaken.

Lucas suggests that meeting the preterm infant's increased requirements may confer long-term benefits. However, this also poses a challenge for the clinicians caring for the neonate in intensive care. The increased requirements may be met by using either fortified breast milk (Kuschel and Harding 2004), preterm formula or a combination of both for enteral feeding (Henderson *et al.* 2007). There is evidence that human milk may have additional benefits in terms of neurocognitive development (Lucas 1993). When a mother's own breast milk is not available for feeding her preterm or low birth weight infant, the alternatives are either formula milk or expressed breast milk from a donor mother ('donor breast milk'). Following a systematic review, Quigley *et al.* (2007) suggest that feeding with formula may increase short-term growth rates but may be associated with a higher risk of developing necrotising enterocolitis. They found no evidence of an effect on longer-term growth, or on development. The choice of milk remains with the clinician, though the mother's choice for her infant must be taken into consideration in any decisions made regarding formula or milk substitutes. Involving the mother in informed discussions is good practice and should occur as part of the partnership in care between parents and staff.

Growth

The assessment of growth parameters remains one of the most practical and valuable tools to estimate the nutritional status in neonates. There are various charts currently used in practice to help determine a neonate's nutritional status. Charts that are suitable for the appropriate clinical, demographic, ethnic and socioeconomic similarities of the population should be used, as growth patterns vary according to the population under review. While there may be differing opinions as to whether to use intra-uterine or extra-uterine growth charts, postnatal growth rates that are comparable to those of the fetus should be used in the nutritional management of preterm infants (American Academy of Pediatrics 1985).

The majority of infants will lose up to 15 per cent of their body weight soon after birth, but can expect to regain their birth weights within 3 weeks of age. The normal intra-uterine growth rate is 15–20g/kg per day for an infant growing around the 50th centile; this is not often achieved postnatally in sick or preterm infants. Many studies have shown that rates of weight gain can exceed these rates by in excess of 50 per cent of the intra-uterine growth trends (Heird *et al.* 1993). The higher growth trends appear to be associated with rates of fat accumulation in excess of the intra-uterine rate. These may be useful in low birth weight infants as a support for their environmental adaptation. However, the effect of increased fat deposits on the long-term well-being of the preterm infant remains unclear.

Preterm infants are born with low body stores of nutrients that would normally accumulate in late gestation. After birth, preterm infants rapidly acquire a pattern of growth together with metabolic and nutrient handling skills which would not be seen at a corresponding post-conceptional age in utero. Preterm infants need to grow at a much faster rate than term infants. To achieve this growth, the recommended nutrient intakes for preterm infants are much higher than those for term infants (Consensus Recommendations 2005). Therefore, preterm infants need to be assessed for their adequate nutritional requirements based on their ability to adapt to their environment and any contributing disease factors that are present.

Postnatal head growth is a strong predictor of early developmental outcome in low birth weight infants and insufficient calories provided to **small for gestational age** (SGA) infants beyond the first two weeks of life may result in failure to initiate catch-up head growth (Tan *et al.* 2008). Adequate nutrition can be estimated by measuring the infant's growth through body weight, length and head circumference. The ponderal index, which is a calculation of body weight and length, gives an indication of the quality of the growth by relating the body weight to the overall length. Length and head circumference are important to measure as they are indices of skeletal and organ growth, whereas weight may change due to fluid balance changes and fat disposition. However, these measures can be inaccurate and care needs to be taken to ensure consistency and skill in taking these measurements in order for them to be meaningful.

The practicalities of weighing a baby in NICU can be a source of concern for nurses caring for these infants. The reliability of weighing sick ventilated infants has not been evaluated and the possible harms of weighing the infant need to be balanced against the accuracy of the technique. The use of in-bed scales has not been adequately tested as a reliable method for assessing growth in sick and/or small infants who are ventilated. However, to provide a good estimate of the trends in the infant's weight the procedure of weighing needs to be meticulous. The infant should be weighed at the same time of the day and the same scales used. The accuracy of the scales should be checked regularly. A documented unit policy on the procedure may be beneficial in achieving some consistency, especially in intensive care, as the infant may have splints, drains and multiple lines to consider in the total weight.

Assessment

Assessment is an important aspect of caring for the infant in NICU, and nutritional assessment and readiness to feed is a pivotal part of the routine assessment made by nurses (Table 12.1). There are numerous assessment tools which have been developed to assist in the evaluation of infant feeding. Howe *et al.* (2008) reviewed seven assessment tools for their psychometric properties and concluded that the NOMAS (Braun and Palmer 1986) demonstrated advantages over other assessment tools. Infants need to be observed for their readiness to feed and tolerance of enteral feeds as well as how they are achieving their nutritional goals. Obvious parameters of weight and corrected age are taken into consideration when making an assessment of the infant's readiness to feed. The infant's behavioural organisation skills, including his or her ability to maintain a quiet alert state and to display clear engagement and disengagement cues should also always be considered. Infants are seen as collaborators in their own care, and provide the best information base from which to design

Table 12.1 Considerations for feeding readiness

Enteral feeds	Sucking feeds	Neuro-behavioural readiness
Age	Age	Neuro-behavioural maturation
Availability of	Weight	■ >32 weeks post
breast milk	Demonstrated	conceptual age
Intra-uterine	sucking behaviours	Physiologic/behavioural
growth restriction	Respiratory stability	stability
Perinatal asphyxia	■ ability to maintain	■ Regular respirations
Respiratory support	oxygenation	■ Physiologic and behavioural
Intestinal motility	■ respiratory rate	cues – signs of stress
	■ apnoeas	■ Approach vs. avoidance
	Work of breathing	cues
	Continuous positive	■ Stable in environment
	airway pressure	Hunger cues
	Tolerance of gastric tube	Behavioural state
	feeds	■ Smooth state transitions
		■ Ability to reach and maintain
		alert state
		Motor development
		■ Tone
		■ Flexed and tucked
		■ Oral-motor development
		■ Good facial tone
		■ Energy resources

Source: Adapted from McGrath (2004).

285

feeding routines (Als and Gilkerson 1997). Due to the wide adoption of the developmental care philosophy, nurses are becoming more proficient in reading the infant's cues and adjusting routines to suit the individual infant (see p. 20). McCain (1997) found that awake behaviour dominated in the successful feeders and concluded that awake and quiet behaviours represent optimal feeding states. By viewing feeding from the infant's perspective, nurses can optimise intake, prevent fatigue and reduce some of the dangers associated with feeding premature infants. The families can be supported and involved from the early stages of feeding so that they can learn to recognise their infant's signs of stability or stress during feeding and intervene appropriately to promote the infant's self-regulation (Shaker 1999).

Part of the nutritional assessment is to determine if the infant is ready to feed and has effective suck and swallow coordination (Table 12.1). Futile attempts to suck and swallow may be due to structural or functional defects, which need to be eliminated before continuing with feeding attempts. Prematurity may contribute to the infant's inability to tolerate enteral feeds and attempts to oral feed should be delayed until the appropriate gestational age of at least 32–34 weeks (Tudehope and Steer 1996).

Once feeds have been commenced, the infant's tolerance of the feeds forms part of the nutritional assessment. In NICU, feed intolerance may indicate a worsening underlying disease or a stress response from noxious causes. Gastric aspirates have been used as an indication of feed tolerance in tube-fed infants. Kirkham (1998), in a randomised controlled trial, found the procedure of gastric aspiration had little influence on the hours of feed interruption. This could relate to the lack of consensus about what is an acceptable volume of aspirate to determine cessation or withholding of feeds. There is, however, no clinical evidence as to what constitutes an acceptable volume of aspirate that may indicate feed intolerance. Thus the monitoring of the trends in volumes of aspirate may be a more useful guide.

In Kirkham's study, stated interruption to feeds was more likely to occur due to abdominal distension. However, the measurement of abdominal distension appears to be a practice based on ritual with no evidence that measurement using a tape is a reliable method. Indeed many texts will recommend the practice without a thorough evaluation of the technique. A more appropriate assessment would be to observe and gently palpate the abdomen to determine an increase in tension and resistance.

The signs of a soft abdomen, the presence of bowel sounds, the passage of stool and minimal gastric aspirates indicate a functioning gastrointestinal tract. Milk feeds may not be tolerated in some infants and when attempts are made to feed, there are increasingly large gastric aspirates and/or vomiting. The use of a prokinitic agent such as metoclopramide may improve feed intolerance by facilitating gastric emptying and motility. Other drugs such as cisipride have been used for feed intolerance, although a systematic review of its use showed there is a lack of conclusive evidence as to its effectiveness from scientific methodological trials (Premji et al. 1997). Thus feed intolerance can be a difficult problem when trying to establish enteral feeds. Patience and perseverance on behalf of the carers and an ability to interpret the infant's cues as to his or her readiness to feed can aid the eventual success of establishing and maintaining feeds.

Feeding the NICU infant

Feeding the preterm infant is not a natural physiological process. None of the current dietary regimes can mimic the transplacental process. Individualisation of nutritional care is important. Two factors are important in the postnatal adaptation to enteral feeding: the gestational age of the infant and the composition of feeds the infant receives. When feedings are delayed, so is the process of intestinal colonisation, leaving the infant more susceptible to enteric pathology and other infection (Yellis 1995; Bedford-Russell 2009).

Requirements

Caloric requirements for full-term infants are based on measurements of basal metabolic rates and estimates of calories required for physiological functioning. Basal metabolic requirements include energy for thermoregulation, respiration, cardiac functioning and cellular activity. Energy requirements increase in disease states such as fever, sepsis and hypoxia. Preterm infants have higher metabolic and growth rates and an increase in insensible water losses, leading to an increase in energy and nutritional requirements to support their higher growth rates. Wahlig and Georgieff (1995) recommend changes in nutritional requirement based on some neonatal diseases (Table 12.2). When the infant requires intensive or special care there is often an increase in their energy expenditure; therefore when providing care nurses should aim to promote energy conservation and growth by implementing practices such as minimal handling, maintaining a neutral thermal environment and providing developmentally supportive environmental care (Darby and Loughead 1996).

Goals for nutritional support during the first few days of life are the maintenance of fluid status, glucose homeostasis, and normal serum electrolytes and mineral concentrations. Extremely premature infants have decreased body stores of nutrients and, consequently, a limited capacity to tolerate starvation, especially if coupled with metabolic demands imposed by illness (Pereira 1995).

The nutritional requirements for the healthy term infant have been fairly well defined. There is less evidence available, however, on the nutritional requirements for the preterm or sick infant requiring intensive care.

Parenteral nutrition

Parenteral nutrition may be used as a supplement to enteral nutrition or it may be used exclusively. It has become a popular choice for providing nutrients to

Table 12.2 Effects of neonatal diseases on specific nutrient requirements

Nutrient	RDS	BPD	CHD Cyanotic	CHF	Sepsis	IUGR
Free H$_2$O	⇓⇓	⇓⇓	⇔	⇓⇓	⇔	⇑
Energy	⇑	⇑⇑	⇑	⇑⇑	⇑	⇑
Fat	⇔	⇑	⇑	⇑	⇔	⇑
CHO	⇑	⇓	⇑	⇑	⇑	⇑
Protein	⇔	⇑	⇑	⇑	⇑⇑	⇑
Calcium	⇔	+⇑	++⇑	++⇑	⇔	⇑
Iron	⇔	*⇑	⇑	⇔	⇓	⇑
Vitamin A	⇑*	*⇑	⇔	⇔	⇔	⇔
Vitamin E	⇔	⇑	⇔	⇔	⇔	⇔

Key: RDS, Respiratory distress syndrome; BPD, bronchopulmonary disease; CHD, (congenital) heart disease; CHF, congestive heart failure; IUGR, intrauterine growth retardation; CHO, carbohydrate.

* = in <1500g infant.

\+ = especially if on calciuric diuretic (furosemide).

++ = especially post-operatively.

Source: Wahlig and Georgieff (1995). Reproduced with permission.

the infant requiring intensive care. It may be administered using a variety of routes, the most popular being via a peripherally inserted central catheter (PICC).

Parenteral nutrition solutions have improved over the past 10 years; however, they are still not perfect. Improved growth patterns for preterm infants have shown that the parenteral nutrition is beneficial if commenced early in post-natal life (Poindexter and Denne 2005). The components of the solutions are protein, energy in the form of glucose and lipids together with electrolytes, minerals, trace elements and vitamins. Several factors will influence the parenteral requirements and these include infant's activity level, body temperature and degree of stress (Kilbride *et al.* 2006). Caloric requirements are approximately 85–100Kcal/kg/day and may be greater for very low birth weight (VLBW) infants, these estimates being based on enteral nutrition requirements. Studies indicate that a minimum of 1–1.5g/Kg/day of protein is needed to achieve protein synthesis. The quantity of nitrogen required by a term infant is based on estimates from breast milk intake, for parenteral protein requirements the estimates are 3g/kg/day of amino acids. Heird *et al.* (1993), through a review of the available clinical trials, have shown that parenterally delivered nutrients support normal to supernormal rates of growth. He recommends daily amino acid intakes of 3g/kg and energy intakes of 80–90kcal/kg for intra-uterine rates of nitrogen retention and weight gain. The pattern of the amino acid mixture is an important determinant of the efficiency of the total mixture. Lipid infusion plays an important role in preventing fatty acid deficiency and in ensuring sufficient non-nitrogen calories without exceeding glucose tolerance. Rates of 2–3g/kg daily appear to be well tolerated when given by continuous infusion. Van Beek *et al.* (1995) recommend starting parenteral feeding in preterm infants, including amino acids and fat as soon as possible after birth; however, they do recommend caution in infants with sepsis, respiratory disease or extreme prematurity. Preterm infants have poor tolerance of both glucose and fat when infused above physiological levels (Jones *et al.* 1993); therefore nurses need to ensure that the infusion rate remains constant and avoid the temptation to 'catch up' with volumes when the infusion has been disrupted.

Despite the available research and evidence for the use of parenteral nutrition for neonates, there remain many unanswered questions (Heird *et al.* 1993). These questions are important for clinicians when making decisions for the use of parenteral nutrition in NICU. Issues such as cost-effectiveness, complications of routes of administration, effect on morbidity, ratio of energy to amino acid requirements, and the relationship of early enteral feeding and necrotising enterocolitis are a few that need to be considered.

When parenteral nutrition is used in NICU, specific care is required to ensure the complications associated with its use are avoided. Infants should be monitored regularly for their fluid intake and output, their tolerance of dextrose by measuring both blood and urine glucose, and their tolerance of lipids by monitoring plasma turbidity, either by observing a sample of settled blood or spinning a sample of blood. If signs of **turbidity** persist, then a sample should be sent for analysis in the laboratory. Other complications include sepsis, metabolic disturbances and catheter-related problems.

Enteral nutrition

Human milk is the preferred diet for enteral feeds. There is wide variation in the nutrient and non-nutrient content of the milks currently available. Formulas designed for preterm use differ in composition from milks designed for term infants. Human milk also varies in composition during the course of lactation, diurnally and during a breastfeed. The milk from mothers who have delivered prematurely has a different composition from mothers who have delivered at term as it is higher in protein (2.4g versus 1.8g/100ml). If formula is to be used for term infants, then standard formulas based on cow's milk with a protein concentration of 13–15g/l provide the best nutritional source (Atkinson 1992).

Atkinson (1992) found that there is a lack of properly controlled randomised trials concerning optimum infant nutrition. Based on a comprehensive review of the literature, Atkinson states that breastfeeding will be most successfully achieved in mothers who receive adequate education and support from knowledgeable health professionals. The breastfed term infant can be adequately nourished for the first six months of life by breast milk alone (Kramer and Kakuma 2002).

Early nutrition of low birth weight infants can influence later neurodevelopment (Lucas 1993) so it remains vital that early nutritional needs are met. Whereas breast milk supplies adequate nutrients to meet the nutritional demands of the term infant, the nutrient component of premature human milk provides insufficient quantities to meet the estimated needs of the premature infant. Fortification of human milk with multicomponent supplementation has been used to increase the rate of growth in very low birth weight infants. Multicomponent fortification of human milk is associated with short-term improvements in weight gain, linear and head growth, however there is no evidence supporting long-term advantages in terms of growth or neuro-developmental outcome (Kuschel and Harding 2004).

Methods

Feeding practices vary between clinicians and institutions and remain an issue for nurses who draw on their experiences when initiating and planning the feeding regime for infants in their care. Feeding the infant in the NICU needs to be planned on an individual basis taking into account the infant's illness, development and family presence.

Infants who are less than 32 weeks' gestation do not effectively suck, lack coordination of sucking, swallowing and breathing, and have delayed gastric emptying which can influence their transition to independent sucking feeds (Dodrill et al. 2008). Non-nutritive sucking (NNS) is often used as part of the process of implementing and establishing sucking feeds. Pinelli and Symington (2005) found that NNS appeared to facilitate the transition to full oral/bottle feeds as well as facilitating behavioural state. Therefore, based on the available evidence, NNS in preterm infants would appear to have some clinical benefit, and additionally does not appear to have any short-term negative effects (ibid.). The use of a pacifier may also be beneficial, as a self-consoling strategy by promoting calming behaviour in an infant unable to take sucking feeds. Non-nutritive sucking can be used during tube feeds when infants are alert or restless to support a calm, organised state prior to attempting sucking feeds.

Another feeding practice is the use of minimal enteral nutrition in parenterally fed neonates (also known as *trophic* feeding). Tyson and Kennedy's (2005) systematic review found the group who received trophic feedings required significantly less time to reach full milk feeds and had a reduction in hospital stay. Once a decision has been made to commence enteral feeds, the frequency and volume of the feeds need to be taken into consideration. Each infant needs to be individually assessed and their underlying disease considered prior to initiating enteral feeds (Miller and Willging 2007). Bombell et al. (2008) found no evidence that delaying progressive enteral feeds affected the incidence of necrotising enterocolitis, mortality or other neonatal morbidities in low birth weight or extremely premature infants. NEC is not associated with a slow increase in volumes of enteral feeds in very low birth weight infants (McGuire et al. 2008). The use of tube feeding is a common practice for preterm, low birth weight and sick infants. However, conflicting results of studies make it difficult to make universal recommendations regarding either continuous or bolus feeds for VLBW infants (Premji and Chessell 2002). In a recent study, Dsilna *et al.* (2008) found that continuous feeding is associated with less behavioural stress than bolus feeds in infants who are less than 1200 grams in the first 15 days of life. Mandich *et al.* (1996) found that apnoea appears to influence the length of time it takes for a premature infant to begin receiving full oral feedings. This may be due to the frequency and the pattern of grading of feeds. The degree of maturity has been shown to influence the transition time to bottle or breastfeeding (Sheppard and Fletcher 2007; Dodrill *et al.* 2008). Clinicians need to use the evidence from these studies to remind them of the caution required when feeding small or sick infants. The use of parenteral nutrition in combination with the slow introduction of enteral feeds may avoid some of the problems previously identified.

There is little evidence to support either the oro-gastric or naso-gastric route for tube placement (Hawes *et al.* 2004). An early study by Van Someran *et al.* (1984) found a decrease in the incidence of central apnoea and periodic breathing in infants with oro-gastric tubes. There was, however, no difference in obstructive apnoea. Although nasal tubes have been considered to be more stable and less prone to displacement than oral tubes, there has been concern that nasal tubes may partially obstruct breathing. Only two small trials were found that compared these two options and these did not find convincing evidence to support routine use of one rather than the other (Hawes *et al.* 2004).Studies have shown that infants with naso-gastric tube placement have lower minute ventilation and tidal volume during continuous and intermittent sucking (Shaio 1994). Therefore, there appear to be fewer benefits for the use of naso-gastric tube placement, although depending on the individual infant the placement of gastric tubes nasally may be more suitable. None of the studies compared different tube sizes and this may be significant for some smaller infants or those with underlying respiratory problems. Very low birth weight infants should be monitored during feeding or breathing pauses, as bradycardia and desaturation have been reported when a nasogastric tube is in place (Shaio 1994).

Another alternative to gastric feeding is transpyloric feeding where a tube is passed via the oesophagus through the pylorus into the distal end of the duodenum or jejunum (see p. 360). This method was popular in the 1970s and is only used for specific conditions such as gastro-oesophageal reflux disease (GORD). The procedure is technically more complex in that a tube cannot always be passed and may result in additional X-rays to verify tube position. Major complications of tube feeding, such as aspiration, necrotising enterocolitis and diarrhoea, are not reduced by using transpyloric tube feeds. A systematic review (McGuire *et al.* 2008) found no evidence of any beneficial effect of transpyloric feeding in preterm infants. However, there is evidence of adverse effects and transpyloric tube feeding as a usual method of enteral cannot be recommended for preterm infants (see p. 333).

Specific problems in NICU

Respiratory disease is a common problem in NICU and infants with an acute respiratory illness require an appropriate nutritional regime due to their increased metabolic demands. Oxygen consumption and therefore energy expenditure are increased (Wahlig and Georgieff 1995). Preterm infants are frequently ill, and this may be a major factor on the practical management of feeding and on nutritional requirements. Infants with respiratory disease often tolerate enteral feeds poorly and feeds may need to be delayed or kept at minimal levels until they have overcome the severity of the disease.

Infants with cardiac disease or failure may require restricted volumes, making it difficult to achieve their nutritional requirements. These infants pose particular difficulties when it comes to establishing a feeding regime as they often require increased energy intake. Pillo-Blocka et al. (2004) found, when higher formula concentrations are advanced quickly, the results of improved energy intake and weight gain enabled these infants to be discharged sooner. A challenge of feeding these infants is to maintain their extra calories while at the same time reducing the energy expenditure of feeding (Wahlig and Georgieff 1995). Complementary feeds of breast and tube may be necessary to ensure the infant receives adequate rest following feeding episodes.

Infants with chronic lung disease (CLD) need more energy and a relatively low carbohydrate to fat ratio to reduce carbon dioxide production and retention (Steer et al. 1992). Ryan (1998) recommends increasing the energy density of the feeds so that sufficient energy is delivered in tolerable volumes. Howe et al. (2007) found that transitional feeding rates may be a better indicator for discharge than sucking pattern in infants with CLD. The sucking pattern for this group remained immature and required prolonged hospital stay.

Necrotising enterocolitis (NEC) is characterised by intense transmural intestinal inflammation, ischaemia, necrosis, and sometimes perforation. NEC affects 1-8 per cent of infants admitted to neonatal intensive care units. Risk factors include low birth weight (<1500g) and prematurity. Several prospective, randomised trials have assessed the preventive effects of early probiotic supplementation of breast milk or formula in premature infants. Despite differences in study design and probiotic strains used (e.g. *L. adicophilus*, *B. bifidum*, *L. rhamnosus* GG, *B. infantis*, *S. thermophilus*), studies have consistently demonstrated a reduced rate of NEC in probiotic-treated infants (reduction by up to 80 per cent) (Al Faleh and Bassler 2008) A systematic review (Henderson et al. 2007) found formula milk may contain more nutrients than maternal breast milk but lacks the antibodies and other substances present in breast milk that protect and develop the immature gut of preterm or low birthweight infants. Supplementation of breast milk or formula with probiotics in very low birth weight infants appears safe, improves feeding tolerance and reduces the rate of NEC and bacterial sepsis (ibid.). The use of IgA was thought to prevent NEC; however, the evidence does not support the administration of oral immunoglobulin for the prevention of NEC (Foster and Cole 2004).

A particular challenge for nurses in the neonatal nursery is the problem feeder. Once enteral feeds have been commenced, several problems may arise that need to be considered and potential complications avoided. Gastro oesophageal reflux has been identified as a fairly common occurrence (Novak 1996) and can be very distressing for the infant, mother and caregiver trying to establish oral feeds. Practices are often based on empirical opinion. There is no evidence to support or refute the efficacy of feed thickeners in newborn infants with GOR (Huang *et al.* 2002). Gastro-oesophageal reflux may be less and of shorter duration in infants who are breastfed compared to formula fed (Tan and Jeffery 1995).

The lack of normal feeding behaviour during critical periods may result in the loss of the ability to feed (Skuse 1993). Therefore encouragement with oral stimulation and pleasant sensations may help the infant to adjust and referral to a speech and language therapist may be of benefit.

Neonatal surgery can have a significant effect on the feeding regimes and patterns in NICU. Infants who have undergone gastrointestinal or other major surgery may have their enteral feeds delayed for several weeks. How the feeds are commenced and increased in volume is often at the discretion of the surgeon. However, nurses can contribute to the discussion and take an active role in the feeding plan to suit infant and family. There remain no hard and fast rules for post-operative feeding, but the resumption of intestinal motility and peristalsis play a vital role in the timing of the commencement of feeding. A more difficult problem concerns the measurement of tolerance and the grading to full oral feeds.

Family support

Many infants are admitted to NICU where feeding routines play an important part in their recovery. It is the role of the nurse to develop a plan of care that includes the infant's nutritional goals. As part of the plan, the mother's preferences and involvement in the feeding schedule are an integral part of the infant's recovery phase.

Families with infants in NICU often become frustrated at the difficulty and time involved in establishing a feeding routine. The delivery of a sick or preterm infant can be an anxiety-producing event, which may physically and psycho-logically impede the mother's ability to breastfeed. Support from well-informed staff can alleviate some of these anxieties and help facilitate a successful breastfeeding experience.

There have been several studies looking at mothers' intention to breastfeed their infants when they are admitted to NICU. Byrne and Hull (1996) found 64 per cent and Griggs *et al.* (2001) found 71 per cent of mothers intending to breastfeed on admission. The breastfeeding rates on discharge were 49 per cent; this drop may reflect their experiences in NICU. Mothers have indicated that a feeling of tenseness rather than embarrassment inhibited lactation (Byrne and Hull 1996). Information on breastfeeding and expressing milk should be clear, simple and unequivocal and, most importantly, should be agreed by all who advise the mothers. Mothers have reported that seeing their infant receive their expressed milk by tube feeds reinforces their breastfeeding efforts (Meier *et al.* 1993).

Mothers have identified an unsupportive environment in NICU, the quality of advice given on breastfeeding, work organisation practices and the behaviours of nurses as inhibitors for the initiation of breastfeeding (Nyqvist and Sjoden 1993). In addition, they felt uncomfortable in the hectic and technological environment with other sick infants, neonatal staff, other parents and equipment (Griggs *et al.* 2001). Practices may vary between units, but nurses need to consider ways of involving the families when feeding is commenced. For example, the feeding schedules could be agreed with the mothers and practical assistance may be offered to encourage the mothers to assist during tube feeds.

Strategies to assist in the successful transition from parenteral to tube to oral feeds include a warm, comfortable and private environment (Byrne and Hull 1996). Meier *et al.* (1993) found the NICU environment influenced the mothers' ability to breastfeed with mothers wanting a quiet room; however, they did not want to be left alone during breastfeeding. Griggs *et al.* (2001) found mothers requested opportunities to live in and be on call for feeding opportunities. The presence of an experienced and supportive nurse would be seen to be of benefit to these already stressed and anxious women.

Breastfeeding is obviously the preferred method of feeding; however, infants who have spent considerable time in NICU may take time to fully establish breastfeeds. Supplementing breastfeeds by cup over bottle feeding gives no benefit to breastfeeding beyond discharge home and delays discharge considerably (Flint *et al.* 2007). There is currently insufficient evidence on which to base recommendations for a tube alone approach to supplementing breastfeeds (Collins *et al.* 2008).

When assessing infant readiness for discharge after a long or complex stay in NICU, the infant needs to maintain a stable cardio-respiratory function during feeding (Dodds and Merle 2005). There remains some controversy regarding discharging preterm infants home on tube feeds or keeping them in hospital until full sucking feeds are established (Collins *et al.* 2003); many units, however, discharge infants still requiring some tube feeds home with appropriate community family support. Infants admitted to NICU come from a diverse range of cultural backgrounds. When initiating feeds, the particular cultural traditions and beliefs may not be able to be met. Nurses working with the families need to be considerate and sympathetic to the possibility of cultural clashes. Western ideals may not be always acceptable, therefore special consideration needs to be given to instructing mothers regarding expressing their milk and breastfeeding in a busy intensive care environment.

Conclusion

Providing adequate nutrition to infants in the neonatal intensive care unit presents a major challenge to the doctors and nurses caring for the infants. The goal of feeding is to meet the metabolic requirements of a number of the developing organ systems. Presently the adequacy of nutrition is measured by plotting the infant's growth. A challenge is to consider other ways of measuring the outcome. Assessment of the infant's readiness for feeds and the infant's ability to feed normally are a major focus of the nursing care in NICU. Nurses are in powerful positions to influence how neonates attain their goals and to assist the infant–mother dyad. By using an evidenced-based approach to their practice, optimal outcomes for each infant and family individual can be achieved.

There has been an abundance of evidence for nutrition and feeding in the past decade; however, much of the evidence on neonatal nutrition and feeding practices dates back several decades. Practices have evolved that are based on tradition, ritual and personal preferences, and nurses need to challenge this approach. Evaluation of the available evidence and literature is necessary in order to change practices and optimise infant nutrition and outcomes.

Case study: nutritional requirements of a preterm infant requiring assisted ventilation

Ahmed was born at 27 weeks' gestation. He was the first child of a young married couple. At birth, Ahmed breathed spontaneously and required minimal resuscitation. He was transferred to NICU. His birth weight was 980g. An arterial blood gas and chest X-ray indicated respiratory distress syndrome and he was intubated, received surfactant and was ventilated. Ahmed required assisted ventilation for the first week of life; he was then extubated and nursed in a double-walled incubator and was receiving supplemental oxygen of 25 per cent.

Ahmed's mother visited each day with her husband and family. During her visits she appeared anxious and often relied on the information concerning Ahmed's progress to be relayed to her by her husband.

Q.1. What would be the most appropriate method to supply Ahmed's nutritional requirements for the first week of his life?

Q.2. Which are the risk factors that may impact on Ahmed commencing enteral feeds?

Q.3. Once Ahmed is to commence enteral feeds, what regime would be appropriate for him?

Q.4. How would you assess the outcome of Ahmed's nutritional goals?

Case study: nutritional requirements of a term infant with a congenital heart defect

Maggie was born at term to a 38-year-old woman. At birth Maggie's Apgar scores were 6 and 8 at one and five minutes. During a breastfeed on the postnatal ward Maggie's mother noticed that she became blue. On examination a heart murmur was present. Further investigation revealed Maggie had a congenital heart defect. She was transferred to NICU and was scheduled for surgery later in the day.

Maggie tolerated her surgery well and was extubated and nursed in an open care system. One week following surgery Maggie remained nil by mouth, had an oro-gastric tube in place and was having 3ml of aspirate every 4 hours. Her mother asked if she could breastfeed Maggie as she had been expressing regular volumes of milk.

Answer the questions below giving a rationale for your choices based on the evidence in the chapter.

Q.1. How does Maggie's disease affect her nutritional needs?

Q.2. How should Maggie be fed?

Q.3. Are there any contributory factors that may complicate Maggie's progression with oral feeds?

Q.4. What assistance may her mother find beneficial?

References

Al Faleh, K.M. and Bassler, D. (2008) 'Probiotics for prevention of necrotizing enterocolitis in preterm infants', *Cochrane Database of Systematic Reviews*, Issue 1, Art. No. CD005496. DOI: 10.1002/14651858.CD005496.pub 2.

Als, H. and Gilkerson, L. (1997) 'The role of relationship-based developmentally supportive newborn intensive care in strengthening outcome of preterm infants', *Seminars in Perinatology* 21(3): 178–89.

American Academy of Pediatrics Committee on Nutrition (1985) 'Nutritional needs of low birth weight infants', *Pediatrics* 75: 976–86.

Atkinson, S.A. (1992) 'Feeding the normal term infant: human milk and formula', in M. Bracken and J. Sinclair (eds) *Effective Care of the Newborn*, New York: Oxford University Press.

Bedford-Russell, A. (2009) 'Neonatal infection – prevention and treatment', Abstract presentation. ReAsoN Conference, 30 June, Warwick, UK.

Berseth, C.L. (2005) 'Developmental anatomy and physiology of the gastrointestinal tract', in H.W. Taeusch, R.A. Ballard and C.A. Gleason (eds) *Avery's Diseases of the Newborn*, 8th edn, Philadelphia, PA: Elsevier Saunders.

Bombell, S. and McGuire, W. (2008) 'Delayed introduction of progressive enteral feeds to prevent necrotising enterocolitis in very low birth weight infants', *Cochrane Database of Systematic Reviews*, Issue 2, Art. No. CD001970.DOI: 10.1002/14651858.CD001970.pub 2.

Braun, M.A. and Palmer, M.M. (1986) 'A pilot study of oral-motor dysfunction in at-risk infants', *Physical and Occupational Therapy in Pediatrics* 5: 13–25.

Byrne, B. and Hull, D. (1996) 'Breast milk for preterm infants', *Professional Care of Mother and Child* 6(2): 39–45.

Collins, C.T., Makrides, M. and McPhee, A.J. (2003) 'Early discharge with home support of gavage feeding for stable preterm infants who have not established full oral feeds', *Cochrane Database of Systematic Reviews*, Issue 4, Art. No. CD003743.DOI: 10.1002/14651858.CD003743.

Collins, C.T., Makrides, M., Gillis, J. and McPhee, A.J. (2008) 'Avoidance of bottles during the establishment of breast feeds in preterm infants', *Cochrane Database of Systematic Reviews*, Issue 4, Art. No. CD005252.DOI: 10.1002/14651858.CD005252.pub 2.

Consensus Recommendations (2005) 'Summary of reasonable nutrient intakes for preterm infants', in R. Tsang, R. Uauy, B. Koletzko and S. Zlotkin (eds) *Nutrition of the Preterm Infant: Scientific Basis and Practical Guidelines*, Cincinnati, OH: Digital Publishing Inc, pp. 415–16.

Cry Tan-Dy and Ohlsson, A. (2005) 'Lactase treated feeds to promote growth and feeding tolerance in preterm infants', *Cochrane Database of Systematic Reviews*, Issue 2, Art. No. CD004591.DOI: 10.1002/14651858.CD004591.pub 2.

Darby, M.K. and Loughead, J.L. (1996) 'Neonatal nutritional requirements and formula composition: a review', *Journal of Obstetric, Gynecologic and Neonatal Nursing* 25(3): 209–17.

Dodds, K.M. and Merle, C. (2005) 'Discharging neonates with congenital heart disease after cardiac surgery: a practical approach', *Clinics in Perinatology* 32: 1031–42.

Dodrill, P., Donovan, T., Cleghorn, G., McMahon, S. and Davies, P. (2008) 'Attainment of early feeding milestones in preterm infants', *Journal of Perinatology* 28(8): 549–55.

Dsilna, A., Christensson, K., Gustafsson, A., Lagercrantz, H. and Alfredsson, L. (2008) 'Behavioral stress is affected by the mode of tube feeding in very low birth weight infants', *Clinical Journal of Pain* 24(5): 447–55.

Flint, A., New, K. and Davies, M.W. (2007) 'Cup feeding versus other forms of supplemental enteral feeding for newborn infants unable to fully breastfeed', *Cochrane Database of Systematic Reviews*, Issue 2, Art. No. CD005092. DOI: 10.1002/14651858.CD005092.pub 2.

Foster, J. and Cole, M. (2004) 'Oral immunoglobulin for preventing necrotizing enterocolitis in preterm and low birth-weight neonates', *Cochrane Database of Systematic Reviews*, Issue 1, Art. No. CD001816.DOI: 10.1002/14651858.CD001816.pub 2.

Griggs, J., Spence, K. and Ellercamp, C. (2001) 'Breastfeeding trends in a children's hospital', *Neonatal, Paediatric and Child Health Nursing* 4(3): 15–22.

Hamosh, M. (1996) 'Digestion in the newborn', *Clinics in Perinatology* 23(2): 191–209.

Hawes, J., McEwan, P. and McGuire, W. (2004) 'Nasal versus oral route for placing feeding tubes in preterm or low birth weight infants', *Cochrane Database of*

Systematic Reviews, Issue 3, Art. No. CD003952.DOI: 10.1002/14651858. CD003952.pub 2.

Heird, W.C., Kashyap, S., Ramakrishnan, R., Schulze, K.F. and Dell, R.B. (1993) 'Nutrition, growth, and body composition', in B.L. Salle and P.R. Swyer (eds) *Nutrition of the Low Birthweight Infant: Nestlé Nutrition Workshop Series, 32*, New York: Vevey/Raven Press.

Henderson, G., Anthony, M.Y. and McGuire, W. (2007) 'Formula milk versus maternal breast milk for feeding preterm or low birth weight infants', *Cochrane Database of Systematic Reviews*, Issue 4, Art. No. CD002972.DOI: 10.1002/14651858. CD002972.pub 2.

Howe, T., Sheu, C. and Holzman, I.R. (2007) 'Bottle-feeding behaviors in preterm infants with and without bronchopulmonary dysplasia', *American Journal of Occupational Therapy* 61(4): 378–83.

Howe, T., Lin, K.C., Fu, C.P., Su, C.T. and Hsieh, C.L. (2008) 'A review of psychometric properties of feeding assessment tools used in neonates', *Journal of Obstetric, Gynecological and Neonatal Nursing* 37(3): 338–49.

Huang, R.C., Forbes, D.A. and Davies, M.W. (2002) 'Feed thickener for newborn infants with gastro-oesophageal reflux', *Cochrane Database of Systematic Reviews*, Issue 3, Art. No. CD003211.DOI: 10.1002/14651858.CD003211.

Jones, M.O., Pierro, A., Hammond, P., Nunn, A. and Lloyd, D.A. (1993) 'Glucose utilization in the surgical newborn infant receiving total parenteral nutrition', *Journal of Pediatric Surgery* 28(9): 1121–5.

Kien, C.L. (1996) 'Digestion, absorption, and fermentation of carbohydrates in the newborn', *Clinics of Perinatology* 23(2): 211–28.

Kilbride, H.W., Leick-Rude, M.K. and Allen, N.H. (2006) 'Total parental nutrition', in G.B. Merenstein and S. Gardner (eds) *Handbook of Neonatal Intensive Care*, 8th edn, St Louis, MO: Mosby.

Kirkham, P. (1998) 'Is there a relationship between feeding intolerance and gastric aspirates? A pilot study', in *Proceedings of the 2nd Annual Congress of the Perinatal Society of Australia and New Zealand*, March (ISSN 1327–6859).

Kramer, M.S. and Kakuma, R. (2002) 'Optimal duration of exclusive breastfeeding', *Cochrane Database of Systematic Reviews* (I) CD003517.

Kuschel, C.A. and Harding, J.W. (2004) 'Multicomponent fortified human milk for promoting growth in preterm infants', *Cochrane Database of Systematic Reviews*, Issue 1, Art. No. CD000343.DOI: 10.1002/14651858.CD000343.pub 2.

Lucas, A. (1993) 'Influence of neonatal nutrition on long-term outcome', in B.L. Salle and P.R. Swyer (eds) *Nutrition of the Low Birthweight Infant: Nestlé Nutrition Workshop Series, 32*, New York: Vevey/Raven Press.

Lucas, A., Morley, R. and Cole, T.J. (1998) 'Randomised trial of early diet in preterm babies and later intelligence quotient', *British Medical Journal* 317: 1481–7.

Mandich, M., Ritchie, S.K. and Mullett, M. (1996) 'Transition times to oral feeding in premature infants with and without apnoea', *Journal of Obstetric, Gynecology and Neonatal Nursing* 25(9): 771–6.

McCain, C.C. (1997) 'Behavioral state activity during nipple feedings for preterm infants', *Neonatal Network* 16(5): 43–7.

McClure, R.J., Chatrath, M.K. and Newell, S.J. (1996) 'Changing trends in feeding policies for ventilated preterm infants', *Acta Paediatrica* 85: 1123–5.

McGrath, J.M. (2004) 'Feeding', in C. Kenner and J. McGrath (eds) *Developmental Care of Newborns and Infants: A Guide for Health Professionals*, St Louis, MO: Mosby.

McGuire, W. and Bombell, S. (2008) 'Slow advancement of enteral feed volumes to prevent necrotising enterocolitis in very low birth weight infants', *Cochrane Database of Systematic Reviews*, Issue 2, Art. No. CD001241.DOI: 10.1002/14651858. CD001241.pub 2.

McGuire, W. and McEwan, P. (2007) 'Transpyloric versus gastric tube feeding for preterm infants', *Cochrane Database of Systematic Reviews* 2007, Issue 3, Art. No. CD003487.DOI: 10.1002/14651858.CD003487.pub 2.

Medoff-Cooper, B., Verklan, T. and Carlson, S. (1993) 'The development of sucking patterns and physiologic correlates in very low birth weight infants', *Nursing Research* 42(2): 100–5.

Meier, P.P., Engstrom, J.L., Mangurten, H.H., Estrada, E., Zimmerman, B. and Kopparthi, R. (1993) 'Breastfeeding support services in the neonatal intensive care unit', *Journal of Obstetric, Gynecology and Neonatal Nursing* 22(4): 338–47.

Miller, C.K. and Willging, P.J. (2007) 'The implications of upper-airway obstruction on successful infant feeding', *Seminars in Speech and Language*, 10th Anniversary Issue 28(3): 190–203.

Nehra, V., Genen, L.H. and Brumberg, H.L. (2002) 'High versus low medium chain triglyceride content of formula for promoting short-term growth of preterm infants', *Cochrane Database of Systematic Reviews*, Issue 3, Art. No. CD002777.DOI: 10.1002/14651858.CD002777.

Novak, D.A. (1996) 'Gastroesophageal reflux in the preterm infant', *Clinics in Perinatology* 23(2): 305–20.

Nyqvist, K.H. and Sjoden, P. (1993) 'Advice concerning breast feeding from mothers of infants admitted to a neonatal intensive care unit: the Roy adaptation model as a conceptual structure', *Journal of Advanced Nursing* 18: 54–63.

Pereira, G.R. (1995) 'Nutritional care of the extremely premature infant', *Clinics in Perinatology* 22(1): 61–75.

Pillo-Blocka, F., Adatia, I., Sharieff, W., McCrindle, B.W. and Zlotkin, S. (2004) 'Rapid advancement to more concentrated formula in infants after surgery for congenital heart disease reduces duration of hospital stay: a randomized controlled trial', *The Journal of Pediatrics* 145: 761–6.

Pinelli, J. and Symington, A. (2005) 'Non-nutritive sucking for promoting physiologic stability and nutrition in preterm infants', *Cochrane Database of Systematic Reviews*, Issue 4, Art. No. CD001071.DOI: 10.1002/14651858.CD001071.pub 2.

Poindexter, B.B. and Denne, S.C. (2005) 'Parental nutrition', in H.W. Taeusch, R.A. Ballard and C.A. Gleason (eds) *Avery's Diseases of the Newborn*, 8th edn, Philadelphia, PA: Elsevier Saunders.

Premji, S.S. and Chessell, L. (2002) 'Continuous nasogastric milk feeding versus intermittent bolus milk feeding for premature infants less than 1500 grams', *Cochrane Database of Systematic Reviews*, Issue 4, Art. No. CD001819.DOI: 10.1002/14651858.CD001819.

Premji, S.S., Wilson, J., Paes, B. and Gray, S. (1997) 'Cisipride: a review of the evidence supporting its use in premature infants with feeding intolerance', *Neonatal Network* 16(7): 17–21.

Quigley, M., Henderson, G., Anthony, M.Y. and McGuire, W. (2007) 'Formula milk versus donor breast milk for feeding preterm or low birth weight infants', *Cochrane Database of Systematic Reviews*, Issue 4, Art. No. CD002971.DOI: 10.1002/14651858.CD002971. pub 2.

Ryan, S. (1998) 'Nutrition in neonatal chronic lung disease', *European Journal of Pediatrics* 157 (Suppl. 1): S19–S22.

Schanler, R. (2005) 'Enteral nutrition for the high-risk neonate', in H.W. Taeusch, R.A. Ballard and C.A. Gleason (eds) *Avery's Diseases of the Newborn*, 8th edn, Philadelphia, PA: Elsevier Saunders.

Shaio, S.P.K. (1994) 'Nasal gastric tube placement: effect on sucking and breathing in very low birth weight infants', PhD dissertation, Case Western Reserve University.

Shaio, S.P.K. and Difore, T.E. (1996) 'A survey of gastric tube practices in Level II and Level III nurseries', *Issues in Comprehensive Pediatric Nursing* 19: 209–20.

Shaker, C.S. (1999) 'Nipple feeding preterm infants: an individualised, developmentally supportive approach', *Neonatal Network* 18(3): 15–22.

Sheppard, J.J. and Fletcher, K.R. (2007) 'Evidence-based interventions for breast and bottle feeding in the Neonatal Intensive Care Unit', *Seminars in Speech and Language* 28(3): 204–12.

Silvestre, M.A., Morbach, C.A., Brans, Y.W. and Shankaran, S. (1996) 'A prospective randomised trial comparing continuous versus intermittent feeding methods in very low birth weight neonates', *Journal of Pediatrics* 128: 748–52.

Simmer, K., Patole, S. and Rao, S.C. (2008a) 'Longchain polyunsaturated fatty acid supplementation in infants born at term', *Cochrane Database of Systematic Reviews*, Issue 1, Art. No. CD000376.DOI: 10.1002/14651858.CD000376.pub 2.

Simmer, K., Schulzke, S. and Patole, S. (2008b) 'Longchain polyunsaturated fatty acid supplementation in preterm infants', *Cochrane Database of Systematic Reviews*, Issue 1, Art. No. CD000375.DOI: 10.1002/14651858.CD000375.pub 3.

Skuse, D. (1993) 'Identification and management of problem eaters', *Archives of Disease in Childhood* 69: 604–8.

Spence, K., Smith, J. and Peat, J. (2003) 'Accuracy of weighing simulated infants with in-bed and freestanding scales while connected and disconnected to a ventilator', *Advances in Neonatal Care* 3(1): 27–36.

Steer, P.A., Lucas, A. and Sinclair, J.C. (1992) 'Feeding the low birthweight infant', in M. Bracken and J. Sinclair (eds) *Effective Care of the Newborn*, New York: Oxford University Press.

Stenson, B.J., Middlemist, L. and Lyon, A.J. (1998) 'Influence of erythromycin on establishment of feeding in preterm infants: observations from a randomised controlled trial', *Archives of Disease in Childhood: Fetal and Neonatal Edition* 79: F212–F214.

Tan, J.C.H. and Jeffery, H.E. (1995) 'Factors that influence the choice of infant feeding', *Journal of Paediatric and Child Health* 31(5): 375–8.

Tan, M., Abernethy, L. and Cooke, R. (2008) 'Improving head growth in preterm infants – a randomised controlled trial II: MRI and developmental outcomes in the first year', *Archives of Disease in Childhood: Fetal and Neonatal Edition* 93(5): F342–F346.

Tudehope, D.I. and Steer, P.A. (1996) 'Which milk for the preterm infant?', *Journal of Paediatric Child Health* 32(4): 275–7.

Tyson, J.E. and Kennedy, K.A. (2005) 'Trophic feedings for parenterally fed infants', *Cochrane Database of Systematic Reviews*, Issue 3, Art. No. CD000504. DOI: 10.1002/14651858.CD000504.pub 2.

Van Beek, R.H.T., Carnielli, V.P. and Sauer, P.J.J. (1995) 'Nutrition in the neonate', *Current Opinion in Pediatrics* 7: 146–51.

Van Someran, V., Linnett, S.J., Stothers, J.K. and Sullivan, P.G. (1984) 'An investigation into the benefits of resiting nasoenteric feeding tubes', *Pediatrics* 74: 379–83.

Wahlig, T.M. and Georgieff, M.K. (1995) 'The effects of illness on neonatal metabolism and nutritional management', *Clinics in Perinatology* 22(1): 77–96.

Yellis, M. (1995) 'Human breast milk and facilitation of gastrointestinal development and maturation', *Gastroenterology Nursing* 18(2): 11–15.

Chapter 13

Neonatal Infection

Glenys Connolly

Contents

Introduction

Infection is an important cause of mortality and morbidity in the newborn period. The incidence of early onset neonatal sepsis is said to have dramatically declined over the past 10 years, due to increased use of antenatal antibiotics and more effective management of premature rupture of membranes (Bedford-Russell 1996), however, there has been an increase in late onset **nosocomial** infection. This increase is due, in part, to the improved survival of extremely low birth weight (ELBW) infants, with its associated immunological incompetence, long stay in hospital, and increased usage of parenteral nutrition through central venous catheters (Philip 1994; Greenough 1996; Avila-Figueroa *et al.* 1998). Nosocomial infection is defined as any infection that is not present or incubating at the time of admission (Parvez and Jarvis 1999); it is a common, costly and clinically important measure of outcome and may be a valuable indicator of performance in neonatal intensive care (Fowlie *et al.* 1996).

This chapter will review the current information regarding neonatal susceptibility to, and acquisition of infection, the organisms commonly implicated and investigation and treatment modalities. It should serve to increase the neonatal nurse's ability to detect and manage the infected infant. Terminology used in the chapter is defined at the outset in Table 13.1.

Acquisition of antenatal infection

The intra-uterine environment should be sterile, with the fetus surrounded by amniotic fluid which has bacteriostatic or bacteriocidal properties against many organisms (Isaacs and Moxon 1999). In addition, enclosure within the amniotic

Table 13.1 Definitions used in neonatal infection

Timing of infection	
Very early onset	< 24 hours
Early onset	< 48 hours
Late onset	>72 hours
Nosocomial infection	Hospital acquired infection
Bacteraemia	The presence of viable bacteria in the blood.
Septicaemia	Systemic disease caused by the multiplication of organisms circulating in the blood
Sepsis	The presence of various pus-forming and other pathogenic organisms, or their toxins in the blood or tissues

Source: Bone (1991), Philip (1994), Berger *et al.* (1998).

membranes serves to provide the fetus with a physical barrier against invading organisms, which may reside in the maternal genital tract.

The consequence of these mechanisms is that most fetuses are effectively protected from infection while in utero. Should an ascending organism breach these defences, amnionitis may occur, which infects the fetus due to the direct aspiration into the bronchial tree initiating pneumonia and bacteraemia (Blumberg and Feldman 1996). The organism group B streptococcus (GBS) is highly implicated in this transmission route, and is the commonest organism for early onset septicaemia and meningitis (Blumberg and Feldman 1996; Greenough 1996; Berger *et al.* 1998; Beardsall *et al.* 2000).

The mycoplasmas, *Mycoplasma hominis* and *Ureaplasma urealyticum*, commonly inhabit the female urogenital tract and have also been implicated in the premature onset of labour and the development of chorioamnionitis. Chorioamnionitis is widely believed to be responsible for premature rupture of membranes and preterm labour (Fox 1993), possibly due to invoking an increase in the synthesis of prostaglandins. The role of *Ureaplasma urealyticum*, specifically in the aetiology of chronic lung disease (CLD), continues to court controversy with more than 30 studies supporting or refuting its role in the evolution of the disease process (Wang *et al.* 1995; Lyon 1996; Castro-Alcaraz *et al.* 2002).

Other organisms that may ascend from the genital tract and contaminate the amniotic fluid are *Bacteroides*, *Escherichia coli*, *Clostridium* and *Peptococcus*. As *E. coli* is highly implicated in the development of neonatal meningitis, suspicion of infection with this organism should be taken seriously.

Infection via the maternal bloodstream (transplacental haematogenous spread) is also recognised, whereby organisms affecting the fetus are present despite intact membranes. *Listeria monocytogenes* causes placentitis (Fox 1993) with the placenta covered with military granulata; this then serves as a focus from which the fetus is subsequently infected. The transplacental mode of spread may also affect placental function, resulting in a growth-restricted fetus. The placental transfer of viruses, for example, cytomegalovirus and rubella, is well documented (Logan 1990; Miller 1990). Their acquisition in the first trimester is associated not only with growth restriction but significant congenital defects. Likewise, documented evidence exists of placental transfer of hepatitis B and herpes simplex and varicella zoster, but these are said to be rarer events, and the more likely source of infection is intrapartum (Logan 1990; Lyall and Tudor-Williams 1997). GBS and mycoplasmas are also thought to have the ability to cross the maternal placenta, or breach the membranes, as they have been isolated when the membranes have been intact.

Intra-uterine infection with parvovirus B19 is associated with severe fetal anaemia and development of hydrops fetalis due to inhibition of the erythroid progenitor cells (Logan 1990). Women presenting with fetal hydrops should have serum screening for this organism antenatally, in order to optimise postnatal management.

The transmission of human immunodeficiency virus (HIV) from mother to fetus is known to involve several routes; transplacental acquisition is well documented, and thought to be related to the maternal viral burden, disease stage and the mother's own immune response (Johnstone and Mok 1990; Mueller and Pizzo 1995; Lindsay and Nesheim 1997).

Acquisition of intrapartum (vertical) infection

Factors that increase the likelihood of transmission of infection during the delivery process are the presence of preterm labour, maternal pyrexia and prolonged rupture of membranes (Rennie 1995). The most commonly acquired organism via this route, again, is GBS, due to the human gastrointestinal tract being the most common reservoir for this organism. Its secondary transmission to the female genito-urinary tract is said to occur in 5–40 per cent (average 20 per cent) of pregnant women (Blumberg and Feldman 1996; Glantz and Kedley 1998). Vertical transmission of GBS can be significantly reduced if the mother is given antibiotics during labour (Beardsall et al. 2000). The acquisition of herpes simplex virus (HSV) infection is highest at this time due to contact with the genital secretions during delivery, with the attack rate for infection being greater if the mother has a primary infection at the time. The risk of infection is lower if recurrent lesions are present (Logan 1990; Kohl 1997). Likewise, hepatitis B virus (HBV) is also more likely to be transmitted around the time of birth by contact with the maternal vaginal secretions (Kane 1997). HIV transmission during delivery is also attributed to contact with the infected secretions. Vertical transmission of HIV is said to have fallen considerably in Europe and the USA following initiation of perinatal antiretroviral therapy and elective Caesarean section in HIV positive mothers (Sharland et al. 2002).

The length of time in contact with the birth canal is implicated in transmission of infection, with studies suggesting that the first-born twin has a 2.8 higher infection rate than the co-twin, due to more prolonged exposure to blood and cervical secretions in the maternal genital tract during delivery (Kline 1996).

Genital chlamydia is recognised as the world's most common sexually transmitted disease (Darville 2005). Transmission to the fetus during vaginal delivery is said to be in the order of 50 per cent. The total number of sexually transmitted infections (syphilis, gonorrhoea and chlamydia) appears to be on the increase in the UK with chlamydia and gonorrhoea rising by 20 per cent and 5 per cent respectively in 1996–1997 (Hughes et al. 1998). This worrying rise in chlamydia has implications for the neonatal population in that chlamydial conjunctivitis is said to occur in 2–4 per 1000 live births in the UK and 10-63 per 1000 live births in the USA. As chlamydial conjunctivitis can present as late as 14 days of age, any infant who develops discharging eyes around this time should be taken seriously, screened and treated accordingly. In congenital infections left undiagnosed, between 10 and 20 per cent of those affected develop pneumonitis which may be severe enough to require ventilation (Issacs and Moxon 1999).

It can be seen then that the vertical transmission of infection from the mother to the fetus is high. Since it remains impossible to detect sero-positivity for HBV and HIV and other organisms, in all women, health care workers who come into contact with patients' (both maternal and infant) blood and body fluids should implement universal precautions routinely as a matter of good practice (DoH 2001).

Late onset and nosocomial infection

Studies suggest that the face of neonatal infection has changed over the past decade, with a discernible decrease in early onset sepsis, to one of late onset which is invariably hospital acquired (Philip 1994; Berger *et al.* 1998). The term nosocomial infection (NI) is defined as 'related to a hospital', or 'hospital acquired'. The source of the infection may be from contact with the mother, hospital personnel, or inanimate objects.

Late onset sepsis may occur due to the invasion of bacteria that have previously colonised the infant's upper respiratory tract, conjunctivae, mucosal surfaces, umbilicus or skin. This process occurs due to alteration in the host's native microflora which is affected by antibiotics, disease processes and reduced host immunity (Greene 1996). The time between colonisation and invasion will vary but predicting when this may occur is an important surveillance challenge to clinicians within neonatal units.

Nosocomial infection in NICU is reported to occur in up to 32 per cent of NICU admissions (Stoll *et al.* 2002) and is most prevalent in the **very low birth weight** (VLBW), with the most common sites for infection being the bloodstream followed by pneumonia and then 'other' sites (Parvez and Jarvis 1999).

The commonest organisms in late onset infection are *Staphylococcus*, *Klebsiella*, *Escherichia coli* and *Pseudomonas* (Greene 1996). More recently a fourfold to sixfold increase in fungal infections has been reported (Hostetter 2001). Coagulase negative staphylococci (CONS) is the most prevalent cause of late onset infection (Stoll *et al.* 2002), it being associated with catheter placement for intravenous feeding (Avila-Figueroa *et al.* 1998; Berger *et al.* 1998; Isaacs 2003), whereby the bacteria attaches to the polymer surface, proliferates forming a protective 'slime' layer and then disseminates. Spafford *et al.* (1994) suggest that this risk may be reduced by the addition of continuous low-dose vancomycin to the parenteral fluids; however, concerns about the emergence of vancomycin-resistant organisms and few clinically important benefits of routine prophylaxis preclude this approach at present (Craft *et al.* 2000). Avila-Figueroa *et al.* (1998) further suggest that it is not necessarily catheter placement that is the issue, but the lipid infusions the infant is receiving, and propose that 'lipid emulsions may fuel a proliferation of colonizing bacteria and facilitate bloodstream invasion'. The two most effective practices to reduce the incidence of catheter-related CONS are effective hand hygiene and disinfection of catheter hubs prior to drug and fluid administration (Kilbride *et al.* 2003).

CONS is not only implicated in central lines and lipid infusion, having been reported to be a significant contaminant of hospital stethoscopes, which may serve as a vector for its transmission around NICU. Wright *et al.* (1995) highlight the fact that VLBW infants have immature, and often abraded, skin with a variety of portals for infection from lines and surgical incisions, and as a consequence have an increased susceptibility to infection from stethoscopes that may be placed near these sites. They report a fall in contamination rates following the instigation of a more rigorous stethoscope-cleaning policy, which reduces the bacterial load to which the infants are exposed. Furthermore application of topical creams to help maintain skin integrity also appears to give infants an increased susceptibility to CONS infection (Conner *et al.* 2003) and should only be used with this borne in mind.

Staphylococcus aureus is another frequently reported pathogen in neonatal nosocomial infection, with the infant less than 1500g, invasive procedures and longer hospitalisation denoting the most 'at-risk' groups (Yamauchi 1995). 'Outbreaks' of infection within NICUs are invariably related to lapses in good infection control procedures. Hand washing is the single most important factor in the prevention of the spread of infection. It is a simple, inexpensive procedure yet non-compliance with hand hygiene techniques remains a worrying facet within neonatal care. Studies suggest that as few as 20 per cent of individuals comply with hand hygiene techniques (Borghesi and Stronati 2008) despite the evidence that poor hand-washing practices contribute to nosocomial infection (Larson 1995; Callaghan 1998; Pessoa-Silva *et al.* 2007). The use of alcohol rubs between patient contacts is thought to be more effective in removing organisms than soap and water alone (Girou *et al.* 2002); however, visible contamination with body fluids should be removed with soap and water prior to its application. Infection control teams will provide local information and guidance as to what should be used in particular circumstances.

Hand washing is not the only area implicated in cross-infection. The laryngoscope has been identified as a potential vector responsible not only for colonisation of infants with *Pseudomonas aeruginosa*, but has also been implicated in the subsequent deaths of five infants in two separately reported outbreaks (Foweraker 1995; Neal *et al.* 1995). This can be avoided by use of single patient-only equipment or strict attention to maintaining cleanliness and decontamination if it is necessary to share equipment.

There is thought to be a substantially greater mortality and morbidity among infants who develop nosocomial infections (Fanaroff *et al.* 1998). Whether this is as a result of the septicaemia or a reflection of infant vulnerability is yet to be determined. Prevention of NI is an important and integral part of the neonatal nurse's role. Its control and incidence may, potentially, be reduced by enforcing strategies that reduce contamination and cross-infection, education of all members of the team and parents regarding hand hygiene techniques, and by liaising with, and taking advice from, the infection control team. The risk factors for hospital acquired infection are listed in Table 13.2.

Table 13.2 Risk factors for nosocomial infection

Infant

Weight <1500g

Depressed immunological function

Presence of underlying disease

Raised gastric pH

Poor nutritional status

Need for total parenteral nutrition (esp. lipids)

Multiple antibiotic usage

Multiple sites of access
    ETT tube
    IV cannulae
    central catheter placement

Long stay in hospital

Environment

Poor compliance with infection-control techniques
    Hand washing
    shared equipment (e.g. laryngoscopes)
    scales
    scanning equipment

Presence of opportunistic organisms

Overcrowding

Inadequate staffing levels

Poor disposal of contaminated waste

Source: Adapted from Sproat and Inglis (1992).

The susceptible host

Infection is more common in the neonatal period due to exposure to a large number of organisms, and also a failure of the host defence mechanisms to clear micro-organisms from the blood and tissues. The 'immune deficiency' of the newborn is relative rather than absolute (Isaacs and Moxon 1999), and is due to its naïveté rather than defects *per se*. The immune system is made up of several component parts which are all necessary to maintain defence mechanisms and recognise invading foreign material. The physical defences include the skin, gastric secretions, tears, intact mucous membranes, ciliated epithelium and urine pH. All, or certainly some of these aspects will be potentially affected in the sick newborn infant by either immaturity due to poor keratinisation of the skin, or by interventions preventing their efficacy. Intravenous cannulas breach skin defences and endotracheal intubation and ventilation which will inhibit mucociliary movement.

Non-specific defences include **phagocytes** (neutrophils, monocytes), natural killer cells (NK), inflammatory responses and the antimicrobial proteins, including complement activation. Phagocytes are derived from a common precursor myeloid stem cell, often referred to as colony-forming units (CFUs). These units are stimulated by colony stimulating factor (CSF) and cytokines. Polymorphonuclear neutrophils are the most numerous of the white blood cells and are chemically attracted to bacteria and fungi which they are able to destroy by first engulfing the organism and then inducing the 'respiratory burst', in which oxygen is actively metabolised to release hydrogen peroxide, hydroxyl radicals and superoxides which are powerful microbiocidal agents (Roitt 1991). This process is dependent on the cells' ability to be able to 'home in' on the organism by chemotaxis with the activation of complement, which amplifies the response and increases adherence to the surface by opsonisation. Serum opsonins are plasma protein substances that enhance phagocytosis by making the organism more visible or 'attractive' to the macrophages, which then allows engulfment and destruction to occur. In the newborn infant this process can be affected, as there is little or no transplacental crossage of complement. While infected newborns do have an ability to release complement, it has both quantitative deficiencies and qualitative differences which affect its function (Lewis and Wilson 1995). Concentration increases postnatally but does not reach adult levels until between 6–18 months of age. It is also recognised that term and preterm infants have a relative deficiency in opsonin activity to a variety of organisms (Crockett 1995). It follows therefore that both phagocytosis and opsonisation are affected, and a study undertaken by Kallman *et al.* (1998) shows this to be particularly pertinent in the case of GBS infection, with the problem being further compounded in the preterm population.

Macrophages develop from monocytes and are crucial to the body's defence system. They reside in specific parts of the body, mainly the alveoli and liver. From these strategic positions, macrophages filter out blood-borne **antigens** and degrade them without producing an immune response. They also serve to provide a further function by becoming antigen presenting cells (APC), whereby a fragment of the antigen is displayed on the macrophages' surface, which the immune system then recognises as non-self and brings into force the cell and antibody mediated immune responses.

NK cells are derived from **lymphocytes**, and are closely related to T lymphocytes. They play an important part in the defence of intracellular pathogens, particularly herpes group viruses. NK cells destroy by the binding to the membrane of the target, and releasing a cytolysin, which destroys by **apoptosis**. **Interferons** augment NK cells' toxicity, and since interferons are produced by virally infected cells, an integrated feedback defence is created (Roitt 1991). Although NK cells are said to appear early to mid-gestation, they are immature and have decreased cytotoxic activity which diminishes their functional ability. This functional ability is further reduced due to the newborn's inability to produce sufficient amounts of γ interferon (Harris 1992).

Specific defence mechanisms involve two distinct lymphocytes. Both of these cell types are generated from bone marrow, but where they gain immuno-competence determines their ultimate development into **T cells**, which are responsible for **cell mediated immunity**, or **B cells**, which confer so-called **humoral immunity**, from which antibodies are produced.

T cells are 'educated' within the thymus gland. During this time they differentiate into three cell types: T helper cells (CD4 cells), T cytotoxic cells (CD8 cells) and T suppressor cells. T helper cells are the most numerous, and their function is to recognise antigens on the surface of APCs and stimulate a proliferation of cytotoxic T cells and B cells by the release of interleukins. Cytotoxic T cells bind to the targeted cell and perforate the cell membrane, which allows for an influx of extracellular calcium, killing it. Suppressor T cells are inhibitory in their action and are thought to suppress activity of both T and B cells once the antigen has been inactivated. This mechanism is also thought to be important in preventing autoimmune disease. While there is no evidence to support maternal transfer of T cell specific immunity to the fetus, the neonate can produce a T cell response to an antigen challenge. However, overall function is impaired due to diminished cytotoxicity and decreased cytokine (interleukin) production (Lewis and Wilson 1995).

Within humoral immunity it is recognised that maternal transfer of some **immunoglobulins** (antibody) does occur, and affords the neonate some pro-tection in the initial stages. Maternal IgG transfer begins at approximately 22 weeks of gestation, transporting larger quantities after 30 weeks (Lewis and Wilson 1995). This is made possible by the presence of receptor sites on the placenta. As the placenta does not have such sites for IgM (the acute phase immunoglobulin), it cannot cross to the fetus, so immunity to acute maternal infection around the time of delivery is not achieved. Elevated IgM levels in the newborn indicate congenital intra-uterine infection.

The more preterm the neonate is, the less placental transfer will have occurred, so passive immunity is diminished. Neonatal resistance to bacterial pathogens to which the mother has little or no IgG is particularly compromised by the inability to produce antibody, due to immaturity or a lack of B cells (Lewis and Wilson 1995). In conjunction with this, passively acquired IgG is rapidly catabolised, with a half-life of approximately 20 days. Losses will occur much more quickly in the sick infant who is repeatedly bled and transfused with washed packed erythrocytes (Lawton 1992), so the benefit of the maternal transport system is quickly lost.

B cells are the antibody-producing component of the immune system. Once an antigen (organism) has been recognised within the body, B cells become activated to produce plasma cells which secrete antibody specific to the antigen. Some B cells differentiate to become memory cells which remain in the system so that a more rapid immune response occurs, should the same antigen present itself at a later date.

The five immunoglobulin types have differing structures depending on their site and function:

- IgG is the most abundant antibody in the plasma. It provides passive immunity to the fetus, it is able to neutralise toxins and bind organisms to enhance phagocytosis. It also activates complement and increases **opsonisation**.
- IgM is the largest immunoglobulin and is an efficient agglutinating and cytolytic agent.
- IgA is secretory in nature and present in saliva, tears, intestinal secretions and maternal colostrum. It inhibits adherence of organisms to the surface of mucosal cells, thereby preventing entry to the body. It also activates complement.
- IgD function appears in the main to be present on the surface of lympho-cytes to control activation and suppression of B cells.
- IgE is present in very low quantities in the serum but is present in higher quantities in certain sites, for example, the respiratory and gastrointestinal tracts. It triggers the release of histamine and other vasoactive agents when presented with antigen and creates the body's 'allergic' responses (Roitt 1991).

It can be seen, therefore, that the newborn infant is equipped with mechanisms to cope with organisms following birth, but the immune system and its responses are restricted by physiological differences and functional deficiencies, which are further compromised in the premature or physiologically stressed infant.

Signs of neonatal sepsis

The neonatal nurse, with expert clinical skills and judgement, is pivotal in the early recognition of sepsis. It is imperative that sepsis is pre-empted or detected as early as possible as the recognised inadequacies of the immune system response, and its inability to contain micro-organisms may lead to rapid proliferation and dissemination of organisms leading to an overwhelming septicaemia or meningitis, or in the worst scenario, death. Indicators for potential infection should be apparent from the maternal history, for example, gestational age, rupture of membranes, maternal pyrexia or infection. These facts can be elicited during a pre-delivery visit to the labour ward, if time allows, or by communication with the delivery unit team.

Despite any overt history, the interventions that most infants receive following admission to NICU increase the likelihood of acquiring infection, by breaches of physical defence systems following intubation and ventilation, the siting of intravenous and arterial lines, and by exposure to multiple members of the NICU team.

Respiratory signs

Infants presenting with tachypnoea, grunting, recession and apnoea (Isaacs and Moxon 1999) may have early onset congenital infection or respiratory distress syndrome. It is impossible to differentiate these conditions clinically or even following chest radiography, as the chest X-ray reveals similar findings. These infants need careful consideration, as both problems may coexist, and without antibiotic therapy the septicaemia can kill in hours (Greenough *et al.* 1992).

The respiratory symptoms from GBS infection are due, in part, to the organism-mediated release of the vasoactive agent thromboxane A_2, which causes severe pulmonary vascular constriction. This combined with the infant's reduced white cell ability to kill the organism leads to rapid dissemination of the disease process and profound generalised physiological instability.

Respiratory distress presenting after 4-6 hours of age is usually due to pneumonia (see p. 128) (Greenhough and Milner 2005).

Late onset sepsis and meningitis may manifest with respiratory signs due to central effects on the respiratory centre leading to tachypnoea or apnoea.

Thermal signs

Temperature instability, after environmental factors have been eliminated, may be an early indicator of infection. Approximately half of the babies with proved sepsis are febrile, one-third are normothermic and 15 per cent have hypothermia (Isaacs and Moxon 1999). The further the deviation from the normal range, be that high or low, the more significant the finding is. A widening toe:core temperature gap (>1.5°C) may also occur as the peripheral perfusion of the infant reduces in response to sepsis.

Cardiovascular signs

Cardiovascular changes of tachycardia, hypotension and poor capillary refill times may indicate sepsis. A heart rate of greater than 160bpm is often present in early sepsis. If cardiac output is compromised or peripheral vasoconstriction is present, the capillary refill time (CRT) may be prolonged. The sites for estimating CRT are optimally the forehead and the sternum, with the refill time being less than 3 seconds (Strozik *et al.* 1998). Pallor or mottling of the skin (cutis marmorata) may also be apparent.

Skin signs

The skin should be carefully scrutinsed for lesions of petechiae, which may result from congenital infection. A raised papular 'pin point' rash (granu-lomatous infantiseptica) can be present in an infant with congenital *Listeria* infection (Isaacs and Moxon 1999). Necrotic skin lesions are associated with *Pseudomonal* sepsis or sepsis due to fungi. Necrotising fasciitis can be caused by *Staphylococcus aureus* and Gram negative bacteria. Disseminated intra-vascular coagulation (see p. 220), with **petechiae** and bleeding from puncture sites, the gut or kidneys, is a rare, late and worrying sign. It is thought to occur following triggering of the clotting cascade as a result of diffuse endothelial damage from the circulating endotoxins (Emer 1992). Jaundice occurs in one-third of septic infants, and is more associated with Gram negative infections, but may occur in GBS. It is probably due to increased haemolysis and endotoxic effects on the liver and is characteristically conjugated (Isaacs and Moxon 1999).

Gastrointestinal signs

Gastrointestinal signs of distension and ileus are a common and important sign of sepsis and need to be differentiated from intestinal obstruction or necrotising enterocolitis (NEC), all of which may present similarly with poor toleration of milk and bile-stained gastric aspirates. While no single organism has been found to be the cause of NEC, *Klebsiella, Clostridium difficile* and *E. coli* have, among others, been implicated in its development. However, 'epidemic' NEC presumed to be infectious agent-related is responsible for only 5 per cent of all cases (Clark and Miller 1996). Tolerance of enteral feeds is generally poor in infection and may be an early sign of sepsis in an infant who has previously been enterally fed.

Blood sugar instability may also be an early sign, with hyperglycaemia requiring insulin therapy a feature of fungal infection (Hostetter 2001).

Neurological signs

Lethargy, irritability or 'not handling' well occurs in approximately one half of infants with sepsis, and should always be further investigated. Meningitis may be heralded by increasing irritability, alterations in consciousness, poor tone and tremors, with up to 75 per cent of infants having some seizure activity (Klein and Marcy 1995a).

Table 13.3 (Radetsky 1995) shows a composite of the overall likelihood ratios of clinical findings for neonatal bacterial infection. This table demonstrates not only the diversity of signs but also how poorly many of them correlate to infection. Given, however, that most infants will present with many of the listed signs, the likelihood of infection increases.

Investigations

Despite the current trend in nursing and medicine towards 'evidence-based' decision-making and management, experience and intuition are often the

Table 13.3 The likelihood ratios of clinical findings for neonatal bacterial infections

Clinical finding	Likelihood ratio
Common signs	
Pallor	14.4
Poor feeding	8.7
Tachycardia/arrhythmia	5.6
Decreased peripheral perfusion	5.4
Unstable blood pressure	4.0
Abdominal distension	3.5
Apnoea	3.1
Lethargy	2.3
Hyperbilirubinaemia	2.0
Retractions	1.7
Grunting	1.6
Abnormal tone	1.6
Tachypnoea	1.3
Cyanosis	0.3
Temperature instability	0.7
Uncommon signs	
Purpura	47.0
Omphalitis	32.5
Vasomotor instability	8.1
Bleeding	6.5
Pustules	6.1
Bulging fontanelle	5.4
Splenomegaly	4.1
Rash	4.0
Diarrhoea	3.6
Seizures	2.3

Source: Radetsky (1995).

precursors of the initiation of screening for infection in an infant who 'doesn't handle well'. This intuitive aspect is probably as effective a screening tool as any when one considers Fowlie and Schmidt's (1998) systematic review of diagnostic tests for bacterial infections which concluded that the reported accuracy of tests is generally poor. There is, of course, a necessity to try to confirm diagnosis and identify the causative organisms in order to ensure that the most appropriate antibiotic therapy is prescribed. Once sepsis is suspected, a battery of laboratory tests can be put in place to confirm or refute suspicions.

Surface swabs and site cultures

Surface swabs and cultures from deeper sites are often obtained initially on admission to NICU or when late onset sepsis is suspected. The sensitivity of surface swabs in the detection is high, in the order of 90 per cent (Thompson *et al.* 1992), but the specificity is said to be poor, at around 50–78 per cent (Evans *et al.* 1988; Thompson *et al.* 1992). There appears to be little value in obtaining swabs on admission from multiple sites, for example, nose, throat or rectum, as the optimal site for culture is reported to be the deep ear swab alone (Evans *et al.* 1988; Thompson *et al.* 1992), and obvious focal lesions in later onset suspected infections.

Gastric aspiration and culture do not help identify which babies are likely to develop infection, as the polymorphonuclear leucocytes and bacterial content of the specimen are of maternal origin and reflect fetal exposure to infection, but not necessarily neonatal infection (Borderon *et al.* 1994; Powell and Marcy 1995).

Tracheal aspirates obtained following long-term ventilation, similarly, may not reflect infection, but rather colonisation of bacteria within the system (Powell and Marcy 1995). The treatment of such cases with antibiotics demands caution as it may contribute to an increase in resistant strains of organisms.

Haematological tests

Blood culture is mandatory before starting treatment with antibiotics (Yoxall *et al.* 1996), and is considered the definitive laboratory test (Radetsky 1995). The blood should be drawn from a peripheral vein or artery following strict cleansing of the overlying skin, or from newly inserted umbilical catheters. Blood taken from indwelling catheters that have been present for some time may reflect contamination or colonisation of the intravascular device (Yoxall *et al.* 1996; Isaacs and Moxon 1999), and as a consequence is not recommended.

Other haematological tests include the total neutrophil count. This test is a more reliable indicator of neonatal sepsis than the total white cell count as the normal range is wide and varies with gestation and postnatal age. Further to this, other pathology such as asphyxia, meconium aspiration, periventricular haemorrhage and pneumothorax can give a raised total count (Powell and Marcy 1995). Both neutropenia (less than $2–2.5 \times 10^9$) and neutrophilia (greater than $7.5–8.0 \times 10^9$) are indicators of infection, with neutropenia being particularly suggestive of severe sepsis as this reflects depletion of the granulocyte pool in the bone marrow (Isaacs and Moxon 1999). Immature neutrophils are seen in the peripheral blood of healthy newborns, but their presence is increased in sepsis as an increased number are released from the bone marrow. This is described as the 'left-shift'. Measuring the immature to total neutrophil ratio (ITR) is said to be a sensitive predictor of sepsis, with a ratio of greater than 0.2 being a good indicator of infection (Roberton 1992).

Measurement of acute phase proteins, especially C-reactive protein (CRP), is often undertaken, with elevated levels being indicative of sepsis. CRP levels also rise in necrotising enterocolitis, meconium aspiration and following surgery. Whether it is a sensitive enough predictor for sepsis, in isolation, is debatable but its value in monitoring the course of infection and infant response to therapy is recognised (Roberton 1992; Powell and Marcy 1995; Benitz *et al.* 1998), as its level should return to normal in less than 2–7 days if the stimulus to its production has been removed (Yoxall *et al.* 1996). In persistently elevated CRP levels, bacterial meningitis or abscess formation in NEC should be suspected.

Platelet count measurement in the newborn is well established, with the normal count, regardless of birthweight, rarely being less than $100 \times 10^9/l$ in the first 10 days of life or less than $150 \times 10^9/l$ during the next three weeks. Thrombocytopenia is very common in infants with candidiasis but also occurs in 50 per cent of cases of bacteraemia (Isaacs and Moxon 1999), but is usually a late finding and not until some time after the infant is obviously septic (Powell and Marcy 1995).

Cerebrospinal fluid

Lumbar puncture (LP) (see p. 349) has been considered mandatory in the evaluation of newborns for infection (Radetsky 1995) to rule out bacterial meningitis, which occurs more frequently in the neonatal period than at any other time in life, and carries a significant morbidity among survivors (Yoxall *et al.* 1996). Positive culture yield is said to be low in infants in whom the procedure is performed on a 'routine' basis as part of admission screening (Klein and Marcy 1995a; Radetsky 1995). This factor, coupled with the technical difficulties, discomfort and potential hypoxia encountered in the ventilated and physiologically unstable infant, means that many units will not perform this procedure unless the infant is manifesting with central nervous system signs. The use of local anaesthesia has been suggested in reducing pain, but this does not prevent the other physiological changes encountered by infants (Klein and Marcy 1995a) and its use potentially increases handling and duration of the procedure. Controlled pre-oxygenation may be employed to ameliorate the hypoxia, but this needs careful assessment and attention by the nurse assisting the procedure.

Some units continue to undertake this procedure despite the associated problems, the opinion being that the high incidence of neonatal meningitis with its associated mortality and morbidity justifies its inclusion in routine infection screening (Yoxall *et al.* 1996).

The obtained cerebrospinal fluid (CSF) should be 'crystal clear'. Yellow coloration (xanthochromia) is often seen on neonatal specimens due to bilirubin staining or old intraventricular haemorrhage. A CSF white cell count of more than 30/mm³ with more than 66 per cent neutrophils, or a CSF protein level greater than 1g/l in a term infant or 2g/l in a preterm infant, are suspicious and meningitis should be seriously considered. A CSF glucose level should also be measured and correlated to the plasma glucose level. The plasma glucose sample should *always* be taken prior to the LP, as the level will probably increase due to stress, which can make the result less easy to interpret. The CSF glucose should be approximately 70–80 per cent of the blood glucose (Rennie 1995), in bacterial meningitis it will be low but in viral meningitis can be normal. CSF protein counts are usually high in both bacterial and viral meningitis.

Urine

Urine should be obtained for culture, but therapy should not be withheld if there is difficulty obtaining the specimen. If a bag is to be used to collect the specimen the surrounding area should be thoroughly cleaned to minimise contamination from organisms colonising on the skin. The bag should be removed as soon as urine is voided for the same reason. Positive bag urine cultures are often viewed with suspicion, and a suprapubic aspiration may be performed. While this procedure often appears drastic (see p. 352), the long-term implications of a urinary tract infection with its potential development of renal scarring and atrophic kidneys in later life (Klein and Marcy 1995b) probably justifies its use.

Urine antigen detection (latex agglutination test) may be available to facilitate early detection of GBS. It is reported to be between 88 and 100 per cent sensitive (Radetsky 1995), but is not available in many hospitals.

Other laboratory tests, including fibronectin levels, which fall in infection, and cytokine concentrations such as IL1β, IL6 and tumor necrosis factor, which are thought to be endogenous mediators of immune response to bacterial infection, are currently being researched but further clinical data are needed to determine whether these are truly useful in diagnosing and following the progress in neonatal infection.

Management of the infected newborn

Supportive therapy and broad spectrum antibiotics should commence as soon as infection is suspected, as a delay can result in mortality or significant morbidity.

General supportive therapy

Ventilatory support

Many babies will become apnoeic when infected. Depending on the underlying cause, respiration may be further compromised due to abdominal distension, which may invoke diaphragmatic splinting, resulting in poor oxygenation and carbon dioxide retention (see p. 394). Elective intubation and ventilation are an important supportive measure that may be neglected, following prescription of antimicrobials in the misguided hope that they will be sufficient, leaving the infant to collapse and require emergency resuscitation later (Isaacs and Moxon 1999).

Ventilation will usually be necessary in the infant with GBS due to its association with pulmonary vasoconstriction and the development of persistent pulmonary hypertension (see pp. 133 and 170).

Cardiovascular support

Maintenance of the circulation cannot be overemphasised. The septicaemic infant is likely to be shocked, so assessment and management of blood pressure and perfusion are of paramount importance. The result of a reduction in circulating blood volume can cause pre-renal renal failure unless aggressive management is adopted.

Peripheral perfusion and capillary refill time needs to be frequently estimated. Blood pressure should be maintained within normal limits for the infant's gestation and age (see p. 168). Both are often compromised due to poor cardiac output, acidaemia and low circulating volume. Volume replacement with blood or fresh frozen plasma (FFP), saline or human albumin solution (HAS) is indicated. Blood and FFP are the most beneficial as they, theoretically, not only replace volume but also contain immunoglobulins and clotting factors (Isaacs and Moxon 1999), but there are no studies providing evidence that the outcome from infection is better if FFP is used (Bedford-Russell 1996). Human albumin solution or normal saline may be given, saline being as effective in treating hypotension as albumin (Osborn and Evans 2004), but neither contains the postulated added value of blood or FFP. The volume replacement should be given at 10–20ml/kg over 30 minutes, being mindful that the hypoxic, acidaemic infant has poor myocardial contractility and is prone to overload and cardiac failure (Roberton 1997), so careful monitoring is required.

If volume replacement is not sufficient to treat the hypotension, an inotropic agent may be included, for example, dopamine or dobutamine (see p. 169).

Acid base balance

The acid base state may be compromised in septic shock. While the instigation of ventilatory support to correct respiratory acidaemia, and support of the cardiovascular system with volume and inotropes should correct the blood pH, further correction may be necessary by the use of intravenous alkali therapy. The use of bicarbonate continues to be contentious (see p. 74), but the effect of acidaemia on myocardial contractility, surfactant production and pulmonary vascular resistance warrants its careful and considered use in the infant with a pH less than 7.25 and a base deficit of greater than 10mmol/l.

Fluid and electrolyte balance

Management of fluids in this infant needs to be meticulous, with a record of intake of all infusions and boluses of colloid and crystalloid being strictly made. Fluid balance may be further complicated in infection due to the inappropriate secretion of antidiuretic hormone (IADH) brought about by severe hypoxia or meningitis (Isaacs and Moxon 1999).

Urine output should be measured by the weighing of nappies, urine collection bags/devices or catheterisation, each having its advantages and disadvantages.

Nappies need frequent changing to prevent evaporative losses, which, though not as much of a problem now with hyper-absorbent disposables, still means more regular handling. Collection devices either fall off if not sufficiently secured or can cause skin excoriation in the very premature or fragile newborn, and catheterisation is usually undertaken with a tube not specifically designed for this purpose, increasing the likelihood of trauma and introduction of infection in this already compromised infant.

Hyponatraemia may also transpire secondary to IADH secretion, and both sodium and potassium losses increase in NEC or the diuretic phase of acute tubular necrosis, which may occur following low renal perfusion states. Hypoglycaemia may occur as a result of increased metabolic demands coupled with low substrate (Karp et al. 1995), so regular monitoring is imperative if acute and long-term sequelae are to be avoided. Fluid volumes and concentrations of dextrose need to be carefully titrated to maintain blood glucose within the acceptable normal range.

Haematological management

A careful running total of blood taken for testing needs to be recorded as sick infants, especially those less than 1500g, tolerate anaemia badly (Greenough et al. 1992). Regular top-up transfusions may be required to correct deficits.

Bruising, oozing and petechiae due to consumptive coagulopathy (see p. 220) need to be promptly recognised and managed with platelet transfusion, fresh frozen plasma, cryoprecipitate and vitamin K, as appropriate.

Exchange transfusion (see p. 216) may be advocated in extreme circumstances, as it corrects bleeding by simultaneously washing out coagulation inhibitors and supplying missing coagulation factors. It is also a source of opsonins and has the potential to increase the oxygen-carrying capacity of the blood (Perez and Weisman 1997). However, the procedure potentially carries with it dramatic haemodynamic changes which may be poorly tolerated.

Antimicrobial therapy

Because of their susceptibility to vertically and nosocomially acquired infection, newborn infants are often prescribed antibiotics on presumptive sepsis before cultures are reported (Saez-Llorens and McCracken 1995). Initially, broad spectrum cover is prescribed, which is usually dependent on local policies and the unit flora, changing to specific antibiotics when dictated by the culture and sensitivity results. While this is accepted as the most appropriate and safe practice for the infant, administration of broad spectrum agents for empirical treatment of presumed sepsis is highly implicated in antimicrobial resistance, which worldwide is a problem reaching crisis dimensions (Goldmann and Huskins 1997).

It has also been postulated that indiscriminate use of antibiotics may actually predispose infants to NEC rather than reducing the risk (Clark and Miller 1996). The use of antibiotic therapy within neonatal units therefore needs to be multidisciplinary, involving the prescribing clinician, clinical microbiologist, the infection control team and the nurse caring for the infant, if potential problems are to be avoided.

In acute infection, intravenous administration of antibiotics is the route of choice. Oral medication is clearly unreliable in babies who are shocked, acidotic and obviously unwell, with the risk of delayed absorption being too great (Neonatal Formulary 2007).

As neonatal nurses are invariably the ones who administer these drugs to this susceptible population, an understanding of the choice of drugs and their potential side-effects needs to be considered if the NMC's *Standards for Medicines Management* (NMC 2008) is to be adhered to. Advice and information should be sought from the unit's pharmacist and reputable texts, for example, *The Neonatal Formulary* (2007), regarding reconstitution solutions, displacement volumes, recommended dosage and storage of individual drugs.

Penicillins

With a 40-year record of safety and efficacy in neonates, penicillin remains the drug of choice for proved infections caused by groups A and B streptococci, susceptible pneumococci, meningococci, gonococci and *Treponema pallidum* (Edwards 1997). Penicillin G does not penetrate CSF well, even in bacterial meningitis, so other antimicrobials are recommended.

Ampicillin is effective against most strains of enterococci and *Listeria monocytogenes*. Despite the increasing prevalence of methicillin-resistant *Staphylococcus aureus* (MRSA), some antistaphylococcal penicillins are useful for infections caused by susceptible *S. aureus* and *S. epidermidis*. The withdrawal of methicillin from commercial use has necessitated substitution with nafcillin (Saez-Llorens and McCracken 1995; Edwards 1997). Ticarcillin, a semi-synthetic penicillin, is useful against *Pseudomonas aeruginosa*.

As penicillins are primarily excreted by the kidneys, renal function should be carefully monitored when the drugs are given parenterally. In high-dose penicillin treatment, bone marrow suppression can occur, so the WBC should also be monitored during treatment (Edwards 1997).

Aminoglycosides

The aminoglycosides – gentamicin, netilmicin, tobramicin – are widely employed in the newborn with a possible or proved infection resulting from Gram-negative enteric pathogens (Isaacs and Moxon 1999; Neonatal Formulary 2007). They are also proposed to have a synergistic effect when used with penicillin against GBS (Saez-Llorens and McCracken 1995).

Adverse effects from aminoglycosides include renal toxicity and **otoxicity,** although the latter is difficult to determine due to other variables within the NICU setting. It is thought that gentamicin toxicity is more likely to occur with a dosage interval of 12 hours, as this leads to many infants having toxic trough levels. Dosage intervals need careful consideration. Intervals of 24 hours in infants older than 32 weeks are recommended. This dosing interval should be increased to 36 hours when less than 32 weeks, in the first week of life (Davies and Cartwright 1998; Nestaas *et al.* 2005). Serum levels should be determined before the third dose (Edwards 1997; Neonatal Formulary 2007) is administered, or earlier if renal function is compromised.

Aztreonam

The aminoglycoside-like activity of aztreonam, with good CSF penetration, and its absence of nephrotoxic or ototoxic effects may make it useful against *E. coli* in the setting of renal compromise.

Cephalosporins

The cephalosporins are grouped into generations based on their spectrum of activity. The third generation cephalosporins (cefotaxime, ceftazidime) are the most useful in the treatment of neonatal infections, with activity against Gram-negative bacilli, meningococci, gonococci and *Haemophilus influenzae.* Ceftazidime is particularly effective against *Pseudomonas*. These drugs are generally well tolerated by neonates (Saez-Llorens and McCracken 1995), but serum creatinine levels, white blood cell counts and differential should be performed regularly to monitor for potential renal or bone marrow toxicity (Edwards 1997).

Vancomycin and teicoplanin

These glycopeptide antibiotics are active against staphylococci, streptococci, enterococci and other Gram-positive bacteria. Too rapid infusion of vancomycin can lead to a dramatic red 'rash' due to histamine release. Infants receiving vancomycin should have renal function monitored and the trough level should be measured after the third to fifth dose as ototoxicity secondary to the drug has been reported. Teicoplanin is not reported to have the same side-effects and as it is given once daily by slow bolus injection confers some benefits over vancomycin.

Metronidazole

Metronidazole has excellent activity against Gram-negative, obligate anaerobic bacilli such as *Bacteroides* and *Clostridium* species. It is particularly useful following gut surgery and in necrotising enterocolitis (Edwards 1997; Neonatal Formulary 2007).

Chloramphenicol

Chloramphenicol has been used for many years in the treatment of meningitis. Due to its toxicity in causing vascular collapse, bone marrow suppression and 'grey baby syndrome', many authors suggest its use should now be abandoned in the treatment of neonatal infection (Saez-Llorens and McCracken 1995; Edwards 1997; Isaacs and Moxon 1999); as much safer and effective drugs are now available, its usage should be confined to exceptional circumstances.

Adjunctive therapies

The use of intravenous immunoglobulins (IVIG) in prevention or treatment of neonatal infection remains controversial (Bedford-Russell 1996). In the 1980s studies suggested that it significantly reduced the incidence of nosocomial infection, mortality and morbidity (Haque *et al.* 1986; Chirico *et al.* 1987), but in a further study Weisman *et al.* (1994) did not see any significant alteration of rate of sepsis or mortality when given prophylactically. Ohlsson and Lacey (2004) also conclude that currently there is insufficient evidence to support the routine administration of IVIG preparations in neonatal infections. There is an international multi-centre trial underway that may conclusively support or refute their use in clinical practice (INIS, NPEU 2008); the results of this trial are due in 2010.

As septic neonates are at risk of neutropenia and storage pool depletion, white blood cell transfusion has been attempted and other developments have centred on the use of granulocyte colony stimulating factor (GCSF), and granulocyte macrophage colony stimulating factor (GMCSF), to enhance endogenous defence mechanisms (Bedford-Russell 1996; Bedford-Russell *et al.* 2001). Again a multi-centre trial is underway (PROGRAMS) to study the efficacy of such interventions. The role of prostaglandin, thromboxane and leukotriene inhibition in the treatment of sepsis has not yet been established. The suggestion that non-steroidal anti-inflammatory agents such as ibuprofen or indomethacin may be utilised in order to ameliorate the effects of thromboxanes and tumour necrosis factor, which contribute to pulmonary hypertension and endotoxaemia (Rennie 1995; Perez and Weisman 1997), is also being further investigated.

Conclusion

Congenital and hospital acquired infection remains a significant cause of neonatal mortality and morbidity. In increasing knowledge of the common causative organisms and the antenatal, intrapartum and postnatal factors associated with their acquisition, the neonatal nurse is well placed to advocate for the most effective management strategies to help optimise the infant's outcome.

Case study: neonatal infection

A 30-year-old woman is admitted to the delivery unit at 29 weeks of gestation with a history of ruptured membranes for 22 hours. In a previous pregnancy it is noted that she had a urinary tract infection with group B haemolytic streptococcus and that infant was treated with antibiotics.

Q.1.   What factors from this history are useful in determining what course of action should be taken both ante- and postnatally in this woman's management?

She progresses through labour and a girl is delivered, within a two-hour period. She cries at delivery, becomes pink and her heart rate is above 100 min. She is given CPAP and transferred to NICU for further assessment and management.

Q.2.   What are the factors that make this infant susceptible to infection?

Q.3.   On admission to NICU, what should the immediate management of this infant be?

Two hours after admission she has increased work of breathing and her mean blood pressure has fallen to 20mmHg.

Q.4.   What are the potential causes of her deterioration, and what management strategies should be instigated in order to stabilise this infant?

Q.5.   On day 2 a central venous catheter is inserted in order to give total parenteral nutrition. Why might this procedure adversely affect this infant's outcome?

References

Avila-Figueroa, C., Goldmann, D.A. and Richardson, D.K. (1998) 'Intravenous lipid emulsions are the major determinant of coagulase-negative staphylococcal bacteraemia in the very low birth weight newborns', *Pediatric Infectious Diseases Journal* 17: 10–17.

Beardsall, K., Thompson, M.H. and Mulla, R.J. (2000) 'Neonatal group B streptococcal infection in South Bedfordshire, 1993–1998', *Archives of Disease in Childhood: Fetal and Neonatal Edition* 82: F205–F207.

Bedford-Russell, A.R. (1996) 'New modalities for treating neonatal infection', *European Journal of Pediatrics* 155 (Suppl. 2): S21–S24.

Bedford-Russell, A.R., Emmerson, A.J.B., Wilkinson, N. *et al.* (2001) 'A trial of recombinant granulocyte colony stimulating factor for the treatment of very low birthweight infants with presumed sepsis and neutropenia', *Archives of Disease in Childhood: Fetal and Neonatal Edition* 84: F172–F176.

Benitz, W.E., Han, M.Y., Madan, A. and Ramachandra, P. (1998) 'Serial serum C-reactive protein levels in the diagnosis of neonatal infection', *Pediatrics* 102(4): E41.

Berger, A., Salzer, H.R., Weninger, M. *et al.* (1998) 'Septicaemia in an Austrian neonatal intensive care unit: a 7-year analysis', *Acta Paediatrica Scandinavica* 87: 1066–9.

Blumberg, R.M. and Feldman, R.G. (1996) 'Neonatal group B streptococcal infection', *Current Paediatrics* 6: 34–7.

Bone, R.C. (1991) 'Let's agree on terminology: definitions of sepsis', *Critical Care Medicine* 19(7): 973–6.

Borderon, E., Desroches, A., Tescher, M. *et al.* (1994) 'Value of examination of the gastric aspirate for the diagnosis of neonatal infection', *Biology of the Neonate* 65: 353–66.

Borghesi, A. and Stronati, M. (2008) 'Strategies for the prevention of hospital-acquired infections in the neonatal intensive care unit', *Journal of Hospital Infection* 68: 293–300.

Callaghan, I. (1998) 'Bacterial contamination of nurses' uniforms: a study', *Nursing Standard* 13(1): 37–42.

Castro-Alcaraz, S., Greenberg, E.M., Bateman, D.A. and Regan, J.A. (2002) 'Patterns of colonization with *Ureaplasma urealyticum* during neonatal intensive care unit hospitalizations of very low birthweight infants and the development of chronic lung disease', *Pediatrics* 110(4).

Chirico, G., Rondini, G., Plebani, A. *et al.* (1987) 'Intravenous gamma globulin therapy for prophylaxis of infection in high risk neonates', *Journal of Pediatrics* 110: 437–42.

Clark, D.A. and Miller, M.J.S. (1996) 'What causes necrotising enterocolitis and how can it be prevented?', in T.N. Hansen and N. McIntosh (eds) *Current Topics in Neonatology 1*, London: W.B. Saunders.

Conner, J.M., Soll, R.F. and Edwards, W.H. (2003) 'Topical ointment for preventing infection in preterm infants', *Cochrane Database of Systematic Reviews* Issue 4, CD001150.

Craft, A.P., Finer, N.N. and Barrington, K.J. (2000) 'Vancomycin for prophylaxis against sepsis in preterm infants', *Cochrane Database of Systematic Reviews* Issue 1, CD001971.

Crockett, M. (1995) 'Physiology of the neonatal immune system', *Journal of Obstetric, Gynecologic and Neonatal Nursing* 24(7): 627–34.

Darville, T. (2005) 'Chlamydia trachomatis infections in neonates and young children', *Seminars in Pediatric Infectious Diseases* 16(4): 235–44.

Davies, M.W. and Cartwright, D.W. (1998) 'Gentamicin dosage intervals in neonates: longer dosage interval – less toxicity', *Journal of Pediatrics and Child Health* 34: 577–80.

DoH (Department of Health) (2001) 'Standard principles for preventing hospital acquired infections', *Journal of Hospital Acquired Infections* 47: S21–S37.

Edwards, M.S. (1997) 'Antibacterial therapy in pregnancy and neonates', *Clinics in Perinatology* 24(1): 251–66.

Emer, M.L. (1992) 'Disseminated intravascular coagulation in the neonate', *Neonatal Network* 11(8): 5–13.

Evans, M.E., Schaffner, W., Federspiel, C.F. *et al.* (1988) 'Sensitivity, specificity, and the predictive value of body surface cultures in a neonatal intensive care unit', *Journal of the American Medical Association* 259: 248–52.

Fanaroff, A.A., Korones, S.B., Wright, L.L. *et al.* (1998) 'Incidence, presenting features, risk factors and significance of late onset septicaemia in very low birth weight infants', *Pediatric Infectious Diseases Journal* 17: 593–8.

Foweraker, J.E. (1995) 'The laryngoscope as a potential source of cross infection', *Journal of Hospital Infection* 29: 315–16.

Fowlie, P.W. and Schmidt, B. (1998) 'Diagnostic tests for bacterial infection from birth to 90 days – a systematic review', *Archives of Disease in Childhood: Fetal and Neonatal Edition* 78: F92–F98.

Fowlie, P.W., Gould, C.R., Parry, G.J. *et al.* (1996) 'CRIB (clinical risk index for babies) in relation to nosocomial bacteraemia in very low birthweight or preterm infants', *Archives of Disease in Childhood: Fetal and Neonatal Edition* 75: F49–F52.

Fox, H. (1993) 'The placenta and infection', in C.W.G. Redman, I.L. Sargent and P.M. Starkey (eds) *The Human Placenta*, Oxford: Blackwell Scientific.

Girou, E., Loyeau, S., Legrand, P. *et al.* (2002) 'Efficacy of handrubbing with alcohol based solutions versus standard handwashing with antiseptic soap; randomised clinical trial', *British Medical Journal* 14: 325–62.

Glantz, J.C. and Kedley, K.E. (1998) 'Concepts and controversies in the management of Group B streptococcus during pregnancy', *Birth* 25(1): 45–53.

Goldmann, D.A. and Huskins, W.C. (1997) 'Control of nosocomial antimicrobial resistant bacteria: a strategic priority for hospitals worldwide', *Clinical Infectious Diseases* 24 (Suppl. 1): S139–S145.

Green, A. (1991) 'Intravenous immunoglobulin for neonates', *Maternal and Child Nursing* 16: 208–11.

Greene, J.N. (1996) 'The microbiology of colonization, including techniques for assessing and measuring colonization', *Infection Control and Hospital Epidemiology* 17: 114–18.

Greenough, A. (1996) 'Neonatal infections', *Current Opinion in Pediatrics* 8: 6–10.

Greenough, A. and Milner, A.D. (2005) 'Pulmonary disease of the newborn', in J.M. Rennie (ed.) *Roberton's Textbook of Neonatology*, 4th edn, London: Churchill Livingstone.

Greenough, A., Morley, C.J. and Roberton, N.R.C. (1992) 'Acute respiratory disease in the newborn', in N.R.C. Roberton (ed.) *Textbook of Neonatology*, 2nd edn, London: Churchill Livingstone.

Haque, K.N., Zaidi, M.H., Haque, S.K. *et al.* (1986) 'Intravenous immunoglobulin for prevention of sepsis in preterm and low birthweight infants', *Pediatric Infectious Diseases Journal* 5: 622–5.

Harris, M.C. (1992) 'The inflammatory response', in R.A. Polin and W.W. Fox (eds) *Fetal and Neonatal Physiology*, Philadelphia, PA: W.B. Saunders.

Hostetter, M.K. (2001) 'Fungal infections in the neonatal intensive care unit', *Seminars in Pediatric Infectious Diseases* 12(4): 296–300.

Hughes, G., Simms, I., Rogers, P.A., Swan, A.V. and Catchpole, M. (1998) *Communicable Disease Report*, London: Public Health Laboratory Service.

Isaacs, D. (1998) 'Prevention of early onset group B streptococcal infection: screen, treat, or observe?', *Archives of Disease in Childhood: Fetal and Neonatal Edition* 79: F81–F82.

Isaacs, D. (2003) 'A ten year multicentre study of coagulase negative staphylococcal infection in Australian neonatal units', *Archives of Disease in Childhood: Fetal and Neonatal Edition* 88: F89–F93.

Isaacs, D. and Moxon, R.E. (1999) *Handbook of Neonatal Infections: A Practical Guide*, London: W.B. Saunders.

Johnson, A., Sendegeya, C., Keany, M. and Thompson, M. (1996) 'An outbreak of *Staphylococcus aureus* on a neonatal unit', *Maternal and Child Health* 21(7): 184–9.

Johnstone, F.D. and Mok, J. (1990) 'Human immunodeficiency virus in pregnancy and the newborn', in G.L. Chamberlain (ed.) *Modern Antenatal Care of the Fetus*, Oxford: Blackwell Scientific.

Kallman, J., Schollin, J. and Schalen, C. (1998) 'Impaired phagocytosis and opsonisation towards group B streptococci in preterm infants', *Archives of Disease in Childhood: Fetal and Neonatal Edition* 78: F46–F50.

Kane, M.A. (1997) 'Hepatitis viruses and the neonate', *Clinics in Perinatology* 24(1): 181–91.

Karp, T.B., Scardino, C. and Butler, L.A. (1995) 'Glucose metabolism in the neonate: the short and sweet of it', *Neonatal Network* 14(8): 17–23.

Kilbride, H.W., Wirtschafter, D.D., Powers, R.J. and Sheehan, M.B. (2003) 'Implementation of evidence-based potentially better practices to decrease nosocomial infections', *Pediatrics* 111(4): e519–e533.

Klein, J.O. and Marcy, S.M. (1995a) 'Bacterial sepsis and meningitis', in J.S. Remington and J.O. Klein (eds) *Infectious Diseases of the Fetus and Newborn*, Philadelphia, PA: W.B. Saunders.

Klein, J.O. and Marcy, S.M. (1995b) 'Bacterial infections of the urinary tract ', in J.S. Remington and J.O. Klein (eds) *Infectious Diseases of the Fetus and Newborn*, Philadelphia, PA: W.B. Saunders.

Kline, M.W. (1996) 'Vertical human immunodeficiency virus infection', in T.N. Hansen and N. McIntosh (eds) *Current Topics in Neonatology*, London: W.B. Saunders.

Kohl, S. (1997) 'Neonatal herpes simplex virus infection', *Clinics in Perinatology* 24(1): 129–50.

Larson, E.L. (1995) 'APIC guideline for handwashing and hand asepsis in health care settings', *American Journal of Infection Control* 23: 251–69.

Lawton, A.R. (1992) 'B-cell development', in R.A. Polin and W.W. Fox (eds) *Fetal and Neonatal Physiology*, Philadelphia, PA: W.B. Saunders.

Lewis, D.B. and Wilson, C.B. (1995) 'Developmental immunology and the role of host defences in neonatal susceptibility to infection', in J.S. Remington and J.O. Klein (eds) *Infectious Diseases of the Fetus and Newborn*, Philadelphia, PA: W.B. Saunders.

Lindsay, M.K. and Nesheim, S.R. (1997) 'Human immunodeficiency virus infection in pregnant women and their newborns', *Clinics in Perinatology* 24(1): 161–80.

Logan, S. (1990) 'Viral infections in pregnancy', in G.L. Chamberlain (ed.) *Modern Antenatal Care of the Fetus*, Oxford: Blackwell Scientific.

Lyall, E.G.H. and Tudor-Williams, G. (1997) 'Perinatal transmission of HIV', *Current Opinion in Infectious Diseases* 10: 239–45.

Lyon, A.J. (1996) 'Genital mycoplasmas and infection in the neonate', in T.N. Hansen and N. McIntosh (eds) *Current Topics in Neonatology*, London: W.B. Saunders.

Miller, E. (1990) 'Rubella infection in pregnancy', in G.L. Chamberlain (ed.) *Modern Antenatal Care of the Fetus*, Oxford: Blackwell Scientific.

Mueller, B.U. and Pizzo, P.A. (1995) 'Acquired immunodeficiency syndrome in the infant', in J.S. Remington and J.O. Klein (eds) *Infectious Diseases of the Fetus and Newborn*, Philadelphia, PA: W.B. Saunders.

Neal, T.J., Hughes, C.R., Rothburn, M.M. and Shaw, N.J. (1995) 'The neonatal laryngoscope as a potential source of cross-infection', *Journal of Hospital Infection* 30: 315–17.

Neonatal Formulary (2007) *Neonatal Formulary*, 5th edn, Oxford: Blackwell Publishing.

Nestaas, E., Bangstad, H.J., Sandvik, L. and Wathne, K.D. (2005) 'Aminoglycoside extended interval dosing in neonates: a meta analysis', *Archives of Disease in Childhood: Fetal and Neonatal Edition* 90: F294–F300.

NPEU (2008) Available at: www.npeu.ox.ac.uk/inis.

Nursing and Midwifery Council (2008) *Standards for Medicines Management*, London: Nursing and Midwifery Council.

Ohlsson, A. and Lacey, J.B. (2004) 'Intravenous immunoglobulins for suspected or subsequently proven infection in neonates', *Cochrane Database of Systematic Reviews* Issue 1, Art No. CD001239.

Osborn, D.A. and Evans, N. (2004) 'Early volume expansion for prevention of morbidity and mortality in very preterm infants', *Cochrane Database of Systematic Reviews* Issue 2, Art No. CD002055.

Parvez, F.M. and Jarvis, W.R. (1999) 'Nosocomial infections in the nursery', *Seminars in Pediatric Infectious Diseases* 10(2): 119–29.

Perez, M.D. and Weisman, L.E. (1997) 'Novel approaches to the prevention and therapy of neonatal bacterial sepsis', *Clinics in Perinatology* 24(1): 213–29.

Pessoa-Silva, L.C., Hugonnet, S., Pfister, R. *et al.* (2007) 'Reduction of health care associated infection risk in neonates by successful hand hygiene promotion', *Pediatrics* 120: e390.

Philip, A.G.S. (1994) 'The changing face of neonatal infection: experience at a regional medical centre', *Pediatric Infectious Diseases Journal* 13: 1098–102.

Powell, K.R. and Marcy, S.M. (1995) 'Laboratory aids for the diagnosis of neonatal sepsis', in J.S. Remington and J.O. Klein (eds) *Infectious Diseases of the Fetus and Newborn*, Philadelphia, PA: W.B. Saunders.

Radetsky, M. (1995) 'The laboratory evaluation of newborn sepsis', *Current Opinion in Infectious Diseases* 8: 191–9.

Rennie, J. (1995) 'Bacterial and fungal infections', in M.I. Levene and J.J. Lilford (eds) *Fetal and Neonatal Neurology and Neurosurgery*, Edinburgh: Churchill Livingstone.

Roberton, N.R.C. (1992) 'Neonatal infection', in N.R.C. Roberton (ed.) *Textbook of Neonatology*, 2nd edn, London: Churchill Livingstone.

Roberton, N.R.C. (1997) 'Use of albumin in resuscitation', *European Journal of Pediatrics* 156: 428–31.

Roitt, I. (1991) *Essential Immunology*, Oxford: Blackwell Scientific.

Royal, J., Halasz, S., Eagles, G. *et al.* (1999) 'Outbreak of extended spectrum β lactamase producing *Klebsiella pneumoniae* in a neonatal unit', *Archives of Disease in Childhood: Fetal and Neonatal Edition* 80: F64–F68.

Saez-Llorens, X. and McCracken, G.H. (1995) 'Clinical pharmacology of antibacterial agents', in J.S. Remington and J.O. Klein (eds) *Infectious Diseases of the Fetus and Newborn*, Philadelphia, PA: W.B. Saunders.

Sharland, M., Gibb, D.M. and Tudor-Williams, G. (2002) 'Advances in the prevention and treatment of paediatric HIV infection in the United Kingdom', *Archives of Disease in Childhood* 87: 178–80.

Spafford, P.S., Sinkin, R.A., Cox, C., Reubens, L. and Powell, K.R. (1994) 'Prevention of central venous catheter-related coagulase-negative staphylococcal sepsis in neonates', *Journal of Pediatrics* 125: 259–63.

Sproat, L.J. and Inglis, T.J.J. (1992) 'Preventing infection in the intensive care unit', *British Journal of Intensive Care* 2(6): 275–85.

Stern, C.M. (1992) 'Neonatal infection', in N.R.C. Roberton (ed.) *Textbook of Neonatology*, 2nd edn, London: Churchill Livingstone.

Stoll, B.J., Hansen, N., Fanaroff, A.A. *et al.* (2002) 'Late onset sepsis in very low birth weight neonates: the experience of the NICHD Neonatal Research Network', *Pediatrics* 110: 285–91.

Strozik, K.S., Pieper, C.H. and Cools, F. (1998) 'Capillary refilling time in newborns – optimal pressing time, sites of testing and normal values', *Acta Paediatrica Scandinavica* 87: 310–12.

Thompson, P.J., Greenough, A., Gamsu, H.R. *et al.* (1992) 'Congenital bacterial sepsis in very preterm infants', *Journal of Medical Microbiology* 36: 117–20.

Wang, E.E.L., Ohlsson, A. and Kellnar, J.D. (1995) 'Association of *Ureaplasma urealyticum* colonization with chronic lung disease of prematurity: results of a meta-analysis', *Journal of Pediatrics* 127: 640–4.

Weisman, L.E., Stoll, B.J., Kueser, T.J. *et al.* (1994) 'Intravenous immune globulin prophylaxis in premature neonates', *Journal of Pediatrics* 125: 922–30.

Wright, I.M.R., Orr, H. and Porter, C. (1995) 'Stethoscope contamination in the neonatal intensive care unit', *Journal of Hospital Infection* 29: 65–8.

Yamauchi, T. (1995) 'Nosocomial infections in the newborn', *Current Opinion in Infectious Diseases* 4: 474–8.

Yoxall, C.W., Isherwood, D.M. and Weindling, A.M. (1996) 'The neonatal infection screen', *Current Paediatrics* 6(1): 16–20.

Chapter 14

Diagnostic and Therapeutic Procedures

Elizabeth Harling and Glenys Connolly

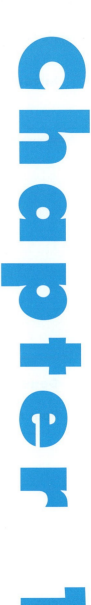

Contents

Introduction

Infants admitted into a neonatal intensive care unit (NICU) will undoubtedly undergo a barrage of interventions in order to stabilise, diagnose and provide ongoing management of specific problems and conditions. A study in 1995 showed that in one cohort of infants (54 in total) over 3000 procedures were undertaken during their time in NICU (Barker and Rutter 1995).

Practitioners need to be mindful that all procedures, no matter how 'routine' or perceivably benign they may seem, carry an element of risk in this vulnerable population and as a consequence the question should always be asked 'Is this procedure really necessary?' before embarking upon it.

This chapter incorporates the most utilised diagnostic and therapeutic procedures that can be undertaken in managing many infants within the NICU setting. Invariably individual NICUs will have their own guidelines for their local practice, but the information in this chapter may assist the development of guidelines where they don't exist, or provide individuals with 'handy hints' on how to be successful when undertaking certain procedures.

General issues surrounding procedures

Pain management

As all of these procedures are potentially painful or will cause some distress to the infant, comfort and safety must be addressed prior to undertaking any of them. The use of pharmacologic and non-pharmacologic therapies should be considered; for example, swaddling, containment holding and administration of oral sucrose (24 per cent) (Gibbins *et al.* 2002; Huang *et al.* 2004) have been shown to be effective in many minor procedures. However, more potent analgesic agents both locally and systemically may be deemed more appropriate for more invasive interventions (see p. 242).

Skin preparation

Skin preparation prior to procedures needs careful consideration if procedure-related sepsis is to be minimised. Pratt *et al.* (2007) recommend 2 per cent chlorhexadine in 70 per cent isopropyl alcohol for skin decontamination prior to insertion of central venous access devices in the adult patient. It has been reported in several case reports (Reynolds *et al.* 2005; Mannan *et al.* 2007) that alcohol-based skin preparation agents are damaging to preterm skin, and as a consequence of this, many units utilise aqueous solutions (Datta and Clarke 2008) or clean off any antimicrobial solution with sterile normal saline following its use. Liberal and excessive use of any cleaning agent may pool under the infant, causing prolonged skin contact during the procedure which may result in burns and great care should be taken to avoid this (Reynolds *et al.* 2005;

Upadhyayula *et al.* 2007). All interventions should be undertaken adhering to an aseptic non-touch technique (ANNT) or sterile procedure in order to reduce the risk of hospital acquired infection.

Gastric tube placement

Naso/oro-gastric tube

This is probably the commonest procedure carried out within NICU as the majority of infants requiring admission will be too sick or too immature to undertake sucking feeds. Other infants may require gastric decompression due to underlying pathology (e.g. intestinal obstruction (see p. 400) or the use of respiratory support such as bi-nasal prong continuous positive end expiratory pressure (CPAP)) (see p. 138). The choice of whether to insert naso- or oro-gastric tube follows careful clinical assessment of the infant.

An infant on bi-nasal prong CPAP will require an oro-gastric tube in order to prevent over-distension of the stomach and facilitate enteral feeding, whereas an infant with a gastrointestinal disorder may tolerate a naso-gastric tube more readily.

The size of tube will vary according to the infant's size and gestation and the reason for placement. For example, an infant with an intestinal obstruction will require a wider bore tube (8fg) to allow for aspiration of refluxed bile and decompression of the stomach, whereas a tube used specifically for feeding should have a narrower bore (5–7fg) to prevent too rapid delivery of milk by gravity.

Indications

- prematurity
- neurological impairment (see p. 191)
- respiratory compromise
- sick term infants
- gastrointestinal anomalies both pre- and post-surgery (see p. 400)

Access to the gastrointestinal tract may be through:

- naso-gastric tube
- oro-gastric tube
- transpyloric tube

Equipment

- appropriate-sized feeding tube
- 5ml syringe

- ■ pH testing strips
- ■ securing tape

Procedure

The length the tube needs to be inserted has to be determined before commencement of the procedure begins (Table 14.1). There is evidence to suggest that insertion of naso-gastric tubes induces the same pain scores equivalent to that of heel pricks and oral sucrose (24 per cent) should be considered prior to the procedure (McCullogh *et al.* 2008).

As infants can become bradycardic during the procedure, due to vagal stimulation (Van Someran *et al.* 1984; Greenspan *et al.* 1990), oxygen and suction should be readily available during the procedure.

For oro-gastric tube placement, put the infant in the **supine** position with the head in the midline and gently pass the tube backwards over the tongue into the oropharynx, advancing slowly until the predetermined length is reached.

For naso-gastric tube placement, put the infant in the position described above with the head slightly extended to push the nose upwards. Directing the tube backwards and downwards through the nostril, advance slowly until the predetermined length is reached.

The tube then needs to be secured effectively by adhesive tape. As facial scarring can occur when tape is removed, consideration of a protective barrier layer (e.g. Cavilon™ or Duoderm™) should be given prior to fixing with adhesive tape.

The tube should be checked for correct position in the stomach by testing for the pH of the fluid aspirated. Historically, litmus paper was used for this purpose but this is no longer deemed suitable; pH strips/paper should now be used, with feeding via the tube only commencing if a pH of <5.5 is recorded (NPSA 2005).

The position of the naso-/oro-gastric tube should be checked prior to any feed or medication and also between times if the securing tape has become loose. Documentation of the length the tube has been inserted to is good practice and this should be checked prior to feeding.

***Table 14.1* Gastric tube length estimation in centimetres**

Orogastric tube	Measure from the bridge of the nose to the **xiphisternum** and add 1 cm
Nasogastric tube	Measure from the xiphisternum to the ear tip and to the bridge of the nose
Transpyloric tube	Measure from the bridge of the nose to the ankle, with the infant supine and legs extended

Additionally, it is recommended that dedicated enteral feeding systems should be used that do not contain ports or connectors that can be connected to intravenous systems (NPSA 2007).

In sick infants who will be requiring early chest X-rays to determine lung pathology the tube should be passed prior to this. This not only helps to determine the position of the tube tip but also helps to exclude **situs inversus**.

Transpyloric tube

Infants suffering from marked gastro-oesophageal reflux may benefit from transpyloric tube feeding. but as they can cause significant gastrointestinal disturbances (McGuire and McEwan 2002) they should only be used following consultation with a medical practitioner.

Equipment

- size 5fg silicone jejunal feeding tube
- size 6fg gastric feeding tube
- 2 × 5ml syringes
- pH testing strips
- sterile water
- securing tape

Procedure

Measure the duodenal tube as per Table 14.1 and follow the procedure for naso-gastric tube placement until fluid is aspirated from the stomach confirming the position by the use of pH paper.

Turn the infant on to its right side and instil 1–2ml of sterile water, to induce peristalsis, and continue to advance the tube until resistance is felt which indicates the pylorus has been reached. The tube can then be gently advanced until bile is aspirated. If bile is not aspirated, the infant should be kept on the right side with an attempt to advance the tube made every 15 minutes. It can take several hours for peristalsis to carry the tube from the pylorus to the jejunum and achieve aspiration of bile. The tube should then be secured. Once achieved, an oro-gastric tube should be passed, and an X-ray taken to confirm position of both tubes before use. The oro-gastric tube serves to ensure the stomach remains decompressed and monitors reflux of milk. In larger infants, a naso-gastric tube can be passed into the same nostril as the transpyloric tube.

Complications

- Vagal stimulation bradycardia is associated with enteral tube placement (Van Someran *et al.* 1984; Greenspan *et al.* 1990)
- Increased work of breathing, especially if nasogastric tubes are used in infants with respiratory compromise, due to infants being obligate nose breathers (Stocks 1980; Van Someran *et al.* 1984).
- **Aspiration** of feed into the lungs through tubes inadvertently dislodged or passed into the lungs or only as far as the **distal** oesophagus. Continuing to administer feeds when there is stasis of milk in the stomach can also lead to aspiration; it is therefore important to check the amount of residual feed in the stomach at regular intervals (see p. 286) for this reason.
- Perforation of the oesophagus, posterior pharynx, stomach or duodenum, though very rare, can occur if the tube is passed too forcefully (Agarwala *et al.* 1998).
- A risk of necrotising enterocolitis has been associated with transpyloric tubes (McGuire and McEwan 2002).

Blood sampling

Obtaining blood samples is an important part of the diagnostic process and the infant's subsequent treatment. Over the course of an infant's stay in NICU many blood tests will be undertaken and as a consequence each and every test should be carefully considered as to its necessity before blood is drawn. What should be borne in mind is that the total volume of blood in an average neonate is 80ml/kg and that a 4ml aliquot of blood taken from a 1kg infant approximates to 5 per cent of its circulating volume.

Additionally, multiple sampling is painful, can lead to anaemia, can cause scarring (Barker and Rutter 1995) and can lead to the infant physiologically deteriorating.

Depending on what the blood is required for, three options are available:

- capillary blood sampling
- venepuncture
- arterial sampling

Capillary blood sampling

Capillary blood sampling is the most common procedure undertaken in NICU. Barker and Rutter (1995) describe 3283 heel pricks performed on just 54 infants during their stay on NICU.

Traditionally blood obtained from the heel was from the areas beyond the **lateral** and **medial** limits of the calcaneus, to reduce the incidence of osteomyelitis (Blumenfeld *et al.* 1979). Further studies using ultrasound now deem it safe to extend the area sampled across the **plantar** surface of the heel but avoiding the posterior aspect, so long as an automated lancet is used to a no greater depth than 2.4mm (Figure 14.1). The reduction in density of the heel pricks in the previous denoted sites should reduce associated pain (Jain and Rutter 1999). The use of an automated device also reduces the risk of secondary injury to the infant if the device is inadvertently dropped into the cot and risk of needle stick injury to the operator.

Indications

- most biochemical and haematological tests requiring less than 1ml of blood;
- metabolic and cytogenetic testing;
- blood glucose analysis;
- acid-base status.

Equipment

- appropriately sized automated lancet device (e.g. Tenderfoot™);
- sample bottles/heparinised capillary tubes;
- alcohol swab (unless blood glucose is to performed when water alone should be used as alcohol affects the result).

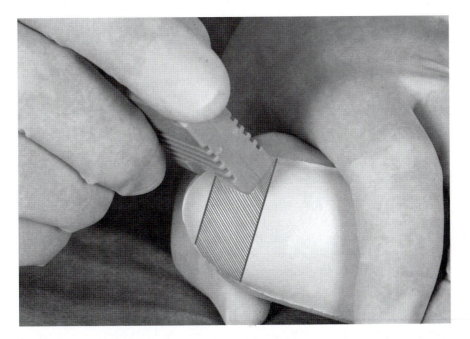

Figure 14.1 Capillary blood sampling; shaded area indicates 'safe' area for heel prick

Procedure

Clean the heel with water or antimicrobial agent and allow it to dry.

Holding the foot firmly but gently, puncture the heel across the plantar surface avoiding the posterior aspect. Gentle squeezing of the heel allows the blood to flow which can then be collected into the blood bottle. The first drop of blood should be wiped away to prevent contamination of sample with serous tissue fluid. Samples for acid base balance gravitate into the heparinised tube by capillary action.

Excessive squeezing should be avoided as this can cause **haemolysis** of the sample leading to inaccurate results and to the test having to be repeated.

Complications

- pain and discomfort;
- infection of puncture sites;
- scarring;
- physiological deterioration in condition;
- haemolysis of sample – platelet counts and creatinine can be unreliably low and potassium levels unreliably high.

Venous blood sampling

Indications

- A larger volume of blood is required.
- A non-haemolysed sample is of utmost importance.
- Poor peripheral perfusion does not permit capillary sampling.
- The sample is required for blood culture (bacterial, fungal or viral).
- Accurate diagnosis of polycythaemia.

Procedure

The most common site for venepuncture is the dorsum of the hand or foot. The veins of the antecubital fossa and long saphenous should be avoided as these are prime sites for long-term cannulation and percutaneous longline placement. The femoral vein should not be used due to the increased risk of damage or infection to the hip joint.

Equipment

- 22G or 23G flanged collection needle
- sample bottles
- alcohol swab

NB: If blood is required for microbiological culture, follow procedure for venous cannulation and collect blood from cannula hub with sterile needle and syringe.

Procedure

Cleanse the skin.

Contain the limb, keeping the skin taut to stabilise the vein and so that blood is static within the vessel.

Gently insert needle into the vein at a 30–45-degree angle, ensuring that the flat aspect of the needle is against the skin and the bevel is facing upwards.

Once blood flow commences, collect the sample into the bottle(s) without any excessive squeezing.

To remove the needle, place a sterile swab over the puncture site as needle is withdrawn.

Apply gentle pressure to achieve haemostasis and prevent bruising.

Complications

- Infection – minimised by aseptic technique.
- Bruising – minimised by application of pressure following needle removal.
- Venous thrombosis – often unavoidable if multiple sampling required from same vessels.
- Physiological destabilisation of baby.
- Scars from skin punctures.

Arterial blood sampling

There may be times when an arterial blood sample is required, usually for an arterial pH when an indwelling line, central or peripheral, is not *in situ*.

The most common sites for sampling are the radial, posterior tibial and the dorsalis pedis arteries. The brachial artery should be avoided due to its poor collateral circulation and its close proximity to the median nerve. Likewise the femoral artery should be avoided due to the risk of trauma and infection of the hip.

This procedure should be used as a 'one-off' sample as repeated sampling from the same artery can lead to spasm and distal ischaemia. Arteriovenous fistulae can also occur.

Equipment

- 25G hypodermic needle
- 1ml heparinised syringe/heparinised capillary tube

Procedure

The radial artery is the most frequently used, and use of the right radial will reflect pre-ductal oxygen content in the blood.

Prior to undertaking the procedure it is imperative to check the collateral circulation is intact. This is achieved by undertaking the Allen's test. To perform this test, elevate the arm and simultaneously apply digital pressure to occlude both the radial and the ulnar arteries. This will cause the hand to blanch; releasing the pressure on the ulnar artery should allow the hand to return to its normal colour evidencing that the collateral circulation is intact.

Locate the artery by gentle palpation in the normal manner or by trans-illumination by the use of a cold light placed on the opposite side of the wrist.

Cleanse the area with an alcohol swab.

Partially extend the wrist and puncture the artery just proximal to the transverse wrist crease, at a 45-degree angle to the skin slowly advancing the needle in the opposite direction of the blood flow (Figure 14.2). Over-extension of the wrist can impeded flow, causing occlusion of the vessel.

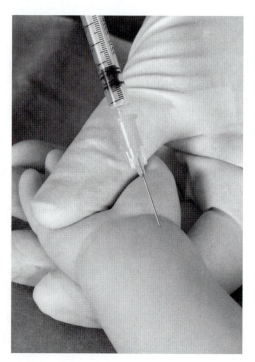

***Figure 14.2* Arterial puncture sampling right radial artery**

Applying gentle suction pressure to the plunger, remove the required amount of blood.

Following removal of the needle, apply a sterile swab and digital pressure for five minutes or until haemostasis is achieved.

If using the dorsalis pedis or posterior tibial arteries, the foot should be partially plantar flexed or **dorsiflexed** respectively.

Complications

- Arteriospasm or ischaemia to the surrounding tissue – minimised by the use of the smallest gauge needle and keeping punctures to a minimum.
- Haematoma or haemorrhage – prevented by correct withdrawal of the needle and digital pressure until haemostasis is achieved.
- Infection – rare and avoided by use of a strict sterile procedure.
- Inaccurate blood gas result; too much heparin may lead to a falsely low pH and PCO_2.
- Intolerance to the procedure can lead to a fall in PO_2 during procedure.

Peripheral artery cannulation

When repeated arterial sampling or invasive blood pressure monitoring is required, insertion of an indwelling line should be undertaken (see p. 345 for UAC). The same sites used for arterial sampling can be used.

Equipment

- 24G cannula
- leur lock extension set, three-way tap and leur lock 2ml syringe primed with 0.9 per cent or 0.45 per cent sodium chloride
- 50ml syringe of heparinised 0.9 per cent or 0.45 per cent sodium chloride (1 unit heparin/ml)
- infusion pump, pressure transducer and manometer line
- skin-cleansing agent
- method of securing and transparent dressing

Procedure

Locate the artery as previously described (p. 337) and verify collateral circulation is evident (Allen's test). Cannulate the artery in the opposite direction to the flow of blood.

A flashback of blood should be immediately evident in the trochar of the cannula; it should then be smoothly advanced into the lumen of the artery removing the stylet as it is passed.

The leur lock extension piece should be carefully and firmly attached and the artery slowly flushed clear of blood, observing for blanching.

Close the three-way tap so that no blood is lost while the cannula is secured in place.

A non-occlusive dressing should be used so that the site of insertion and surrounding area can be inspected regularly.

A splint may be used to stabilise the limb but the digits should be clearly visible.

The infusate should be securely connected and commenced at 0.5–1ml/hour, ensuring all connections are secure and open.

Attach to the transducer to enable invasive blood pressure monitoring to be commenced.

Complications

- Arterial spasm – prevented by avoidance of excessive suction pressure on syringe when sampling. Allow the blood to flow back freely if possible.
- Persistent blanching of the surrounding tissues or extremities requires the cannula to be removed immediately to avoid loss of tissue integrity.
- Vessel damage – slow infusion of an isotonic solution will help minimise damage to the tunica intima of the artery and reduce thrombus and emboli formation.
- Infection – avoided by use of aseptic technique during procedure.
- Haemorrhage – avoided by ensuring cannula firmly secured and all leur lock connections secured.

Removal of the catheter requires digital pressure with a sterile swab for five minutes or until haemostasis is achieved.

Peripheral vein cannulation

This is the most commonly used method of access to the circulatory system. Any superficial vein can be cannulated; the veins of the antecubital fossa and long saphenous should be reserved for percutaneous longline insertion.

The preferred sites are those of the dorsum of the hand or foot; scalp veins provide the same access but are usually used when other peripheral veins are not accessible.

Indications

- Administration of intravenous fluids, drugs, blood and blood products.

Equipment

- 22G or 24G cannula
- extension set with leur lock primed by 2ml syringe with 0.45 per cent or 0.9 per cent sodium chloride
- cleansing agent with sterile cotton wool or alcohol swabs
- Cavilon™ dressing
- sterile tape for securing (e.g. steri-strips)
- sterile gauze swab
- sterile transparent dressing
- splint

Procedure

The procedure should be undertaken observing aseptic technique.

Prepare all the equipment beforehand ensuring that the needle runs down the centre of the cannula and easily pulls out before attempting to use it.

Identify the vein and cleanse the skin of the overlying area thoroughly.

Hold the skin taut to immobilise the vein, then puncture the skin, a few millimetres proximal to the vein ensuring that the tip of the needle is protruding out from the end of the cannula and that the bevel is facing upwards (Figure 14.3).

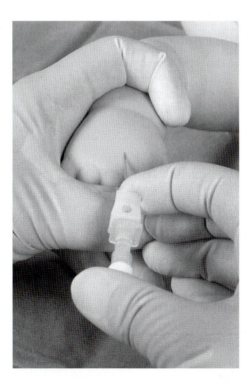

Figure 14.3 **Venous cannulation dorsum of left hand**

Enter the vein from the anterior surface or from the side advancing the needle 1–2mm in the direction of the flow of blood; this ensures the cannula is within the vein lumen. A flashback of blood into the needle hub confirms the position.

Hold the hub of the needle with the thumb and third finger and gently ease the cannula off the needle into the vein with the index finger.

Once the cannula is in position, the needle can be completely removed; this should be accompanied by the flow of blood into the cannula hub.

The primed extension set should now be firmly secured in place, and the cannula flushed observing for blanching or extravasation. Resistance to flow indicates the cannula has been misplaced and it should be removed.

Before securing with steri-strips and transparent dressing, apply cavilon to the surrounding skin, and place a small square of gauze under the hub of the cannula to prevent skin damage. Immobilise the limb with a splint if necessary.

The cannulated limb should be left visible to allow for close observation of the site. The intravenous pump pressure should be recorded immediately following insertion and hourly subsequent to this. The pump pressure alarm should be set slightly higher than the infusing pressure (e.g. 30cm H_2O) to allow for movement artefact increases in pressure but not too high so as not to alarm if occlusion of the cannula is occurring.

Increasing pressure readings suggests that infiltration and **extravasation** may be occurring and warrants further investigation.

Complications

- Infiltration of the subcutaneous tissue following rupture of the vessel due to advancing the cannula with the needle still protruding through the end or by infusion of **hypertonic** solutions causing irritation to the vessel wall.
- Emboli or thrombosis – avoided by flushing the cannula via a primed extension set.
- Air emboli – avoided by vigilant observation of the infusing fluid giving set for bubbles.
- Haematoma caused by damage to the vessel wall during cannulation – avoided by gentle advancement of the cannula and firm digital pressure over site following removal of the cannula.
- Vasospasm occurs occasionally but usually resolves spontaneously.
- Infection minimised by adequate cleaning and aseptic technique.
- Phlebitis can occur when irritant intravenous fluids and drugs are given or when cannula is in situ for a protracted length of time. Avoided by giving highly irritant fluids (e.g. total parenteral nutrition (TPN) via percutaneous longline and recording clearly when cannula are inserted).

Percutaneous venous longline

Percutaneous venous longline access is usually required in the very preterm or sick infants or infants who will require long-term TPN following gut surgery. Their advantage is that they last longer than peripheral venous lines and can be safely used for infusion of fluids known to have a local irritation or sclerosing effect.

There are several lines available, the smallest of which (27G) comes with a guide wire and can be inserted via a 22G cannula or 22G with a splitting cannula. A large vein should be used; those of the long saphenous, medial and lateral antecubital veins or the superficial temple vein are used most frequently.

Indications

- administration of inotropic medication
- administration of total parenteral nutrition (TPN)
- administration of hypertonic solutions (e.g. 15 per cent dextrose)
- administration of long-term therapies (e.g. antifungal medication)

Equipment

- sterile pack of instruments
- sterile gown and sterile gloves
- longline of choice (e.g. with wire or splitting needle)
- 22G cannula if using wired variety
- cleansing agent
- 10ml syringe with 0.9 per cent or 0.45 per cent sodium chloride
- steri-strips
- sterile transparent dressing

Procedure

Prior to commencing the procedure, identify the vein to be used and estimate the length of insertion (Table 14.2).

Adopting a strict aseptic technique, thoroughly cleanse the area over and around the site of insertion which should include any area that will ultimately lie under the sterile transparent dressing. Drape the surrounding area.

Table 14.2 Percutaneous longline length measured in centimetres

Measure from the site of insertion to the approximate position in vena cava outside of the right atrium

Access the vein via either a 22G cannula or splitting needle. Blood flow is usually brisk; apply gentle pressure to the vein to overcome this, and thread the primed line gently through the needle introducer using fine non-toothed forceps.

Be aware that the dead space of the needle is approximately 5cm and this needs to be taken into account when advancing the line.

Once the line has been inserted to the desired length, disconnect the line from the blue compression mounting and carefully slide the butterfly out of the vein and off the line. If using a splitting cannula, gently pull it out of the vein and carefully split it to remove it from the line. Applying gentle pressure to the site of insertion will prevent accidental removal of the line as the device is removed. Assemble the connections and flush the line to ensure the line has not become impacted during the insertion.

Coil the remaining line into loops on the skin putting a small sterile gauze dressing under the compression mounting before securing with steri-strips and transparent dressing. Care should be taken not to kink the line.

If using a wired line, this should not be primed prior to insertion as this necessitates the removal of the guide wire. The line is inserted via a 22G cannula in the same way; the cannula should be removed from the vein and pulled loosely up the line and on to the hub before securing it under the transparent dressing.

Isotonic infusion fluid should be started immediately to prevent line occlusion, but the line position should be verified radiologically prior to the commencement of TPN or inotropic agents. Lines are generally radio-opaque but contrast medium may be given prior to X-ray to check line tip position.

The line tip should be outwith the intracardiac chambers (DoH 2001) and should lie 0.5–1cm outside the right atrium in either the inferior or superior vena cava, depending on the size of the infant (Darling *et al.* 2001). If the line is in too far it should be withdrawn following an aseptic technique.

Line tips at the shoulder or groin may be used but there is a higher risk of extravasation injury.

Complications

- Infection especially with coagulase negative staphylococcus aureus (CONS) when lines are used for TPN (Avila-Figuero *et al.* 1998; Berger *et al.* 1998; see p. 306). This is avoided by strict asepsis during line insertion and utilising a non-touch technique when changing fluids and giving drugs. In cases of suspected or proven sepsis, the line should be removed.
- Prolonged bleeding from the insertion site – haemostasis by gentle pressure must be achieved before the dressing is applied.
- Shearing off of the line on the point of the butterfly – never pull the line back with the butterfly in situ.
- Cardiac arrhythmias, pericardial effusion and cardiac tamponade – avoided by having the line tip outwith the cardiac chambers (Darling 2001; DoH 2001).
- **Thrombus** formation – avoided by continuous infusion of fluid.

Umbilical vessel catheterisation

The newborn infant is in a unique position in that it has direct access to its central circulation and the body's great vessels in the guise of its umbilical arteries and vein.

Cannulation of these vessels allows ease of access for arterial blood sampling, monitoring blood pressure and central venous pressure, administration of blood and blood products and administration of irritant drugs such as hyperosmolar solutions and inotropes.

Umbilical artery catheterisation

Umbilical artery catheters (UACs) are among the most commonly used invasive lines within the NICU environment, allowing for continuous invasive blood pressure monitoring and sampling of arterial blood. Depending on type of catheter used continuous reading of PaO_2 and $PaCO_2$ levels can also be achieved.

The size of the catheter used depends on the size of the infant and varies from 3.5–5.0fg. Catheters should have leur locking connectors to reduce the risk of accidental disconnection and exsanguination. The catheter should have a single end hole rather than side holes as this reduces the risk of aortic thrombosis (Barrington 1999a).

Indications

- frequent arterial blood gas and pH estimation
- continuous arterial blood pressure monitoring
- exchange transfusion (p. 216)
- fluid infusion

Equipment

- umbilical vessel catheterisation pack containing instruments and cord ligature
- sterile gown and gloves
- scalpel and blade
- umbilical catheters size 3.5fg–5.0 fg attached via a leur lock to a three-way tap and primed with 0.9 per cent or 0.45 per cent sodium chloride and a 10ml syringe. Mark the tap with the red flag. Close the three-way tap to the catheter before insertion.
- cleansing agent
- suture
- pressure transducer and monitoring set up
- 50ml syringe and leur locked line primed with 0.45 per cent or 0.9 per cent sodium chloride with 1 unit/ml of heparin added

345

Calculate the insertion length of the catheter by multiplying the infant's weight by three and adding nine. At the point of insertion add the length of the remaining cord stump to the total (Table 14.3).

Table 14.3 Umbilical arterial catheter length estimation (in centimetres) for high position

3 × wt in kg + 9 + length of cord stump

The catheter tip should sit above the diaphragm at **thoracic vertebrae** T6–T10. This *high* position is said to be preferable to the *low* position, lumbar vertebrae L3–L5 as it has a lower incidence of vascular complications (Barrington 1999b).

Measuring from the umbilicus to the shoulder tip will also give an approximate catheter length for the high position.

Procedure

The infant should be in the supine position; a second person may be useful to contain the infant during the procedure or ensure that adequate sedation/analgesia is given prior to commencement. The infant should have ECG and oxygen saturation monitoring in place prior to commencing. Ensure that there is a good lighting source to illuminate the area.

Utilising an aseptic technique at all times, prepare the equipment, attach the catheter to the three-way tap, flush the catheter and turn the tap to the off position to prevent accidental air embolus.

Clean around the cord, cord clamp and umbilical area with an antimicrobial agent. Holding the cord clamp in sterile gauze, drape the infant's chest and abdomen.

Tie a cord ligature around the base of the cord stump and tighten sufficiently to stem any oozing from the cord. If pulled too tightly it can damage the vessels.

Apply an artery forceps across the cord approximately 2 centimetres from the base and cut across the cord on its underside with one smooth cut of the scalpel.

The vessels run in a spiral route down the cord which makes them difficult to access if the cord is left too long. Identify the two arteries but only attempt to catheterise one; this will allow a second person to make an attempt if the first is unsuccessful.

The umbilical vein is found at 12 o'clock; it is the largest vessel with a gaping appearance, the arteries lie inferior to the vein at 4 o'clock and 8 o'clock, and they are smaller and whiter in appearance.

Stabilise the cord on each side with the artery forceps, ensuring that they do not impinge on any of the vessels.

Gently tease open the lumen of the chosen artery with the non-toothed forceps followed by an artery probe. Patience is required as too forceful probing will lead to damage of the intima and to a false passage.

Once the vessel is sufficiently dilated, the tip of the primed catheter can be introduced and gently but firmly advanced to the estimated position. It is normal to feel resistance at the level of the umbilical ring and the internal iliac junction; sustained but gentle pressure helps to overcome this.

Once in place, the three-way tap can be opened and the catheter aspirated; the presence of pulsating blood in the catheter confirms that it is in an artery. The catheter then needs to be secured in place. There are several techniques and the one described here ensures that no tape is attached to the infant's skin reducing potential skin damage and epidermal stripping.

Secure the catheter by putting a stitch on either side of the catheter leaving long tails. Line the stitch ends up with the catheter, then loop the catheter back on itself and tape it all together. Commence the infusion of heparinised solution and transduced monitoring as soon as possible.

The line position should be checked on chest and abdominal X-rays, where it should be seen to pass down the anterior abdominal wall into the pelvis before ascending the abdominal and thoracic aorta to the left-hand side of the vertebrae. The exact tip position can be identified by counting down the thoracic vertebrae.

The procedure, including equipment numbers and catheter size and position, should be documented in the infant's case notes.

The lower limbs and buttocks should be checked for colour and perfusion at regular intervals; any concerns should be reported immediately and if blanching or discoloration persists, the catheter should be removed to avoid ischaemic injury.

Regular zeroing of the transducer and ensuring that it is at the approximate level of the heart will ensure accurate recordings of blood pressure. Observation of the transduced wave form is helpful in underfilling of the heart, widened pulse pressure may indicate a patent ductus arteriosus (see p. 166) and a dampened trace may indicate partial occlusion of the line.

Complications

- Vascular accidents – vasospasm and thrombosis lead to ischaemic limbs and buttocks, resulting in loss of limbs.
- Haemorrhage – loose connections in the line can lead to immediate and torrential exsanguination; leur lock line should always be used. The infant should be nursed in the supine position with the catheter clearly visible at all times. If the infant's condition warrants prone nursing, then this can be undertaken once the catheter is known to be secure and stable and with caution.
- Vessel perforation – never force a catheter into position; the infant may become hypotensive from hypovolaemia and surgical intervention may be required to ligate the bleeding vessel once immediate resuscitation with blood and fluids has been undertaken.

■ Infection – always insert the catheter using an aseptic technique. If the catheter is not in the correct position (e.g. too low), it should not be advanced as this represents an infection risk. It should either be withdrawn to a low position L3 to L5 or removed completely and replaced.

Umbilical vein catheterisation

Indications

■ during emergency resuscitation at delivery for administration of drugs and fluids
■ exchange transfusion (see p. 216)
■ administration of drugs and fluids not suitable for peripheral administration, e.g. inotropes
■ central venous pressure monitoring

Equipment

■ umbilical vessel catheterisation pack containing instruments and cord ligature
■ sterile gown and gloves
■ scalpel and blade
■ umbilical catheters size 4 or 5fg, single or double lumen attached to a three-way tap and primed with 0.9 per cent or 0.45 per cent sodium chloride and a 5ml syringe
■ cleansing agent
■ 0.9 per cent sodium chloride/sterile water
■ suture and tape to secure
■ 50ml syringe and leur locked line primed with 0.45 per cent or 0.9 per cent sodium chloride.

Procedure

Calculate the insertion length of the catheter by multiplying the infant's weight by three and adding nine and dividing by two. At the point of insertion, add the length of the remaining cord stump to the total (Table 14.4).

Table 14.4 Umbilical venous catheter length estimation (in centimetres)

$$\frac{3 \times \text{wt in kg} + 9 + \text{length of cord stump}}{2}$$

This calculation will place the catheter tip in the vena cava above the diaphragm but not into the right side of the heart.

Follow the procedure as for UAC insertion. Identify the vein which is found at 12 o'clock; it is the largest vessel which often does not require dilatation.

Stabilise the cord with the artery forceps and apply gentle **caudal** traction.

Place the tip of the primed catheter into the vein and advance in an upwards direction through the ductus venosus into the inferior vena cava. If resistance is felt, the catheter may have entered the portal system. Withdraw the catheter 1–2cm, twist it and re-advance. Once the catheter is in to the desired length, blood should be able to be freely aspirated. The catheter can then be secured utilising the same technique described for UAC.

The infusing fluid should be commenced as soon as possible and once position has been checked to be safe, on chest and abdominal X-rays, TPN or inotropes may be commenced as required.

Complications

- Air embolus can occur if the line is not primed fully or if the catheter is left open to the atmosphere.
- Thrombosis can be reduced by the heparinisation of the infusing fluid.
- Hyperosmolar solutions (>300mOsmol/kg/H_2O) can cause hepatic necrosis, thrombosis and portal hypertension if infused into the liver. A UVC placed in the liver should be removed (Wilkinson and Calvert 1992).

Lumbar puncture

Controversy surrounds the use of lumbar puncture. Some units undertake the procedure every time an infection screen is performed, others only when central nervous system infection or disorder is suspected.

Indications

- diagnostic purposes for central nervous system disorders, e.g. subarachnoid haemorrhage
- to confirm a diagnosis of suspected meningitis
- to reduce intracranial pressure by drainage of cerebrospinal fluid (CSF) in communicating hydrocephalus
- to measure intracranial pressure

Equipment

- sterile dressing pack
- sterile gloves
- cleansing agent

- spinal needle, 22G × 1.5' or 25G x 1'
- plain sterile bottles × 3, fluoride bottle for glucose analysis
- transparent spray dressing

Procedure

The success of a lumbar puncture is directly proportional to the person holding the infant, therefore use an experienced assistant! The infant should be held in the left lateral position, with head and knees flexed while keeping the back as vertical as possible. If the infant is unable to tolerate this position, a 'sitting' position can be adopted.

With the infant in this position, the interspace between lumbar vertebrae 4 and 5 can be identified by following a line down from the iliac crest to lumbar vertebra 4.

Using an aseptic technique, clean the area in a widening circle, starting at the identified site of insertion and taking it up over the iliac crest. Drape the area leaving only the selected interspace exposed identifying the interspace again.

Infiltrative local anaesthesia can be used (Lidocaine 1 per cent 0.3ml/kg) but there is little evidence that it reduces distress in the situation (Neonatal Formulary 2007) and may be more painful than a well-performed procedure.

To insert the needle, hold the tip of the thumb of the left hand on L4 and insert the needle into the midline of the space below. With a steady pressure, direct it slowly towards the umbilicus. The 'give' as the ligamantum flavum and the dura are penetrated are not always evident in the neonate and this necessitates frequent withdrawal of the stylet from the needle to ensure that it has not been advanced too far, leading to a bloody specimen. Once CSF is seen, remove the stylet fully and collect three serial specimens of 5–6 drops in each of the plain bottles for microscopy, culture and sensitivity, cell count and differentials, and a further 3 drops into the fluoride tube for CSF glucose.

Replace the stylet and withdraw the needle. Use a sterile swab over the area applying gentle pressure until any flow of CSF has stopped; transparent spray dressing can then be applied.

Complications

- Hypoxia, apnoea and bradycardia resulting from holding in the required position – may be reduced by holding the (non-ventilated) infant in a sitting position.
- Infection – reduce by using strict asepsis but there is a risk of introducing micro-organisms in the blood into the CSF during sampling.
- Blood in sample – if it clears as CSF flows indicates a traumatic tap; persisting blood indicates a blood vessel has been punctured.
- Interspinal epidermoid tumour – results from using a needle without a stylet. The needle displaces a plug of epithelial tissue into the dura as it is advanced.

- Herniation of cerebral tissue through the foramen magnum – uncommon in neonates due to the open fontanelle.
- Spinal cord and nerve damage – prevented by using the interspace below L4.

Urine sample collection

Urine can be obtained in one of several ways depending on what it is needed for:

- aspirated from cotton wool balls placed in the nappy
- sterile adhesive urine collection bag
- 'clean catch' straight into container
- urethral catheterisation
- suprapubic aspiration

Indications

- Cotton wool ball sample is sufficient for urinalysis testing for glucose ketones, urobilinogen, reducing substances, bilirubin, blood, pH, leucocytes.
- 'Clean catch' can be used for microscopy culture and sensitivity, osmolality and urea and electrolytes. A bag specimen can also be used but contamination can occur.
- A sterile collection bag can be used. When applying the bag, ensure the area is clean and dry. Application of a barrier film spray may help prevent skin damage when removing the bag.
- Urethral catheterisation used for accurate measurement of urine output when weighing of nappies is not thought to be accurate enough and in urine retention not amenable to bladder expression, e.g. posterior urethral valves.
- Suprapubic aspiration is the best method of avoiding a non-contaminated specimen for microscopy.

Urethral catheterisation

Equipment

- sterile dressing pack
- sterile gloves
- cleansing agent
- 4fg feeding tube
- sterile lubricating jelly

Procedure

Place infant in supine position with thighs abducted. Using an aseptic technique cleanse the penis from the meatus and down the shaft, or separate labia and cleanse vulval area anterior to posterior. Lubricate the outside of the feeding tube.

Stabilise the penis with the non-dominant hand and insert lubricated tube gently until urine is visible in the tube, or separate labia and gently insert into urethra. If tube is inadvertently placed in vagina, leave it in situ while a clean tube is placed anterior to it and remove once urine is visible in the second tube.

Secure to the penis with steri-strips around the tube and then to lower abdomen. In female infants, secure to the upper thigh with steri-strips. Attach to sterile collection device.

Urinary catheters should be removed as soon as no longer required to reduce incidence of infection.

Complications

- Infection due to not adhering to strict asepsis.
- Trauma from using rigid feeding tube and putting tube in too far.
- Kinking of catheter from inserting it too far, leading to obstructed flow and can lead to knotting of catheter.

Suprapubic aspiration

Equipment

- sterile dressing pack
- sterile gloves
- 2ml or 5ml syringe
- cleansing agent
- sterile container

Procedure

Ensure that the infant has a full bladder and not recently voided prior to procedure; undertaking an abdominal ultrasound will be helpful. As the lubricating jelly and pressure from the probe may invoke spontaneous micturition, have a pot available to obtain a clean catch!

Put the infant into the supine position and abduct the thighs. Cleanse the area above the symphysis pubis to the umbilicus. With the needle and syringe held at a 90-degree angle puncture the skin 0.5–1cm in the midline above the symphysis pubis advancing to a depth of 1–2cm while aspirating the syringe.

Once urine is visible in the syringe stop advancing to avoid perforation of the posterior bladder wall.

Once sample is collected, withdraw needle and apply pressure with sterile gauze before covering with sterile dressing. Send the fresh sample to the laboratory immediately.

Complications

- Transient microscopic haematuria.
- Bowel perforation can occur if needle advanced through the posterior bladder wall with faecal matter becoming evident on aspiration. The procedure should not be carried out on an infant with abdominal distension or dilated loops of bowel.

Table 14.5 shows the anatomical reference points seen on chest and abdominal X-rays relevant to the procedures discussed in the case study (p. 359).

Endotracheal tube placement

Endotracheal tube (ETT) intubation may be approached from the orotracheal or nasotracheal route; while these routes achieve the same end, they require slightly different techniques.

Table 14.5 Anatomical reference points seen on chest and abdominal X-rays relevant to the procedures

Structure	Vertebral level
Vocal cords	Cervical 1–2
Carina	Thoracic 3– 4
Ductus arteriosus	Thoracic 4–5
Coeliac axis	Thoracic 12
Superior mesenteric artery	Thoracic 12–Lumbar 1
Renal artery	Lumbar 1
End of conus medullaris	Lumbar 2
Inferior mesenteric artery	Lumbar 3
Aortic bifurcation	Lumbar 3–4
Iliac crests	Lumbar 3–4
End of subarachnoid space	Sacral 1–2

Indications

- to provide artificial mechanical respiratory support
- to remove meconium or particulate matter from the trachea
- to instil exogenous surfactant
- to ensure airway security during prolonged resuscitation or transfer of infants between neonatal units

Equipment

- paediatric laryngoscope with straight blade (size 0 and 1)
- endotracheal tubes (see Table 14.6 for size and length)
- Magill forceps (if nasal route is being used)
- stethoscope
- suction apparatus
- self-inflating bag and mask/T-piece resuscitation equipment

Procedure

It is recognised that intubation of the awake, conscious infant is a potentially painful and distressing procedure; Byrne and MacKinnon (2006) suggest that such physiological distress may increase neonatal morbidity. Prior to the procedure the infant should be premedicated in order to facilitate a more effective technique with less harmful fluctuations in physiological parameters in routine semi-urgent intubations (ibid.).

Place the infant in the supine position with the head in the mid-line and slightly extended – 'sniffing the air' position. The head should not be over-extended as this will narrow the airway and make the cords difficult to visualise.

Hold the laryngoscope in the left hand and with the right hand gently open the infant's mouth inserting the blade of the laryngoscope to the right side of the mouth sweeping the tongue to the left (Figure 14.4). Advance the blade a

Table 14.6 Endotracheal tube size estimation

Tube size (mm)	Infant weight (g)	Infant gestation
2.5	< 1000	< 29 weeks
3.0	1000–3000	28–34 weeks
3.5	> 3000	34 weeks–Term

Note: The 'tip to lip' length of an oral tube should be estimated as the weight in kilograms plus 6cm (e.g. 2kg infant tube length 8cm at lips). For nasal tubes, add 2cm to account for nasopharyngeal anatomy.

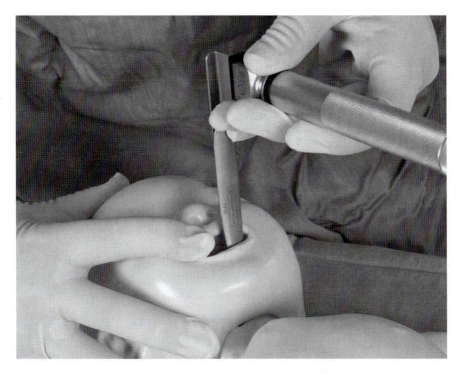

Figure 14.4 Endotracheal intubation, head in mid-line with slight extension. Note delicate holding of laryngoscope and operator's finger protecting infant's upper lip.

few millimetres into the **vallecula** and by lifting the blade vertically, elevate the **epiglottis** to bring the entrance to the larynx and the vocal cords into view. The view can be enhanced by exerting pressure on the thyroid cartilage with the ring or little finger of the left hand. Cautious suction at this point will ensure that all of the landmarks are clearly visible. Insert the oral tracheal tube into the right side of the mouth and through the vocal cords. If a nasal tube is used, it should be lubricated and passed through the nostril until visible in the pharynx. It is then guided through the vocal cords with Magill forceps.

The tip of the ETT is then advanced 1–1.5cm below the vocal cords to position it midway between the thoracic inlet and the **carina**; this approximates to the second thoracic vertebra.

Hold the ETT firmly in place and confirm its position by giving positive pressure ventilation by bag or T-piece and observing for chest movement. The chest should be auscultated, listening for equal air entry on both sides.

The most common problem is a tube advanced too far and placed into the right main bronchus; to overcome this, slowly withdraw the ETT until equal breath sounds are heard. Auscultation over the stomach will help identify a tube inadvertently passed into the stomach. The tube should then be secured in place taking care to protect the underlying skin with a barrier layer such as Cavilon™ or Duoderm™.

A chest X-ray taken in the **anteroposterior** view will confirm the position of the ETT. When undertaking the chest film, care must be taken to hold the head in the mid-line and not flexed so that there is correct centring of the X-ray beam on to the chest to ensure satisfactory location of the tube. An X-ray taken with the head deviated to the side or with the beam centred on the abdomen, especially in term infants, may distort the position of the tube or make it appear marginally higher than it is (Meerstadt and Gyll 1994). When viewing the X-ray, count down the vertebrae from where the posterior ribs arise, commencing at the first thoracic vertebrae (T1); the tip of the ETT should lie at T2.

Following verification of the ETT position, its length in centimetres at lips or nose and size of the tube used should be clearly documented so that in the case of subsequent re-intubations the information is readily available. Should the tube be repositioned post-X-ray, that too should be clearly documented.

Stylets can be used to aid oral intubations with softer tubes as they keep the tube more rigid. If using, caution should be exercised so that it does not protrude beyond the tip of the ETT where it could cause damage to, or even perforation of the trachea or oesophagus if misplaced. Care also needs to be exercised when removing the stylet from the ETT as accidental extubation can occur.

Complications

- Tracheal perforation – a rare complication avoided by careful use of the laryngoscope, ETT and stylet.
- Oesophageal perforation – the result of traumatic intubation which can lead to stricture formation and require surgical correction.
- Laryngeal oedema – apparent after extubation and may require re-intubation and a short course of steroids to be given to reduce oedema and inflammation.
- Subglottic stenosis – associated with long-term intubations and multiple re-intubations, may require surgical correction.
- Palatal grooves – the result of long-term oral intubation and pressure on the palate.
- Brain penetration – a complication of nasal intubation whereby the ETT is passed through the cribriform plate (Cameron and Lupton 1993).

Chest drain placement

Indications

- pneumothorax
- pleural effusion

Pneumothorax is reported to occur in 5–10 per cent of ventilated babies (Greenough and Milner 2005) and may constitute a medical emergency, and requires expeditious action with the insertion of a chest drain. **Pneumothorax** leads to increased work of breathing, hypoxia and hypercapnia. A **tension pneumothorax** not only compromises the respiratory status but leads to a decreased cardiac output resulting in hypotension and cardiovascular instability which may result in intraventricular haemorrhage (p. 187).

Tension pneumothorax can be temporarily relieved by insertion of size 21G butterfly attached to a 10ml syringe via a three-way tap into the second intercostal space in the midclavicular line. This type of aspiration is undertaken in an emergency only and should be followed by insertion of a chest drain.

Pleural effusion can seriously impede lung inflation and requires drainage.

Equipment

- sterile chest drain pack
- sterile gown and gloves
- cleansing agent
- 1 per cent Lidocaine
- 2ml syringe and 25G needle
- size 10 or 12fg plural drain
- underwater seal drain or **Heimlich valve**
- suture
- sterile transparent dressing
- low-grade suction equipment

Procedure

This procedure should be undertaken following strict aseptic technique.

Position the infant in the supine position with the affected side tipped up to approximately 45° and the arm positioned to an angle of 90°. The infant should be given sufficient analgesia prior to commencement of the procedure. A chest drain should never be inserted without local anaesthesia, Lidocaine 1 per cent (0.3ml/kg) infiltrated into the tissues at the site of insertion will be effective within one to two minutes and last for one to two hours (Neonatal Formulary 2007).

The site of insertion is usually the fourth intercostal space in the anterior axillary line. The second intercostal space in the mid-clavicular line is best avoided especially in girls for cosmetic reasons. The nipple and areolar lie at the fourth rib in this line and are not always evident in the very preterm infant.

Once local anaesthesia has been achieved, make an incision in the skin and into the intercostal muscle no wider than the width of the drain. Be aware that the intercostal artery, vein and nerve run just beneath the rib; by working above the superior aspect of the lower rib, this neurovascular structure is avoided.

Using fine blunt forceps separate the muscle fibres with a dissecting action until the pleural space is entered. The trochar within the drain should not be used to dissect the muscle or pierce the pleura. It should be withdrawn 0.5cm

357

into the drain and clamped into position before insertion. Gently ease the drain in along the track that has been created, keeping it tangential to the lung and guiding it anteriorly to where the air tends to accumulate in a supine infant. Insert the drain 2–3cm in the small preterm infant and 3–4cm in the term infant. Ensure that the drain's side holes are within the pleural space.

When the drain is in place the trochar can be withdrawn until there is sufficient space to clamp the drain close to the skin, after which it can be removed completely. Misting of the lumen of the drain indicates it is within the plural space. The clamp should remain in situ until an underwater seal drain or Heimlich valve is attached to prevent air from entering the pleural space. If required, suction can be applied at a negative pressure of 5–10cm water.

Secure the drain in position by placing a suture on either side of the incision and securing the tails to tape placed as close to the skin as possible. A sterile transparent dressing should then be applied over the entire site. Purse string sutures should not be used as they increase the risk of scarring.

To drain a pleural effusion, the same technique is used, but as fluid is heavier than air it gravitates to a lower dependent area of the lung; as a consequence, the drain is directed posteriorly towards the base of the lung in order to achieve drainage.

The movement of air through the drain should be observed and recorded hourly to help determine tube patency and efficacy. Once the drain is no longer deemed necessary, the suction can be discontinued; if then there is no clinical deterioration, it can be removed.

Complications

- Bleeding from damaged intercostal, mammory, pulmonary or axillary vessels.
- Intercostal nerve damage.
- Phrenic nerve damage leading to **eventration** of the diaphragm.
- Thoracic duct injury.
- Lung damage – a drain wrongly inserted to remove pleural effusion can cause pneumothorax or a brochopleural fistula.
- **Syncope** – rare but can occur if fluid is removed too quickly.
- Infection – avoided by use of aseptic technique.
- Scarring and altered breast tissue development – reduced by not using purse string sutures and avoiding drain placement on the anterior chest wall.

Case study: UAC and UVC insertion

Robert is a 25-week gestation infant delivered to a primigravid mother following spontaneous onset of preterm labour. His mother had received one dose of antenatal steroids prior to delivery. At birth, he was in good condition. He was put into a polythene bag (see pp. 69 and 101), transferred to the resuscitaire and electively intubated to receive exogenous surfactant. His heart rate was greater than 100 throughout. Robert was transferred to NICU where he continued to be ventilated and had a UAC inserted for arterial access to allow blood sampling for gas analysis, etc. and blood pressure monitoring. He had a UVC inserted for fluid and drug therapy.

His initial chest X-ray (Figure 14.5 (a)) shows the following:

■ Chest expansion to eight posterior ribs with evidence of respiratory distress syndrome (surfactant deficiency). Air bronchogram seen at carina. Left heart border not clearly defined (but a slightly rotated film).
■ Endotracheal tube tip (a) at T3–4 (withdrawn to T2).
■ Nasogastric tube is in stomach (b).
■ UAC tip (c) is at T6 (to the left side of spinal column).
■ UVC tip (d) is appropriately placed, e.g. not in liver (to the right side of spinal column).
■ Abdominal temperature probe is also in situ.

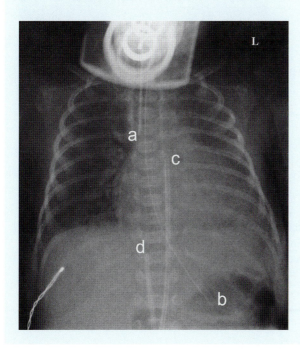

Figure 14.5
(a) Chest X-ray

Robert was introduced to enteral feeding with maternal breast milk at 24 hours of age and was graduated to full enteral feeds over the next two weeks. During this time he had episodes of desaturations and bradycardia which was thought to be reflux related (p. 333). He commenced anti-reflux medication. Despite this he continued to reflux and could not tolerate increases in his feed volume. Following clinical discussion it was decided to jejunally feed Robert.

The tube was measured (see p. 333) and gradually passed.

His abdominal X-ray (Figure 14.5 (b)) shows:

- Gastric tube (a) in stomach, necessary to keep stomach decompressed and check for refluxing of milk.
- Transpyloric tube in jejunum (b).
- There is presence of gas throughout the gut.
- ECG electrodes can also be seen as can abdominal temperature probe.

Figure 14.5 (b) Abdominal X-ray

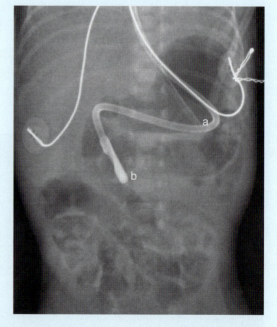

Robert tolerated an increase in volume to 180ml/kg and gained weight. After two weeks of jejunal feeding he was recommenced on gastric feeding which was well tolerated.

Acknowledgements

Elizabeth Harling was the author of this chapter in the first edition. Thank you to Debbie Eadie (ANNP) and Department of Medical Photography, Derriford Hospital, Plymouth, for their help with the photographs in this chapter.

References

Agarwala, S., Dave, S., Gupta, A.K. and Mitra, A.K. (1998) 'Duodenal–renal fistula due to naso gastric tube in a neonate', *Paediatric Surgery International* 14: 102–3.

Avila-Figueroa, C., Goldmann, D.A. and Richardson, D.K. (1998) 'Intravenous lipid emulsions are a major determinant of coagulase – negative staphylococcal bacteraemia in the very low birth weight newborns', *Pediatric Infectious Diseases Journal* 17: 10–17.

Barker, D.P. and Rutter, N. (1995) 'Exposure to invasive procedures in neonatal intensive care unit admissions', *Archives of Disease in Childhood: Fetal and Neonatal Edition* 72: F47–F48.

Barrington, K.J. (1999a) 'Umbilical arterial catheters in the newborn: effects in the catheter design (end vs side hole)', *Cochrane Database of Systematic Reviews*, Issue 1, Art. No. CD5000508.DOI.1002/14651858. CD000508.

Barrington, K.J. (1999b) 'Umbilical arterial catheters in the newborn: effects of positioning of the catheter tip', *Cochrane Database of Systematic Reviews*, Issue 1, Art. No. CD5000505.DOI.1002/14651858 CD000508.

Berger, A., Salzer, H.R., Weninger, M. *et al.* (1998) 'Septicaemia in an Austrian neonatal intensive care unit; a seven year analysis', *Acta Paediatrica Scandaniavia* 87: 1066–9.

Blumenfeld, T.A., Turi, G. and Blanc, W.A. (1979) 'Recommended site and depth of newborn heelstick punctures based on anatomical measurements and histopathology', *Lancet* i: 230–3.

Byrne, E. and Mackinnon, R. (2006) 'Should premedication be used for semi urgent or elective intubation in neonates?', *Archives of Disease in Childhood* 91: 79–83.

Cameron, D. and Lupton, B.A. (1993) 'Inadvertent brain penetration during neonatal nasotracheal intubation', *Archives of Disease in Childhood* 69: 79–80.

Darling, J.C., Newell, S.J., Mohandee, O., Uzan, O., Cullinane, C.J. and Dear, P.R.F. (2001) 'Central venous catheter tip in the right atrium: a risk factor for neonatal cardiac tamponade', *Journal of Perinatology* 21: 461–4.

Datta, M.K. and Clarke, P. (2008) 'Current practices in skin antiseptics for central venous catheterisation in UK tertiary level neonatal units', *Archives of Disease in Childhood: Fetal and Neonatal Edition* 93: F328.

Department of Health (2001) *Review of Four Neonatal Deaths due to Cardiac Tamponade Associated with the Presence of Central Venous Catheters*. Available at: www.dh.gov.uk/en/PublicationsandStatistics/PublicationsPolicyandGuidance/DH400 9584, downloaded 07/04/08.

Gibbins, S., Stevens, B., Hodnett, E., Pinelli, J., Ohlsson, A. and Darlington, G. (2002) 'Efficacy and safety of sucrose for procedural pain relief in preterm and term neonates', *Nursing Research* 51: 375–82.

Greenhough, A. and Milner, A.D. (2005) 'Acute respiratory disease', in J.M. Rennie (ed.) *Roberton's Textbook of Neonatology*, 4th edn, Philadelphia, PA: Elsevier.

Greenspan, J.S., Wolfson, M.R. and Holt, W.J. (1990) 'Neonatal gastric intubation: differential respiratory effects between nasogastric and orogastric tubes', *Pediatric Pulmonology* 8: 254–8.

Huang, C.M., Tung, W.S., Kuo, L.L. and Ying-Ju, C. (2004) 'Comparison of pain responses of premature infants to the heelstick between containment and swaddling', *Journal of Nursing Research* 12: 31–40.

Jain, A. and Rutter, N. (1999) 'Ultrasound study of heel to calcaeum in neonates', *Archives of Disease in Childhood: Fetal and Neonatal Edition* 180: F243–F245.

Mannan, I., Chow, P., Lissauer, T. *et al.* (2007) 'Mistaken identity of skin cleansing solution leading to extensive burns in an extremely preterm infant', *Acta Paediatrica* 96: 1536–7.

McCullough, S., Halton, T., Mowbray, D. and Macfarlane, P.I. (2008) 'Lingual sucrose reduces pain response to naso gastric tube insertion: a randomised clinical trial', *Archives of Disease in Childhood: Fetal and Neonatal Edition* 93: F100–F103.

McGuire, W. and McEwan, P. (2002) 'Transpyloric versus gastric tube feeding for preterm infants', *Cochrane Database of Systematic Reviews*, Issue 3, Art. No. CD003487.

Meerstadt, P.W.D. and Gyll, C. (1994) *A Manual of Neonatal Emergency X-Ray Interpretation*, London: W.B. Saunders.

Neonatal Formulary (2007) *Neonatal Formulary*, Oxford: Blackwell Publishing.

NPSA (2005) 'Reducing the harm caused by misplaced naso and orogastric feeding tubes in babies under the care of neonatal units', *Patient Safety Alert*, London: National Patient Safety Agency.

NPSA (2007) 'Promoting safer measurement and administration of liquid medicines via oral and other enteral routes', *Patient Safety Alert*, London: National Patient Safety Agency.

Pratt, R.J., Pellowe, C.M., Wilson, J.A. *et al.* (2007) 'epic2: national evidence based guidelines for preventing healthcare associated infections in NHS hospitals in England', *Journal of Hospital Infection* 65S: S1 – S64. Available at: www,epic.tvi.ac.uk (accessed 30 June 2008).

Resuscitation Council (UK) (2006) *Newborn Life Support*, 2nd edn, London: Resuscitation Council (UK),

Reynolds, P.R., Banerjee, S. and Meek, J.H. (2005) 'Alcohol burns in extremely low birth weight infants: still occurring', *Archives of Disease in Childhood: Fetal and Neonatal Edition* 90: F10.

Stocks, J. (1980) 'Effects of nasogastric tubes on nasal resistance during infancy', *Archives of Disease in Childhood* 55: 17–21.

Upadhyayula, S., Kambalapalli, M. and Harrison, C.J. (2007) 'Safety of anti infective agents for skin preparation in premature infants', *Archives of Disease in Childhood* 92: 646–7.

Van Someran, V., Linnett, S.J. and Stothers, J.R. (1984) 'An investigation into the benefits of resisting nasoenteric feeding tubes', *Pediatrics* 14: 379–83.

Wilkinson, A. and Calvert, S. (1992) 'Procedures in neonatal intensive care', in N.R.C. Roberton (ed.) *Textbook of Neonatology*, 2nd edn, London: Churchill Livingstone.

Chapter 15

Neonatal Anaesthesia

Beverley Guard, Liam Brennan and Rachel Homer

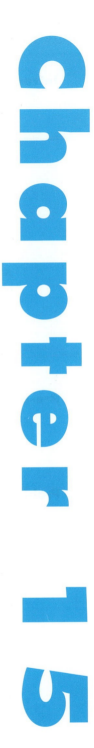

Contents

Introduction

The demand for neonatal anaesthesia has grown enormously in recent decades due to the increased survival of premature infants and developments in surgical techniques for congenital malformations previously considered inoperable.

The technical skills required to anaesthetise a neonate safely are very demanding and difficult to acquire: only a minority of anaesthetists possess such skills. Following the 1989 report of the National Confidential Enquiry into Perioperative Deaths (NCEPOD), and more recently the Tanner Report, there is an increasing trend towards centralisation of paediatric surgical services in specialist centres, and mounting evidence that occasional paediatric practice is unsafe leading to worse outcomes (Campling *et al.* 1990; Tanner 2007). In addition, there are marked differences in the anatomy, physiology and pharmacology of neonates compared to adults or even older children. The neonatal anaesthetist needs to have technical skills, specialist knowledge and be thoroughly acquainted with the differing patterns of disease in the neonatal age group. This chapter hopes to assist the neonatal nurses' knowledge and understanding of anaesthesia in this vulnerable population.

Pre-operative assessment

All neonates must be carefully assessed pre-operatively by the anaesthetist, with the emphasis on detection of the following problems.

Problems of prematurity affecting anaesthesia

Pulmonary disease

The incidence of respiratory distress syndrome (RDS) and chronic lung disease increases with decreasing gestational age at birth, with infants of less than 32 weeks' gestation being at particular risk. Occasionally it is necessary to perform urgent surgery on an infant during the initial respiratory illness. Many of these infants will be on mechanical ventilation, continuous positive airway pressure (CPAP) or require oxygen supplementation pre-operatively. Careful note should be made of mechanical ventilatory settings, since minor ventilatory changes peri-operatively can result in serious sequelae such as **pneumothorax** and pulmonary hypertensive crises. Even after minor surgery, infants with lesser degrees of RDS may require a period of post-operative ventilation.

Ex-premature infants with chronic lung disease may require pre-operative physiotherapy, and as they are prone to bronchoconstriction may benefit from pre-operative inhaled bronchodilators or steroids. In addition, they may have subglottic stenosis as a complication of long-term intubation and in particular recurrent intubations (Leung and Berkowitz 2007); evidence of inspiratory stridor or upper airway obstruction may suggest this problem. The incidence of this problem is said to be reducing as practitioners are more aware of the possibility of intubation-related airway trauma and the increased use of nasal prong CPAP (Wain 2003; Greenough 2008).

Cardiovascular disease

There is an increasing incidence of patent ductus arteriosus (PDA) with decreasing birth weight and with decreasing gestational age, with an incidence of 70 per cent in preterm infants born at 25 weeks' gestation (Dagle *et al.* 2009). Clinical features include a **dynamic precordium**, a systolic murmur and signs of congestive cardiac failure. A significant PDA, that is, one associated with heart failure and/or pulmonary oedema, should be treated before surgery for other conditions where at all possible (see p. 166).

Persistent pulmonary hypertension results from constriction of the pulmonary vascular bed causing a delay or reversal of the transition from fetal to adult circulation. It most frequently occurs in response to acidosis, hypoxaemia or hypotension, all common in the sick surgical neonate (Friesen and Williams 2008). The result is a right-to-left shunt of blood at atrial and ductal level leading to worsening hypoxaemia and acidosis. Attempts should be made to reduce pulmonary vascular resistance before surgery by treating the underlying causes and by using pulmonary vasodilators if necessary.

Glycaemic control

Carbohydrate reserves in all neonates are low but preterm infants have particularly poor reserves because glycogen is not stored significantly until 36 weeks' gestation. Hypoglycaemia is therefore likely to accompany any significant period of pre-operative starvation and must be avoided. In preterm infants normoglycaemia is maintained by commencing an intravenous glucose infusion at the commencement of the starvation period.

Thermoregulation

The ability of neonates to maintain a normal core temperature is limited by a large surface area:volume ratio, immature sweating, poor insulation (due to less body fat) and a high basal metabolic rate, with preterm infants being at greatest risk of developing hypothermia (Ibrahim and Yoxall 2009). The range of ambient temperatures over which the core temperature of the infant is maintained at between 36.7 and 37.3°C while metabolic heat production is kept at a minimum is known as the neutral thermal environment (Hackman 2001). The lower limit of the neutral thermal environment may be as high as 36°C in a 1000g infant soon after birth (see p. 101).

Associated congenital/chromosomal anomalies

Surgery in the neonatal period is frequently for the correction of congenital anomalies. Many of these may be associated with other abnormalities, which should be actively sought pre-operatively. The following are of particular relevance to the anaesthetist.

Congenital heart disease

Some cardiac abnormalities may not present until several days or even weeks after birth, with symptoms often arising following closure of the ductus arteriosus. A high index of suspicion is therefore necessary, particularly if a heart murmur is detected on clinical examination and there are accompanying signs of cardiorespiratory impairment.

Important considerations in a baby with congenital heart disease include the direction of any intracardiac shunt, the presence of cyanosis or cardiac failure, the dependence of the circulation on flow through the ductus arteriosus and drug therapy. The baby's condition should be optimised before surgery in conjunction with neonatologists and paediatric cardiologists if necessary (see p. 173).

Airway abnormalities

The presence of a cleft lip and palate or of a more severe facial abnormality such as Pierre-Robin syndrome or cystic hygroma (see p. 415) may make tracheal intubation difficult (Figure 15.1).

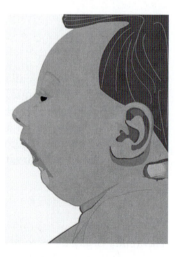

Down's syndrome (trisomy 21)

Common abnormalities include congenital heart disease, upper cervical spine instability and a large tongue, which may make airway management difficult (Mitchell *et al.* 1995).

Figure 15.1
Profile view of an infant
with Pierre-Robin syndrome

Familial anaesthetic problems

Most neonates will be undergoing their first anaesthetic. A history of any familial anaesthetic complications – particularly the development of malignant hyperpyrexia or suxamethonium apnoea under anaesthesia – should therefore be sought by the anaesthetist.

Pre-operative investigations and preparation

Investigations

The need for pre-operative investigations will depend on the age and clinical condition of the baby and the nature of the proposed surgery.

Weight

An accurate weight pre-operatively is essential in order to calculate appropriate drug doses, fluid volumes and ventilatory parameters.

Haemoglobin

The haemoglobin concentration (Hb) should be measured in all infants except healthy term babies undergoing minor surgery. The Hb at birth varies with gestational age (Roberton and Rennie 2001), with a normal value of 14.5g/dl at 28 weeks rising to 15.5–17.0g/dl at term. The Hb subsequently declines, the fall being greater in preterm babies due to lower red cell survival and poorer production of red cells (Proytcheva 2009). Transfusion practices are changing with an increasing appreciation of the risks involved, such as new variant Creutzfeld-Jacob Disease (nvCJD). Whereas previously it was unquestioned that an Hb less than 10g/dl was abnormal and should be corrected before surgery, some anaesthetists now tolerate an Hb as low as 8g/dl for minor surgery (Murray and Roberts 2004), even though anaemia in preterm infants may be associated with an increased incidence of post-operative apnoea.

Clotting studies

These should be carried out in neonates with sepsis, for example, necrotising enterocolitis or jaundice, and abnormalities corrected where possible pre-operatively.

Blood electrolytes

Serum sodium and potassium concentrations should be measured in any infant receiving intravenous fluids or diuretic therapy. Ionised calcium levels fall during the first week of life with a slow rise to adult levels during the second week. The fall is greatest in low birth weight infants. Calcium levels should be checked pre-operatively in any preterm or sick infant and levels below 1.75mmol/l corrected as severe hypocalcaemia can cause generalised hypotonia, jitteriness and seizures.

Blood glucose

Blood glucose concentration should be monitored closely peri-operatively and then at least four-hourly until satisfactory glucose homeostasis is achieved.

Blood cross-match

This is essential if major surgery is proposed for any infant and even for minor surgery in very low birth weight infants, in whom small amounts of intra-operative blood loss may be very significant. Cytomegalovirus-seronegative blood is recommended by the British Committee for Standards in Haematology (BCSH) Transfusion Task Force.

Oxygen saturation and blood gas analysis

Oxygen saturation is easily measured non-invasively with a pulse oximeter and should be recorded in all infants pre-operatively. Blood gas analysis should be performed in babies with severe cardiorespiratory disease or with sepsis.

Chest X-ray

A chest X-ray is required in babies with cardiorespiratory disease, those on mechanical ventilation and those with a tracheo-oesophageal fistula or a diaphragmatic hernia.

Echocardiography

Should be performed pre-operatively in any neonate or infant with a heart murmur, regardless of the presence or the absence of signs of cardiorespiratory impairment and particularly children with conditions that are known to be associated with congenital heart lesions, e.g. Down's syndrome (Birch *et al.* 1995).

Preparation

The baby's condition should be optimised before surgery, with correction of fluid deficits, electrolyte, acid base and haematological abnormalities wherever possible. In conditions associated with intestinal obstruction, a nasogastric tube should be inserted and aspirated at frequent intervals to minimise the risk of pulmonary aspiration of gastric contents. Babies with lung disease may benefit from pre-operative physiotherapy.

Prolonged pre-operative starvation is dangerous in neonates as they are at increased risk of hypoglycaemia (see above). Appropriate exclusion periods for milk feeds and clear liquids are now well defined (Table 15.1).

Premedication

Atropine

This drug is rarely if ever used as a routine premedicant now that the inhalational anaesthetic agent halothane has largely fallen out of use. However, it should still be kept immediately available to treat **bradyarrhythmias** and excessive airway secretions (which can produce troublesome airway complications during the peri-operative period). The dose is 20mcg/kg intravenously or intramuscularly.

Sedatives

These drugs are unnecessary in the neonatal age group in whom pre-operative anxiety is not a factor. Prolonged effects of sedative drugs may be hazardous in this age group (see below).

Caffeine

Intravenous caffeine has been shown to reduce the incidence of post-operative apnoea in former preterm infants and has been advocated pre-operatively by some authorities (Wellborn *et al.* 1989).

Table 15.1 Pre-operative fasting times for neonates and infants

Type of feed	Duration of fast (hours)	
	Neonates	Infants
Clear fluid	2	2
Breast milk	4	4
Formula milk	4	6
Solids	N/A	6

Source: Adapted from Emerson *et al.* (1998).

Transfer to the operating theatre

Neonates should be transported to the operating theatre in a warm incubator, with monitoring appropriate to the severity of illness. All neonatal intensive care units should have a transport incubator equipped with an appropriate ventilator and the capability to monitor oxygen saturation, ECG and arterial blood pressure. It should also carry all drugs and equipment required for neonatal resuscitation.

The operating theatre environment

It is essential to maintain a baby in an environment that limits heat loss and thus reduces metabolic heat production. Morbidity and mortality have been shown to increase if a baby cools, with increased tendency to hypoxaemia, acidosis, coagulopathy and intraventricular haemorrhage (Laptook and Watkinson 2008). The operating theatre should therefore be warmer than for adult surgery, with a temperature of 25°C and humidity of 50 per cent. (Additional measures that may be taken to reduce thermal stress are discussed in the section on anaesthetic equipment.)

Intra-operative management

Induction of anaesthesia

Anaesthesia should be induced in the operating theatre to improve safety and to avoid unmonitored transfers (however brief) of the anaesthetised infant. Parental presence is not necessary for the infant, as such young babies are not obviously disturbed by separation; however, if parents express a desire to be present at induction their wishes should be respected. The majority of infants will already have intravenous access in situ before arrival in the operating theatre or will have a cannula inserted on arrival to facilitate intravenous induction of anaesthesia. More robust neonates may be induced via the inhalational route and vascular access obtained after the child is asleep. The decision between an inhalation or intravenous induction rests with the anaesthetist managing the case.

Intravenous induction

This is the preferred method for induction of anaesthesia in most infants. Following intravenous cannulation, but before giving any drugs, the baby is given 100 per cent oxygen via a face mask. This reduces the possibility of the baby becoming hypoxaemic when apnoeic, the risk of which greatly outweighs the risk of oxygen toxicity at this time (see below). A sleep dose of an induction agent is then given, typically thiopental 2–3mg/kg. Propofol is popular as an induction agent in general paediatric anaesthesia, but is not licensed for use in infants under one month of age. Sleep doses are smaller in neonates due to increased endorphin and progesterone levels and a deficient blood–brain barrier.

Following induction of anaesthesia, muscle relaxants may be given to facilitate tracheal intubation. If rapid intubation is required, for example, in babies at risk of aspiration of gastric contents, suxamethonium 2–3mg/kg is used. In other situations, muscle relaxants with a slower onset of action such as atracurium or vecuronium are commonly used, whereas the longer-acting pancuronium is rarely indicated for peri-operative use.

Inhalation induction

This is a useful alternative to intravenous induction, particularly in vigorous babies in whom intravenous cannulation may prove difficult. Sevoflurane is the volatile anaesthetic agent of choice for inhalational induction of anaesthesia in infants. Halothane is now virtually obsolete, at least in Europe and North America. Sleep is achieved smoothly and rapidly (within 60 seconds) and there is minimal tendency for a bradycardia to occur. Sevoflurane is added to oxygen or an equal mixture of oxygen and nitrous oxide and administered via an anaesthetic face mask in concentrations of up to 8 per cent until the baby is deeply enough anaesthetised to tolerate intravenous cannulation. Muscle relaxants may then be administered to facilitate tracheal intubation.

Airway management

During general anaesthesia for neonates it is usual to intubate the trachea and use positive-pressure ventilation during all but the shortest surgical procedures. The airway may be difficult to maintain using a face mask and inhalational anaesthetic agents produce marked respiratory depression in this age group. Hypoxaemia due to reduced lung volumes and inefficient ventilation is therefore likely to occur unless controlled ventilation is used. In addition, gastric dilatation occurs following assisted ventilation using a face mask. The laryngeal mask airway (LMA) may be useful in the case of a difficult airway, such as Pierre-Robin syndrome, but is not otherwise used to substitute for tracheal intubation in the neonatal age group.

Awake intubation in anaesthetic practice is virtually obsolete. It has been demonstrated that it is associated with a higher incidence of significant desaturation than intubation following induction of anaesthesia (Kong et al. 1992). In addition, awake intubation produces a significantly greater rise in anterior fontanelle pressure than following general anaesthesia and theoretically carries a risk of causing an intraventricular haemorrhage in high-risk babies (Millar and Bissonnette 1994). It is, therefore, nowadays accepted that tracheal intubation should generally take place after induction of anaesthesia.

Maintenance of anaesthesia

Adequate anaesthesia during surgery has been demonstrated to reduce the infant's stress response and may improve outcome (Anand *et al.* 1988). High inspired concentrations of inhalational anaesthetics often cause severe cardiovascular depression in neonates. Consequently, a 'balanced' technique is usually favoured, combining a low concentration of inhalational anaesthetic in nitrous oxide and oxygen or an air–oxygen mixture to ensure that the infant is anaesthetised. This is combined with muscle relaxants and adequate analgesia (see below). Ventilation is maintained intra-operatively, either manually or via a mechanical ventilator.

Oxygen and retinopathy of prematurity

The use of oxygen during anaesthesia in preterm neonates should be carefully controlled. Preterm babies are at risk of developing retinopathy of prematurity if blood oxygen levels are too high, even for short periods of time (Finer and Leone 2009). Hyperoxia causes vasoconstriction and allows the release of angiogenic substances and oxygen-free radicals which may be toxic to many body systems. It is wise, therefore, to limit the inspired oxygen concentration to give a partial pressure of oxygen in arterial blood (PaO_2) of between 7 and 10kPa. Pulse oximetry does not accurately detect hyperoxia but can be used as a guide (Brockway and Hay 1998); the lowest inspired oxygen concentration that maintains an oxygen saturation of 90–94 per cent should be used.

Emergence from anaesthesia and extubation

If extubation is anticipated, the inhaled anaesthetic should be discontinued shortly before completion of surgery. When the surgical drapes are removed, the infant should be kept warm. The effects of muscle relaxants should be reversed completely and ventilation maintained with an air–oxygen mixture until the infant awakens and re-establishes spontaneous ventilation. The nose and mouth should be cleared of secretions and the nasogastric tube aspirated and removed if not required post-operatively. Extubation should only take place once the infant is fully awake and breathing regularly and adequately. After extubation, oxygen should continue to be delivered via a face mask.

Analgesia

Historically, post-operative paediatric analgesia was poorly managed. Neonates in particular were assumed to be incapable of perceiving pain and were seldom given adequate post-operative analgesia. However, advances in neonatal neurobiology have prompted a reconsideration of this approach (see p. 232).

There is now no doubt that even the most premature infants respond to noxious stimuli, with well-developed physiological and behavioural responses (Anand and Hickey 1987). The modern view is that all infants must receive appropriate pain relief after surgery. Most of the methods of pain control used in adults can be modified for neonatal use; a multimodal regimen using paracetamol, local anaesthesia and opioids is central to this approach.

Opioids

The term 'opioid' is used to describe a group of drugs which act at specific receptors in the central nervous system resulting in profound analgesia. The most commonly used drugs in neonatal anaesthesia are morphine and fentanyl while the ultra-short-acting remifentanil has attractive potential for intra-operative use.

Opioids must be used cautiously in neonates because immature metabolic pathways, particularly in the liver, may result in very unpredictable or prolonged responses to these drugs. The most major concern is the risk of opioid-induced respiratory depression. If the neonate is to receive respiratory support post-operatively then morphine or fentanyl can be used quite safely. Indeed, many paediatric anaesthetists would plan to electively ventilate a neonate after major surgery that necessitated ongoing opioid analgesia. Whether ventilated or breathing spontaneously, all neonates who have received opioids must be managed in a high dependency environment, with continuous pulse oximetry and apnoea monitoring being mandatory (Pounder and Steward 1992).

Morphine

Morphine has a longer duration of action and greater potency in neonates than in older children and adults (Lynn and Slattery 1987) (see p. 448). This is mainly because of immature hepatic function resulting in delayed metabolism of opioid drugs. It should therefore be given less frequently and in a smaller dose. If post-operative ventilation is planned, then up to 50mg/kg may be given intra-operatively. Post-operatively, up to 20mcg/kg of morphine per hour may be used by continuous intravenous infusion but most neonates are well analgesed by 5–10mcg/kg per hour (Purcell-Jones et al. 1987). Morphine should be used with extreme caution in neonates who are breathing spontaneously after surgery. Many authorities avoid morphine in this situation or limit the infusion to 5mcg/kg per hour.

Fentanyl

This synthetic opioid is useful in neonates with haemodynamic instability, particularly those with pulmonary vascular problems. It is a much more potent drug than morphine but has a shorter duration of action after a single bolus dose. After prolonged infusions, however, the drug will accumulate, resulting in excessive sedation, hypoventilation and risk of apnoeic episodes. For intra-operative use during major neonatal surgery, up to 10mcg/kg is commonly used, necessitating post-operative respiratory support. Larger doses may be used but can potentially induce chest rigidity, particularly in preterm infants. Post-operatively an infusion of 4–8mcg/kg per hour may be used in ventilated neonates, but fentanyl should not be used in spontaneously breathing babies (see p. 448).

Remifentanil

This newer synthetic opioid is useful when profound analgesia is required intra-operatively but ongoing analgesia will be provided by other means. With both a rapid onset and an ultra-short half-life it is readily titrated to changes in levels of surgical stimulus, and is thus especially useful in neonates with haemodynamic instability. It is given by infusion at doses up to 0.25mcg/kg/minute; the dose is limited by potential for chest wall rigidity. However, unlike fentanyl, remifentanil will not accumulate even in renal or liver failure.

Paracetamol

Paracetamol has been safely used in preterm and term babies and is a useful adjunct to opioid analgesia and nerve blockade after both major and minor surgery. Its analgesic effects are due to the inhibition of prostaglandin synthesis in the central nervous system. Single doses of 15mg/kg orally or intravenously achieve therapeutic serum concentrations and may be repeated six-hourly (Hopkins *et al.* 1990), but rectally a loading dose of 40mg/kg is required followed by 30mg/kg 12-hourly if adequate serum levels are to be achieved (Anderson *et al.* 2002). Total dose should not exceed 40-60mg/kg per 24-hour period. Doses should be further reduced in neonates with evidence of impaired hepatic function, particularly those with significant jaundice.

Non-steroidal anti-inflammatory drugs

These drugs are not recommended in the neonatal period as they can interfere with platelet function and hence blood-clotting mechanisms, and can also compromise renal function.

Local anaesthesia

Local anaesthetic techniques are invaluable in neonates, reducing or avoiding the need for opioids with their attendant risks in this high-risk group. All of the local anaesthetic techniques utilised in adults are feasible in neonates. The free (biologically active) fraction of local anaesthetic drugs is higher than in older infants due to a reduced concentration of plasma-binding proteins; doses should thus be adjusted accordingly. Levo-bupivacaine is the most commonly used drug, for which the dose should not exceed 1.5mg/kg. Levo-bupivacaine is considered safer than bupivacaine because of its lower potential to cause cardiac arrythmias in overdose or when inadvertently injected into a blood vessel.

Wound infiltration

Wound infiltration is a simple and safe method of providing post-operative analgesia. It has been found to be effective following pyloromyotomy (McNicol *et al*. 1990) and is a useful alternative to ilio-inguinal nerve block for inguinal herniotomy (Reid *et al*. 1987). The opportunity to use this valuable technique in neonatal surgery should never be neglected.

Peripheral nerve blocks

A wide range of peripheral nerve blocks are potentially applicable to neonatal surgery but in practice only a few are commonly utilised. They are commonly used in conjunction with general anaesthesia and can provide very effective, long-lasting post-operative analgesia. Dorsal penile nerve block is very useful for penile surgery, especially circumcision, and has in fact been used as the sole anaesthetic technique for this procedure (Stang *et al*. 1988). Blockade of the ilio-inguinal nerve provides very effective analgesia after groin surgery, particularly inguinal herniotomy (Reid *et al*. 1987).

Central (neuro-axial) blocks

Local anaesthetic drugs introduced into the epidural or subarachnoid space can produce anaesthesia and analgesia of the lower limbs, abdomen and even thorax depending on the technique and the dose and volume of local anaesthetic used.

Such techniques are becoming increasingly popular in neonates as they allow major surgery to be undertaken under very light or even without general anaesthesia (Williams *et al*. 1997). In addition, they provide excellent post-operative analgesia, eliminating or reducing the need for opioid analgesia and thus potentially avoiding mechanical ventilation after surgery (Bosenberg *et al*. 1992).

Caudal epidural anaesthesia

Single-shot caudal anaesthesia is suitable for all surgical procedures below the umbilicus, and is mainly indicated in neonates for inguinal herniotomy, lower limb surgery and genito-urinary surgery (Figure 15.2). It is a very simple technique and major complications are rare.

Continuous caudal epidural anaesthesia involves the insertion of a catheter into the caudal space. The catheter may be threaded in a **cephalad** direction to a lumbar or thoracic level. An infusion of local anaesthetic can then be used to provide analgesia following major abdominal and thoracic surgery (Bosenberg *et al.* 1988). The limitation of this technique is the proximity of the caudal catheter to the anus, which has raised concerns with regard to infection when this route is used for continuous post-operative analgesia.

Lumbar and thoracic epidural anaesthesia

Lumbar and thoracic epidural blockade is less popular than the caudal block because it is technically more difficult to perform, needs specially designed equipment and has the potential for more serious complications. These complications include inadvertent total spinal anaesthesia or intravenous injection of local anaesthetic with the potential for convulsions and profound cardiovascular collapse. Other rare complications include epidural haematoma or abscess. The UK national paediatric epidural audit revealed 96 complications out of 10,633 epidurals performed during a five-year period; of these, only five were classed as serious, and only one child had lasting effects 12 months later (Llewellyn and Moriarty 2007).

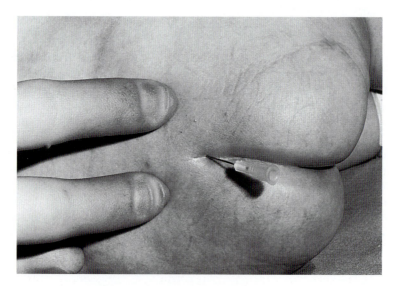

Figure 15.2 Insertion of a caudal epidural block

The haemodynamic instability commonly seen with epidural anaesthesia in adult practice (especially hypotension due to sympathetic nervous system blockade) is very unusual in the infant age group. This has been attributed to incomplete maturation of the sympathetic nervous system in the newborn resulting in very low levels of basal vascular tone. Epidural analgesia is now being increasingly used to provide excellent analgesia after abdominal and thoracic surgery. Though it is difficult to assess accurately the level of sensory block in a neonate, an adequate level can be assumed if the infant appears comfortable, while an excessively high block may be associated with an increased incidence of bradycardia or respiratory impairment.

Spinal anaesthesia

Spinal anaesthesia involves performing a lumbar puncture followed by injection of local anaesthetic into the subarachnoid space. It is technically easier than an epidural, has a rapid onset and provides complete motor and sensory blockade. The main disadvantages are a short and variable duration of action, which is no more than one hour.

Spinal blockade is a useful technique for inguinal herniotomy in ex-preterm neonates where it is associated with a lower incidence of post-operative bradycardia and desaturation than following general anaesthesia (Krane *et al.* 1995). It may also be used in combination with epidural anaesthesia for major abdominal surgery (Williams *et al.* 1997).

Fluid therapy

Fluid administration during surgery must take into account the maintenance requirements of the infant, the loss of fluid from sequestration and evaporation, and blood loss. The goal of intra-operative fluid replacement is to maintain cardiovascular stability and organ perfusion, though caution should be taken to prevent fluid overload as this could potentially cause cardiac failure secondary to the reopening of a PDA.

Maintenance of fluid

The fluid deficit generated during the fasting period should be replaced during surgery in addition to ongoing maintenance requirements (Cunliffe *et al.* 2007). Opinions vary as to the best intravenous fluid to use, with much debate surrounding the problem of hyponatraemia caused or exacerbated by overzealous peri-operative administration of hypotonic fluids such as 4 per cent glucose + 0.18 per cent sodium chloride (Paut and Lacroix 2006). In UK practice, very premature infants would generally be maintained on 10 per cent glucose solutions with sodium supplements guided by serum sodium levels. Five per cent glucose + 0.45 per cent saline is in general use for older infants. However, the hormonal stress response to surgery usually raises blood glucose concentrations in neonates (Sandstrom *et al.* 1995) and hyperglycaemia may occur with glucose-containing fluids. Hyper- and hypoglycaemia are hazardous for the neonatal brain and so intravenous fluid therapy should always be guided by regular blood glucose monitoring.

Replacement of fluid lost by evaporation/sequestration

During surgery, water is lost by evaporation from the operative site and protein-rich fluid is sequestered in the surrounding tissues as a result of surgical trauma, depleting the intravascular fluid volume. In infants, these fluid losses during abdominal surgery are estimated to be between 6 and 10ml/kg per hour, 4–7ml/kg per hour in thoracic surgery and only 1–2ml/kg per hour in superficial procedures (including neurosurgery) (Cunliffe *et al.* 2007). This should be replaced by Hartmann's solution or 0.9 per cent sodium chloride.

Replacement of blood loss

The pre-operative haemoglobin concentration (Hb) and blood loss peri-operatively will determine whether blood loss is replaced by blood or non-sanguinous fluid. The estimated blood volume (EBV) should be calculated (90ml/kg for a preterm baby, 85ml/kg for a term baby). The maximal allowable blood loss (ABL) can then be calculated from the formula:

$$ABL = EBV \times \frac{\text{initial Hb} - \text{lowest acceptable Hb}}{\text{initial Hb}}$$

The lowest acceptable Hb will depend on clinical circumstances. Blood loss can be determined by accurate weighing of surgical swabs and noting suction losses and replaced with a colloid solution until the maximal ABL is reached. Thereafter blood should be used. The most commonly used colloid in neonates is still 4.5 per cent human albumin solution, although controversy regarding its safety has led to the increased use of other synthetic colloids, including Gelofusine® and Haemaccel®. Synthetic starches might also be used, although their sequestration within the reticuloendothelial system is a cause for concern. Replacement of clotting factors by the use of fresh frozen plasma (FFP) should commence earlier rather than later due to the relatively deficient clotting systems in neonates. Platelet infusions may be required in cases of massive blood transfusion.

Assessment of the adequacy of volume replacement can be gauged clinically. Changes in pulse and blood pressure are both unreliable guides to hypovolaemia in neonates. Assessment of the peripheral circulation gives far more information:

capillary refill time should be rapid (less than two seconds) and extremities should be pink and warm. Prolonged refill time and increased core–peripheral temperature gradient are important clinical signs, suggesting volume depletion (Lambert *et al.* 1998). Measurement of urine output and central venous pressure (CVP) may also provide useful information, particularly during prolonged surgery or where large blood and fluid losses are anticipated.

Anaesthetic equipment

Neonatal anaesthesia requires specialised equipment. All equipment should be thoroughly checked before commencing any anaesthetic.

Airway equipment

Many of the items of equipment required for airway maintenance are available in a variety of sizes to suit all infants. It is not always possible to predict which will be appropriate, so a full range should be immediately available for every case.

Face masks

Face masks should have a low dead space to prevent rebreathing of expired gases. Several types are available: the Rendell–Baker mask has become obsolete as it can be difficult to obtain a good seal on the face in order to inflate the lungs without leakage of gases (Palme *et al.* 1985). Nowadays a circular cushioned-rim-type face mask is used which many anaesthetists (and neonatal intensive care staff) find easier to manipulate in small infants (Figure 15.3). Care must be taken that the mask is not covering the baby's eyes, as there is a risk of causing corneal abrasions.

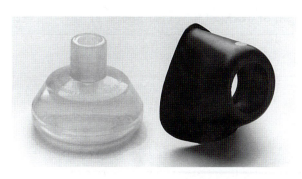

Figure 15.3 Anaesthetic face masks. The cushioned rim silicone mask (*left*) has now superseded the black rubber Rendell-Baker version (*right*) in neonatal practice.

Oral airways

Difficulties maintaining the airway in an anaesthetised neonate may be lessened if an oral airway is used, but will be increased if one of an incorrect size is chosen. Too small an airway may fail to overcome airway obstruction due to the tongue falling backwards whereas too large an airway may produce airway obstruction itself or induce laryngospasm or vomiting in a semi-conscious baby. The size is estimated by placing the airway against the baby's chin; with the flange at the middle of the baby's lips with the tip of the airway reaching the angle of the mandible.

Laryngoscopes

The infant larynx lies higher and more **anteriorly** than in older children or adults. In addition, the epiglottis is large and leaf-shaped and can obscure the laryngeal inlet. The best view of the larynx is obtained by using a laryngoscope with a short, straight blade.

Tracheal tubes

These should be parallel-sided, uncuffed, radio-opaque and marked at 1cm intervals from the tip. Each tube is sized according to the internal diameter. The approximate sizes and lengths of tracheal tubes according to the weight of the infant are shown in Table 15.2. Plain tubes are suitable for most procedures and can be used via the oral or nasal route (see p. 353), though 'south-facing' preformed RAE™ oral tubes are popular for orofacial and neurosurgery and 'north-facing' preformed RAE™ oral tubes are often used for other procedures because they are easy to secure in position and are less likely to kink (Figure 15.4).

Table 15.2 Size and length of tracheal tubes for neonates

Body weight (kg)	Internal diameter (mm)	External diameter (mm)	Length at lip (cm)	Length at nares (cm)
< 0.7	2.0	2.9	5.0	6.0
0.7 – 1	2.5	3.7	5.5	7.0
1.1 – 2	3.0	4.4	6.0	7.5
2.1 – 3	3.0	4.4	7.0	9.0
3.1 – 3.5	3.0	4.4	8.5	10.5
> 3.5	3.5	4.8	9.0	11.0

Source: Adapted from: Peutrell and Weir (1996: 180).

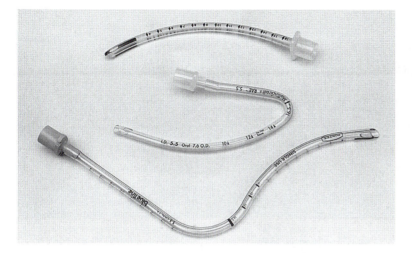

Figure 15.4 Tracheal tubes. Uncuffed tubes are appropriate for neonates, familiar straight tube (top). Preformed tubes (middle and bottom) are useful during head and neck surgery

Other equipment

In addition to the equipment mentioned above, small Magill forceps should be available for insertion of nasal tracheal tubes or throat packs and intubation stylets narrow enough to fit through the smallest tracheal tube should be available to aid a difficult intubation. Nasal intubation is rarely performed; although the chance of tube dislodgement or kinking is lower with this route, the risk of causing troublesome sinusitis is increased.

Breathing systems

The breathing system provides the means of delivering the anaesthetic gases and vapours to the patient. In a neonate, it should be lightweight, easy to assemble, present minimal resistance to breathing and have as small a dead space as possible. The most popular system in the UK is the Jackson–Rees modification of the Ayre's T-piece (Figure 15.5). This can be used for spontaneous or positive-pressure ventilation. It can also be used to apply positive end-expiratory pressure (PEEP) or continuous positive airway pressure (CPAP), manoeuvres which are essential in neonates to prevent collapse of the small airways and improve oxygenation.

Ventilators

Neonates are ventilated intra-operatively either by hand or by attachment to a mechanical ventilator. Manual ventilation is popular in neonates as it provides the anaesthetist with a 'feel' of the compliance of the lungs. There is a danger,

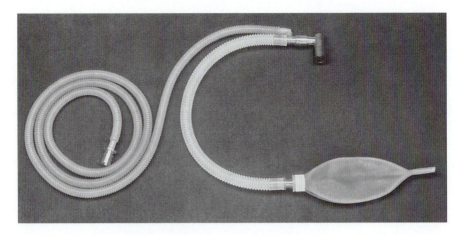

Figure 15.5 T-piece breathing system

however, of applying too much pressure and causing pulmonary barotrauma or even a pneumothorax. T-piece occluding ventilators which are pressure-limited (including the majority of those used on a neonatal intensive care unit) can be used in the very sick neonate with respiratory disease. More popular in the operating theatre setting is the 'bag squeezer'-type ventilator which essentially replaces the anaesthetist's hand squeezing the bag. These produce a constant flow and tidal volume unless higher pressures are required, when most become pressure-limited. For reasons already mentioned, an additional feature required of all neonatal ventilators is the facility to apply PEEP.

Equipment for maintenance of body temperature

The importance of maintaining an infant's body temperature cannot be over-emphasised (see Chapter 5). In addition to a warm operating theatre, the following measures can be utilised.

Overhead radiant heater

This should be used during both induction of anaesthesia and application of the skin preparation. It can also be used during emergence from anaesthesia.

Warming mattresses

These are essential to reduce conductive heat loss through a cold operating table. The surface temperature should not exceed 39°C to prevent skin burns. An alternative is the hot air mattress, which surrounds the infant in a microclimate of warm air.

Body temperature must be monitored whenever active warming is used, to avoid hyperthermia.

Humidifiers

Humidification of inspired anaesthetic gases reduces evaporative heat loss from the respiratory tract and may be either active or passive. Active humidification requires a water bath with careful temperature control. This method is commonly used in the neonatal intensive care unit. Passive humidifiers are devices with a high surface area that allow an exchange of heat and moisture from exhalation to inhalation. They are included in the anaesthetic breathing system in close proximity to the tracheal tube. They have been shown to be as efficient as a heated humidifier when used in ventilated neonates over a six-hour period (Schiffmann *et al.* 1997).

Other methods

All fluids administered should be warmed to 37°C. In addition, the infant can be wrapped in cotton wool, aluminium foil or plastic sheets (such as food grade plastic wrap) to prevent radiant and convective heat loss. Particular attention should be paid to the head, which is relatively larger in neonates and exposes a big surface area for heat loss.

Equipment for intravenous fluid administration

Intravenous cannulae

For reliable venous access an over-the-needle, plastic cannula should be used. These are available in sizes as small as 24G. For all but the most minor surgical procedures most neonatal anaesthetists would ensure that there are two functioning intravenous cannulae in situ.

Fluid administration sets

The small volume of infusate required by neonates makes syringe pumps and other sorts of infusion devices preferable for the administration of maintenance fluids. They should have a volume limiter and a pressure alarm. Other devices include giving sets with a micro-drop outlet and a burette, which can be filled with a predetermined volume of fluid (for example, one hour's requirements) to prevent inadvertent overload.

Administration of fluid boluses including colloid and blood product is most easily achieved manually by a syringe attached via a three-way tap, provided care is taken not to introduce any bubbles, which could traverse the still-patent foramen ovale causing systemic air **emboli.** This is particularly the case if nitrous oxide is used during the anaesthetic as this gas will cause expansion of any air bubbles and exacerbate the potential for embolisation.

Anaesthetic monitoring

Although there is no substitute for the continuous presence of a well-trained anaesthetist, there is evidence to suggest that intra-operative adverse events can be avoided by physiological monitoring of the neonate (Cote *et al.* 1988). Minimal monitoring in any baby undergoing surgery should include the following.

Cardiovascular monitoring

Electrocardiography (ECG)

Cardiac output in neonates is rate-dependent. Bradycardia leads to a fall in cardiac output and hypotension, whereas tachycardia may be a sign of hypovolaemia, pain or inadequate anaesthesia. Although a very useful monitor, the ECG does not give any indication of the adequacy of vital organ perfusion.

Blood pressure

The oscillometric method and Doppler method of non-invasive blood pressure measurement are most commonly used in neonatal practice. The oscillometric method measures mean blood pressure accurately and derives systolic and diastolic pressure using a computer algorithm. It is a reliable method in neonates provided the correct cuff size is used (cuff width to arm circumference ratio should be approximately 0.5). The Doppler method uses an arm cuff and an ultrasonic transducer. This is placed over the radial or brachial artery and detects changes in vessel wall movement to record systolic and diastolic blood pressure.

Invasive arterial pressure should be measured via a catheter inserted into the umbilical artery or a peripheral artery when rapid fluid shifts, particularly large blood losses or sudden haemodynamic changes, are anticipated (for example, during cardiac surgery). Indwelling arterial access also allows blood gases and other parameters such as blood glucose and haematocrit to be easily monitored during major and prolonged surgery. Limb perfusion must be closely monitored when arterial catheters are in situ.

Precordial and oesophageal stethoscope

A precordial stethoscope is a device secured over the left sternal border. An oesophageal stethoscope is a soft catheter with holes in its distal end positioned in the mid-oesophagus. Both allow continuous monitoring of heart and breath sounds though they do not give accurate information about the adequacy of cardiac output or pulmonary ventilation. Neither of these devices is in common use in contemporary UK practice.

Respiratory monitoring

Pulse oximetry

Pulse oximetry is essential in the monitoring of neonates. It provides continuous, non-invasive beat-to-beat monitoring of oxygen saturation and heart rate. Positioned in neonates over the lateral border of the foot or medial border of the hand, it also provides information about peripheral perfusion and therefore cardiac output and volume status.

Limitations of pulse oximetry are interference from diathermy and motion. It does not accurately detect hyperoxia and is inaccurate at oxygen saturations below 75 per cent (Cote *et al.* 1988).

Capnography

A capnograph measures the change in carbon dioxide (CO_2) with each breath by sampling expired gas. In healthy neonates the end-tidal CO_2 concentration closely approximates arterial PCO_2. The value of end-tidal CO_2 is influenced not only by arterial PCO_2 but also by cardiac output and ventilation. It is, therefore, a useful monitor of cardiovascular status in addition to the adequacy of ventilation, including inadvertent disconnection from mechanical ventilation.

Temperature monitoring

Temperature should be monitored in all neonates undergoing surgery. Core temperature can be estimated at several sites, including oesophagus, rectum, tympanic membrane or nasopharynx. Oesophageal probes are the most convenient. Skin temperature should also be measured because the gradient between core and peripheral temperature gives a useful indication of the adequacy of cardiac output (Lambert *et al.* 1998).

Post-operative care

All small infants require close observation and monitoring in the post-operative period. This may be in a high dependency area or in an intensive care unit, depending on the prematurity of the infant, the surgical condition and other coexisting medical problems. As with all post-operative patients, adequate analgesia must be provided; this may be achieved by several methods which have already been described. Fluid administration should be tailored to the needs of the infant and measures taken to maintain body and peripheral temperature (Lee *et al.* 2008).

There are certain post-operative problems that are encountered far more frequently in infants. These include apnoeic episodes, extubation stridor and respiratory insufficiency requiring ventilatory support.

Post-operative apnoeas

The neonate, particularly the preterm infant, breathes irregularly. Periodic respiration in which breathing and apnoea alternate is common; however, cessation of breathing for longer than 15 seconds (or less if associated with bradycardia or desaturation) is significant and abnormal. Neonates are prone to develop apnoeas following general anaesthesia, the risk rising with increasing prematurity and with the use of intra-operative opioids (Walther-Larsen and Rasmussen 2006). Regional anaesthesia without sedation reduces the risk significantly (Wellborn 1992). High-dose caffeine (10mg/kg IV) may also be protective (Wellborn et al. 1989) although this is not a common practice in the child managed post-operatively on a NICU. Most apnoeas can be treated successfully with stimulation and oxygen. Rarely, CPAP or mechanical ventilation is necessary if apnoeic episodes are recurrent in the post-operative period.

Post-extubation stridor

Stridor may rarely occur either immediately or within a few hours of tracheal extubation. It is usually due to subglottic oedema caused by trauma exerted on the tracheal mucosa at the level of the cricoid cartilage by an oversized tracheal tube. The risk is greatest if there is no leak around the tracheal tube following insertion, if the tube moves within the trachea during surgery and if multiple intubation attempts were necessary.

Possible therapies include inhalation of nebulised adrenaline, intravenous dexamethasone or the provision of CPAP via a nasal prong. If reintubation is required, a smaller tracheal tube should be used and an audible gas leak around the tube should be present before it is subsequently removed.

Assessing the need for post-operative ventilation

A key issue in early post-operative management is the increased need for post-operative ventilatory support. Both pre- and post-operative factors are important in assessing the need for post-operative ventilation.

Pre-operative factors

Ventilatory drive is immature in neonates and puts the premature infant at increased risk of post-operative apnoeas; for the term infant this risk applies up to 46 weeks' postconceptual age and for the ex-premature infant for as much as 60 weeks' postconceptual age. Infants who have had repeated problems with apnoeic spells are more likely to require respiratory support post-operatively. In addition, common problems of prematurity such as respiratory distress syndrome and persisting patent ductus arteriosus affect the efficiency of pulmonary gas exchange and make post-operative respiratory support more likely (Stewart 1982). Other pre-existing problems such as congenital heart disease and airway problems such as laryngomalacia ('floppy larynx') make post-operative respiratory insufficiency more likely.

Post-operative factors

Respiratory insufficiency is likely to occur following a prolonged anaesthetic due to the residual effects of anaesthetic and analgesic drugs (particularly opioids) on ventilatory drive. Abdominal distension following abdominal surgery may compromise diaphragmatic function and therefore effective spontaneous ventilation. Other factors, including hypothermia, acidosis and anaemia, may also be indications for a period of post-operative ventilation.

Signs of respiratory distress

The assessment of post-operative respiratory distress is largely clinical. A respiratory rate of greater than 60 breaths per minute should alert the anaesthetist to the possibility of respiratory insufficiency, particularly if associated with signs of increased work of breathing demonstrated by grunting respiration, nasal flaring and the presence of subcostal, intercostal and substernal recession. Restlessness, irritability, apnoeic episodes or failure to regain consciousness may also reflect hypoxaemia or hypercarbia.

Blood gas and acid base analysis should follow any suspicion of respiratory insufficiency. Other investigations, including chest radiography, may be indicated but if there is any suggestion that ventilatory support is required on clinical grounds this should be instituted without delay. This may initially be by bag and mask ventilation and subsequently nasal CPAP or reintubation and mechanical ventilation.

Conclusion

Many full-term neonates undergo anaesthesia and surgery uneventfully. The greatest problems are seen in sick and premature infants, particularly if cardio-respiratory insufficiency is present pre-operatively. Care of these infants requires a multidisciplinary approach by skilled personnel. The importance of communication between the anaesthetist and the neonatal nursing and medical team cannot be overemphasised and is essential if the best possible outcome is to be achieved.

Case study: premature infant with necrotising enterocolitis

Holly is a 9-week-old infant who was born at 26 weeks' gestation. She required ventilation for six weeks and is still receiving nasal CPAP. Over the past 48 hours her condition has deteriorated with abdominal distension, increasing oxygen requirements and deranged blood-clotting indices. A presumptive diagnosis of necrotising enterocolitis has been made and she now requires a laparotomy at the regional paediatric surgical centre 40 miles away.

Q.1. What additional ventilatory support is likely to be required for transport of this infant?

Q.2. What blood products will need to be ordered prior to her going to theatre?

Q.3. What are the problems for the anaesthetist in the intra-operative management of this case?

Q.4. Is any special monitoring required in the post-operative period?

Q.5. What methods may be used to provide adequate pain relief in the post-operative period?

Acknowledgements

Beverley Guard was the co-author of this chapter with Liam Brennan in the first edition.

References

Anand, K.J.S. and Hickey, P.R. (1987) 'Pain and its effect in the human neonate and fetus', *New England Journal of Medicine* 317: 1321–9.

Anand, K.J.S., Sippell, W.G. and Aynsley-Green, A. (1988) 'Does halothane anaesthesia decrease the metabolic and endocrine stress responses of newborn infants undergoing operation?', *British Medical Journal* 296: 668–72.

Anderson, B.J., van Lingen, R.A., Hansen, T.G., Lin, Y.C. and Holford, N.H.G. (2002) 'Acetaminophen developmental pharmacokinetics in premature neonates and infants', *Anesthesiology* 96: 1336–45.

Bosenberg, A.T. (1998) 'Epidural analgesia for major neonatal surgery', *Paediatric Anaesthesia* 8: 479–83.

Bosenberg, A.T., Bland, B.A.R. and Schulte-Steinberg, O. (1988) 'Thoracic epidural anaesthesia via caudal route in infants', *Anesthesiology* 69: 265–9.

Bosenberg, A.T., Wiersma, R. and Hadley, G.P. (1992) 'Oesophageal atresia: caudo-thoracic epidural anesthesia reduces the need for postoperative ventilatory support', *Pediatric Surgery International* 7: 289–91.

British Committee for Standards in Haematology. Available at: www.bcshguidelines.com.

Brockway, J. and Hay, W.W. Jr (1998) 'Prediction of arterial partial pressure of oxygen with pulse oxygen saturation measurements', *Journal of Pediatrics* 133(1): 63–6.

Campling, E.A., Devlin, H.B. and Lunn, J.N. (1990) *The Report of the National Enquiry into Perioperative Deaths 1989*, London: NCEPOD.

Cote, C.J., Golstein, E.A., Cote, M.A., Hoaglin, D.C. and Ryan, J.F. (1988) 'A single blind study of pulse oximetry in children', *Anesthesiology* 68: 184–8.

Cunliffe, M. *et al.* (2007) 'APA Consensus Guideline on Perioperative Fluid Management in Children'. Available at: www.apagbi.org.uk/docs/Perioperative_Fluid_Management_2007.pdf.

Dagle, J.M., Lepp, N.T., Cooper, M.E., Schaa, K.L., Kelsey, K.J., Orr, K.L., Caprau, D., Zimmerman, C.R., Steffen, K.M., Johnson, K.J., Marazita, M.L. and Murray, J.C. (2009) 'Determination of genetic predisposition to patent ductus arteriosus in preterm infants', *Pediatrics* 123(4): 1116–23.

Emerson, B.M., Wrigley, S.R. and Newton, M. (1998) 'Pre-operative fasting for paediatric anaesthesia: a survey of current practice', *Anaesthesia* 53(4): 326–30.

Finer, N. and Leone, T. (2009) 'Oxygen saturation monitoring for the preterm infant: the evidence basis for current practice', *Pediatric Research* 65(4): 375–80.

Friesen, R. and Williams, G.D. (2008) 'Anesthetic management of children with pulmonary arterial hypertension', *Paediatric Anaesthesia* 18: 208–16.

Greenough, A., Premkumar, M. and Patel, D. (2008) 'Ventilatory strategies for the extremely premature infant', *Paediatric Anaesthesia* 18: 371–7.

Hackman, P.S. (2001) 'Recognizing and understanding the cold-stressed term infant', *Journal of Neonatal Nursing* 20(8): 35–41.

Hopkins, C.S., Underhill, S. and Booker, P.D. (1990) 'Pharmacokinetics of paracetamol after cardiac surgery', *Archives of Disease in Childhood* 65: 971–6.

Ibrahim, C.P. and Yoxall, C.W. (2009) 'Use of plastic bags to prevent hypothermia at birth in preterm infants: do they work at lower gestations?', *Acta Paediatrica* 98(2): 256–60.

Kong, A.S., Brennan, L., Bingham, R. and Morgan-Hughes, J. (1992) 'An audit of induction of anaesthesia in neonates and small infants using pulse oximetry', *Anaesthesia* 47: 896–9.

Krane, E.J., Haberkern, C.M. and Jacobson, L.E. (1995) 'Postoperative apnea, bradycardia and oxygen desaturation in formerly premature infants: prospective comparison of spinal and general anesthesia', *Anesthesia and Analgesia* 80: 7–13.

Lambert, H.J., Baylis, P.H. and Coulthard, M.G. (1998) 'Central–peripheral temperature difference, blood pressure, and arginine vasopressin in preterm neonates undergoing volume expansion', *Archives of Disease in Childhood: Fetal and Neonatal Edition* 78(1): F43–F45.

Laptook, A.R. and Watkinson, M. (2008) 'Temperature management in the delivery room', *Seminars in Fetal and Neonatal Medicine* 13(6): 383–91.

Lee, H.C., Ho, Q.T. and Rhine, W.D. (2008) 'A quality improvement project to improve admission temperatures in very low birth weight infants', *Journal of Perinatology* 28(11): 754–8.

Lerman, J., Sikich, N., Kleinman, S. and Yentis, S. (1994) 'The pharmacology of sevoflurane in infants and children', *Anesthesiology* 80: 814–24.

Leung, R. and Berkowitz, R.G. (2007) 'Incidence of severe acquired subglottic stenosis in newborns', *International Journal of Pediatric Otorhinolaryngology* 71(5): 763–8.

Llewellyn, N. and Moriarty, A. (2007) 'The national pediatric epidural audit', *Paediatric Anaesthesia* 17(6): 520–33.

Lynn, A.M. and Slattery, J.T. (1987) 'Morphine pharmacokinetics in early infancy', *Anesthesiology* 66: 136–9.

McEwan, A.I., Birch, M. and Bingham, R. (1995) 'The preoperative management of the child with a heart murmur', *Paediatric Anaesthesia* 5(3): 151–6.

McNicol, L.R., Martin, C.S., Smart, N.G. and Logan, R.W. (1990) 'Perioperative bupivacaine for pyloromyotomy pain', *Lancet* 335(i): 54–5.

Millar, C. and Bissonnette, B. (1994) 'Awake intubation increases intracranial pressure without affecting cerebral blood flow velocity in infants', *Canadian Journal of Anaesthesia* 41(4): 281–7.

Mitchell, V., Howard, R. and Facer, E. (1995) 'Down's syndrome and anaesthesia', *Paediatric Anaesthesia* 5: 379–84.

Murray, N.A. and Roberts, I.A.G. (2004) 'Neonatal transfusion practice', *Archives of Disease in Childhood: Fetal and Neonatal Edition* 89: F101.

Palme, C., Nystrom, B. and Tunell, R. (1985) 'An evaluation of the efficiency of face masks in the resuscitation of newborn infants', *Lancet* i: 207–10.

Parnis, S.J. and van-der-Valt, J.H. (1994) 'A national survey of atropine use by Australian anaesthetists', *Anaesthesia and Intensive Care* 22(1): 61–5.

Paut, O. and Lacroix, F. (2006) 'Recent developments in the perioperative fluid management for the paediatric patient', *Current Opinion in Anaesthesiology* 19(3): 268–77.

Peutrell, J.M. and Weir, P. (1996) 'Basic principles of neonatal anaesthesia', in D.G. Hughes, S.J. Mather and A.R. Wolf (eds) *Handbook of Neonatal Anaesthesia*, London: W.B. Saunders.

Pounder, D.R. and Steward, D.J. (1992) 'Postoperative anaesthesia: opioid infusions in infants and children', *Canadian Journal of Anaesthesia* 39: 969–74.

Proytcheva, M.A. (2009) 'Issues in neonatal cellular analysis', *American Journal of Clinical Pathology* 131(4): 560–73.

Purcell-Jones, G., Dormon, F. and Sumner, E. (1987) 'The use of opioids in neonates', *Anaesthesia* 42: 1316–20.

Reid, M.F., Harris, R., Phillips, P.D., Barker, I., Periera, N.H. and Bennett, N.R. (1987) 'Day-case herniotomy in children: a comparison of ilio-inguinal nerve block and nerve block for postoperative analgesia', *Anaesthesia* 42: 658–61.

Roberton, N.R.C. and Rennie, J. (2001) *A Manual of Neonatal Intensive Care*, 4th edn, London: Hodder Arnold.

Sandstrom, K., Nilsson, K., Andreasson, S., Niklasson, A. and Larsson, L.E. (1995) 'Metabolic consequences of different perioperative fluid therapies in the neonatal period', *Acta Anaesthesiologica Scandinavica* 37(2): 170–5.

Schiffmann, H., Rathgeber, J., Singer, D., Harms, K., Bolli, A. and Zuchner, K. (1997) 'Airway humidification in mechanically ventilated neonates and infants: a comparative study of heat and moisture exchanger vs. a heated humidifier using a new fast-response capacitive humidity sensor', *Critical Care Medicine* 25(10): 1755–60.

Stang, H.J., Gunnar, M.R., Snellman, L., Condon, L.M. and Kestenbaum, R. (1988) 'Local anesthesia for neonatal circumcision: effects on distress and cortisol response', *Journal of the American Medical Association* 259: 1507–11.

Tanner, S. (2007) 'Trends in children's surgery in England', *Archives of Disease in Childhood* 92: 664–7.

Wain, J.C. (2003) 'Postintubation tracheal stenosis', *Chest Surgery Clinics of North America* 13(2): 305–14.

Walther-Larsen, S. and Rasmussen, L.S. (2006) 'The former preterm infant and risk of post-operative apnoea: recommendations for management', *Acta Anaesthesiologica Scandinavica* 50(7): 888–93.

Wellborn, L.G. (1992) 'Post-operative apnoea in the former preterm infant', *Paediatric Anaesthesia* 2: 37–44.

Wellborn, L.G., Hannallah, R.S., Fink, R., Ruttimann, U.E. and Hicks, J.M. (1989) 'High-dose caffeine suppresses postoperative apnea in former preterm infants', *Anesthesiology* 71: 347–9.

Wellborn, L.G., Rice, L.J., Hannallah, R.S., Broadman, L.M., Ruttimann, U.E. and Fink, R. (1990) 'Postoperative apnea in former preterm infants: prospective comparison of spinal and general anaesthesia', *Anesthesiology* 72: 838–42.

Williams, R.K., McBride, W.J. and Abajian, J.C. (1997) 'Combined spinal and epidural anaesthesia for major abdominal surgery in infants', *Canadian Journal of Anaesthesia* 44(5 part 1): 511–14.

Chapter 16

Neonatal Surgery

Stevie Boyd and Anne Aspin

Contents

Introduction

Neonatal surgery has evolved rapidly over the past 50 years, its success contributing to a reduction in neonatal mortality. Sophisticated antenatal screening and fetal anomaly apperception have led to a changing pattern of operable malformations, and the delivery of a baby with an undiagnosed major structural anomaly is now rare.

Although fetal intervention remains in the experimental arena, there are recent positive advantages indicated in feto-endoscopic surgery in areas such as cleft lip and palate (Papadopulus *et al*. 2005), nephrectomy due to inferior vena cava and renal thrombosis (El-Saify *et al*. 2007), urinary tract obstruction (Biard *et al*. 2005), congenital diaphragmatic hernia (Harrison *et al*. 2003), congenital cystic adenomatoid malformation (CCAM) (Wilson *et al*. 2006) and extralobar pulmonary sequestration, sacrococygeal teratoma (Hedrick *et al*. 2004) and myelomeningocele (Johnson *et al*. 2003).

Antenatal diagnosis of surgically correctable malformations will allow for in-utero transfer and planned delivery in a specialist centre. Regionalisation secures exemplary utilisation of resources and the expertise of the multidisciplinary team (MDT). The surgeon apart, neonatologists, specialist anaesthetists, laboratory technicians, physiotherapists and pharmacists are all crucial to the peri-operative care and recovery of these small, vulnerable, but surprisingly resilient patients.

Parents should meet with the surgeon as soon as the diagnosis is made. They need patient, expansive verbal, written and pictorial information (Johnson and Sandford 2004) about the anomaly, its short-term management and the possible long-term sequelae. Meeting NICU staff, other parents and early receipt of specialist information booklets may help to avoid long periods of uncertainty, especially when the diagnosis is made antenatally.

Multiple defects can be associated with chromosomal abnormalities; therefore it is important to differentiate between examphalos and gastroschisis; and between duodenal and jejunal obstruction, as there may be associated cardiac anomalies and Down's Syndrome. If a chromosomal anomaly is found in the fetus or neonate, the parents should be offered genetic counselling.

The timing and mode of delivery should be a joint decision between the obstetrician and the neonatal team. Although many conditions are managed with a natural birth, occasionally a Caesarean section might be safer with an anomaly such as gross hydrocephalus. In infants with known congenital anomalies, appropriately skilled personnel should be present at the delivery.

General principles of management

The main goal on the arrival of a baby into NICU is expedient stabilisation. Skilful assessment and management pre-operatively should determine how well the baby will cope with surgery. While the surgery may be relatively short, its success will depend upon the calibre of both pre- and post-operative care.

Thermoregulation

Prevention of hypothermia is imperative (Meyer and Bold 2006). This is well recognised and compensated for in NICU, but transportation vehicles and operating theatres may not be so well adapted and the temperature will need adjustment. The baby's core temperature should be maintained at 37°C with peripheral temperature maintained at 36°C; a wider toe:core gap may indicate under-perfusion possibly due to hypovolaemia or infection. Infants undergoing laparotomy are at increased risk from heat loss directly from exposed bowel. Aqueous rather than alcohol-based skin preparations should be used to reduce evaporative heat loss.

Respiratory function

Assessment of respiratory function is a prerequisite for all surgical neonates as urgent intervention may be required. Anatomical abnormalities or increasing abdominal distension may compromise ventilation. Additionally, some of these infants may be further compromised from surfactant deficiency or aspiration pneumonia. The extent of respiratory support they require will depend upon clinical and radiological findings and blood gas analysis (see p. 135).

Gastric decompression

Intestinal obstruction and/or sepsis predispose the infant to increased gastric secretions whether it is bile, gastric juices or blood. Gastric decompression is necessary to avoid vomiting and aspiration pneumonia; it will also reduce splinting of the diaphragm and aid ventilation. Gastric decompression is achieved with a correctly positioned naso-gastric tube large enough to prevent blockage (8fg or greater) (see p. 331). The tip of the tube should be in the stomach confirmed by pH paper (Phang *et al.* 2004) and left on continuous open drainage with gentle intermittent aspiration.

Fluid and electrolyte balance

Surgery can exacerbate physiological imbalances in the newborn. It is essential, therefore, for continuous assessment and monitoring of perfusion, parenteral fluid and electrolyte requirements and metabolic response to surgical trauma. Some infants will need fluid resuscitation pre-operatively – hypovolaemia can result from continuous loss of fluid from, for example, the exposed viscera in gastroschisis and examphalos. Losses via the naso-gastric tube should be measured and may need replacement with normal saline with added potassium.

Alterations in acid base balance can be caused by several factors. Respiratory acidosis occurs with inadequate ventilation, for example, in pulmonary hypoplasia secondary to congenital diaphragmatic hernia. Metabolic acidosis can occur when bicarbonate losses are increased or with poor tissue perfusion, tissue necrosis, infection, hypovolaemia and as a result of intestinal fistulas and necrotising enterocolitis (NEC). The commonest cause in the 'surgical neonate' is hypovolaemia which requires fluid replacement for its correction. Correction with bicarbonate should be cautious, as it may cause hypocalcaemia (Haycock 2003).

During prolonged pre-operative stabilisation, and conditions predisposing paralytic ileus, total parenteral nutrition allows delivery of nutritional substrates directly into the circulation. It promotes anabolism and provides for normal growth and development until gut function is restored. The stimulus of surgery and intermittent positive-pressure ventilation (IPPV) lead to increased aldosterone and antidiuretic (ADH) secretion resulting in water and sodium retention. It may therefore be pertinent to restrict fluid and sodium post-operatively (see p. 258).

Glycogen is a skeletal muscle and hepatic storage carbohydrate and is metabolised when blood glucose falls outside the homeostatic range (Kotoulas et al. 2006). Neonates have poor glycogen stores due to decreased availability of substrate in utero, and therefore need a constant glucose intake. It is essential that dextrose should be administered and the blood glucose monitored frequently, maintaining a level of 2.6–5.0mmol/L (Nicholl 2003).

A neonate's blood volume is approximately 80ml per kilogram body weight. A 2kg infant therefore has a circulating volume equivalent to the average loss during minor adult surgery! It is vital that operations are performed by specialist paediatric surgeons (Royal College of Surgeons 1999) as their techniques have evolved to limit blood loss.

Coagulation status should be assessed pre-operatively and treated accordingly. The neonate is deficient in vitamin K and if required to be nil by mouth, a dose should be given either subcutaneously or intramuscularly; however, in an emergency, it can be given intravenously but close observation will be required for anaphylaxis (Beers et al. 2006).

Neonates with severe sepsis or NEC may develop disseminated intravascular coagulation (DIC) (see p. 220) with associated thrombocytopenia (Puri and Sureed 1996; Stokowski 2006). Clotting factors should be replaced by transfusion with appropriate blood products.

A central venous line is highly recommended for prolonged venous access (see p. 343), and peripheral cannulae for administration of medications (see p. 340) and blood product transfusion when necessary. Arterial access is also helpful to monitor haemodynamic, biochemical and respiratory status.

Pharmacological support

There is a risk of sepsis whenever surgery is performed, especially in intra-uterine growth restriction (IUGR) and preterm babies with immature immune systems. Untreated infection promotes deterioration of the respiratory and cardiovascular systems and prophylactic antibiotic therapy can reduce this risk. However, continual review of the course of treatment is essential to minimise the eventual microbial resistance to antibiotic therapy over time (Kolleff and Fraser 2001).

Inotropes are often necessary to improve cardiac function, thus improving organ perfusion (see p. 169).

Pain relief is an important consideration both pre- and post-operatively. Cellular damage, particularly in cases of NEC, release pain-producing substances, augmenting the perception of pain (Brophy 2007).

Intubation and ventilation are usually necessary for the facilitation of adequate pain relief, as neonates are sensitive to the respiratory depressant effects of opiates. Effective analgesia via an epidural catheter can be provided without depressing respiration, providing toxic doses of regional bupivicaine are avoided (see p. 376) (Reynolds 2005).

Transportation

The critically ill neonate can make several potentially hazardous journeys – from the delivery room to NICU, possibly to a regional surgical centre, as well as to and from the operating theatre. Safe transportation demands collaboration between a doctor and nurse experienced in neonatal intensive care, and a specialist anaesthetist for the return journey from theatre.

It is suggested that utilisation of specialist staff at this time reduces 'disasters' such as aspiration, hypothermia and airway obstruction (Puri 1996a) even on these short journeys within a hospital (Chapter 17).

Post-operative considerations

Management in the post-operative period mirrors the pre-operative care in achieving and maintaining physiological stability, but in addition the factors listed in Figure 16.1 need careful consideration.

Most commonly encountered congenital disorders

Oesophageal atresia (OA) and tracheo-oesophageal fistula (TOF)

The oesophagus and trachea have a common embryological origin. Initially they are fused, but a septal separation occurs by week 6 and failure of complete separation will result in **fistula** formation. The oesophagus should re-canalise and become patent by week 10; failure to do this results in **atresia** (Merei *et al.* 1998). Thus TOF and atresia can occur as separate entities but more frequently occur concurrently.

The commonest form, constituting 85 per cent, is a blind proximal oesophageal pouch with a 1–2cm gap, and a distal TOF (Kuo and Urma 2006).

- Do not leave the operating theatre until the baby is stable. Ideally a doctor and anaesthetist should be in attendance on the return journey to NICU
- Before returning the baby to the incubator and ventilator, check the settings, then reconnect fluids and monitor leads to static equipment
- Adjust maintenance and arterial line fluids. Commence NG replacement losses if necessary. Titrate sedation and epidural infusions as appropriate. Observe entry sites
- Attach naso-gastric tube to drainage bag
- As soon as possible record:

core temperature	then 4-hourly until stable
blood sugar	then 1–2-hourly until stable
ventilator settings	then 1-hourly until stable
blood pressure	continuous read-out, but record hourly
heart/respiratory rate	

- Attach peripheral temperature probe and maintain temperature above 34°C
- Organise a chest X-ray if the baby was intubated in theatre, there is a chest drain in situ and following diaphragmatic hernia repair
- Check blood gas and repeat as necessary
- Record urinary output – attach urine bag or weigh nappies – expect 1ml/kg per hour after the first 24 hours
- Check biochemical and haematological status
- Maintain adequate pain relief
- Carefully observe wounds, stomas, etc., recording any losses
- Tailor endotracheal suction to each individual's needs – pre-oxygenating if necessary
- Encourage parental involvement in care as appropriate, remembering that minimal handling is essential to recovery. Apart from babies who are electively paralysed, who must have eye care, passive movements and a change of position every 4 hours – 6- to 8-hourly care is adequate (see p. 337)

Figure 16.1 **General post-operative considerations following major surgery**

Variations relate to the width of the gap, which may extend to a 'long gap' greater than 2cm, or just consist of membrane.

There are four less common types of this condition: pure atresia with no fistula; a **proximal** and **distal** fistula together; a fistula with no atresia (H-TOF); and a proximal fistula. Associated anatomical features include a hypertrophied proximal oesophageal pouch – a result of fetal swallowing amniotic fluid. If the pouch is not hypertrophied, a fistula should be suspected.

There is an association with other abnormalities, including VATER, VACTERL and CHARGE syndromes (see p. xxvii) (Kaplan and Hudgins 2008) and it is important to recognise the association with Potters and Edwards Syndrome – in which the poor prognosis may not justify surgical repair (Shaw-Smith 2006).

Maternal **polyhydramnios** is usually present because amniotic fluid is unable to pass into the gastrointestinal tract for absorption and subsequent transfer to the placenta. The anomaly may be diagnosed by ultrasound – the inability to demonstrate a fetal stomach in the presence of normal or increased amniotic fluid is highly suggestive of OA, allowing appropriate measures to be taken at birth. However, there is often no antenatal diagnosis and symptoms present in the early postnatal hours. The neonate will cough and choke on excessive saliva in the mouth and upper respiratory tract. If enteral feeds are offered, the oesophageal pouch will fill, followed by regurgitation. Gastric contents can also reflux from the stomach through the fistula into the respiratory tract, presenting danger of aspiration and pneumonitis. The abdomen will rapidly distend as the intestines fill with air.

The accurate evaluation of a fistula requires special investigation, but the diagnosis of a proximal atresia is confirmed by passing a radio-opaque tube size 8–10fg through a nostril until resistance is felt and by X-ray of the neck, chest and abdomen. The tube will sit in the oesophageal pouch or be coiled if too small a tube is used. Although infants with an H-type fistula may have early signs of respiratory distress, aggravated by feeding orally, the diagnosis is not often confirmed in the early neonatal period (Tarcon *et al.* 2003; Ng *et al.* 2006).

At birth, these neonates should be positioned with the head elevated at 45°, or prone to prevent aspiration pneumonia. A double-lumen Replogle tube (Replogle 1963) placed in the upper pouch and connected to low pressure continuous suction will minimise this risk. Continuous monitoring and close observation are paramount, to ensure the Replogle tube does not block with thick, tenacious secretions. Instillation of 0.5ml saline down the large bore each hour and 0.25–0.5ml down the small bore every 15 minutes help to maintain tube patency and keep the pouch clear.

Endotracheal intubation is not usually necessary; indeed, with a distal fistula it is possible to rupture the stomach with mechanical ventilation.

The timing of operative intervention, which involves the repair of any fistula and the establishment of oesophageal continuity, depends on the width of the oesophageal gap. Repair of the atresia is not an emergency, but disconnection of the distal fistula into the stomach is essential. It is important to optimise the infant's clinical status and this may be achieved by chest physiotherapy and antibiotics particularly if aspiration has occurred.

Associated anomalies should be identified pre-operatively by undertaking ultrasound scans of the abdomen and cardiac echocardiography.

Fistulae are usually repaired within hours of birth, with ideally end-to-end primary **anastomosis** of the oesophagus performed at the same time. A right posterolateral transpleural thoracotomy may be used. More recently repairs have been made via less invasive thoracoscopy (Allal *et al.* 2005). The distal fistula and oesophagus are often hypoplastic due to the absence of functional challenge making the repair difficult.

A 'long gap' requires staged surgery involving a six-week to three-month period for growth of the oesophagus (Spitz 2007). Purposeful stretching of the upper pouch can be achieved by intermittent bougé insertion and, following insertion of a gastrostomy, stretching of the lower pouch can be achieved by initiating gastro-oesophageal reflux. Other options include electromagnetic stimulation or graded tension that is applied to the disconnected oesophageal segment (Goyal *et al.* 2006).

Surgery to divert the upper oesophagus to the neck as a cervical oesophagostomy and insertion of a gastrostomy tube is another option. This allows the baby to go home with its family 'sham feeding' until major reconstruction is undertaken.

It is essential to maintain the sucking reflux while awaiting corrective surgery. A Teat-Replogle device (Boyd and Tsang 1996) provides oral comfort, keeps the pouch clear and encourages sucking. It is also well tolerated for long periods.

Although the ideal oesophagus is the patient's own and every effort should be made towards oesophageal preservation, sometimes the gap never shortens to an operable length and it is necessary to perform a colonic, jejunal or gastric interposition. However, this is a huge undertaking with potential serious complications, and should only be considered if the condition is irremediable.

The need for post-operative ventilatory support not only depends on the infant's respiratory but also the tightness of the repair. If the anastomosis is under tension, the baby will need to be given muscle relaxants and nursed with the neck flexed for five days while healing takes place.

A transanastomotic tube (TAT) will be in situ to minimise the potential for oesophageal **stenosis** and allow early enteral feeding post surgery. It is essential that the TAT is securely fixed and labelled '**DO NOT REMOVE**' and the baby wears mittens in the early post-operative period. Unplanned removal and replacement of the TAT can seriously damage the surgical site. A chest drain is usual, and antibiotics are continued until it is removed.

If a primary anastomosis has been performed, a barium contrast swallow checks for an anastomotic leak. However, some centres consider routine contrast studies inappropriate as a minor leak is insignificant and will heal spontaneously, and a major leak will present with a tension pneumothorax or frothy blood-stained secretions from the chest drain. These complications are recognised as serious causes of post-operative morbidity and mortality.

Gastro-oesophageal reflux is one of the most common long-term problems in repairs that have been tight initially or reconstructed and is thought to be due to disordered oesophageal motility and presence of a small volume stomach.

Treatment may involve non-invasive measures such as positioning and by thickened feeds, medications such as H_2 antagonists, proton pump inhibitors and **prokinetics.** Anti-reflux surgical procedure (**fundoplication**) may be necessary. Feeding difficulties and vomiting, which may last for years, especially following tight repairs, are common and often relate to oesophageal strictures (Paran *et al.* 2007). Frequent oesophageal dilations may be necessary to enable normal eating and swallowing. Parents should be given detailed information and advice about this; it is useful to put them in contact with another TOF family, and local support group.

Tracheomalacia can be serious enough to progress to respiratory distress with obstruction, cyanosis, bradycardia respiratory and even cardiac arrest, and also causes the characteristic 'TOF' cough or 'seal bark' (Guiney 1996).

Repeated chest infections are a concern for the family at home. Instruction on chest physiotherapy and positioning may be applicable to those who have thick tenacious secretions which are difficult to 'cough up' and occasionally the use of a nebuliser in the winter months helps to loosen secretions.

Fistular regrowth may occur and should be suspected in the child who develops frequent respiratory infections, with gagging, cyanosis and apnoea.

Early diagnosis, improved surgical techniques, and sophisticated intensive care have positively influenced survival. One of the most common major congenital abnormalities has progressed from being incompatible with life to one with a mortality limited to those associated with extreme prematurity, or other life-threatening anomalies (Spitz and Hancock 1994).

Mechanical intestinal obstruction

Many babies vomit, but this is not necessarily serious and may simply be due to gastro-oesophageal reflux, especially if the vomit is milk with most of the feed retained. Pyloric stenosis usually presents with projectile, non-bilious vomiting at around two to four weeks. Yellow vomit may not be serious as bile in the gall bladder and duodenum is yellow. However, if it becomes combined with digestive juices, indicating gastric stasis, it turns green and this should always be taken seriously. Other signs of obstruction include abdominal distension, failure to pass meconium and lethargy.

Approximately one-third of cases of obstruction in the neonatal period are suspected antenatally with ultrasound demonstration of dilated bowel (Speidel *et al.* 1998); the remainder may be missed unless there is a high level of clinical awareness. All incidences may be associated with maternal polyhydramines, fetal growth restriction and prematurity.

Obstruction can occur as a result of paralytic ileus in septicaemia, or in the extremely premature infant with an immature gut, but more importantly as a result of mechanical intestinal obstruction, of which there are numerous causes, necessitating urgent treatment.

There are three common causes in the upper part of the gastro-intestinal tract, and three in the lower part (Table 16.1); an abdominal X-ray will highlight the position of the obstruction. Less common causes of bilious vomiting are incarcerated inguinal hernia, imperforate anus and necrotising enterocolitis.

In general, the lower down the small intestine the defect, the later the presentation after birth. Irrespective of the cause, if obstruction is suspected, a size 8fg–10fg naso-gastric tube should be passed, aspirated regularly and left on free drainage. This will decompress the gut and prevent aspiration of gastro-intestinal contents. Intravenous therapy should be commenced and fluid and electrolytes imbalances corrected.

Table 16.1 Causes of intestinal obstruction

Upper	Lower
Duodenal atresia	Low small bowel atresia
High small bowel atresia	Meconium ileus
Malrotation with volvulus	Hirschsprung's disease

Duodenal atresia

The duodenum begins its development in the fourth week of gestation. Epithelial proliferation is so abundant that at five to six weeks there is temporary duodenal occlusion, and its failure to become recanalised by the end of the embryonic period (nine weeks) results in one of two main groups of atresia. In the first type, the proximal and distal segments of the duodenum end blindly and are either separate or joined by a fibrous cord; the second type consists of partial or complete duodenal webs (Calkins and Karrer 2006). Infants with the latter anomaly may feed normally, until a milk curd gets stuck in a partial web and causes obstruction.

Vomiting is the most common symptom of complete atresia, and is usually present on the first day of life and is usually bilious, as 80 per cent of the obstructions are in the post-ampullary region. The high level of obstruction reduces the likelihood of abdominal distension. Meconium may be passed in the first 24 hours, followed by constipation. Fluid and electrolyte imbalance will occur if a diagnosis is not made with the infant becoming dehydrated, hungry and distressed. An X-ray shows high intestinal obstruction with the classic 'double bubble' – fluid in the lower part of the stomach and the duodenum proximal to the obstruction (Figure 16.2).

The principle of the repair (duodenoduodenostomy) is the same for both anomalies, as it is not possible to remove the web, the bile duct often opening on to it. Parallel incisions are made above and below the web or atresia, and the two ends are anastomosed.

Approximately 30 per cent of neonates with duodenal obstruction also have Down's syndrome, and the incidence of prematurity is as high as 60 per cent (Mustafawi and Hassan 2008). There is also an association with VATER and VACTERL syndromes.

Small bowel atresia

Jejuno-ileal atresia is a common cause of intestinal obstruction in the newborn, and is thought to be due to localised intra-uterine vascular accident with ischaemic necrosis of the bowel and subsequent reabsorption of the affected segment (Riego de Rios and Chung 2006; Rode and Millar 2006).

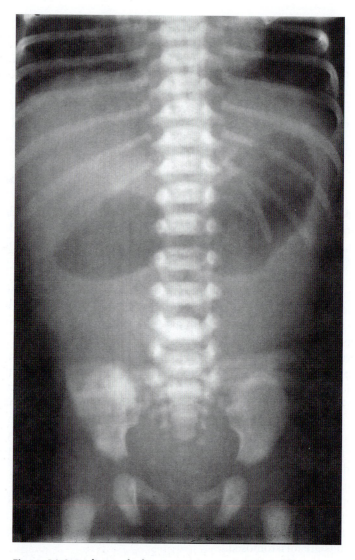

Figure 16.2 **Radiograph showing a classic 'double bubble'**

At delivery, green liquor should alert the suspicion of obstruction. In the post-natal period gastric aspirates exceeding 25ml and persistent bilious vomiting are of concern. Progressive abdominal distension and delay in passing meconium are later presenting symptoms.

At operation the appearances are similar to duodenal atresia with either a complete atresia or a web. Surgery entails resection of the atresia/web. Intestinal continuity is restored with an end-to-end/end-to-side anastomosis. If there is sufficient length of bowel, the adjacent distended and collapsed segments should also be resected. The proximal bowel has been dilated, hypertrophied and atonic for many weeks in utero; if it is not possible to remove it, there may be a few weeks before tone and peristalsis are restored – the higher the atresia, the longer the period of intestinal dysfunction. When appropriate, gradual weaning from parenteral to enteral feeding can take place. Insufficient bowel length either as a result of the primary insult, excessive removal of residual bowel, or post-operative complications can lead to short gut syndrome necessitating long-term parenteral nutrition (TPN).

As there is an association with cystic fibrosis, all infants with small bowel atresia should have a serum immunoreactive trypsin test, gene depletion assay or a sweat test to exclude it (Cywes *et al.* 1994).

Malrotation with volvulus

Development of the midgut results in rapid growth and physiological umbilical herniation during the sixth week of gestation. At 10 to 11 weeks, the gut begins a 270-degree counter-clockwise rotation around the superior mesenteric artery. The bowel destined to be the caecum re-enters the abdomen descending to the right ileac fossa, where fixation followed by closure of the abdomen occurs around the twelfth week (Bass *et al.* 1998). The duodenum with the duodeno-jejunal flexure (DJF) in the midline or to its left, and the proximal colon, are attached to the posterior abdominal wall. The small bowel is suspended **posteriorly** by **mesenteries** which carry blood, lymphatic vessels and nerves, and extends from the DJF to the ileocaecal region.

Normally the mesentery has a broad base and cannot undergo **torsion**. Malrotation occurs when development is halted and the caecum ends up adjacent to the duodenum. The mesenteries fail to undergo normal fixation, so the small intestines are suspended by a narrow stalk, which is able to twist into a volvulus, causing an obstruction. All green bilious vomiting should arouse the suspicion of volvulus. The X-ray will look similar to the 'double bubble' of duodenal atresia. Unless surgery is carried out promptly, the volvulus continues to twist a few more degrees, the superior mesenteric artery becomes linked and the midgut becomes infarcted. Gangrene will then develop with loss of small bowel and part of the colon. The only chance of long-term survival, if this occurs, would be a small bowel transplant, which may work in a few select cases.

Surgery involves untwisting the volvulus as soon as possible. Frequently Ladd's bands are found between the caecum and the peritoneum causing further obstruction by compressing the duodenum. These are divided and the gut is mobilised and returned to the abdomen with the caecum on the left and the duodenum on the right, broadening the base of the mesentery, preventing the tendency to further twisting. Malrotation is thus changed into non-rotation (Ladd's procedure). If the infant's general condition is satisfactory and the caecal area shows no signs of inflammation or pathological changes, an appendice-tomy is performed (Kluth and Lambrect 1994). With the ileocaecal valve in the left upper quadrant, appendicitis in later life could pose considerable diagnostic difficulty.

Meconium ileus

Meconium is a dark mucilaginous material that is a mixture of secretions of the maturing intestinal glands, ingested amniotic fluid and the debris of proliferative epithelial cells. It begins to fill the lower ileum and colon late in the fourth month of gestation and continues until the time of birth. Meconium ileus is caused by abnormal meconium blocking the terminal ileum (Yoo *et al.* 2002).

Meconium-stained liquor is often reported which actually represents bilious vomiting in utero. At birth, the infant usually has abdominal distension and continues to vomit bile. On examination, loops of gut may be visible or palpable, and meconium plugs may be passed following rectal examination. The X-ray appearance is that of a low obstruction.

Perforation and meconium peritonitis may occur, but providing there is no evidence of this and the infant is stable, this obstruction can often be relieved with a gastrografin enema. Gastrografin is radio-opaque and will demonstrate a micro colon with dilated small bowel proximal to the obstructing segment (Kiely 1996). However, it is a quiescently dangerous substance; its hydroscopic action draws large quantities of fluid out of a baby's circulation into the intestinal lumen, causing transient osmotic diarrhoea. While having the advantage of lubricating the abnormal meconium which is then spontaneously evacuated, it can cause severe fluid depletion and cardiovascular collapse. It is therefore crucial that these babies have intravenous access, a good circulating blood volume and that they are carefully monitored during and following the procedure. There is the added risk of intestinal perforation if excessive pressure on the enema syringe is transferred to the bowel (Ein 1994).

If gastrografin is contraindicated or several enemas fail to relieve the obstruction, surgery may be necessary. At laparotomy an incision is made into the bowel just above the obstruction and the abnormal meconium is washed out with gastrografin and normal saline. The dilated bowel is resected if there is sufficient intestinal length, and continuity is restored with end-to-end anastomosis, or a stoma is formed if the neonate's condition is grossly unstable.

Some 90–95 per cent of neonates with meconium ileus have cystic fibrosis, and 8–10 per cent of these present in the neonatal period with obstruction caused by the tenacious meconium (Rivosecchi 2006).

Hirschsprung's disease

Hirschsprung's disease occurs due to an absence of enteric ganglion cells in the submucosa of the distal bowel. They first appear in the developing oesophagus at five weeks and migrate down to the ano-rectal junction by 12 weeks. Their absence is attributed to the failure of migration, and the earlier the arrest of migration, the longer the affected segment of bowel. The **aganglionic** segment always includes the rectum, and the total colon is affected in 8 per cent of cases (Puri 1996b). The aganglionic segment is collapsed, and non-peristaltic, causing functional intestinal obstruction. Abdominal distension, bile-stained vomiting and failure to pass meconium are presenting signs. On abdominal X-ray, the normal bowel appears as mega colon with dilated small bowel proximal to the aganglionosis. When gentle rectal examination is performed, the rectal wall always appears tight and resists further probing. This may cause the explosive passage of meconium and flatus followed by normal bowel movements for a few days before signs of obstruction recur. Hirschsprung's enterocolitis – indicated by the presence of foul-smelling diarrhoea, abdominal distension, bile vomiting and potential perforation – may occur and, if undiagnosed, can be fatal. The diagnosis of Hirschsprung's is confirmed with suction biopsies of the colorectal mucosa, which is a simple and apparently painless procedure. Daily rectal washouts with warm normal saline (Coran and Teitelbaum 2000) should be undertaken by the family/carer for a few weeks at home prior to definitive surgery. A stoma is fashioned at the most distal part of the normal innervation to decompress the bowel, while allowing the neonate to feed and grow. Surgery should be carried out with a pathologist available to examine frozen section samples. Research is ongoing in stem cell therapy in Hirschsprung's disease which has the potential to generate new nerves capable of stimulating gut motility (Edgar *et al*. 2006).

Anorectal anomalies

Anorectal abnormalities result from anomalous development of the urorectal septum, causing incomplete separation into urogenital and anorectal sections, and an aberrant anal orifice (Moore and Persaud 2003). They present with a spectrum of defects – from minor malformations requiring minimal treatment, to a very sick infant with intestinal obstruction and complex life-threatening defects (Pena 1996). Anomalies of the upper urinary tract, cardiovascular system and sacrum are associated, as are atresias of the gastrointestinal tract.

Lesions are classified depending on whether the rectum ends superior or inferior to the puborectalis sling. High lesions present as anorectal agenesis or rectal atresia, frequently associated with recto-urethral, -vestibular or -vaginal fistulae. Alternatively, low lesions are classified as anal agenesis, stenosis or an imperforate anus (which may be just a thin membrane through which meconium can be excreted).

Low lesions are associated with anocutaneous fistulae, and in girls, an ectopic stenotic anus. All neonates should have a full clinical examination after birth to exclude anomalies such as imperforate anus. A lateral X-ray with the neonate laid prone and head down, with a radio-opaque marker over the skin dimple (at 24 hours of age to allow air to reach the large bowel), will identify the level of obstruction, while revealing any associated sacral abnormalities.

Low lesions require division of fistula or anoplasty, and may need frequent subsequent anal dilatations, but the prospects of long-term faecal continence are good.

High lesions require formation of a dysfunctional sigmoid colostomy, anorectoplasty at several months of age, followed by anal dilatations and subsequent closure of colostomy. Some of these infants never achieve reasonable continence (Speidel *et al.* 1998) and long-term enema management may be necessary. Urinary tract infections are common, especially with high lesions, and delayed treatment when there is a fistula can lead to progressive rectal distension and rectal inertia.

Congenital diaphragmatic hernia (CDH)

During embryological development the thoracic and abdominal portions of the body cavity move freely until the diaphragm develops to separate them (Jesudason *et al.* 2000). CDH results from defective fusion of the pleuro-peritoneal membrane when the intestines return to the abdomen from the umbilical cord, and allows the abdominal viscera to slip into the thorax. It usually occurs on the left side (8:1), through the posterior foramen of Bochdalek, but can also occur near the xiphisternum through the foramen of Morgagni, or on the right.

CDH is considered to be a syndrome and it is thought (Thebaud *et al.* 1998; Steinharn *et al.* 1999) that an insult at a critical time of embryological development leads to varying degrees of:

- Pulmonary hypoplasia, resulting from impaired lung growth and bronchial division. As terminal bronchi can only support a limited number of alveoli, there is a reduction in the gas exchange area. The compressed lung may also show changes.
- Lung 'immaturity', which is further compounded by surfactant dysfunction.
- Abnormally thick-walled pulmonary arterioles massively constrict, following hypoxia at birth, resulting in persistent pulmonary hypertension of the newborn (PPHN) (see pp. 131 and 170).
- Left heart hypoplasia caused by mechanical compression by the herniated organs, or altered haemodynamics because development of the heart chambers is dependent on the blood flow they received.

These factors decrease gaseous exchange across the alveolar capillary membrane and lead to progressive hypoxia and hypercarbia. If they are not dealt with, decreased cardiac output and oxygen delivery become insufficient to sustain life. The mortality rate (50–60 per cent) is associated with the hypoplastic lungs, cardiac malformations and hypoxia-induced intraventricular haemorrhage (Rana *et al.* 2008).

CDH accounts for 8 per cent of all major congenital abnormalities. It can occur singly or as part of multiple malformation syndromes such as Fryn's (Steinhorn *et al.* 1997), and the pentralogy of Cantrell (Cantrell *et al.* 1958). The association with congenital heart and renal malformations is especially high.

Infants with a left-sided defect, especially if preterm, usually present with respiratory distress. This can range in severity from cyanosis totally unresponsive to intervention and incompatible with life, through tachypnoea, nasal flaring, recession and cyanosis not improved with supplemental oxygen. Some infants can be asymptomatic or have mild symptoms not diagnosed for hours, days or even months.

Other clinical signs include a scaphoid abdomen with increased chest diameter, a shift in the trachea and cardiac impulse, and decreased breath sounds – but with bowel sounds in the chest on the ipsilateral side. Radiologically, there is bowel in the thorax and an absent diaphragm (Figure 16.3). Malrotation may coexist. The main differential diagnosis is congenital cystic adenomatous malformation of the lung (CCAM).

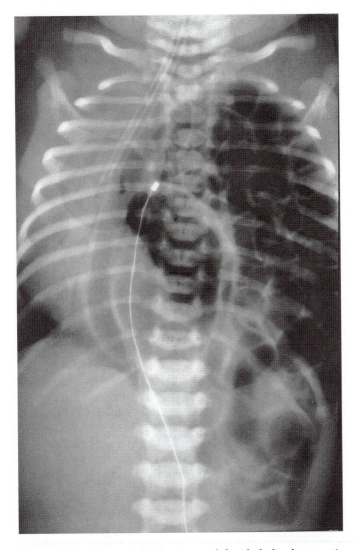

Figure 16.3 Radiograph showing a left-sided diaphragmatic hernia shortly after birth

Management is aimed at correcting the abnormality antenatally (rare) or ameliorating its devastating effects by preventing PPHN postnatally (see pp. 131 and 170). There is minimal evidence to support fetal surgical intervention as mortality is high. Decreased surfactant activity in these infants suggests maternal antenatal steroids may be of value.

Some of these infants may be critically ill at birth and recovery can be a lengthy, precarious process. At delivery, it is important to avoid mask ventilation; if air is forced into the gastrointestinal tract in the thorax, ventilation will be further compromised.

Gastrointestinal decompression with a large bore naso-gastric tube on continuous drainage with intermittent aspiration is of the utmost importance.

Early intubation to maintain adequate oxygenation is necessary with IPPV or HFO ventilation. HFO maintains lung volume, permits adequate gaseous exchange with small tidal volumes, and has been shown to recruit collapsed alveoli. Exogenous surfactant may be of value (Steinhorn et al. 1997). Placement of an umbilical arterial catheter or a preductal peripheral artery cannula (more accurate when measuring Po_2 in PPHN) is crucial for determination of blood gas values.

Intravenous access is a priority to maintain adequate perfusion, although fluid restriction may be necessary. These infants do not tolerate positive fluid balance; increased circulatory volume could lead to pulmonary oedema, worsening the respiratory status.

Support with inotropic agents, nitric oxide and infusions of prostaglandin may be used to optimise ventilation (Shiyanagi 2008).

Inhaled nitric oxide is not universally effective in improving oxygenation in CDH infants, unless used in conjunction with extracorporeal membrane oxygenation (ECMO) (Steinhorn et al. 1997). ECMO (see p. 133) provides partial cardiopulmonary bypass in infants who have failed other modalities of respiratory and cardiac support, but have reversible cardiopulmonary failure.

Repair of the diaphragm and reduction of herniated viscera were performed as an emergency in the past but today, a delayed approach (up to seven to ten days) allows for adequate pre-operative stabilisation, and improves survival.

The optimal time for surgery is considered to be after 24 hours of stability with a PaO_2 of more than 8kpa in less than 50 per cent supplemental oxygen, with low rates and pressures (Davenport 1999; Shiyanagi et al. 2008). Surgery involves reduction of the viscera and repair of the defect through a subcostal incision (Figure 16.4). Rarely, the defect is repaired with a synthetic patch, or transposed latissimus dorsi or abdominal oblique muscle flaps. A chest drain with underwater seal is sometimes inserted on the ipsilateral side to drain air or fluid. This remains controversial but if one is in place the fluid loss should be measured and recorded and the bottle placed in a safe area below the baby to avoid accidental knocks. Chest drain clamps should be readily available should they be required.

Initial post-operative care is not significantly different from pre-operative management: the goal is still to avoid PPHN and associated shunting; if there are still major problems, in most cases, surgery was performed too early.

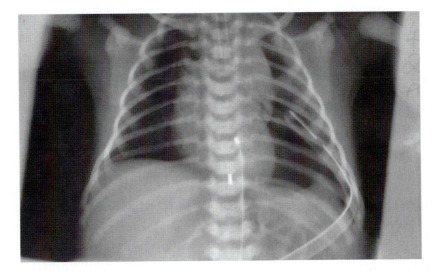

Figure 16.4 Chest radiograph following surgical repair of diaphragmatic hernia

Ventilation may be difficult due to the tight abdominal closure, as well as the mediastinal shift splinting the contralateral lung in an overinflated, non-compliant state. High inspiratory pressures are necessary to maintain adequate oxygenation, and the FiO_2 should always be increased prior to endotracheal suction to prevent oxygen-deficit pulmonary vasoconstriction. Pneumothorax may occur in the immediate post-operative period due to the high ventilatory pressures despite the use of muscle relaxants and should be drained expediently. Ventilatory support can be weaned when the infant is stable, with normalised blood gases.

Pain control should be managed as per individual unit protocol – either by morphine (see p. 373) or epidural infusion (see p. 376) and intravenous Paracetamol. Calorific requirements for healing, growth and development are maintained with TPN until the gastrointestinal tract has recovered from the effects of surgery, analgesia and paralysis.

Apart from post-operative complications of infection, fluid and electrolyte imbalance and haemorrhage, there may be long-term decreased lung function. Diaphragmatic eventration can occur as a separate entity, or occasionally after thoracic surgery, and requires plication. Chylothorax is a rare complication, and following thoracentesis and recovery, the infant will require semi-elemental milk (Greenough and Roberton 1999). Gastro-oesophageal reflux occurs in approximately 40 per cent of cases (10–20 per cent requiring fundoplication). Some 5–10 per cent will have a neurological handicap presumed to be due to the hypoxia and cardiovascular instability, or as a complication of ECMO (Davenport 1999).

Abdominal wall defects

Exomphalos and gastroschisis

The embryology of normal abdominal wall closure, and the sequence of events leading to umbilical and para-umbilical defects, are speculative. Some researchers feel that gastroschisis is the end result of a ruptured exomphalos, while others feel these two conditions have different pathology and embryology (Anveden-Hertzberg and Gauderer 1996).

The most popular description of exomphalos is a developmental arrest resulting in failure of the midgut to return to the abdominal cavity. The amount of herniated intestine varies from a small umbilical hernia-like lesion, to a huge anomaly, containing the entire midgut and liver. Unless ruptured, it is covered with a sac consisting of peritoneum and amnion, the umbilical cord emerging from the caudal part. Eviscerated bowel in exomphalos is usually normal in appearance.

Gastroschisis is due to incomplete closure of the lateral abdominal folds, leading to a defect in or near the median plane of the ventral wall leading to protrusion of the intra-abdominal viscera. There is no membrane covering the herniated bowel, and the cord is intact. The eviscerated bowel is often foreshortened, inflamed, thickened and matted with serosal peel. Clinical research suggests that this damage is caused by prolonged exposure to urine in the amniotic fluid, and/or progressive constriction on the intestine and its blood supply by the umbilical ring (Simmons and Georgeson 1996).

Accurate antenatal diagnosis can be made as early as 12 weeks of gestation, as an exomphalos in its sac is distinguishable from gastroschisis, the ultrasound appearance of which has been likened to a honeycomb due to the freely floating, thickened bowel loops in amniotic fluid (Molenaar 1996).

Malformations associated with gastroschisis are uncommon, apart from relatively few instances of coincidental intestinal atresia or stenosis. It can, however, be complicated by oligohydramnios severe enough to put the fetus at risk of pulmonary hypoplasia, deterioration of the bowel in utero leading to reabsorption of some of the bowel (Snyder et al. 2001;Winter et al. 2005), limb deformities and fetal distress, and is common in premature infants of young mothers.

The affiliation of chromosomal and cardiac anomalies with exomphalos is well recognised (Groves et al. 2006).

There remains much debate surrounding the issues of early versus late delivery, and Caesarean section versus vaginal delivery for these infants (Cusick et al. 1997). Some authors feel there is no evidence that the mode of delivery improves the final outcome (Salihu 2004), with infants with unsuspected exomphalos being delivered vaginally with the sac intact.

Following delivery, the priority is protecting the sac from rupture and infection. Large amounts of heat may be lost from the exposed bowel in gastroschisis, or through the amnion covering the exomphalos. The lesion should be immediately covered with cling-film to protect it from trauma, contamination, and to prevent traction on the mesentery. This also allows for easier observation of the viscera and keeps the lesion covered with the infant's own body fluids.

A naso-gastric tube left on free drainage with intermittent suction or low wall continuous suction will decompress the gut and prevent aspiration. Respiratory distress should be managed as necessary, and all infants should have chest and abdominal X-rays to evaluate the lungs, heart, diaphragm, the air pattern in the bowel and the position of the naso-gastric tube. Antibiotics should be commenced as soon as intravenous access is established.

Significant protein and insensible fluid losses from the abnormal bowel in gastroschisis are unavoidable, and should be supplemented parenterally. Perfusion and blood pressure should be carefully monitored to ensure stability and prevent hypotension. As there is an association between exomphalos and Beckwith–Wiedemann syndrome (Speidel *et al.* 1998), blood sugar levels should be monitored.

Surgery is not always necessary, and while primary closure is preferred, the intestines may be encased within a silo or an entire closure undertaken on the neonatal unit. Post-operative ventilation with initial muscle relaxation may be required.

For those infants born prematurely, necrotising enterocolitis remains a risk. Advancing practices of silo application, keen monitoring and specialist milks appear to have reduced this risk in the early days, but it can still present weeks later (Chabra 2006). However, sepsis is a continuing risk, and antibiotics should be continued for 7–10 days.

A large exomphalos containing centrally herniated liver poses challenges – the most significant being space limitations of the abdominal cavity, and hypotension as well as respiratory distress from diaphragmatic splinting. In addition, the liver may exert pressure on the vena cava creating acute hepatic vascular outflow obstruction and renal compromise (Skarsgard and Barth 1997). If primary closure is not feasible, a Silastic silo is an option; however, in a number of neonates, conservative treatment with Flamazine may be an option with skin grafting later. These procedures avoid the respiratory distress and caval vein obstruction associated with primary closure. Granulation, epitheliasation and contraction of the sac size occur, allowing for reconstruction of the abdominal wall some months later (Molenaar 1996).

The prognosis of infants with gastroschisis is infinitely better than those with exomphalos (Molenaar 1996). Ischaemic changes in the wall of the damaged intestine in gastroschisis may cause absorption and motility disturbances for some infants (Simmons and Georgeson 1996), and mortality is usually due to short-gut syndrome, or complications of long-term parenteral nutrition. Prognosis of exomphalos is dependent on the severity of associated anomalies.

Umbilical hernia

This is due to a protrusion of a loop of bowel through the linea alba into a patent umbilicus. Unlike exomphalos, it is covered by subcutaneous tissue and skin. It ranges in size from 1 to 5cm, reaching a maximum by the end of the first month, and distends during crying. It is relatively common, complications are rare and the deficit will often close by cicatrisation during the early years of life, umbilical herniorrhaphy being safely reserved for persistent lesions (Johnstone 1994).

Inguinal hernia

An inguinal hernia develops, often bilaterally, due to the processus vaginalis remaining patent after birth (Tovar 2003). It is one of the most common surgical conditions in infancy, the incidence increasing rapidly in preterm and small for gestational age (SGA) infants (Johnstone 1994), presumably precipitated by respiratory effort and artificial ventilation. It is more common in males, often associated with undescended testes (Moore and Persaud 2003), and can be secondary to increased abdominal pressure with necrotising enterocolitis and tight gastroschisis/exomphalos repairs.

Presentation is a swelling in the groin, extending to the scrotum or the labia. It is usually first noticed by the parents, and may only be visible while the infant is crying, feeding or straining to pass a stool.

The hernia can usually be reduced initially by gentle pressure, when it will return to the abdomen with a characteristic 'gurgle' (Johnstone 1994). While it remains reducible and asymptomatic, most centres delay definitive surgery until the preterm infant is ready for discharge. Uemura *et al.* (1999), however, recommend earlier repair to avoid operative difficulties. Although the premature infant may be at risk, warranting intensive care, the sac is small and easier to separate from the cord; and incarceration and gonadal ischaemia are prevented.

Inguinal herniotomy consists of reduction of the contents into the abdomen, reconstruction of the posterior wall of the inguinal canal, ligation of the hernial sac and return of the testes to the scrotum (Wright 1994). Much controversy surrounds the question of surgical exploration contralaterally.

Repair of a simple hernia in a term infant is safe in an appropriate environment, with few complications. Wound infiltration with local anaesthetic and rectal or intravenous Paracetamol are effective as post-operative pain relief.

If the hernia is not easily reducible, it can become incarcerated or strangulated with vascular compromise of the sac contents. If this occurs, the baby will be in pain, and show signs of toxicity and shock, abdominal distension and constipation, and possibly bloody stools. Abdominal X-ray will show bowel, fluid levels and abdominal gas within the hernia. The infant should be nursed with the buttocks elevated until a surgical opinion can be sought. Ideally, if the infant is stable, non-operative reduction under sedation is preferred as there is a high risk of complications with surgery at this stage (Tovar 2003).

If the hernia strangulates, haematological and biochemical assessment, and stabilisation, are necessary, prior to laparotomy and repair. Resection and anastomosis may be necessary if the affected bowel is non-viable. Post-operatively, intravenous fluids, naso-gastric aspiration and antibiotics will be necessary until peristalsis is established.

Hydrocoele

Occasionally the abdominal end of the processus vaginalis remains open but is too small to permit herniation of the intestine. Peritoneal fluid passes into it and forms a hydrocoele – a painless collection of fluid around the testicle, presenting as a soft, non-tender, translucent swelling. Hydrocoeles are very common, usually resolve spontaneously, and are of no significance unless they become very large and tense, when a surgical opinion should be sought, to avert torsion of the testes. Hydrocoele is sometimes difficult to differentiate from an incarcerated hernia; a rectal examination will exclude the latter (Puri and Surana 1996).

Most commonly encountered acquired disorders

Necrotising enterocolitis (NEC)

NEC is an inflammatory disease of the bowel, predominantly affecting pre-mature infants, but it sometimes occurs in 'cohorts' (Sankaran *et al.* 2004). The specific cause remains enigmatic, but several risk factors have been identified which suggest the pathophysiology is multifactorial. Epidemiological studies reveal that most aetiological factors describe events in a population of physically stressed high-risk neonates. There appears to be a complex relationship between mucosal injury, infection and hyperosmolar enteral feeds.

Mucosal injury

Hypoxia and systemic hypotension lead to sparing of the vital organs at the expense of the gut, which is vulnerable to under-perfusion and ischaemic damage. Factors associated with hypoxic stress include prolonged rupture of membranes, placental abruption, low Apgar scores, RDS and apnoea. Left-to-right shunting through a PDA compromises blood flow to the gut, and the presence of umbilical catheters is also implicated.

Microbial infection

There is little evidence that infection is the cause of NEC, but it is an important factor in the pathogenesis. Damaged or immature epithelium may lead to a leaky mucosal barrier allowing hydrogen and toxin-producing micro-organisms to invade the gut wall, with decreased levels of IgG contributing to the mucosal damage (Hebra and Ross 1996). Although no single organism is consistently associated with NEC, blood cultures may be positive in 20–30 per cent of cases (Kliegman and Walsh 1992).

Enteral feeds

Hyperosmolar feeds, or a too rapid increase in volume, can damage the mucosa (Lin and Stoll 2006), with intra-mural milk providing a substrate for bacteria. Ninety per cent of infants with NEC have received enteral feeds. Breast milk, however, has been shown to have a protective effect (Chauhan *et al.* 2008). Milk distending the stomach can lead to a reduction in lung volume with a consequent fall in PaO$_2$ and vascular compromise.

NEC can affect any part of the gastrointestinal tract, but the most frequently affected are the terminal ileum and the splenic flexure. It has a variable course, ranging from mild abdominal distension without systemic symptoms, to gradual clinical deterioration with lethargy, thermal instability and apnoeic episodes. Severe signs of sepsis may follow, with bradycardia, pallor, skin mottling, jaundice and haemorrhaging secondary to DIC (see p. 220). There is usually an absence of bowel sounds, abdominal tenderness, a palpable mass with distended loops of bowel and a red indurated abdomen with periumbilical flaring. The classic 'triad of signs' is abdominal distension, bloody mucousy stools and bilious aspirate. Fulminant sepsis, multi-system failure and death may ensue quickly.

Abdominal X-ray confirms the diagnosis, showing distended loops of oedematous bowel and pneumotosis intestinalis. Serial films may reveal fixed distended loops of bowel and progressive ascites. If perforated, pneumoperitoneum and gas in the portal vein may occur. Other investigations should include biochemical and haematological assays, blood gases and a septic screen.

Treatment for mild to moderate NEC is with antibiotics, intravenous feeding and naso-gastric decompression for up to 10 days. Sicker infants may require platelet transfusion, supplemental oxygen, analgesia and, in severe cases, full respiratory support, inotropes, fluid resuscitation and blood transfusion, with operative intervention as a lifesaving measure.

Although it is not established practice, clinical trials have shown that intravenous IgG combats established infection, by exerting an immuno-protective effect on the gastrointestinal tract if given pre-operatively to infants with NEC (Chauhan *et al.* 2008).

Surgery is required when there is continued clinical deterioration, and drainage of the peritoneal cavity – although of debatable value – may be a first step for severely ill infants who would not survive anaesthesia and operative intervention (Laxman 2006). A drain is inserted percutaneously under local anaesthesia, for the evacuation of gas, exudate, pus and faeces.

Definitive surgery is usually necessary if perforation occurs. Laparotomy and peritoneal toilet are performed, with further surgery aimed at preserving the maximum length of intestine while removing the source of sepsis. The affected gut may be just a punched-out perforation, or a much larger area which is dilated and discoloured, with denuded areas of mucosa, but still viable. Alternatively there may be patchy, necrotic or totally disintegrated areas. If resection and anastomosis of the gut are not possible, formation of one or more stomas will be necessary. These can be closed at a later date providing there are no strictures, but a permanent proximal stoma may be the only treatment for NEC-totalis.

Post-operatively, the stoma should be observed closely for deterioration in perfusion and that it is red and healthy, and that the skin around it shows no sign of irritation. Initially, a non-adherent dressing may be used, but when the stoma begins to function, a suitable-sized bag should be applied, and kept in situ for as long as there is no leakage, thus preserving skin integrity.

There is a risk of recurrence of NEC if enteral feeds are introduced too early. Strictures are the main concern, and rarely fistulae occur and are thought to follow subacute intestinal perforation. Malabsorption, failure-to-thrive and weight loss may be related to the mucosal injury, and short-gut syndrome may follow extensive resection (Castanon *et al*. 2006). Despite improved prognosis, the aggressive form of the disease has not decreased and is still associated with significant rates of morbidity and mortality (Ade-Ajayi *et al*. 1996).

Spontaneous bowel perforation

Small infants continue to have a high mortality rate after spontaneous gastro-intestinal perforation and subsequent development of peritonitis and sepsis, despite advances in perinatal care (Singh *et al*. 2003).

There are mutifactorial associated factors. Perforation can occur following hypoxic, ischaemic challenges to the fetus, e.g. reverse or end diastolic flow or exposure to indometacin via the placenta. This depresses prostaglandin synthesis, leading to premature closure of the ductus arteriosus (Tarrado *et al*. 2005) and reduced gut perfusion.

High-pressure IPPV, congenital defects of the intestinal musculature, infection and postnatal dexamethasone and indomethacin therapy are recognised causes of spontaneous perforation. Nasal-prong and face-mask ventilation are implicated in a disproportionately high number of cases. Other causes are a result of intraventricular haemorrhage, hypotension and dehydration. Umbilical catheters have also been implicated, as they can develop adherent thrombi, and focal perforations could be a result of subsequent small septic emboli to the bowel. The ileum is the most commonly affected part of the bowel.

These infants usually present with a bluish/purple discoloration of the abdomen, and abdominal X-ray shows pneumoperitoneum, but no pneumatosis or portal vein gas as in NEC (Tarrado *et al*. 2005). Surgical reports typically describe normal-looking bowel, apart from localised focal perforation, which can be resected and anastomosed (Singh *et al*. 2003). *Staphylococcus epidermdisis* or *Candida* are commonly grown on peritoneal fluid culture.

Miscellaneous disorders

Cystic hygroma

The fetal lymphatic system develops at around five weeks' gestation. Hygroma results from failure of the establishment of lymphatic drainage leading to pathological accumulations of fluid close to large veins and lymphatic ducts. A generalised lymphatic obstruction sequence may develop into progressive hydrops which may result in fetal demise (Goldstein *et al*. 1994).

Detection of fetal cystic hygroma in the second trimester of pregnancy is associated with an increased frequency of chromosomal anomalies, so termination of the pregnancy may be discussed at this point (Trauffer *et al*. 1994). If it proceeds, vaginal delivery may be possible, but Caesarean section should be considered for major lesions. Respiratory distress is the most significant complication, with very large masses compromising the airway. Facilities for immediate intubation and ventilation (with the possibility of tracheostomy) are mandatory (Goldstein *et al*. 1994).

Some 50–60 per cent of cystic hygromas are identified at birth, with a discrete, soft, mobile, non-tender transilluminable mass. Their size varies from a few millimetres to several centimetres, and they will continue to enlarge due to continued lymph production (Nazir *et al*. 2008).

Spontaneous regression is rare, and aspiration of the fluid is usually followed by reoccurrence, haemorrhage and infection. Infants with large lesions causing tracheal compression require urgent resection. Other methods of management include injections of OK432 (lyophilised mixture of Group A Streptococcus pyogenes) (Mahomed 2003) or laser surgery.

Hygromas are benign, so although every effort should be made to excise the cyst completely, no major nerves or vessels should be sacrificed.

Teratoma

Teratomas are neoplasms containing derivatives of one or more of the embryonic germ layers. Sacro-coccygeal teratomas are the commonest extra-gonadal tumour in neonates, especially in girls. They may be identified antenatally, and planned Caesarean section will avoid dystocia, rupture or haemorrhage, as some are highly vascular. These lesions should be protected following delivery, to prevent erosion of the surface; and blood for transfusion should be readily available.

On examination, there is a large skin-covered mass overlying the sacrum and coccyx, frequently displaying the anus anteriorly, palpable abdominally. Large lesions require early surgical referral, as untreated they can cause pain, constipation and urinary tract infections, and intra-spinal extension can cause lower motor neurone damage (Pollak *et al*. 1996). The important differential diagnosis is from a skin-covered spina bifida. Post-operatively the infant should be ventilated and nursed prone, with a urinary catheter in situ.

Teratoma of the cervical region is one of the rarest causes of neonatal respiratory distress, and requires urgent intervention. Complete excision is required, and delayed surgery is only feasible in unstable patients.

The majority of teratomas occurring in neonates are benign and surgical removal is imperative before 3 months of age; after this there is an increased risk of malignancy (Moore and Plaschkes 2003).

Ovarian cyst

The typical neonatal and infant ovary is heterogeneous and cystic. Neonatal cysts are primarily of follicular origin and probably result from disordered folliculogenesis. The incidence is increased in neonates of mothers who have toxaemia. Maternal diabetes and Rhesus incompatibility are also thought to increase the risk of ovarian cyst formation due to increased placental transfer of maternal hormones (Sanjay *et al.* 2005). With improved imaging techniques, antenatal diagnosis is now more common.

Postpartum management is contentious, because of potential malignancy. Cysts of less than 4cm that are uncomplicated (without solid components, septa, or debris) can be managed conservatively in the hope that they will resolve after cessation of hormonal stimulation. Surgical removal should be performed if the cyst increases in size, develops complications, or fails to resolve. Laparoscopy is well tolerated by newborns and will allow for diagnostic visualisation, biopsy and therapeutic intervention of the cyst if necessary (ibid.).

Torsion is the most common complication and can occur antenatally. Post-natally, torsion may be accompanied by pain, vomiting, fever, abdominal distension and peritonitis. Gastrointestinal obstruction, urinary tract obstruction and rupture can also occur (Aslam *et al.* 1995).

Testicular torsion

Testicular **torsion** commonly occurs antenatally (Azmy 1994). The neonatal testis may be prone to torsion because of its extreme mobility within the scrotum. It is generally a condition of large term babies (Burge 1996).

On examination, the scrotum is swollen (two to three times larger than the other side), firm, discoloured and painless if antenatal torsion has already led to testicular necrosis. There is oedema, erythema and a distinct fixation to overlying skin. The swelling will not transilluminate but sonography is a reliable method of early diagnosis (Traubici *et al.* 2003). Following excision of the affected testis, the contralateral side is usually explored prior to fixation.

Biliary atresia

Biliary atresia occurs due to failure of recanalisation of biliary ducts, or liver infection in late fetal life. The diagnosis is usually made from the recognition of prolonged jaundice in the first few weeks of life, followed by the development of pale stools and hepatomegaly. Haematological studies are mandatory for an overall evaluation. Although rarely significant in the differential diagnosis from other non-surgical causes of jaundice, it is important to distinguish biliary atresia from neonatal hepatitis. Accurate and rapid diagnosis is crucial if surgery, to avoid irreversible liver damage, is to be undertaken before 8 weeks of age (Kimura 1996). After this time, liver damage is progressive and the infant will require liver transplantation in order to survive.

Conclusion

In today's climate, prenatal diagnosis of malformations requiring surgery is possible, and represents a major advance in their management. Neonatal surgery has reached a high degree of sophistication and demands centralisation in designated centres with the expertise of a full range of specialist personnel. The fetus is usually in no danger until delivery, so negotiating intra-uterine transfer to such a centre is safer than the resuscitation and transport of a decompensating neonate (Theorell 1990). Family counselling and the timing and mode of delivery can be optimised at the tertiary centre. Consequent to this, maternal–infant bonding can take place without the disruption of an emergency transfer.

However, neonates, particularly preterm infants, have little tolerance to changes in normal physiological parameters, especially when in a compromised state. Accordingly, they endure surgery much better after punctilious pre-operative stabilisation. Compounded complications can be avoided with more delicate surgical techniques, effective and safe pain relief, improved antibiotics and sophisticated respiratory support.

Surgery is traditionally carried out in the operating theatre; associated with this is transportation with its potentially hazardous manipulation of ventilation and interruption of the continuity of care. Gavilanes *et al.* (1997) found that the NICU could be a suitable place for major surgery, with no increase in infection or peri-operative mortality rates. However, a footnote to this study delineates the difficulties of performing intricate surgery without adequate lighting.

Neonatal surgery presents a multidimensional challenge, and unequivocal outcome exacts the coordinated, cooperative and complementary skills of the surgeon, the specialist anaesthetist and the neonatologist. Together with the nursing staff, they can improve both the survival and the quality of life of these tiny patients.

Case study: neonatal surgery

Alex is now 1 week old following delivery at 28/40 weeks' gestation weighing 1.2kg. He was established on feeds of expressed breast milk at 180ml/kg when he became unwell with apnoeas and bradycardia associated with colour changes.

On examination he was lethargic, pale and possited his recent feed which was lightly bile stained.

Q.1. What do you do?

His condition quickly deteriorates and he needs to go to theatre as he has a perforation near the terminal ileum.

Q.2. How can you optimise his condition in preparation for theatre?

It is now two and a half weeks post surgery after resection and formation of an ileostomy. He is receiving breast-milk feeds at 150ml/kg but is not gaining weight.

Q.3. What is your management strategy?

Q.4. What are the potential future risks?

Acknowledgements

Stevie Boyd was the author of this chapter in the first edition.

References

Ade-Ajayi, N., Spitz, L., Kiely, E. *et al.* (1996) 'Intestinal glycos-aminoglycans in neonatal necrotising enterocolitis', *British Journal of Surgery* 83(3): 415–18.

Allal, H., Kalfa, W., Lopez, M., Forgues, D., Guibal, M., Raux, O., Picaud, J. and Galifer, R. (2005) 'Benefits of the thoracoscopic approach for short and long gap esophageal atresia', *Journal of Lapaoendoscopic Advanced Surgery Techniques Advancement* 15(6): 673–7.

Anveden-Hertzberg, L. and Gauderer, M.W.L. (1996) 'Paraumbilical intestinal remnant, closed abdominal wall and midgut loss in a neonate', *Journal of Pediatric Surgery* 31(6): 862–3.

Aslam, A., Wong, C., Haworth, J.M. and Noblett, H.R. (1995) 'Autoamputation of ovarian cyst in an infant', *Journal of Pediatric Surgery* 30(1): 1609–10.

Azmy, A.A.F. (1994) 'Acute penile and scrotal conditions', in P.A.M. Raine and A.A.F. Azmy (eds) *Surgical Emergencies in Children*, Oxford: Butterworth-Heinemann.

Bass, K.D., Rothenberg, S.S. and Chang, J.H.T. (1998) 'Laparoscopic Ladd's procedure in infants with malrotation', *Journal of Pediatric Surgery* 33(2): 279–81.

Beers, H., Porter, R., Jones, T.V., Kaplan, J. and Berkwits, M. (2006) 'Trustworthy information written by medical experts', in *The Merck Manual of Diagnosis and Therapy*, 18th edn, New York: Merck Publishing.

Biard, J., Johnson, M., Carr, M.C. *et al.* (2005) 'Long-term outcomes in children treated by prenatal vesicoamniotic shunting for lower urinary tract obstruction', *Obstetrics and Gynecology* 106(3): 503–8.

Boyd, S.C. and Tsang, T. (1996) 'Teat–Replogle device for oesophageal atresia', *Journal of Neonatal Nursing* 2(2): 24.

Brophy, K. (2007) 'Opioid analgesics and opioid antagonists', in *Clinical Drug Therapy for Canada Practice*, Philadelphia, PA: Lippincott, Chapter 6.

Brown, R.L. and Azizkhan, R.G. (1998) 'Pediatric head and neck lesions', *Pediatric Clinics of North America* 45(4): 889–905.

Burge, D.M. (1996) 'Neonatal testicular torsion', in P. Puri (ed.) *Newborn Surgery*, Oxford: Butterworth-heinemann.

Calkins, C. and Karrer, F. (2006) 'Duodenal atresia', available at: www.emedicine.com/ped/topic2776.htm.

Cantrell, J.R., Haller, J.A. and Ravitch, M.A. (1958) 'A syndrome of congenital defects involving the abdominal wall, sternum, diaphragm, pericardium, and heart', *Surgery, Gynecology and Obstetrics* 107: 602–14.

Castanon, M., Prat, J., Saura, L., Gomez, L., Tarrado, X., Iriondo, M. and Morales, L. (2006) 'Nutritional and surgical management of short bowel syndrome. Our last six patients' experience', *Cir Pediatric* 19(3): 151–5.

Chabra, S. (2006) 'American Academy of Challenges in the prenatal and post-natal diagnosis of mediastinal cystic hygroma', *NeoReviews* 7(8): e419.

Chauhan, M., Henderson, G. and McGuire, W. (2008) 'Enteral feeding for very low birth weight infants: reducing the risk of necrotizing enterocolitis', *Archives of Disease in Childhood: Fetal and Neonatal Edition* 93: F162–F166.

Coran, A.G. and Teitelbaum, D.H. (2000) 'Recent advances in the management of Hirschsprung's disease', *American Journal of Surgery* 180: 382–7.

Cusick, E., Spicer, R.D. and Beck, J.M. (1997) 'Small bowel continuity: a crucial factor in determining survival in gastroschisis', *Pediatric Surgery International* 12: 34–7.

Cywes, S., Rode, H. and Millar, A.J.W. (1994) 'Jejunal-ileal atresia and stenosis', in N.V. Freeman, D.M. Burge, M. Griffiths and P.S.J. Malone (eds) *Surgery of the Newborn*, London: Churchill Livingstone.

Davenport, M. (1999) 'Advances in management of congenital diaphragmatic hernia', paper presented at King's College Hospital, Neonatal Study Day.

Drewett, M., Michailidis, G. and Burge, D. (2006) 'The perinatal management of gastroschisis', 82(5): 305–12. Epub: www.ncbi.nlm.nih.gov/pubmed/16563666.

Duck, S.L. and Bloom, B.T. (1995) 'Spontaneous bowel perforations', *Neonatal Intensive Care* Sept/Oct: 48–52.

Edgar, D., Hawcutt, C., Kenny, S. and Lindley, R. (2006) 'Stem cell therapy in Hirschsprung's disease', University of Liverpool. Available at: www.liv.ac.uk/ulscc/projects/hirschprungs.html.

Ein, S.H. (1994) 'Meconium ileus', in N.V. Freeman, D.M. Burge, M. Griffiths and P.S.J. Malone (eds) *Surgery of the Newborn*, London: Churchill Livingstone.

El-Saify, W., El-Saify, M., Tsang, T., Mathur, A. and Kulkarni, M. (2007) 'Factor V Leiden mutation, in-utero inferior vena cava and renal vein thrombosis: report of successful retroperitoneoscopic nephrectomy. Case report No. 1', *European Surgery* 39(5), October.

Gavilanes, A., Heineman, E., Herpers, M. *et al.* (1997) 'Use of NICU as a safe place for surgery', *Archives of Disease in Childhood: Fetal and Neonatal Edition* 76: F51–F53.

Goldstein, I., Jakobi, P., Shoshany, G. *et al.* (1994) 'Late-onset isolated cystic hygroma: the obstetrical significance, management, and outcome', *Prenatal Diagnosis* 14(8): 757–61.

Goyal, A., Jones, M., Couriel, J. and Losty, P. (2006) 'Oesophageal atresia and tracheoesophageal fistula', *Archives of Disease in Childhood: Fetal and Neonatal Edition*. 91: F381–F384.

Greenough, A. and Roberton, N.R.C. (1999) 'Acute respiratory disease in the newborn', in J.M. Rennie and N.R.C. Roberton (eds) *Textbook of Neonatology*, Edinburgh: Churchill Livingstone.

Groves, R., Sunderajan, L., Khan, A., Parikh, D., Brain, J. and Samuel, M. (2006)

'Congenital anomalies are commonly associated with exomphalos minor', *Journal of Pediatric Surgery* 41(2): 358–61.

Guiney, E.J. (1996) 'Oesophageal atresia and tracheo-oesophageal fistula', in P. Puri (ed.) *Newborn Surgery*, Oxford: Butterworth-Heinemann.

Harrison, M., Keller, R. Hawgood, S. *et al.* (2003) 'A randomized trial of fetal endoscopic tracheal occlusion for severe fetal congenital diaphragmatic hernia', *New England Journal of Medicine* 349(20): 1916–24.

Haycock, G. (2003) 'Management of acute and chronic renal failure in the newborn', *Seminars in Neonatology* 8(4): 325.

Hebra, A. and Ross, A.J. (1996) 'Necrotising enterocolitis', in A.R. Spitzer (ed.) *Intensive Care of the Fetus and Neonate*, St Louis, MO: Mosby.

Hedrick, H., Flake, A., Cromblehome, T. *et al.* (2004) 'Sacrococcygeal teratoma: prenatal assessment, fetal intervention and outcomes', *Journal of Pediatric Surgery* 39(3): 430–8.

Jesudason, E., Connell, M., Fernig, D., Lloyd, D. and Losty, P. (2000) 'Early lung malformations in congenital diaphragmatic hernia', *Journal of Pediatric Surgery* 35(1): 124–8.

Johnson, A. and Sandford, J. (2005) 'Written and verbal information versus verbal information only for patients being discharged from acute hospital settings to home: systematic review', *Health Education Research* 20(4): 423–9.

Johnson, M., Sutton, L., Rintoul, N. *et al.* (2003) 'Fetal myelomenigocele repair: short-term clinical outcomes', *American Journal of Obstetrics and Gynecology* 189(2): 482–7.

Johnstone, J.M.S. (1994) 'Hernia in the neonate', in N.V. Freeman, D.M. Burge, M. Griffiths and P.S.J. Malone (eds) *Surgery of the Newborn*, London: Churchill Livingstone.

Kaplan, J. and Hudgins, L. (2008) 'Vater. Vacterl. Neoreviews', *American Academy of Pediatrics* 9(7): e299.

Kiely, E.M. (1996) 'Meconium ileus', in P. Puri (ed.) *Newborn Surgery*, Oxford: Butterworth-Heinemann.

Kimura, K. (1996) 'Biliary atresia', in P. Puri (ed.) *Newborn Surgery*, Oxford: Butterworth-Heinemann.

Kliegman, R.M. and Walsh, M.C. (1992) 'Pathophysiology and epidemiology of necrotising enterocolitis', in R.A. Polin and W.W. Fox (eds) *Fetal and Neonatal Physiology*, Philadelphia, PA: W.B. Saunders.

Kluth, D. and Lambrect, W. (1994) 'Disorders of intestinal rotation', in N.V. Freeman, D.M. Burge, M. Griffiths and P.S.J. Malone (eds) *Surgery of the Newborn*, London: Churchill Livingstone.

Kollef, M.H. and Fraser, V.J. (2001) 'Antimicrobial resistance has emerged as an important determinant', *Antibiotic Resistance in the Intensive Care Unit* 134(4): 298–314.

Kotoulas, O.B., Kalamidas, S.A. and Kondomerkos, D.J. (2006) 'Glycogen autophagy in glucose homeostasis', *Pathology: Research and Practice* 202(9): 631–8.

Kuo, B. and Urma, D. (2006) 'Esophagus-anatomy and development', *G.I. Motility online* (accessed 3 November 2009).

Laxman, B. (2006) 'Peritoneal drainage versus laparotomy as initial surgical treatment for perforated necrotising enterocolitis in preterm and LBWB', in *The Cochrane Collaboration*, Chichester: John Wiley & Sons.

Lin, P. and Stoll, B. (2006) 'Necrotising enterocolitis', *Lancet* 368: 1271–83.

Mahomed, A. (2003) 'Miscellaneous conditions of the neck and oral cavity', in P. Puri (ed.) *Newborn Surgery*, Oxford: Butterworth-Heinemann.

Merei, J.M., Farmer, P., Hasthorpe, S., Qi, B.Q., Beasley, S.W., Myers, N.A. and Hutson, J. (1998) 'Timing and embryology of oesophageal atresia and tracheo-oesophageal fistula', *Developmental Biology* 249(2): 240–8.

Meyer, M. and Bold, G. (2006) 'Admission temperatures following radiant warmer or incubator transport for preterm infants <28 weeks: a randomised study', *Archives of Disease in Childhood: Fetal and Neonatal Edition* 92: F295–F297.

Mintz, A.C. and Applebaum, H. (1993) 'Focal gastrointestinal perforations not associated with necrotising enterocolitis in very low birth weight neonates', *Journal of Pediatric Surgery* 28: 857–60.

Molenaar, J.C. (1996) 'Exomphalos and gastroschisis', in P. Puri (ed.) *Newborn Surgery*, Oxford: Butterworth-Heinemann.

Monnery-Noché, M., Auber, F., Jouannic, J., Bénifla, J., Carbonne, B., Dommergues, M., Lenoir, M., Lepointe, H., Larroquet, M., Grapin, C., Audry, G. and Helardot, G. (2008) 'Fetal and neonatal varian cysts: is surgery indicated?', *Prenatal Diagnosis* 28(1): 15–20.

Moore, K.L. and Persaud, T.V.N. (2003) *The Developing Human: Clinical Oriented Embryology*, 5th edn, Philadelphia, PA: W.B. Saunders.

Moore, S. and Plaschkes, J. (2003) 'Epidemiology and genetic associations of neonatal tumors', in P. Puri (ed.) *Newborn Surgery*, Oxford: Butterworth-Heinemann.

Mustafawi, A. and Hassan, M. (2008) 'Congenital duodenal obstruction in children: a decade of experience', *European Journal of Pediatric Surgery* 18: 93–7.

Nazir, S., Raza, S., Nazir, S., Sherwood, W., Bowker, C. and Lakhoo, K. (2008) 'Challenges in prenatal and postnatal diagnosis of mediastinal cystic hygroma: a case report', *Journal Medical Case Reports* 2: 256, 366–72.

Ng, J., Antao, B., Bartram, J., Raghavana, A. and Shawis, R. (2006) 'Diagnostic difficulties in the management of H type fistula', *Acta radiological* 47(8): 801–5.

Nicholl, R. (2003) 'What is the normal range of blood glucose concentration in healthy term newborns?', *Archives of Disease in Childhood* 88: 238–9.

Oak, S., Parelkar, S., Akhtar, T., Pathak, R., Vishwanath, N., Satish, K. and Kiran, R. (2005) 'Laparoscopic management of neonatal ovarian cysts', *Journal of Indian Association of Pediatric Surgeons* 10(2): 100–2.

Papadopulos, N., Papadopoulos, M., Kovacs, L., Zeilhofer, H., Henke, J., Boettcher, P. and Biemer, E. (2005) *Fetal Surgery and Cleft Lip and Palate: Current Status and New Perspectives*, The British Association of Plastic Surgeons, New York: Elsevier.

Paran, T., Decaluwe, D., Corbally, M. and Puri, P.(2007) 'Long term results of delayed primary anastomosis for pure oesophageal atresia: a 27 year follow up', *Pediatric Surgery International* 23(7): 647–51.

Pena, A. (1996) 'Anorectal anomalies', in P. Puri (ed.) *Newborn Surgery*, Oxford: Butterworth-Heinemann.

Phang, J., Marsh, W., Barlows, T. and Schwartz, H. (2004) 'Determining feeding tube location by gastric and intestinal pH values', *Nutrition in Clinical Practice* 19(6): 640–4.

Pollak, L., Schiffer, J., Rochkind, S. and Rothman, S. (1996) 'Giant thoracolumbosacral teratoma in an infant', *Pediatric Surgery International* 11: 206–7.

Puri, P. (1996a) 'Transport of the sick neonate', in P. Puri (ed.) *Newborn Surgery*, Oxford: Butterworth-Heinemann.

Puri, P. (1996b) 'Hirschsprung's disease', in P. Puri (ed.) *Newborn Surgery*, Oxford: Butterworth-Heinemann.

Puri, P. (ed.) (2003) *Newborn Surgery*, Oxford: Butterworth-Heinemann.

Puri, P. and Surana, R. (1996) 'Inguinal hernia', in P. Puri (ed.) *Newborn Surgery*, Oxford: Butterworth-Heinemann.

Puri, P. and Sureed, Y. (1996) 'Preoperative assessment', in P. Puri (ed.) *Newborn Surgery*, Oxford: Butterworth-Heinemann.

Rana, A., Khouri, J., Teitelbaum, D., Drongowski, R., Hirshi, R. and Mychaliska, G. (2008) 'Salvaging the severe congenital diaphragmatic hernia patient: is a silo the solution?', *Journal of Pediatric Surgery* 43(5): 788–91.

Replogle, R. (1963) 'Esophageal atresia – plastic sump catheter for drainage of the proximal pouch', *Surgery* 54: 296–7.

Reynolds, F. (2005) 'Maximum recommended doses of local anaesthetics: a constant cause of confusion', *Regional Anaesthesia and Pain Medicine* 30(3): 314–16.

Riego de Dios, R. and Chung, E. (2006) 'Ileal atresia', available at: www.emedicine. com/RADIO/topic359.html.

Rivosecchi, M. (2006) 'Meconium ileus', in P. Puri and M. Hollworth (eds) *Pediatric Surgery, Diagnostics and Management*, New York: Springer.

Rode, H. and Millar, A.J.W. (2006) 'Jejunoileal atresia', in P. Puri and M. Hollworth (eds) *Pediatric Surgery, Diagnostics and Management*, New York: Springer.

Royal College of Surgeons of England (1999) *Surgical Services for the Newborn*, 2nd edn, London: author.

Salihu, H., Emusa, D., Aliyu, Z., Pierre-Louis, B., Duschell, C. and Kirby, R. (2004) 'Mode of delivery and neonatal survival of infants with isolated gastroschisis', *Obstetrics and Gynecology* 104(4): 678–83.

Sanjay, N.O., Parelkar, S.V., Akhtar, T., Pathak, R., Vishwanath, N., Satish, K.V., and Kiran, R. (2005) 'Laparoscopic management of neonatal ovarian cysts', *Journal of Indian Association of Paediatric Surgeons* 10(2): 100–2.

Sankaran, K., Puckett, B., Lee, D., Seshia, M., Boulton, J., Qui, Z. and Lee, S. (2004) 'Variations in incidence of necrotising enterocolitis in Canadian Intensive Care Units', *Journal of Pediatric Gastroenterology Nutrition* 39: 366–72.

Shaw-Smith, C. (2006) 'Oesophageal atresia, tracheoesphageal fistula, and the VACTERL association: review of genetics and epidemiology', *Journal of Medical Genetics* 43: 545–54.

Shiyanagi, S., Okazaki, T., Shoji, H., Shimizu, T., Tanaka, T., Takeda, S., Kawashima, K., Lane, G. and Yamataka, A. (2008) 'Management of pulmonary hypertension in congenital diaphragmatic hernia: nitric oxide with prostaglandin-E1 versus nitric oxide alone', *Pediatric Surgery International* 24(10): 1101–4.

Simmons, M. and Georgeson, K.E. (1996) 'The effect of gestational age at birth on morbidity in patients with gastroschisis', *Journal of Pediatric Surgery* 31(8): 1060–2.

Singh, M., Owen, A., Gull, S., Morabito, A. and Bianchi, A. (2003) 'Surgery for intestinal perforation in preterm neonates: anastomosis vs stoma', *Journal of Pediatric Surgery* 41(4): 725–9.

Skarsgard, E.D. and Barth, R.A. (1997) 'Use of Doppler ultrasonography in the evaluation of liver blood flow during silo reduction of a giant omphalocele', *Journal of Pediatric Surgery* 32(5): 733–5.

Snyder, C., Miller, K., Sharp, R., Murphy, J., Andrews, W., Ill, G., Gittes, G. and Ashcraft, K. (2001) 'Management of intestinal atresia in patients with gastroschisis', *Journal of Pediatric Surgery* 36(10): 1542–5.

Speidel, B., Fleming, P., Henderson, J. *et al.* (1998) *A Neonatal Vade Mecum*, London: Arnold.

Spitz, L. (2007) 'Oesophageal atresia', *Orphanet Journal of Rare Diseases* 2(24). Available at: http://www.ojrd.com/content/2/1/24.

Spitz, L. and Hancock, R.J. (1994) 'Oesophageal atresia and tracheo-oesophageal fistula', in N.V. Freeman, D.M. Burge, M. Griffiths and P.S.J. Malone (eds) *Surgery of the Newborn*, London: Churchill Livingstone.

Steinhorn, R.H., Glick, P.L., O'Toole, S. *et al.* (1997) 'Contemporary understanding of the pathophysiology and management of congenital diaphragmatic hernia', in T.N. Hanson and N. McIntosh (eds) *Current Topics in Neonatology*, London: W.B. Saunders.

Stokowski, L.A. (2006) 'Thrombocytopenia in the neonate: a common clinical problem', *Neonatal Thrombocytopenia: Evaluation and Management CE*, Tennessee: Medscape.

Tarcon, A., Gurakan, B., Arda, S. and Boybat, F. (2003) 'H-type fistula', *Journal of Maternal, Fetal and Neonatal Medicine* 13(4): 279–80.

Tarrado, X., Castañón, M., Thió, M., Valderas, J.M., Garcia Aparicio, L. and Morales, L. (2005) 'Comparative study between isolated intestinal perforation and necrotizing enterocolitis', *European Journal of Pediatric Surgery* 15(2): 88–94.

Thebaud, B., Mercier, J.C. and Dinh-Xuan, A.T. (1998) 'Congenital diaphragmatic hernia', *Biology of the Neonate* 74: 323–36.

Theorell, C.J. (1990) 'Congenital diaphragmatic hernia: a physiological approach to management', *Journal of Perinatal and Neonatal Nursing* 3(3): 66–79.

Tovar, J. (2003) 'Inguinal hernia', in P. Puri (ed.) *Newborn Surgery*, Oxford: Butterworth-Heinemann.

Traubici, J., Daneman, A., Navarro, O., Mohanta, A. and Garcia, C. (2003) 'Testicular torsion in neonates and infants: sonographic features in 30 patients', *American Journal of Radiology* 180: 1143–5.

Trauffer, P.M., Anderson, C.E., Johnson, A. *et al.* (1994) 'The natural history of euploid pregnancies with first-trimester cystic hygromas', *American Journal of Obstetrics and Gynecology* 170: 1279–84.

Tsao, K. and Lee, H. (2005) 'Extrapleural thoracoscopic repair of esophageal atresia with tracheo eosophageal fistula', *Pediatric Surgery International* 21(4): 308–10.

Uemura, S., Woodward, A.A., Amerena, R. and Drew, J. (1999) 'Early repair of inguinal hernia in premature infants', *Pediatric Surgery International* 15: 36–9.

Wilson, R., Hedrick, H., Liechty, K. *et al.* (2006) 'Cystic adenomatoid malformation of the lung: review of genetics, prenatal diagnosis, and in utero treatment', *American Journal of Med Genet A* 140(2): 151–5.

Winter, L., Giuseppetti, M. and Breuer, M. (2005) 'A case report of midgut atresia and spontaneous closure of gastroschisis', *Pediatric Surgery International* 21(5): 415–16.

Wright, J.E. (1994) 'Recurrent inguinal hernia in infancy and childhood', *Pediatric Surgery International* 9: 164–6.

Yoo, S., Jung, S., Eom, M., Kim, I. and Han, A. (2002) 'Delayed maturation of interstitial cells of Cajal in meconium obstruction', *Journal of Pediatric Surgery* 37(12): 1758–61.

Chapter 17

Neonatal Transport

Stevie Boyd and Anne Mitchell

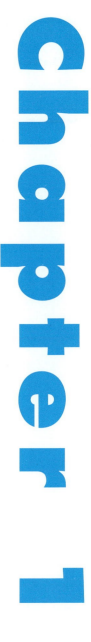

Contents

Introduction

Until comparatively recently in the UK, transfer was largely the responsibility of a locally organised *ad hoc* team who happened to be on duty but who commonly had inadequate training, resources and equipment (Krug 1995). Staff were not in an optimal position to manage the infant en route, nor to deal with emergencies such as physiological deterioration, loss of intravenous access or endotracheal tube misplacement (Kelly *et al.* 1996). By undertaking the transfer, staffing within the neonatal intensive care unit (NICU) was depleted.

As centralised specialist neonatal intensive care units providing complex care to sick newborn infants have developed, there has been recognition that the transport of neonates is an equally highly specialised service, and that this service should only be undertaken by trained neonatal staff who are also trained in the issues associated with the transfer of these vulnerable infants.

Every ill neonate should have access to neonatal intensive care and a reliable, trained service is required to transfer them expediently to the most appropriate facility. Unfortunately the transport service within the UK at present does not always achieve this standard. The review of maternity services in England found that only half of transport services operate on a 24/7 availability, and more concerning is that 5 per cent of hospitals providing neonatal care stated that they did not have access to a dedicated transport service (Commission for Healthcare 2008).

Neonatal transport teams appear to have a wider remit than either adult or paediatric transfer teams, undertaking many transfers that are not deemed to be intensive care retrievals. This wider role is due to the vulnerability of the unique population that they serve.

Transfers can be broken down into several categories:

- Transfer of patients to another hospital for specialist management. These transfers are occurring more frequently due to lack of cot spaces or staffing issues in tertiary units (Commission for Healthcare 2008).
- Retrieval of patients in level 1 or 2 special care baby units for intensive care. Studies indicate that transferring sick infants to a specialist unit will improve the outcome for these infants and provide lower mortality rates (Lyall 1993).
- Back transport to the referring hospital for continuing care once intensive care is no longer required. It is this aspect that few other speciality teams undertake. This may be the transfer of a baby as small as 1kg or requiring nasal CPAP and is perceived to be an important aspect of the neonatal transport service role. This aspect of transport contributes a significant amount to the workload of the transport service and will vary depending on the rate of in-utero transfers within the area covered.
- Internal transport may also be viewed as the remit of the transport service. This includes the transfer of babies to the operating theatre and for imaging. The creation of specialist transport teams has decreased the exposure of NICU staff to transportation of infants, and consequently they are becoming

unfamiliar with the equipment used to transport a baby. Wallen *et al.* (1995) reviewed 180 paediatric intra-hospital transfers and found that there was a significant change in at least one physiological variable in 71.7 per cent of patients transferred to and from the intensive care unit. This has implications for staff training if a dedicated transport team is not available.

It is not cost-effective either fiscally or for staffing resources for each NICU in the UK to have a dedicated inter-hospital retrieval team. The number of journeys for each team would not be sufficient to ensure adequate exposure to transport. This has led to the development of transport teams being based geographically rather than each hospital having to release specifically trained staff.

More sick newborns are transferred for specialist care than any other group of intensive care patients (Major 1996). There is no doubt that in-utero transfer is generally safer for the baby; however, prior to moving a pregnant woman, there should be discussion between both the obstetric and neonatal teams at both receiving and referring units to ascertain that this is the optimal care for the individuals involved (Field 1999). If transfer puts the mother at risk or is over a long distance with a risk of delivery en route, then, with current standards, a neonatal transfer may be safer.

Personnel and training

The majority of acute neonatal transfers were traditionally undertaken by both a doctor and a nurse. Leslie (1997) suggests there are wide local variations in the current compositions of teams, as well as the grade, experience and training of these staff.

The doctor who traditionally undertook neonatal transfers was often a junior member of medical staff who was undertaking a neonatal rotation and had no previous exposure to transport. In many areas, however, the Advanced Neonatal Nurse Practitioner (ANNP) is replacing the doctor's role within the transport team. This practitioner will have specialised in both intensive care of the newborn and neonatal transport (Watts 2001). Independent nurse prescribing has greatly facilitated this career progression for ANNPs.

The transport team nurse will be a neonatally trained member of staff and ideally rostered outwith the NICU staffing to cover transport and in many cases employed as a dedicated neonatal transport specialist. There is much discussion currently around the concept of nurse-led transfers. Many nurses specialising in neonatal transport already regularly undertake planned cases, particularly back transfers, on their own with telephone support if required. While teams have been based within tertiary units, it has been easy to assess infants prior to transfer, and to decide upon the most suitable team composition for individual infants. This, however, is not as easily achieved when the team is based elsewhere and have to rely on other people's judgement as to the team required. Cheema *et al.* (2007) looked at this issue and created guidelines for staff to help decide which transfers are suitable for nurse-only transfers. In other areas, neonatal transport practitioners from both paramedic and nursing backgrounds are successfully being trained to undertake practitioner-led transfers (Fenton and Mitchell 2007).

Irrespective of the background of the personnel involved, the Transport of Neonates in Ambulances (TINA) report (Medical Devices Agency 1995) made several recommendations regarding staff undertaking neonatal transfers. Personnel should have adequate training and experience, including regular exposure to critically ill infants being transferred, in order to become expert in this role. It is not acceptable to send staff on transfers so infrequently that skills cannot be sustained.

Neonatal transport is a complex task and caring for a critically ill infant during a journey is very different from caring for a baby in the stable environment of an intensive care unit where more equipment and staff are available. The two retrieval staff are often the only personnel present once in the back of the ambulance, where the environment is even more challenging with excessive noise, vehicle vibration, restricted lighting, limited work space and immediate support from senior colleagues is not readily available, except at the end of a telephone!

The back of an ambulance or an aircraft are highly unsuitable places in which to perform resuscitative procedures, with small infants becoming cold very quickly. Training for transport staff should build on existing neonatal skills (for non-neonatal staff such as paramedics, this baseline knowledge will need to be included) and include an action plan of what to do in specific emergencies. While it is laudable for staff to respond efficiently to problems en route, even better is for the problems to have been pre-empted and thus prevented. Staff should be competent in providing advanced life support – including airway and ventilation management, vascular access and drainage of pneumothoraces. These skills may be needed, either in the controlled environment of the referring hospital, or during the journey to the receiving unit. During an emergency retrieval, transport staff will need to have the skills required to complete stabilisation of the infant prior to transfer; it is no longer appropriate to 'scoop and run' hoping that the baby will remain stable until they reach the receiving unit. The goal of the transport team should be to effectively stabilise the neonate prior to transfer and to transfer the patient in optimal condition, while providing a level of care indistinguishable from that available in NICU (BPA 1993). This is the gold standard of neonatal transfer and, given the hostile environment in which this care is being delivered, it is indeed a high standard to achieve.

Many common incidents on transport are due to equipment malfunction (Bourchier 1994). Familiarity and confidence in trouble-shooting equipment failure form one of the steepest learning curves for staff undertaking transports as the support of the medical physics team is not readily available.

Irrespective of what qualifications the transport team members hold, it is essential that they are skilled communicators who believe in teamwork and diplomacy (Bloodworth 1995). As 'guests' in the referring unit, these skills will often be as important as their clinical expertise in order not to undermine the staff in the referring unit and ease the transition of care of the infant from one team to the other.

Equipment

Reliable equipment, preferably designed for use on transport, needs to be robust yet lightweight with long battery life and be able to be secured while in use (Wallen *et al.* 1995). It is essential that all equipment is checked by the team before and after each journey and if mechanical, regularly maintained and serviced by the hospital's medical engineering department. Much of the equipment carried will be able to be powered either by mains electricity or by battery and should be plugged into a mains source as much as possible, allowing the battery life to be conserved for periods where mains power is unavailable.

The term 'transport incubator' is loosely used, not only to describe an enclosed, heated, illuminated environment for the infant, but often encompasses the other equipment such as ventilator, multiparameter monitor, intravenous pumps and gas sources which are secured to its frame. Weight must be borne in mind when purchasing new equipment. There is no point in saying that the incubator only weighs 50kg if the frame and all the equipment added on bring this weight up to 200kg. Many current transport systems within the UK weigh more than European guidelines suggest. Current transport incubators are not suitable for infants weighing more than 4.5kg and it can be difficult accessing a larger baby through the portholes. Access to the infant's head, that also allows maintenance of body temperature, is vital for the staff to carry out effective resuscitation. The team needs to carry supplies of any disposables needed for supplemental equipment carried. While transport teams can use disposables available in the referring unit, there is no guarantee that everything required will be available or compatible with the transport equipment.

All equipment must be secured en route but be readily available; resuscitation equipment must be available – most teams will have a stethoscope as well as bag and mask system set up on the incubator along with an oxygen source. Staff must be aware that they are as vulnerable as any other road user and for their own safety must wear seat belts. The baby is often viewed as safe within the incubator but how secure are they to stop them hitting the walls of the incubator during an accident? Safety guidance for parents travelling with their own infant in a car or pram is to use a five-point harness, yet transport systems are sold with velcro straps to cross the body of the baby. Everything in the ambulance (e.g. equipment bags and incubator) should be secured so that it does not become a lethal projectile if the vehicle has to stop suddenly. Team safety must be considered through use of high visibility and safety clothing as well as adherence to lifting and handling guidelines

Each team will have decided on the equipment that they carry according to the service and area that they provide transport for. What is physically carried will depend on whether the team is using a dedicated vehicle or having to take equipment for all contingencies with them. Handheld blood gas analysers are available and blood sugar analysers are carried by most teams but are known to be inaccurate at low blood sugar levels. A relatively new device for use during transport is in line end tidal CO_2 monitoring. Chemical gel mattresses are a useful adjunct to temperature control.

The drugs carried will vary between teams but there must be guidelines available for the use of each drug that is taken out. It is essential to carry drugs and fluids of resuscitation (as well as needles and syringes) which are easily accessible. Other drugs carried may include surfactant, inotropes, muscle-relaxing agents, analgesia and Dinoprostone. It must be remembered to carry adequate diluents and syringe labels. There are cool boxes designed to keep drugs at recommended temperatures for several hours – unfortunately they are often bulky and still need to be secured in the ambulance. It is possible to provide inhaled nitric oxide en route and staff should be aware that most frontline vehicles do have a gas extraction system (normally used during Entonox administration) minimising the risks of exposure to the gas for staff.

It is essential to have a means of direct communication with the team – liaising through a third party is not helpful (Macrae 1994). Telephones need to be charged regularly and any numbers likely to be needed stored in the phone for immediate access en route. It is wise to have a paper copy of telephone numbers in case of battery failure.

The team should take with them a copy of the referral documentation along with any advice/requests given to the referring unit, an observation chart (perhaps with supplemental pages for long transfers), suitable charts for prescribing drugs and fluids and documentation for clinical notes. Many teams have managed to combine several of these into one document which is often in duplicate or triplicate form.

Mode of transport

Those with the luxury of being able to design a dedicated neonatal vehicle should consider the following:

- Space for two intensive care patients being transferred simultaneously with seating for two staff for each baby. One patient can travel in the preferred horizontal position while the other is in the more traditional longitudinal position.
- A bank of batteries built into the chassis which recharge when the vehicle is parked and are plugged into the main hospital supply.
- At least two size F air cylinders plus three size F oxygen cylinders piped to both spaces plus a gas extraction system.
- Year-round means of heating the vehicle when not in use.
- Inclusion of noise dampening for patients and staff.
- A loading device so that it does not rely on staff lifting a transport system into the vehicle.
- Cupboard space and layout.
- Methods of securing the incubator, e.g., 'tite lock' which has been crash-tested.

In reality, many teams have to rely on the frontline vehicles provided by their local ambulance service, while a few have the luxury of a dedicated vehicle;

rarer still is a dedicated driver! The frontline vehicle design can vary tremendously within a region and is not built with neonatal transport in mind. This can influence the team composition and the ability to take parents with the team due to inadequate seating. There is rarely a need to have an air gas supply in these vehicles, therefore the team must either carry sufficient amounts (which need to be secured) or have a ventilator that can entrain air. Power supply will vary from one 12V DC point requiring spade connections in older vehicles to 3-pin plugs in others.

Securing the transport system needs careful consideration. Traditionally the York fitting inside the ambulance was all that held the incubator in place but following investigation into a road traffic accident during a transfer, this was found to be woefully inadequate (Madar and Milligan 1994). The means of fixing incubators into ambulances changed following publication of the TINA report (Medical Devices Agency 1995) but these are not always compatible. It is well worth establishing a good rapport with the local ambulance service to ensure that the needs of the neonatal service are included in future plans for their service.

Most neonatal transport in the UK is undertaken by road, although teams who cover the remote and rural communities regularly travel by air.

Using road vehicles has the advantage of:

- relatively rapid mobilisation;
- ability to travel in most weather conditions;
- covering a wide geographical area without refuelling;
- the option to alter the destination;
- stopping if procedures need to be carried out.

Disadvantages include longer transit times and traffic-related delays.

Both fixed-wing aircraft and helicopters can be utilised for journeys that are long or cannot be accessed easily by road. Teams that use these vehicles regularly need to have worked with the ambulance service and aircraft providers to develop a safe means of loading both the EC135 helicopter and the King Air fixed-wing aircraft without lifting the transport system into or out of the craft.

However, flying is expensive and a lack of appropriate landing sites near most hospitals means that an ambulance is still needed at both ends of the journey to move the baby between the airport and the hospital.

There is little room to manoeuvre when in the aircraft and it must be remembered that even if the patient's condition warrants landing, the pilot cannot land except at an airport. A helicopter is limited by the amount of fuel it can carry but is an ideal means to reach otherwise inaccessible areas. The helicopter is noisy, very small with cramped working space and noticeable vibration as well as having a weight limitation for the combination of staff and equipment. If using a military helicopter, it is also extremely cold and loading involves using a winch. Military aircraft are extremely expensive to use and, as for all flights, health boards will need to authorise this cost. Flying will be limited by inclement weather.

Altitude has an effect on the patient's gas exchange. With increasing altitude, there is a fall in the ambient oxygen tension and an inverse relationship between altitude and barometric pressure (Bourchier 1994). If an infant requires an FiO_2 of 0.50 (50 per cent) at ground level to maintain an adequate physiological PaO_2, a simple equation can determine the required increased FiO_2 at 2500m (Barry and Leslie 2003):

Oxygen requirement at sea level (0.5 for this patient) × barometric pressure at sea level (760mmHg)

divide by barometric pressure at actual altitude (565mmHg at 2500m)

$$\frac{0.5 \times 760}{565} = FiO_2\ 0.67\ (67\ \text{per cent})$$

Both ventilation and optimising haemoglobin need to be considered prior to flying with a sick infant. As air pressure falls, there is an associated expansion of gas within body compartments. Hence all infants undergoing air transport must have a wide-bore nasogastric tube on free drainage. Patients with a pneumothorax should have it drained and chest drain inserted with a **Heimlich valve** (or similar) attached (Bourchier 1994). Infants with a diaphragmatic hernia are at particular risk during flight as bowel gas within the thorax expands causing further ventilatory compromise. Cabin pressurisation reduces these effects by maintaining a preset barometric pressure regardless of the actual altitude (Aoki and McCloskey 1992).

Risk management

Transferring a baby between hospitals is not without risk, but with care, sophisticated monitoring equipment and the skills of a trained team, this risk can be minimised (Cooke 1992). The incidence of iatrogenic and secondary insults, occurring during transport, is directly related to the level of training of the staff (Macrae 1994). Transport-specific training and experience mean that staff undertaking transport as part of a dedicated team are far more likely to anticipate and indeed pre-empt incidents during transport than those who undertake transfers on an *ad hoc* basis. Clinical outcome for the baby depends on how well the transport team prepares prior to undertaking the transfer.

Transport teams are becoming more willing to share information about incidents that have occurred in their area in order for others to learn and avoid the same incident happening to another baby. Local incident reviews are raising safety standards.

Documented avoidable clinical incidents include failure to resuscitate and stabilise shocked infants adequately, failure to assess and manage the airway appropriately and failure to detect and treat changes in vital signs (Macrae 1994). Reliable multiparameter monitoring with visual alarms is essential as audible alarms may be undetected against background noise. Any equipment can fail to function; however, incidents have been greatly reduced by the introduction of dedicated transport teams who have a vested interest in the equipment's efficiency and will often be responsible for daily checks of equipment carried.

Insufficient gas supply is a major potential problem for transport staff. It is recommended to carry twice as much oxygen as the estimated journey time requires and patient condition indicates in order to anticipate changes in ventilation requirements, to cover delays/breakdowns and cylinder leakage.

To calculate the oxygen requirements of a patient:

Patient flow rate (l/min) × Journey time (mins) × 2 (margin of error)

To ensure adequate gas supply:

Divide total oxygen requirements calculated above by the contents of each cylinder (litres)

Contents of a cylinder depend on the cylinder size and are documented on the side of the cylinder (assuming that the cylinder is full) (adapted from Barry and Leslie 2003).

The emergency transport process

A seamless transport episode starts with the daily checks of equipment by the team; the knowledge that everything is present and working makes for an efficient response to any transport request. A dedicated telephone line may be used for this initial contact or it may come via the receiving tertiary unit. During this initial call the degree of urgency required must be ascertained together with clinical details, including provisional diagnosis and current management as well as the basic information of name, age, gestation and birth weight. Many teams have developed referral documentation to be used during this call to enable a standard approach and information exchange to occur. This information will form the basis for both the advice given by the team (if required) and the response time. The advice given will vary depending on from whom the referral is from; a tertiary unit asking for a transfer because of bed availability will not require the same advice and support as a community midwifery unit with no paediatric cover. With the information gained, the team can optimise their plan of management of the baby at the referring unit. If they have the weight of the baby, both drugs and fluids can be calculated in advance. Additionally, extra equipment such as nitric oxide should also be considered at this time. Ideally an ambulance would be immediately available but in reality there is often a delay while vehicle and crew are assembled. Spending time building relationships with the local ambulance control staff has huge benefits as a better understanding of the work undertaken by both groups can impact on the workload and efficiency of each other's service provision.

At the referring unit

Unless the baby is requiring immediate resuscitation on the arrival of the team, it is essential that time is taken to introduce themselves to the staff caring for the baby and to listen courteously to the handover and care the baby has received to date. Failure to address the way in which the handover is paced and integrated with the resident team's care is likely to cause hostility (Leslie and Middleton 1995), and implies criticism of their clinical management. The patient is under the care of the referring unit and the transfer team are there to provide ongoing care and transfer. In a smaller unit with less exposure to sick infants, the team may be viewed as helpful and more skilled; perhaps even essential to stabilisation, but in a tertiary unit any changes in management may be seen as criticism of their care, and skills of tact and diplomacy will be required of all team members to ensure that the baby is stabilised and fit for transfer.

It is essential to obtain (and document) a baseline set of observations on arrival and pre departure. Practice varies between teams as to where observations are documented during the time between these; many continue to use unit documentation (which is photocopied prior to transfer); others have spare sheets to supplement standard documentation during prolonged periods of stabilisation.

Stabilisation of the acutely ill baby must be carried out prior to transfer. This may take several hours if the infant is particularly ill. The presence of hypothermia, hypotension, hypoglycaemia and acidosis before transport has significant negative outcomes and should be corrected prior to moving the infant (Major 1996). If there is any suggestion of respiratory compromise and the infant is not already ventilated, it is prudent to secure an airway prior to the journey. Hand-ventilation en route is likely to be inconsistent, erratic and potentially ineffective, while increasing the risk of dislodging the endotracheal tube and compromising thermal stability. The position of the endotracheal tube and central lines must be checked radiologically before departure.

Diagnostic X-rays and haematological and biochemical results carried out by the referring hospital should be checked, acted on and documented.

Consideration must be given to the need for sedation or muscle relaxants to ensure both the comfort and safety of the baby. The patency and security of lines should be checked, as should the doses and dilutions of drugs and fluids being administered. There should always be spare, secure venous access during an emergency retrieval. Haemodynamically unstable infants should have arterial access to facilitate invasive blood pressure monitoring.

As already highlighted, good communication skills are vital in a successful transport team; this is particularly pertinent where the parents are concerned. Dodds et al. (1995) found that parental stress was directly related to lack of communication between parents and health professionals regarding the infant's transfer, as well as to differences in care practice. Parents are often present on the unit at the time that the team is stabilising the baby for transfer (Leslie and Middleton 1995), and staff need to appreciate the extra anxiety brought about by the transfer (Alfonso et al. 1992). Parents will already be suffering acute emotional stress associated with the birth of their sick baby, and the fact that the baby has to be moved to a specialist unit is an added stressor.

It is vital that one of the transport team takes the time to speak to the parents and appraise them of the situation, as if clear explanations are given as to the need for transfer, parental anxiety can be lessened (ALSG 1997). Additionally, staff may have been so busy with the baby's stabilisation that no one has had time to obtain an accurate maternal medical history which may impact on the future care of the baby. Photographs or video of the infant should be taken for the parents.

If the baby is being transferred due to a need for surgery, consent needs to be obtained. Surgical consent should be obtained by the surgeon undertaking the surgery but when this has to be done by telephone, it is very helpful for a team member to be present during the discussion to give a more detailed explanation of what is required. If the parents are not married, the father cannot give consent for surgery until his name is registered on the birth certificate which some families will find distressing.

A further stressor for the father is having to potentially choose between staying with his newly delivered and perhaps sick partner or visiting his new baby who has been transferred several miles away.

When the mother is fit for transfer, the distance she has to travel to see her baby may cause both emotional conflict or financial hardship, particularly if she has other children to care for (Wilman 1997). If the mother is moved near the baby, she may well be distanced from her usual support system from family and friends (Bose 1989; Coffman et al. 1993).

Only when stabilisation is complete should the infant be transferred to the prepared transport incubator. This is the most likely point in time for lines or endotracheal tubes to be dislodged and the condition of the sick baby compromised. The team needs to discuss this move in advance, identifying:

- What equipment or infusions can be disconnected in advance.
- Who is responsible for the transfer of infusions that need to continue unbroken.
- Who will be responsible for airway management.
- Who will facilitate the move by opening incubator doors and moving equipment as necessary.

This move needs to as expedient as possible in order to maintain the stability gained and lessen thermal stresses to the infant.

As soon as the baby is in the transport incubator, air entry should be re-checked, monitoring resumed, alarms set and all lines are infusing as prescribed. Only when the team are satisfied that the infant is stable in the transport incubator are they ready to leave for the receiving unit, which should be contacted and appraised of the baby's current clinical status and their estimated time of arrival.

The team should ensure that parents have directions/maps and the contact telephone number for the receiving unit. The team must ensure that they have a means of contacting the family while en route as the baby's condition may change or in rare circumstances the final destination may be changed. Currently there is much discussion as to whether a parent should accompany the baby. Most teams do not have a midwife team member and do not feel competent to look after a newly delivered mother who has not been discharged from midwifery care. Staff may feel that they cannot concentrate on the care of a critically ill baby while the father is in the vehicle with them and worry about the father's need for support should the baby deteriorate en route (Melville and Print 1996). Others have concerns that in a stressful situation the father may be aggressive, leaving the staff in a vulnerable situation.

The decision surrounding this must rest with the retrieval team not unit staff as they are the ones who will be responsible for the baby and any fall-out that may arise from parental presence. Some teams are much more relaxed about parents accompanying their infant on the less acute, repatriation back transfers so long as any luggage they have can be securely stowed in the ambulance.

If parents are travelling by car, they should be reminded not to follow the ambulance and that unlike emergency vehicle drivers, they are not permitted to disregard traffic regulations. Disregarding this advice can be a risk to both themselves and other road users.

The speed of the journey to transfer the baby needs to be discussed with the crew prior to commencing the journey. Many ill babies cope better with a smooth, slower journey than one under blue light conditions involving fast driving and braking to avoid hazards. Using ambulance blue lights and sirens is more useful in built-up areas during rush hour than on the open road. It must be remembered that using these is not without risk to staff, baby and other road users. A police presence may be helpful in extremely busy conditions.

During transport, vital signs and oxygenation, fluid rate, gas consumption and incubator temperature should be monitored regularly. While hourly observations and continuous monitoring are standard within NICU, during transport it is more common to document observations every 15 minutes. If the patient has been well prepared for transfer, it is unlikely that procedures other than monitoring will be required, even over long distances. Should interventions be required during the journey, the ambulance should stop in a safe place, as undertaking procedures in the back of a moving vehicle compromises the safety of both the infant and the staff. Unlike care within a hospital there is no definitive documentation legally obligatory; however, the Nursing and Midwifery Code (2008) expects accurate records of all interventions and management strategies to be clearly documented.

In the receiving unit

A comprehensive handover needs to be given to appropriate medical and nursing staff prior to the transfer of care. A final set of observations should be obtained before moving the baby from the transport system into the cot in the receiving unit. This needs to be done in as controlled and thought-out manner as occurred in the referring unit. Results of arrival blood gas and blood sugar should also be part of the documentation. Both the referring unit and the parents should be contacted and updated with the baby's condition. The work of the team is not complete until the equipment has been cleaned, checked, restocked and ready for the next journey.

Legal aspects of transport

For staff used to working within one set environment, there is usually little confusion as to who is legally accountable for the care of an infant within the hospital. However, staff undertaking neonatal transport have raised concerns about vicarious liability when moving an infant between Trusts when neither Trust may be the employer of the transport team. Legal responsibility for the transported patient represents a continuum (Melville and Print 1996). The receiving hospital's responsibility begins when the referring hospital makes the phone call and the patient is accepted. The referring hospital's liability diminishes in proportion to the involvement of the receiving hospital, once that initial phone call has been made and the receiving hospital starts to guide the clinical management of the baby (Aoki and McCloskey 1992). The team's actions should be guided by the consultant accepting the baby. Although no regulations apply directly to intensive care transport in the United Kingdom, there is no substitute for professional accountability and responsibility. The Nursing and Midwifery Council (NMC 2008) states that nurses are personally accountable for their practice and are therefore responsible for their actions and omissions, regardless of advice or directions from another professional. If harm occurs to the patient due to lack of skill, knowledge or competence of a transport nurse, that nurse will be liable, and the nurse's employer vicariously liable (Melville and Print 1996). If the team members are working as stated within their job description, then the employer should provide vicarious liability.

Areas for development

Neonatal transport is a rapidly developing speciality with many changes and challenges ahead. There is a suggestion that combined NICU/PICU teams may be the way forward but as these are very different populations, it may not be appropriate. Cooling is a new treatment modality that may become a standard of care in term infants and teams need to know that they can deliver this therapy safely between hospitals. In Canada, transport teams are offering a further service to smaller units, that of resuscitation, and this may be a development in service provision in the UK.

Conclusion

Neonatal transport in the UK has evolved from an *ad hoc* basis in the 1950s, where a midwife was expected to transfer an infant in an incubator with supplemental oxygen by taxi, into a subspecialty in its own right, with the goal of providing high-standard, timely and safe transport of sick infants. The basic principles of good transport should be applied to all sick patients moved within or between hospitals, whether or not a specialist team is involved. Conscientious initial assessment, resuscitation and prompt, appropriate emergency management should minimise the risks of transport-related morbidity and mortality (ALSG 1997). Effective communication between the referring hospital, NICU and the team is a crucial element in the provision of optimal patient care during neonatal transport (Finterswald 1998). As Leslie and Middleton (1995) conclude, 'Transfer is more than the movement of the baby and associated information, it involves the meshing together of two networks of care.'

Case study: neonatal transport

Nathanial is a post-term infant. This is his mother, Julia's, first pregnancy. She cohabits with her partner Robert. She has booked for delivery in her local hospital which has level 2 neonatal care facilities. During her labour Nathanial became increasingly distressed developing a suboptimal cardiotocograph (CTG) which necessitated his delivery by emergency Caesarean section. He is resuscitated at birth and is transferred to the Special Care Baby Unit in ambient oxygen for respiratory distress and grunting.

His first capillary blood gas shows pH 7.1, PCO_2 8.4, PO_2 4.2, BE 9.0, Bicarbonate 17.3 in 40 per cent oxygen. It is decided to put him on to nasal continuous positive airway pressure (NCPAP) and a gas repeated in 30 minutes. His repeated gas shows no improvement and the tertiary level unit is contacted.

Following discussion, it is decided that Nathanial needs to have is respiratory support escalated and he requires intubation and ventilation.

Q.1. What information needs to exchange between the two units at this time?

On the advice of the tertiary unit, Nathanial is intubated and ventilated and central lines (UAC and UVC) are inserted. His arterial blood gas on pressures 22/5, rate 40, 75 per cent oxygen is pH 7.1, PCO_2 8.0, PO_2 3.1, BE 3.0, Bicarbonate 18.9.

The tertiary unit is contacted again and the decision is made to retrieve Nathanial for further management in a level 3 neonatal unit 50 miles away.

Q.2. What further information needs to be exchanged at this point?

Q.3. What does the tertiary unit's transport team need to organise and prepare at this point?

Q.4. What extra equipment might be required to stabilise and transfer Nathanial?

Q.5. How would the transport team calculate the amount of oxygen that needs to be carried for this transfer?

On the team's arrival in the referring unit, Robert is present but Julia is still in the recovery area of the delivery unit.

Q.6. What are the aspects of this situation that the retrieving team need to consider?

Q.7. What are the major factors that need to be considered when moving Nathanial from his cot space into the transport incubator?

Q.8. Who has legal responsibility for Nathanial's care and treatment at this time?

Acknowledgements

Stevie Boyd was the author of this chapter in the first edition.

References

Alfonso, D., Hurst, I., Mayberry, L. *et al.* (1992) 'Stressors reported by mothers of hospitalised premature infants', *Neonatal Network* 11(6): 63–9.

ALSG (Advanced Life Support Group) (1997) 'Transport of children', in *Advanced Paediatric Life Support: The Practical Approach*, London: BMJ Publishing Group.

Aoki, B.Y. and McCloskey, K. (1992) 'Physiology of air transport', in B.Y. Aoki and K. McCloskey (eds) *Evaluation, Stabilisation and Transport of the Critically Ill Child*, St Louis, MO: Mosby.

Barry, P. and Leslie, A. (2003) *Paediatric and Neonatal Critical Care Transport*, London: BMJ Books.

Bloodworth, K. (1995) 'Neonatal flying squads', *Child Health* 2(5): 192–3.

Bose, C. (1989) 'Organisation and administration of a perinatal transport service', in M. MacDonald (ed.) *Transport of the Perinatal Patient*, Boston: Little, Brown.

Bourchier, D. (1994) 'The transport of surgical neonates', in N.V. Freeman, D.M. Burge, M. Griffiths and P.S.J. Malone (eds) *Surgery of the Newborn*, London: Churchill Livingstone.

BPA (British Paediatric Association) (1993) *The Transfer of Infants and Children for Surgery*, London: BPA.

Cheema, I.U., Bomont, R.K. and Hare, A.B. (2007) 'Planned neonatal transfers by a centralised nurse-led team', *Infant* 3(3): 112–15.

Coffman, S., Levitt, M. and Guacci-Franco, N. (1993) 'Mother's stress and close relationships correlates with infant health status', *Pediatric Nursing* 19(2): 135–40.

Commission for Healthcare Audit and Inspection July (2008) *Towards Better Births: A Review of Maternity Services in England*, London: author.

Cooke, R.W.L. (1992) 'In utero transfer to specialist centres', *Archives of Disease in Childhood* 58: 483–4.

Dodds-Azzopardi, S.E. and Chapman, J.S. (1995) 'Parents' perceptions of stress associated with premature infant transfer among hospital environments', *Journal of Perinatal and Neonatal Nursing* 8(4): 39–46.

Fenton, A.C. and Mitchell, K. (2007) 'Neonatal transport practitioners: a viable alternative to traditional transfer teams?', *Infant* 3(5): 202.

Field, D.J. (1999) 'Organisation of perinatal care', in J.M. Rennie and N.R.C. Roberton (eds) *Textbook of Neonatology*, Edinburgh: Livingstone.

Finterswald, W. (1998) 'Neonatal transport: communication: the essential element', *Journal of Perinatology* 8(4): 358–60.

Kelly, M., Ferguson-Clarke, L. and Marsh, M.J. (1996) 'A new retrieval service', *Paediatric Nursing* 8(6): 18–20.

Krug, S.E. (1995) 'Principles and philosophy of transport stabilisation', in K. McCloskey and R. Orr (eds) *Pediatric Transport Medicine*, London: C.V. Mosby.

Leslie, A. (1997) 'Transferring sick babies: the new practicalities', *Journal of Neonatal Nursing* 6(7): 10–12.

Leslie, A. and Middleton, D. (1995) 'Give and take in neonatal transport', *Journal of Neonatal Nursing* 1(5): 27–31.

Lyall, J. (1993) 'Risk factors', *Nursing Times* 89(31): 23.

Macrae, D.J. (1994) 'Paediatric intensive care transport', *Archives of Disease in Childhood* 71: 175–8.

Madar, R.J. and Milligan, D.W.A. (1994) 'Neonatal transport: safety and security' (Letter), *Archives of Disease in Childhood: Fetal and Neonatal Edition* 71: F147–F148.

Major, C.W. (1996) 'Organisation of a neonatal transport programme', in D.G. Jaimovitch and D. Vidyasagar (eds) *Pediatric and Neonatal Transport Medicine*, Philadelphia, PA: Hanley & Belfus Inc.

Medical Devices Agency (1995) *Transport of Neonates in Ambulances*, London: Department of Health.

Melville, M. and Print, M. (1996) 'Legal issues surrounding neonatal emergency transport: minimising the risk of litigation', *Journal of Neonatal Nursing* 2(4): 18–22.

Nursing and Midwifery Council (2008) *The Code*, London: NMC.

Wallen, E., Venkataraman, S.T., Grosso, M.J. *et al.* (1995) 'Intrahospital transport of critically ill pediatric patients', *Critical Care Medicine* 23(9): 1588–95.

Watts, C. (2001) 'The role of the ANNP: nurse-led neonatal transport', *Journal of Neonatal Nursing* 7(6): 196–200.

Watts, C., Trim, E., Metherall, J. and Lightfoot, E. (2008) 'Neonatal transport: the comfort zone', *Infant* 4(1): 27–30.

Wilman, D. (1997) 'Neonatal transport: the effect on parents', *Journal of Neonatal Nursing* 3(5): 16–22.

Chapter 18

Medication in the Newborn

**Catherine Hall and
Peter Mulholland**

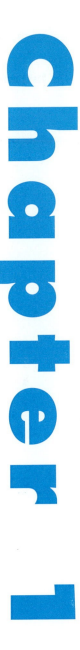

Contents

Introduction

The interest in the use of medicines in children has grown considerably over the last few years, with neonates being a unique group within this population. They have altered renal and hepatic function in comparison with adults and older children. They also have limited ability to absorb medicines enterally, particularly when they are sick. It is rarely appropriate to prescribe medicines to neonates purely as a proportion of the adult dose. Medicines tend not to be manufactured with the neonate in mind and are frequently supplied in a form that makes administration difficult, both in calculation and delivery of the dose. This creates problems for the staff on the neonatal unit in terms of the administration and economic use of drugs. Many medicines used in neonates are either not licensed, or used off-label, i.e. outside the terms of the marketing authorisation (previously known as the product licence). This may be a matter of great concern to staff working in a neonatal intensive care unit as information is often collected in infants after the drug has been used in adults. It is the responsibility of health professionals to ensure that toxicity of medicines is kept to a minimum but that children are not denied appropriate medicines (Choonara *et al.* 1996). In order for nurses to both safely administer drugs to neonates and monitor their effects, it is important that they have an understanding of the way that the body deals with drugs.

This chapter will not attempt to provide comprehensive guidance on dosage and specific details of drug administration; it will, however, aim to provide information on the way in which neonates handle drugs in the body (**pharmacokinetics**) and the importance of this information in both the calculation of drug doses and drug monitoring. The use of unlicensed medicines will also be considered.

Nurses have a professional responsibility to have an understanding of medications they administer (NMC 2008) and most units will have guidelines and policies which should be followed. Since 2005, the *British National Formulary for Children* (*BNF for Children*) (Joint Formulary Committee 2008) has been published in the UK providing prescribers, pharmacists and other health professionals with up-to-date information on medicines for children, including advice that goes beyond that included in marketing authorisations. The 2008 edition now includes additional information on the use of medicines in neonates. Other texts which also contain detailed drug information include *Medicines for Children* (RCPCH 2003) and *The Neonatal Formulary* (Northern Neonatal Network 2007).

Unlicensed medicines

In 1968, the Medicines Act was introduced to provide legislation covering licensing of medicines to try to ensure safety, quality and efficacy. The Act was in response to drug-related toxicities which occurred with thalidomide (**phocomelia**) in the developing fetus and chloramphenicol ('grey baby syndrome') in neonates (Mulhall *et al.* 1983). Despite this legislation, infants and children continue to receive medicines that have not been subject to the licensing system (Choonara and Dunne 1998). In the United Kingdom, most medicines have a Marketing Authorisation issued by the Medicines and Healthcare Products Regulatory Agency (MHRA) which delineates the indications for which a medicine can be prescribed and the recommended dose. Currently, many medicines used in children and neonates are not covered by the Marketing Authorisation – that is, their safety and efficacy have not been endorsed by the manufacturers. Medicines that are used which have a Marketing Authorisation but do not have an indication for use in children are said to be used 'off-label'.

Similarly the formulations available of many medicines are not suitable for administration to children. It may be necessary for the pharmacist to manipulate the medicine in some way to enable it to be administered to a child (Nahata 1999). Tablets that may need to be crushed to form a suspension, injections or parenteral nutrition which are provided in a ready-to-administer form by a pharmacy aseptic unit, and medicines that are imported from another country are all examples of unlicensed use of medicines.

It is not illegal for a prescriber to prescribe, a pharmacist to dispense and a nurse to administer an off-label or unlicensed medicine, as the Medicines Act 1968 makes provision for this to take place. The licence prevents pharmaceutical companies from promoting an unlicensed product or an unlicensed use of a product. The prescriber carries responsibility for the prescribing of the medication. The standard reference texts which provide drug information are often of little use in neonatal prescribing and it is necessary to refer to more specialist paediatric or neonatal formularies, for example, *British National Formulary for Children (BNF-C)*, published in the UK each year (Joint Formulary Committee 2008).

A study carried out in a neonatal intensive care unit by Conroy *et al.* (1999) demonstrated that 90 per cent of patients were given a drug that was either unlicensed or used off-label. Nearly 55 per cent of prescriptions were off-label and 10 per cent were unlicensed.

In May 1996, a joint working party between the British Paediatric Association (BPA), now known as the Royal College of Paediatrics and Child Health (RCPCH) and the Association of the British Pharmaceutical Industry (ABPI) published a report on the licensing of medicines in children (Working Party of the BPA and ABPI 1996). In 1997, European guidelines were published on the clinical investigation of medicines in children. This document (European Agency for the Evaluation of Medicinal Products 1997) states: 'There is a responsibility shared by applicants and the competent authorities to ensure that children have timely access to safe and effective medicines which have accurate, scientifically justified, prescribing information.' The problem has been addressed in the United States of America by establishing several paediatric research units to set up clinical trials to investigate drug use in children.

In 1999, the Standing Committee on Medicines, a joint committee of the Royal College of Paediatrics and Child Health and the Neonatal and Paediatric

Pharmacists Group issued a statement entitled 'The Use of Unlicensed Medicines or Licensed Medicines for Unlicensed Applications in Paediatric Practice', which aimed to inform and guide health professionals and parents who prescribe, dispense or administer medicines for children, and health service managers who have a responsibility to support them, on the use of unlicensed medicines in neonates and children.

In 2004, the European Commission made proposals to tackle the problem of unlicensed medicines in children in a draft Regulation. In 2006, the European Medicines Agency (EMEA) introduced a 'Guideline on Conduct of Pharmacovigilance for Medicines Used by the Paediatric Population' (Doc. Ref. EMEA/CHMP/PhVWP/235910/2005).

Nurse prescribing

The primary legislation to enable nurses and midwives to prescribe is the Medicinal Products prescription by Nurses and Others Act 1992. Since then, there have been several legislative changes to widen the scope of non-medical prescribing. Recent legislation was enacted to enable nurses and midwives to prescribe independently and as supplementary prescribers.

Independent prescribers are expected to prescribe only within their competence and to understand that they are accountable and responsible for their prescribing regardless of the advice they receive prior to writing a prescription. Non-medical prescribers are accountable for their acts and omissions and cannot delegate this accountability to any other person.

Prescribing outside the legal parameters of either supplementary or independent prescribing is a criminal offence.

Non-medical prescribers are responsible for ensuring they work within their profession's standards and keep up to date with these standards.

Pharmacokinetics

Pharmacokinetics is a mathematical way of describing the way in which the body handles a drug. The most important processes involved are *bioavailability*, *distribution* and *clearance*, as defined below. These factors vary between individuals and need to be considered when determining a dosage regimen.

Neonates are a diverse group in terms of their renal and hepatic maturity, making it extremely difficult to predict how an individual infant will respond to a drug.

Bioavailability describes the extent of the administered dose which is available unchanged in the body to exert a pharmacological action. If a drug is given by the intravenous route, the entire dose is available; in other words, it is 100 per cent bioavailable or has a bioavailabilty of 1.0. Medicines given by the enteral route may be incompletely absorbed or be partially metabolised by the gut or liver before entering the systemic circulation – hence they have a bioavailability of less than 100 per cent;. a drug that is only 80 per cent absorbed has a bioavailability of 0.8; drugs given by other routes, including rectal, percutaneous, intramuscular and subcutaneous, usually have reduced bio-availability compared with the intravenous route. Chemical properties of the drug, such as formulation, will also determine the rate and extent of absorption.

Several factors affect the absorption from the gastrointestinal tract. The most relevant are *gastric emptying* and *gastric pH* – both of which continue to change with maturation of the infant. In the term infant, gastric pH is neutral at birth, drops to 1.5–3.0 during the first few hours, returning to neutral over the next 24 hours. For the following two weeks of life there is relative achlorhydria (production of gastric acid in the stomach is absent or low). In the preterm infant there is no initial fall in pH because of immature secretory mechanisms (Morselli 1989). The gastric emptying rate is prolonged in neonates compared with older infants; it is further delayed in premature neonates compared with term infants. Gastrointestinal transit time and peristalsis are increased in infants; these are also influenced by the type of feed the infant receives. For example, prolonged gastric emptying times were demonstrated with feeds of increasing calorie density (Siegal *et al*. 1984). The delay in gastric emptying may decrease or delay the peak concentration of a drug which is given by the oral route, although the clinical significance of this is not known.

A combination of these factors contributes to the erratic and unpredictable gastrointestinal absorption. In infants who are shocked, acidotic or obviously unwell, there is a risk of paralytic ileus and delayed absorption with enteral medication.

After the drug has entered the systemic circulation by whatever route, it has to be distributed throughout the body. *Distribution* is influenced by chemical properties of the drug, route of administration and patient variability. Many of the factors that influence drug distribution change markedly as the neonate matures. For the purposes of simplification, the body can be described in terms of an extracellular and an intracellular compartment, the extracellular compart-ment being the greater. Water-soluble drugs are distributed mainly in this compartment. This process is described by the *one-compartment model*. It is assumed that after the drug appears in the blood it quickly distributes within the body tissues so that the rate of change of the concentration of the drug in the blood is equivalent to the rate of change of the concentration in all body tissues. It is important to remember, however, that many drugs distribute in more than one compartment – for example, two compartments, where one is a small compartment made up of the plasma and well-perfused organs (brain, liver, gastrointestinal system, heart and kidneys) and a second compartment is made up of the rest of the body. The drug concentration in each compartment will vary at any given time (Roberts 1984). The apparent space into which the drug distributes is described by the *volume of distribution*. It does not actually refer to a physiological volume but does indicate the total amount of drug in the body relative to the concentration in the blood. In neonates, total body water makes up to 75 per cent of the total body weight and it may be as high as 85 per cent in preterm infants. Water-soluble drugs that distribute into body water, such as furosemide, therefore, have a greater volume of distribution in neonates compared with adults. This means that for a given dose of drug the total concentration in neonates is lower.

Fat only contributes about 20 per cent of body weight in children, and is further reduced in the neonate compared to older children.

After a drug has been absorbed into the systemic circulation, it is either a free drug or bound to plasma proteins. Only free drugs are active and can exert a therapeutic effect. Plasma proteins are relatively large molecules with binding sites on the surface. A circulating free drug attaches to the binding site, becomes bound and therefore inactive. Drug-protein binding is a reversible process. Drugs have differing affinities for plasma proteins. Any factor that affects the extent of binding to plasma proteins will affect the amount of active drug in the body. These factors include administration of other plasma proteins (such as albumin), presence of other drugs which have a stronger affinity for plasma proteins, and other compounds, such as bilirubin, which bind to plasma proteins. For example, phenytoin is highly protein bound (~90 per cent) and most biochemical assays only report total phenytoin levels (bound + unbound). Where protein binding is altered, total phenytoin levels are misleading as no account is made of the 'free' fraction that is available. Thus corrections may need to be made in periods of hypoalbuminaemia to account for the proportion of 'free' phenytoin available to exert effect.

Acidic drugs tend to bind primarily to albumin compared with basic drugs, which have a greater affinity for other proteins – alpha-1 acid glycoprotein and lipoprotein. These proteins are different in infants from adults, both in the concentration in the body and in their affinity for drugs. Neonatal albumin has a reduced binding capacity for drugs compared with adult albumin. For example, greater concentrations of free drug were found in cord blood (which contains fetal albumin) compared with concentrations found in adult plasma for several drugs including phenobarbital, penicillins and morphine (Reed and Besunder 1989). There is a theoretical risk that there will be competition for albumin binding sites between drugs and bilirubin. Displacement of bilirubin from albumin by drugs could result in bilirubin encephalopathy. This is historically reported with sulphonamides which resulted in many babies suffering brain damage as a result of their antibiotic medication (Silverman *et al.* 1956). There is only likely to be a significant problem with displacement of bilirubin with drugs which are more than 90 per cent protein bound (Rylance 1991). The affinity for binding to albumin by bilirubin is considerably greater than most drugs and therefore the clinical significance of this is still not known.

Clearance describes the rate of drug removal and can be described in terms of plasma clearance, organ clearance or total body clearance. There are two main processes involved in the clearance of drugs from the body – metabolism, primarily in the liver, and excretion by the kidney. Lipid-soluble drugs need to be converted into more water-soluble compounds in the liver before being removed by the kidney. Total body clearance is the sum of these processes.

The processes by which drugs are modified in the liver are known as *biotransformation reactions*, which can be subdivided into phase I (non-synthetic)

446

and phase II (synthetic) reactions. Phase I reactions include oxidation, reduction and hydrolysis which result in the formation of inactive compounds or alternatively active metabolites. These compounds are usually more water-soluble than the original drug and hence can be removed more easily by the kidney. This group of reactions depends on enzyme systems in the membranes of the hepatic microsomal endoplasmic reticulum or enzymes present in other parts of the liver (deaminases) or the blood (esterases). Phase II reactions involve conjugation with glucuronic acid or glycine and sulphate production. These reactions involve liver microsomal pathways (e.g. **cytochrome** P 450) and take place in the mitochondria and in solution in the cell cytoplasm. The drug molecule is rendered inactive as a result of the attached group (e.g. glucuronide) preventing it from crossing biological membranes (Ohning 1995b).

In neonates, these metabolic processes are immature, the extent of which depends on the gestational and postnatal age of the infant. The different metabolic reactions mature at different rates. Cytochrome P 450 activity is about half the adult capacity in term infants. Sulphation and glycination occur at similar rates to adults but glucuronidation is reduced (Rylance 1991).

Removal of drugs and their metabolites may also be performed by the kidney. The factors which effect elimination are blood flow to the kidneys, glomerular filtration and tubular secretion and reabsorption.

Premature infants have a reduced degree of glomerular filtration compared with babies born at term and the rate of maturation is correspondingly slower. It reaches similar rates to adults at around 5 months of age. Glomeruli continue to be produced up to 35 weeks' gestation so it follows that a baby born preterm will have a reduced number of glomeruli and therefore a lower **glomerular filtration rate** (GFR).

Glomerular filtration in the kidney allows removal of small molecules, which include most drugs, but not large plasma proteins. The free drug molecules are transferred into the renal tubules by glomerular filtration. This process cannot remove protein-bound drug molecules. If the infant becomes hypotensive, the GFR will fall and the rate of removal of drugs by the kidney will be reduced. If this is not taken into account when calculating a suitable dose of a drug, it may result in drug accumulation and toxicity. Any process which affects renal blood flow will influence drug clearance by the kidney.

Most drugs are removed by the liver, the kidney or a combination of the two. Gentamicin is excreted purely by the kidney and because of its potential toxicity should be closely monitored, particularly in babies with impaired renal function. Paracetamol and morphine are examples of drugs that are mainly metabolised by the liver. In adults and children, paracetamol is metabolised by glucuronidation. In preterm infants, however, this pathway is immature, so the sulphation pathway is utilised. This mechanism is only used in preterm infants. Phenobarbital is removed from the body by a mixture of renal and hepatic mechanisms. This is a much slower process in a neonate compared with an older child and explains the prolonged neonatal half-life of phenobarbital, which may be up to 200 hours compared with around 70 hours in children.

It is clear that it is important to know how the body deals with drug elimination when prescribing for neonates. The rate at which a drug is removed from the body is described by the pharmacokinetic term *elimination half-life*, which can be defined as the time it takes for the concentration of drug in the blood to fall by a half. The maturity of the infant will affect the pathways available for drug metabolism and excretion. As such, dosage regimens should be adjusted to take into account the gestational and postnatal age of the infant. As the baby matures, the metabolic processes used may change, as with paracetamol. If a drug is given to an infant where there is not a mature metabolic pathway capable of handling the drug, accumulation and toxicity may develop.

The different pharmacokinetic parameters illustrate the different clinical effects of drugs. Morphine has a prolonged half-life in preterm infants of 6–14 hours compared with 2–11 hours in term babies. Morphine is metabolised by glucuronidation in the liver to form two metabolites – morphine-6-glucuronide (M6G) and morphine-3-glucuronide (M3G). M6G is a potent analgesic itself and also is a respiratory depressant but M3G antagonises the analgesic effects of both morphine and M6G and stimulates respiration. M3G has been found to be the predominant metabolite in sick preterm infants with M6G being present to a variable extent because of the reduced ability by premature neonates to convert morphine to M6G (Hartley *et al.* 1993). The variability in clinical response to morphine may be explained by the variability in morphine metabolism in sick neonates. Infants who produce significant amounts of M6G experience a greater analgesic and sedative effect than those who are able to conjugate M6G to a lesser extent (Bhat *et al.* 1992).

Diamorphine (diacetylmorphine) is a semi-synthetic derivative of morphine which is metabolised to morphine. It, like morphine, is given as a loading dose followed by a continuous infusion (Barker *et al.* 1995). It has little to offer over morphine with the exception that it causes less histamine release and may cause less hypotension. The hypotension which occurs may be due to a reduction in stress in the infant as a result of the analgesic and sedative effect (Elias-Jones *et al.* 1991). Diamorphine has similar effects to morphine on respiration and the gut. It is more lipid-soluble than morphine, which may cause sedation more quickly than morphine (Wood *et al.* 1998).

Fentanyl is also used as an analgesic and sedative in neonatal intensive care. It has a shorter duration of action than morphine and is 50–100 times more potent, primarily as a result of its greater lipid solubility. It has a half-life of 6–32 hours in neonates (Koehntop *et al.* 1986) which is prolonged in babies undergoing ligation of a patent ductus arteriosus (Olkkola *et al.* 1995). It is eliminated almost entirely by metabolism in the liver. Fentanyl is given as a loading dose followed by a continuous infusion. The main advantage of fentanyl over other opiates is that it rarely causes haemodynamic instability since it is unlikely to cause histamine release. One study in neonates has also indicated that fentanyl may cause fewer problems with gastrointestinal motility and therefore enteral feeding (Saarenmaa *et al.* 1999). Its disadvantage is that it can cause severe muscle rigidity that may require muscle relaxants to counteract.

Chloral hydrate is a sedative with no analgesic properties. It is usually given orally, although it can also be given rectally. Chloral hydrate has a long but variable half-life, particularly in preterm infants and those with impaired renal and hepatic function. It may also displace bilirubin from its binding sites and long-term use may cause hyperbilirubinaemia. Chloral hydrate is metabolised in the liver to trichloroacetic acid and trichloroethanol, which also has sedative properties (Alexander and Todres 1998). The main side-effect is gastric irritation and it has been associated with paradoxical agitation. There is a risk of accumulation of chloral hydrate because of its long half-life which has been associated with toxicity. Long-term use should be avoided.

Therapeutic drug monitoring (TDM)

TDM is necessary in neonates because doses required are often very different from those used in children and adults. It is usually used when the therapeutic concentration of a drug and the toxic concentration are close together. This type of drug is said to have a *narrow therapeutic index*. The drugs which are most commonly monitored in neonates include the aminoglycosides (gentamicin, netilmicin, amikacin, tobramycin), vancomycin, phenobarbital, phenytoin and theophylline (Patrick 1995). The drug levels required in neonates may be different from those in older children or adults. A good example of this is theophylline (Table 18.1).

The main problem with TDM in neonates is that it usually requires blood samples. Not only is this painful for the infant but due to a low circulating blood volume, it can also contribute to iatrogenic anaemia necessitating blood transfusions (Gilman 1990). With a blood volume of 80–100ml/kg, a premature neonate weighing 500g will only have a total blood volume of 40–50ml. Laboratories that have microassay techniques available should be used for TDM in infants (Koren 1997). Some drugs will require both trough levels (blood taken immediately before a dose when the concentration is at its lowest) and peak levels (blood taken at a specified time after a dose when the concentration is thought to be at its highest) and some may only require trough levels to be measured. It is important that levels are measured at the correct time, and this varies from drug to drug, otherwise the information could at best be meaningless and at worst be dangerous. Serum concentrations have been determined for the narrow therapeutic

Table 18.1 A comparison of serum theophylline in children and adults

Desired therapeutic range (mg/L)

Neonates	Children and adults
8–12	10–20

Source: Adapted from BNF-C (2008).

Table 18.2 Plasma elimination half-lives (in hours) of some drugs given to neonates

Drug	Preterm infants	Term infants
Caffeine	31–132	26–231
Gentamicin	3.5–16.1	2.3–5.9
Phenobarbital	60–200	41–120
Phenytoin	60–130	10–100

Source: Adapted from Rylance (1991).

index drugs which relate concentration to therapeutic effect and toxicity (Sagraves 1995).

Drug levels are usually taken when it is expected that the drug will have reached a steady state within the body; that is, when the rate of absorption is equal to the rate of elimination. This is usually taken as four to five times the half-life of the drug. The half-life will vary between individuals and is also influenced by the age of the patient. Some examples are shown in Table 18.2. For drugs that have a long half-life, such as phenobarbital, it can take many hours or even days to reach the desired therapeutic blood level. It is for this reason that loading doses are given with these drugs at the beginning of a course of treatment before dropping down to a lower maintenance dose, to enable therapeutic drug levels to be reached more quickly.

Drug administration

In many situations in neonatal practice, the choice of formulations available may be as important as drug selection. A dearth of suitable preparations available for administration to neonates can cause problems for the neonatal nurse. As a result of this, there is an increased risk of medication errors taking place (Koren *et al.* 1986). Many drugs will need to be diluted prior to administration purely to allow accurate measurement of the required dose (Northern Neonatal Network 2007).

It is clear that dose selection is a complex issue in the neonate. It is important to remember that as well as the rapid changes that occur in renal and hepatic function, the baby's weight can also change quite rapidly. The dose of a drug may need to be adjusted to take this into account (Walson *et al.* 1993). It is not sensible to adjust doses on a daily weight change but doses should be reviewed on a weekly basis depending on the drugs prescribed and the patient involved. Similarly, as the infant matures, the dosage frequency may need to be increased, for example, with penicillin.

Particularly in babies who are very sick and requiring intensive care, vascular ccess and fluid volumes may become a problem. It may be necessary to infuse more than one drug in the same line. Although this should be avoided wherever possible, there will be situations where it is unavoidable. Some drugs can be given together via a Y-connector which is placed as near to the patient as is possible to minimise the contact time between the drugs (Trissel 2007; Zenk 2003). Drug compatibilities should always be confirmed with a pharmacist. If drugs are considered to be incompatible, then they should be separated by a bolus injection of sodium chloride or glucose depending on the drugs involved. Compatibility of the drug with the infusate must also be established. Drugs should not be co-infused with blood or other blood products, for example, albumin and platelets.

The type of line used for access may influence how a drug is given. It may often be possible for a drug to be given in more concentrated solutions if it is administered via a central venous catheter than if it were given via a peripheral cannula. Concentrated glucose solutions (greater than 10 per cent) should not be given via a peripheral cannula as there is an increased risk of phlebitis and extravasation injury due to the increased osmolarity of the solution (Duck 1997; RCN 2007).

Conclusion

The use of medicines in the neonatal population is a complex issue. Neonates should no longer be considered as 'therapeutic orphans', as they have been described in the past. Drug therapy is increasingly complicated and the neonatal nurse needs to have a good grasp of the basic pharmacokinetic principles to allow the safe administration of medicines and monitoring of the prescribed treatment. It is important that there is a team approach to the use of medicines in neonates; the doctor, nurse and pharmacist all have a role to play.

Case study: prescription of medication for a baby born at 24 weeks' gestation

Baby Kim weighed 650g when born at 24 weeks' gestation. Her mother had ruptured membranes at 21 weeks and received one course of betamethasone. At birth the baby was floppy, bradycardic and gave a single gasp. She was ventilated and had one dose of surfactant, followed 12 hours later by a second dose.

Plan for Kim

Day 1   FBC, blood culture. Double dose benzylpenicillin + gentamicin, im vitamin K.

Day 2   TPN ordered and enteral feeds started at 0.5ml/h.

Day 3   Bile-stained aspirates, feeds stopped. Benzylpenicillin stopped, amoxycillin and metronidazole added.

Day 4   Hypernatraemic dehydration, sodium = 160mmol/l.

Day 5   Abdominal distension, bile-stained aspirates.

Further investigations revealed necrotising enterocolitis.

Q.1.   What factors do you need to consider when prescribing medication for a baby born at 24 weeks' gestation?

Q.2.   Which of the medicines prescribed warrant special monitoring? Would this present any problems?

Q.3.   The baby suffered from hypernatraemic dehydration. Would this affect the likelihood of toxicity developing with any of the medication?

Q.4.   Could any of the antibiotics prescribed be given orally? What are the important points to consider?

Acknowledgements

Catherine Hall was the author of this chapter in the first edition.

References

Alexander, S.M. and Todres, I.D. (1998) 'The use of sedation and muscle relaxation in the ventilated infant', *Clinics in Perinatology* 25(1): 63–78.

Barker, D.P., Simpson, J., Pawula, M., Barrett, D.A., Shaw, P.N. and Rutter, N. (1995) 'Randomised, double blind trial of two loading dose regimens of diamorphine in ventilated newborn infants', *Archives of Disease in Childhood: Fetal and Neonatal Edition* 73: F22–F26.

Bhat, R., Abu-Harb, M., Chari, G. and Gulati, A. (1992) 'Morphine metabolism in acutely ill preterm newborn infants', *Journal of Pediatrics* 120(5): 795–9.

Chay, P.C.W., Duffy, B.J. and Walker, J.S. (1992) 'Pharmacokinetic–pharmacodynamic relationships of morphine in neonates', *Clinical Pharmacology and Therapeutics* 51(3): 334–42.

Choonara, I. and Dunne, J. (1998) 'Licensing of medicines', *Archives of Disease in Childhood* 78: 402–3.

Choonara, I., Gill, A. and Nunn, A. (1996) 'Drug toxicity and surveillance in children', *British Journal of Clinical Pharmacology* 42: 407–10.

Conroy, S., McIntyre, J. and Choonara, I. (1999) 'Unlicensed and off label drug use in neonates', *Archives of Disease in Childhood: Fetal and Neonatal Edition* 80: F142–F145.

Duck, S. (1997) 'Neonatal intravenous therapy', *Journal of Intravenous Nursing* 20(3): 121–8.

Elias-Jones, A.C., Barrett, D.A., Rutter, N., Shaw, P.N. and Davis, S.S. (1991) 'Diamorphine infusion in the preterm neonate', *Archives of Disease in Childhood* 66: 1155–7.

European Agency for the Evaluation of Medicinal Products (1997) *Note for Guidance on Clinical Investigation of Medicinal Products in Children*, London: EAEMP.

European Agency for the Evaluation of Medicinal Products (2006) *Guideline on Conduct of Pharmacovigilance for Medicines Used by the Paediatric Population*, London: EMEA.

Gilman, J.T. (1990) 'Therapeutic drug monitoring in the neonate and paediatric age group: problems and clinical pharmacokinetic implications', *Clinical Pharmacokinetics* 19(1): 1–10.

Hartley, R., Green, M., Quinn, M. and Levene, M.I. (1993) 'Pharmacokinetics of morphine infusion in premature neonates', *Archives of Disease in Childhood: Fetal and Neonatal Edition* 69: F55–F58.

Joint Formulary Committee (2007) *British National Formulary for Children*, London: British Medical Association, Royal Pharmaceutical Society of Great Britain, Royal College of Paediatrics and Child Health and Neonatal and Paediatric Pharmacists Group.

Koehntop, D.E., Rodman, J.H., Brundage, D.M., Hegland, M.G. and Buckley, J.J. (1986) 'Pharmacokinetics of fentanyl in neonates', *Anesthesia and Analgesia* 65: 227–32.

Koren, G. (1997) 'Therapeutic drug monitoring principles in the neonate', *Clinical Chemistry* 43(1): 222–7.

Koren, G., Barzilay, Z. and Greenwald, M. (1986) 'Tenfold errors in administration of drug doses: a neglected iatrogenic disease in pediatrics', *Pediatrics* 77: 848–9.

Morselli, P.L. (1989) 'Clinical pharmacology of the perinatal period and early infancy', *Clinical Pharmacokinetics* 17: 13–28.

Mulhall, A., de Louvois, J. and Hurley, R. (1983) 'Chloramphenicol toxicity in the neonate: its incidence and prevention', *British Medical Journal* 287: 1424–7.

Nahata, M.C. (1999) 'Pediatric drug formulations: challenges and potential solutions', *Annals of Pharmacotherapy* 33: 247–9.

Northern Neonatal Network (2007) *The Neonatal Formulary*, London: BMJ.

Nursing and Midwifery Council (2008) *Standards for Medicines Management*, London: NMC.

Ohning, B.L. (1995a) 'Neonatal pharmacodynamics – basic principles I: Drug delivery', *Neonatal Network* 14(2): 7–12.

Ohning, B.L. (1995b) 'Neonatal pharmacodynamics – basic principles II: Drug action and elimination', *Neonatal Network* 14(2): 15–19.

Olkkola, K.Y., Hamunen, K. and Maunuksela, E. (1995) 'Clinical pharmacokinetics and pharmacodynamics of opioid analgesics in infants and children', *Clinical Pharmacokinetics* 28(5): 385–404.

Patrick, C.H. (1995) 'Therapeutic drug monitoring in neonates', *Neonatal Network* 14(2): 21–6.

RCPCH (2003) *Medicines for Children*, London: Royal College of Paediatrics and Child Health.

Reed, M.D. and Besunder, J.B. (1989) 'Developmental pharmacology: ontogenic basis of drug disposition', *Pediatric Clinics of North America* 36(5): 1053–74.

Roberts, R.J. (1984) 'Pharmacokinetics: basic principles and clinical application', in *Drug Therapy in Infants: Pharmacologic Principles and Clinical Experience*, Philadelphia, PA: Saunders, pp. 13–24.

Royal College of Nursing (2007) *Standards for Infusion Therapy*, reprint, London: RCN.

Rylance, G. (1991) 'Pharmacological principles and kinetics', in G. Rylance, D. Harvey and J. Aranda (eds) *Neonatal Clinical Pharmacology and Therapeutics*, Oxford: Butterworth-Heinemann, pp. 1–25.

Saarenmaa, E., Huttunen, P., Leppaluoto, J., Meretoja, O. and Fellman, V. (1999)· 'Advantages of fentanyl over morphine in analgesia for ventilated newborn infants after birth: a randomized trial', *Journal of Pediatrics* 134(2): 144–50.

Sagraves, R. (1995) 'Pediatric dosing information for health care providers', *Journal of Pediatric Health Care* 9: 272–7.

Saint-Raymond, A. and Seigneuret, N. (2005) 'Medicines for children: time for Europe to act', *Paediatric and Perinatal Drug Therapy* 6: 142–6.

Siegal, M., Lebenthal, E. and Krantz, B. (1984) 'Effect of caloric density on gastric emptying in premature infants', *Journal of Pediatrics* 104: 118–22.

Silverman, W.A., Anderson, T.H., Blanc, W.A. and Crozier, D.N. (1956) 'A difference in mortality rate and incidence of kernicterus among premature infants allotted to two prophylactic antibacterial regimens', *Pediatrics* 18: 614–25.

Trissel, L.A. (2007) *Handbook on Injectable Drugs*, 14th edn, Maryland: American Society of Health-System Pharmacists.

Walson, P.D. (1997) 'Paediatric clinical pharmacology and therapeutics', in T.M. Speight and N.H.G. Holford (eds) *Avery's Drug Treatment*, Auckland: Adis International.

Walson, P.D., Getschman, S. and Koren, G. (1993) 'Principles of drug prescribing in infants and children', *Drugs* 46(2): 281–8.

Wood, C.M., Rushforth, J.A., Hartley, R., Dean, H., Wild, J. and Levene, M.I. (1998) 'Randomised double blind trial of morphine versus diamorphine for sedation of preterm neonates', *Archives of Disease in Childhood: Fetal and Neonatal Edition* 79: F34–F39.

Working Party of the British Paediatric Association and the Association of the British Pharmaceutical Industry (1996) *Licensing Medicines for Children*, London: British Paediatric Association.

Zenk, K.E. (2003) 'Y-site compatibility of common NICU drugs', in K.E. Zenk, J. Sills and R. Koeppel (eds) *Neonatal Medications and Nutrition: A Comprehensive Guide*, Santa Rosa, CA: NICU Inc.

Chapter 19

Bereavement in NICU

Joan Cameron

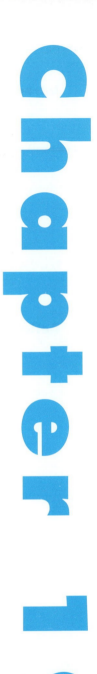

Contents

Introduction

Neonatal loss covers a range of issues from neonatal death to preterm birth and loss of function associated with the outcomes of neonatal care. Neonatal nurses and midwives are closely involved with vulnerable babies and their families and provide care in situations where loss features prominently. Neonatal loss is also linked with complex ethical, legal and professional issues when decisions need to be made about 'best interests' (see p. 478) and withholding or withdrawal of care. The rituals and practices surrounding loss are rooted in culture and neonatal staff must be able to deal with the complex emotional and social issues facing families experiencing neonatal loss. This chapter addresses the important challenges relating to neonatal loss facing neonatal staff and focuses specifically on neonatal death.

Defining loss

Neonatal loss is complex and can be experienced in different ways. A woman giving birth before term may experience a form of loss as she is denied the remainder of her pregnancy to prepare herself for the birth of her baby. Parents of babies who have physical or developmental anomalies may grieve for the loss of the 'normal' baby they were expecting.

The separation necessitated by the admission of the baby to the Neonatal Intensive Care Unit (NICU) can be experienced by parents as a form of loss. Neonatal death can occur soon after birth or may come after many months of neonatal intensive care. Parents may experience multiple instances of loss from the birth of a very preterm baby who then goes on to develop significant problems and who dies after a prolonged period of neonatal intensive care. Parents whose baby has a significant health problem, but survives, may find that the additional care their baby requires means that one or both parents have to relinquish paid employment to provide the care needed. This can lead to loss of status, as well as loss of income. Sometimes these two losses also lead to the loss of friends and social networks as parents no longer share common bonds.

In order to assist parents experiencing loss, neonatal nurses first have to accept that different forms of loss exist and they may be experienced in many ways by parents. Loss is therefore defined by the person experiencing the loss.

Context of neonatal loss in the UK

The incidence of neonatal and post-neonatal death rates (deaths between birth and 12 months) have continued to decrease in the UK. This means that it is relatively uncommon for parents to face the death of a baby. However, as increasing numbers of immature babies survive, parents are more likely to experience loss as a result of morbidity. The 'heroic' stories of tiny babies who survive which appear in the media rarely mention the chronic and sometimes life-limiting conditions which these tiny babies endure. Parents and their families may be completely unprepared for the loss of function and potential their baby may experience.

Babies who die and those who suffer from long-term morbidity are more likely to be born to mothers who register the birth on their own and are more likely to be born to parents from manual social classes (Acolet 2008). Parents from black and minority ethnic communities are also more likely to experience neonatal loss (ibid.). As life expectancy in the UK increases, parents may find that the death of their baby is their first experience of death. This may add to their sense of bewilderment as they try to cope with the emotional impact of the loss while negotiating the legal and social rituals that death necessitates. Neonatal nurses can assist parents by providing support and information at this time.

Grief, bereavement and mourning

Terms such as grief, mourning and bereavement may be used interchangeably but it is important to be clear about what we are saying when we use phrases that may be loaded with meaning. By clarifying our understanding confusion can be avoided.

Bereavement

Bereavement is an objective fact. It is the state of having lost something. In some societies it may be accompanied by a change in status. Neonatal nurses may come across parents wondering if the loss of their baby – especially if it is their only child – means that they are no longer considered as parents in the eyes of society. This change in status may be especially painful because it minimises or denies their loss.

Mourning

Mourning is a signal of distress caused by loss. Most societies have rituals that they follow as part of the mourning process. This may include wearing specific clothes, withdrawing from everyday life and adopting forms of behaviour to indicate that they have experienced a loss. In many westernised societies, mourning rituals have become restricted to the wearing of dark clothes at funerals. Mourning may be difficult for parents who have experienced neonatal loss. Family and friends may find it difficult to recognise the fact that the loss of a baby experienced by the parents is as profound as the loss of an adult. Neonatal nurses can help parents develop ways of indicating their distress to family and friends so that they can provide support.

Grief

Grief is a painful emotion that may be experienced physically, emotionally and behaviourally. Grief can manifest itself in many different ways. People experiencing grief may withdraw from the company of other people; they may deny themselves food; they may experience physical pain sometimes described as 'emptiness'. People who are grieving may experience sleep disturbances and loss of self-esteem. Some women describe how they 'ache' to hold a baby in their arms.

Grief is intensely personal and there is no right or wrong way to experience grief. However, there is some evidence to suggest that grieving parents find it helpful to have information about the range of feelings they may experience (Schott *et al.* 2007). This helps them cope as it 'normalises' the myriad emotions they may encounter and helps them to realise that they are not alone in their suffering. In particular, parents may seek reassurance that their feelings are not signs of madness.

Cultural and personal factors may be very influential in determining how people demonstrate their feelings towards the loss of a baby. It is clear that for the majority of people, grief is at its most intense in the immediate period following the loss but this is not true in all cases. Parkes (1972) and Lake *et al.* (1983) suggest that the normal period of mourning for the loss of a baby is six months to a year. De Frain *et al.* (1991) interviewed parents who had experienced a stillbirth. The parents in this study felt that it took two to three years to recover from the loss but for some it took up to eight years. In multiple births parents may have to deal with the death of one baby while caring for surviving infants. A mother who has been acutely unwell at the time of the birth may be unaware of the death of her infant.

It has been suggested that absence of a grief reaction is pathological. However, there is uncertainty over this. Zeanah *et al.* (1995) use the term 'minimisers' to describe the reactions of people who show a minimal response to loss. These individuals do not appear to show the 'expected' response to loss and appear to suffer no long-term psychological consequences. Some people have attempted to define grief as acute, chronic or complicated but there is little empirical evidence to support these definitions. Although parents may grieve for a long time after the death of their baby, it would seem sensible to suggest that they should seek professional help if their grief prevents them from participating in everyday activities after six months.

Fathers' experience of loss

Men are often expected to suppress their grief in order to support their partner who, it is assumed, will suffer more intensely from the loss of the baby. Men may also find that the need for them to return to work means that they have to suppress feelings of grief in order to take their place in the everyday world. Some research suggests the possibility of asynchronous grieving – where men appear to recover from the loss of the baby faster than their partner (Oliver 1999; Murray *et al.* 2000). However, most studies involving men have small samples and high drop-out rates so it is impossible to generalise these findings (Badenhorst *et al.* 2006). Mekosh-Rosenbaum and Lasker (1995) found that men and women had different ways of coping with the loss of a baby with men more likely to report the use of alcohol and women more likely to report the use of sedatives.

The death of a baby is a traumatic period for families and it has been reported that parents are more likely to divorce or separate after the death of a baby (Oliver 1999). While neonatal nurses cannot be expected to prevent relationship breakups, making parents aware of the possible stresses on their relationship and encouraging them to seek assistance may help them cope with the situation.

Grandparents, siblings and other family members and close friends may also experience loss and grief reactions. Their response to the loss depends on a number of factors: their relationship with the parents, their relationship with the baby and their previous experience of loss. With the permission of the parents, family and friends may be involved in some of the rituals and practices to say goodbye to the baby. They can also be given information about how they can support the baby's parents.

Parents may find their grief overwhelming and this may isolate them from family and friends. Within western societies people are generally given a few weeks to make the transition from bereavement to normal everyday life. Where an infant has spent all his or her life in a neonatal unit, their existence may not be acknowledged by the wider society. Parents have reported friends and family suggesting that the loss may have 'been for the best', or the best way to come to terms with the loss is to have another baby as soon as possible. When a baby dies, the parents may find that they are no longer regarded by family and friends as parents – especially if they have no living children. Their experience of caring for a baby in a neonatal intensive care unit is negated because there is no visible proof of the existence of the baby to the outside world. This lack of recognition of the baby as an individual in their own right may impact on how others respond to the needs of the parents to mourn and grieve their loss. Neonatal staff cannot prevent these situations from occurring but they can help prepare parents for the possibility that well-meaning people may make unhelpful comments and assist them in finding ways to respond to these comments constructively.

Anticipatory grief

Anticipatory grief is used to describe a situation where parents are aware of impending loss (Rando 1986). This may occur when parents have been told that their baby has a condition that is untreatable or where parents are convinced that their baby will die. Anticipating loss may be beneficial, as it can allow the parents to plan for the loss of their baby. This may include planning specific rituals to say goodbye to their baby and include family and friends. Sometimes anticipatory grief may be used as a protective mechanism by parents where they try to distance themselves from the baby in an effort to reduce the pain they may feel should the baby die. It has been suggested that this actually increases the parents' distress should the baby die as they feel guilty for not caring enough about the baby. There is little evidence to support this theory but neonatal nurses should be aware that some parents may find it difficult to form attachments with their baby if they believe that the baby will die and need help to explore and understand the complexity of their feelings.

Remembering anniversaries

Anniversaries are especially poignant for bereaved parents. These may include the expected date of the baby's birth, the baby's birthday and the anniversary of the baby's death. Peppers and Knapp (1980) referred to 'shadow grief' – meaning the memories stirred up on certain dates and times that can last a lifetime. However, they were careful to describe this as a part of normal behaviour and emphasised that remembrance of anniversaries should not be regarded as morbid or abnormal. If family and friends expect the bereaved couple to have 'moved on', anniversaries may be difficult to mark and may be lonely experiences. Again neonatal nurses can help by preparing parents for the potential impact of anniversaries. Parents may decide to mark the occasions and include family and friends. Alternatively, they may decide to withdraw and keep their memories private.

Theory and loss

The purpose of theory in relation to loss is to provide a framework for under-standing loss. Theories can help health professionals and parents come to terms with feelings and experiences relating to neonatal loss. It is important to recognise that loss theories are not 'facts' and that the theories cannot prescribe a right or wrong way to experience loss.

'Stages' or 'phase' models

Neonatal nurses may be aware of models of grief that involve a series of stages. Bowlby (1973) and Parkes (1972) developed models which suggest that the response to loss is in the form of orderly stages or phases as people adjust to the grief caused by separation. The model developed by Kübler Ross (1970) proposed stages including: denial, anger, bargaining, and depression as the inevitability of the loss is recognised. This is finally followed by acceptance of the loss. Although this model is quoted widely in texts relating to neonatal loss, it is important to recognise that the model was derived from a study looking at the reactions of a small group of people who had been given life-limiting diagnoses, rather than bereaved parents. While the model may help parents understand that it is normal to feel angry or isolated when they are bereaved, it may also result in stereotyping and inhibit appropriate responses from staff. For example, a parent who is justifiably angry may find that their feelings are dismissed by describing them as 'being in the anger phase of their grief cycle' rather than dealing with the cause of the anger.

'Grief work' models

Several theorists have produced models that incorporate the concept of grief work (Freud 1957; Worden 1991). These models typically involve confronting the reality of the loss, working through the grief and finally achieving resolution. These models inform some of the procedures that may be used in neonatal units where parents hold and photograph their dead baby. By seeing and holding their dead baby, the parents are able to recognise the finality of death. Grief work models also focus on encouraging parents to acknowledge their feelings and emotions and try to work through how they can resolve the emotional turmoil they are experiencing.

These models can be useful in enabling parents to understand their feelings and to enlist strategies to help them address their emotions. The final element of the grief work model, as in the stages models, is acceptance and 'moving on'. This can be problematic for some parents as it can lead to assumptions on the part of professionals and friends that there is a time when the bereaved parents will have 'recovered' and have put their loss behind them, when it is often the case that parents will remember their loss and the pain of bereavement for a lifetime.

'Continuing bonds' model

More recently models have emerged that focus on continuing bonds. These models challenge the assumption that the bereaved should relinquish their bonds with the dead baby and 'put the past behind them'. Klass *et al.* (1996) and Klass and Walter (2001) have based their theory of continuing bonds on the narratives of bereaved individuals who have related how they use the memory of the dead person to comfort them. The memories are dynamic and change over time and relate to the relationship the person had with the dead person. For example, the parents of a baby who died may imagine them going to school or playing with friends of a similar age in the playground. Klass and Walter (2001) contend that if this practice provides solace, then it is perfectly acceptable.

Because of the dominant role of models that emphasise the need to 'let go and move on' bereaved parents may be reluctant to share their thoughts and feelings about holding on to the memory of their dead baby. Neonatal nurses can use the continuing bonds theory to reassure parents that their desire to maintain a relationship with their dead baby is normal.

Cultural elements of loss

Many of the interventions relating to neonatal loss used in neonatal units are based on European and North American beliefs and practices. There is little information available about their use and acceptability within minority cultures. The evidence base for most of the practices is based on anecdotal evidence rather than robust studies and this, too, means that neonatal nurses must be careful in suggesting interventions for which there is a very limited evidence base and where negative effects may not be recognised (Lang *et al.* 2005; Gold 2007).

Caring for the dying baby

Interventions

The desire of parents and extended families to participate in the care of a dying baby may be influenced by their personal values and beliefs, the society in which they live and the environment in which care is being provided for the baby. It is important to ensure that parents are informed about options for care and their decisions are respected. Using phrases such as 'parents usually want . . .' or 'parents normally do this . . .' may make parents feel that they are obliged to do something they might otherwise not wish to do. McHaffie (2001) described how some parents in her study felt that they ought to participate in some of the rituals suggested by staff because they wanted to fit in with the culture of the neonatal unit. The parents were also worried that some healthcare staff might consider them to be 'bad' parents and uncaring if they did not want to participate in the caregiving activities.

Seeing and holding babies after death has become common practice in many neonatal units. There is evidence that some parents benefit from this but others do not wish to hold their baby and 'encouraging' them to do so in the belief that it will facilitate the grieving process is unhelpful and unkind (Turton *et al.* 2001). Some parents appreciate it when staff treat their baby's body as though the baby were still alive, while others find it disrespectful (McHaffie 2001). There is no easy solution to this situation but staff must be sensitive to the parents' emotions. If they speak to the baby as though they were still alive, the staff may follow their example.

Some cultures have specific rituals relating to the care of the dead. This may include who should handle them and how they may be washed and dressed. Parents of babies dealing with death for the first time may be unsure of rituals relating to their social customs and may look to staff in the neonatal unit to help inform them of the requirements. Having links with a range of faith and social communities can be helpful at this time.

Parents may wish to have photographs of their baby. The hospital staff may take the photographs or the parents may wish to do this themselves. In some units it has become customary to photograph the baby, even if the parents do not wish to have a photograph. This is then kept on file and the parents may access it later if they wish. While the intentions of staff participating in this practice are good, it has to be acknowledged that it may be seen as denying the autonomy of the parents in making decisions. It may also be perceived by some parents as offensive and patronising. Other mementoes parents can be offered include foot and hand prints (specialised paper is now available which avoids ink staining), keeping the cot card or blankets that the baby has been wrapped in, or taking a lock of hair. However, it is recommended that parents are fully informed of all that is available to them and that their decisions are respected and recorded accordingly.

Parents should be offered choices assured that staff will respect their wishes. In most situations, it is possible to reassure parents that they can change their minds. For example, they may decide not to hold their dead baby initially but decide later that they do wish to do this. Staff need to be aware of the changes that take place in bodies after they die and alert parents to these, otherwise this can cause distress (McHaffie 2001). For example, the most obvious change in a baby whose body has been in the mortuary is that it will feel very cold. It may be possible to place the baby under a radiant warmer to remove the chill before the parents hold the baby. Where the environmental temperature is high, changes in the baby's body take place more rapidly. Advice should be sought from a mortuary technician about how long the baby's body can remain out of the mortuary before noticeable changes take place. This is particularly important if the parents want to take their baby home.

Cosmetic changes take place in the baby's body after death. One example of this is lividity – a discoloration caused by the pooling of blood in the veins and capillaries. This may make the skin appear very pink or blue. If parents request to see their baby several hours after the death, these changes will have taken place. Parents need to be advised of any changes in their baby's appearance so that they are prepared for them. Not to do this can cause extreme distress (ibid.).

Special circumstances

Multiple births

Multiple births, especially higher order multiple births, are increasing in the UK. Part of this is attributed to the fact that women conceive later and older women are more likely to have twins than younger women. Higher order multiple births are more likely to be associated with fertility treatment. Issues such as infertility and delayed childbearing may complicate the process of grieving. Some parents may be faced with the loss of a baby after making the decision to reduce the number of fetuses during pregnancy to try to ensure the viability of the pregnancy. They may feel that any sequelae such as preterm birth or the death of a baby is 'punishment' for interfering in the pregnancy. Understanding the difficult choices facing parents who have taken these decisions can help neonatal nurses provide more effective support.

It is important to recognise that parents lose individual babies and not a 'collective' baby. The deaths of babies may not occur simultaneously but happen over a period of months. Parents may be faced with mourning for a dead baby while caring for live babies. This can have the effect of delaying mourning for the dead baby and parents may find that they have profound feelings of loss months after the death of the baby. Parents may also find it difficult to form a relationship with the surviving baby as they try to protect themselves from feelings of grief should another baby die.

If parents wish, the dead baby may be placed alongside the living baby for photographs so that they have a memento of both babies together. Staff should also ascertain from the parents what information should be displayed on the cot card. Some parents may want the cot card to reflect that the baby was a survivor of a multiple birth, while other parents may not want to have this reminder of their loss displayed prominently in the neonatal unit.

Withholding and withdrawing active treatment

Neonatal nurses are sometimes faced with situations where, despite the availability of best possible care, recovery is not possible. The Royal College of Paediatrics and Child Health (RCPCH) suggests that where death is inevitable and treatment will only prolong suffering, or where the baby may survive but would have a physical or mental impairment that would be unbearable, then it may be legally and ethically permissible to withdraw or withhold care (RCPCH 2004).

When making decisions about withholding and withdrawing care, the fundamental principle underpinning decision-making is that any decision must be in the baby's 'best interests' (see p. 478). The concept of best interests is complex and parents and health professionals may hold different views. Research carried out in the UK, however, shows that there is generally agreement between parents and professionals about when care should be withheld or withdrawn (McHaffie 2001). Where there is conflict, it is generally best to try to resolve the situation using mediation, rather than resorting to the law. However, some situations are so complex that legal means may be the only way of achieving resolution. This can lead to tense relationships between the parents and the professionals but it is important to try to understand the parents' perspective. Neonatal nurses have to be extremely careful in these situations to ensure that they continue to support the parents while acknowledging the different viewpoints.

Making the decision to withdraw or withhold invasive treatment can be very difficult for parents and staff. McHaffie and Fowlie (1996) carried out a study investigating parents' and professionals' experiences of withdrawing care and found that in all cases bar one, parents were sure that the timing of the decision was right. The one parent who disagreed felt that the decision should have been made earlier.

In some cases the baby may have been receiving care for many weeks or months and it may be apparent to all involved with the care of the baby that all avenues have been exhausted and that it is kinder to withdraw intervention or withhold invasive forms of treatment and allow the baby to die peacefully. Sometimes, however, the decision may be made either at the time of birth or soon afterwards. For example, a decision may be made not to resuscitate very preterm infants or to withdraw care early from a term baby with severe brain injury following birth. In these situations, parents may have had little time to come to terms with the situation.

Withholding or withdrawing care does not mean that no care is given. The aim of care moves from cure to comfort. Palliative neonatal care is a relatively new concept in neonatal care. A report into the care of critically ill neonates highlighted the fact that most staff working in neonatal units do not have any education or training in palliative care (Nuffield Council on Bioethics 2006). The importance of the need for formal palliative care training for neonatal staff is highlighted by McHaffie's research into withdrawing and withholding care in neonatal units which demonstrated the anguish of parents when they realised that it could take several days for a baby to die after curative treatment had been withdrawn (McHaffie 2001).

Leuthner and Pierucci (2001) suggest that the principles of neonatal palliative care fall into four categories: advance directive planning; the environment for supporting neonatal death; comfort and medical care; and psychosocial support. Catlin and Carter (2002) emphasise that palliative care is as resource-intensive as providing intensive care. Staff caring for the baby and their family must have skills in assessing the baby and managing symptoms. This may include providing pain relief, nutrition, and airway management, including suction and oxygen to ensure that the baby remains comfortable.

Parents require information and support and should be assisted to make meaningful choices at this time. Parents should be facilitated to be as fully involved in their baby's care as they wish. This period can also be used to enable them to create memories of their baby. It may include visits from other family members and friends, the taking of photographs and video recording. Providing privacy in some neonatal units can be problematic. Many units are designed to facilitate maximum observation. This can make it very difficult for families to have private space and time with their dying baby. Sometimes, it may be possible for the baby to be moved to a side room or family room. If this is not possible, then screens and blinds can be used to create privacy for the family. Some parents may wish, with community support, to take their baby home or to a different location to die.

It is not possible to predict how long a baby may survive once active treatment is withdrawn. Changes may take place once treatment, especially ventilatory support, is withdrawn and staff should explain these changes to parents. For example, the baby may change colour or exhibit signs of respiratory distress such as nasal flaring or grunting. Parents can find the lack of certainty very challenging and emotionally exhausting. Where the process of dying is prolonged, neonatal staff should ensure that the parents have access to refreshments and offer to care for the baby while parents take breaks or rest.

Some parents may make a decision not to be present when care is withdrawn or not to participate in caregiving activities. It does not mean that the parents care any less about their baby and they should not be obliged to justify their rationale for not wishing to be involved in palliative care. Staff need to remain sensitive to the parents' right to make decisions and should ensure that they are fully informed about what is happening to their baby. Taking photographs and other mementoes should be carried out only after the parents have given their consent.

Sharing information

Confidentiality is an important aspect of neonatal care and this is especially true in neonatal loss situations. Some parents may choose to withhold full details of the circumstances surrounding their baby's death from other family members. The death may be presented as occurring naturally, rather than as a result of a decision that has been made. Their wishes should be respected and staff should be careful not to reveal the circumstances of the baby's death.

Supporting parents

There is little evidence that routine counselling benefits parents experiencing neonatal loss (Murray *et al.* 2000; Neimeyer 2000). However, some parents are more at risk of developing long-term problems such as stress and depression. Parents who appear to be most at risk of developing problems are those from lower socio-economic groups and parents with limited or no social support (Larson and Hoyt 2007). Part of the role of the neonatal nurse is to elicit through sensitive questioning the support available to the parents and to ensure that they are aware of formal and informal support networks.

Many neonatal units will have specialised staff to help parents experiencing bereavement. This may include bereavement nurses or midwives or psychologists. Information about support groups such as the Stillbirth and Neonatal Death Society (SANDS) and the Child Bereavement Charity should be given to parents. However, it must be remembered that not all parents wish to access these services and neonatal units should continue to provide support for parents who cannot or do not want to use the services of voluntary groups.

Parents, especially mothers, are often invited to provide information about the birth of their baby by manufacturers who will then use this as an opportunity to send marketing materials. If parents do not wish to receive this information, they can use the Baby Mail Preference Service to cancel marketing information.

Staff in neonatal units should also remember to provide appropriate information about the baby's death to other health professionals such as community midwives, health visitors and General Practitioners so that they are fully informed about the circumstances of the baby's death and can offer support to the parents.

Registering the birth and death

The baby's birth and death must be registered. In England and Wales the birth must be registered within 42 days of the baby's birth. In Scotland, the birth must be registered within 21 days of the birth. If the parents are not married, the mother must register the birth. If the father wishes to have his name on the baby's birth certificate, he must accompany the mother to the registry office or sign a statutory declaration form.

When a baby dies, the death should be registered within five days in England and Wales and eight days in Scotland. The death can be registered by either of the parents but they must have a copy of the medical certificate of death. Some registry offices operate an appointments system. This can be helpful for some parents as it eliminates the need to wait in a public place. The appointments system may cause frustration for parents by delaying the registration of the death. It is important that members of staff caring for bereaved parents are aware of local arrangements and give accurate information. Some faiths require that a funeral should take place as quickly as possible after death and this may cause further anxiety; requesting support and advice from the spiritual leader of particular faiths is useful at this time.

When the baby's death is registered, the Registrar collects information about the parents. This can seem very intrusive and unnecessary to bereaved parents (McHaffie 2001) but it is a statutory data collection requirement. By fore-warning parents about the questions, staff can help them cope with the experience. Once the baby's death has been registered, the parents will receive a certificate which is given to the funeral directors to enable them to make arrangements for the baby's funeral. Parents can also obtain a copy of the death certificate. Payment is required for this in England and Wales. In Scotland, an abbreviated extract is given free of charge.

Perinatal autopsy

The perinatal autopsy can help provide a definitive diagnosis after the death of a baby. In the UK, perinatal autopsy rates have fallen. Lyon (2004) suggests that there are two reasons for this: the first is that health professionals believe that better investigative techniques before death have reduced the value of the perinatal autopsy. The second reason relates to the controversy over organ harvesting and storing in the UK which has made health professionals reluctant to approach parents to seek consent. However, there is some evidence that perinatal autopsy can provide new information in about a quarter of all cases (ibid.).

The Royal College of Pathologists (RCP) recommends that a senior member of medical staff, preferably a consultant, should obtain informed consent from the parents (RCP 2000a, 2000b). The parents should be given information about the possible advantages of a post-mortem examination, including the implications for future pregnancies and children. McHaffie (2001) found that the approach of the consultant was very important in obtaining consent for the examination and that the most important reason for parents withholding consent was the fear of mutilation.

The information given to parents should include an explanation of what is involved in the examination, along with an assurance that it will be respectful and that they may have the opportunity to see and hold the baby afterwards. Parents can limit the extent of the post-mortem examination but they do need to be aware that this might limit the information obtained from the examination. The RCP states that parents need to be aware of what happens to organs and tissue samples and allowed to decide if they wish to wait until all the examinations have been completed and the organs returned to the baby before having a funeral. Specific consent needs to be obtained if a request is being made to store the organs or tissue samples for research or education.

When making an appointment for parents to meet to discuss the results of the autopsy, it is important to check that all the examinations have been completed. It can take up to six weeks and sometimes longer to obtain the results. The choice of venue for the meeting should be considered beforehand. Some parents will want to return to the neonatal unit to visit staff, while others may find the experience too overwhelming and will want to have the consultation away from the unit.

Funerals

Funeral directors can help parents plan the baby's funeral. Parents can make their own arrangements if they wish. Most hospitals have an arrangement with funeral directors to provide a funeral for any baby who dies at no cost to the parents. The funeral provided is described as a 'simple' funeral. This includes a coffin and a hearse. Funerals are very expensive and parents may not be able to afford a headstone or permanent memorial. Many neonatal units provide meaningful memorials for all parents such as a book of remembrance to help them record the life of their baby.

It has become common practice for parents and family to attend the baby's funeral. Many parents recount how participating in the event enabled them to say 'goodbye' to their baby. However, neonatal staff must be sensitive to personal beliefs and preferences and refrain from 'encouraging' parents to attend if it is clear that they would rather not do this. Some cultures and religions have only the male relatives attend the funeral and trying to force a woman to go against these norms may increase the distress of the family.

Remembering

Some neonatal units hold remembrance services for parents and their families and there is evidence that many parents find this helpful. When organising events, it is important to take into account the range of beliefs in the community as a whole. Some neonatal units may unintentionally exclude parents whose beliefs conflict with a specific form of ceremony.

Parents may find it helpful to be sent a card on the anniversary of their baby's death. However, McHaffie's (2001) study established that this was only the case if they believed that the card had some meaning for the sender. When the card was sent from a member of staff who wasn't known to the parents, the action was perceived to be formulaic and part of the routine of the unit, and less likely to be viewed as helpful. In units with high staff turnover, this needs to be taken into account and some form of wording used that conveys the genuine sympathy and understanding of the staff for the parents' loss.

Conclusion

Perinatal loss is a very real and important part of neonatal nursing care. The skills needed to provide care for grieving parents are complex and require neonatal nurses to be empathetic, compassionate and reflective. This chapter has highlighted some of the elements involved in the provision of care to dying babies and their families. The increasing emphasis on the provision of palliative care for the dying neonate requires the acquisition of additional caring skills. These skills can be developed through self-reflection and consideration of the theories and evidence base that exists surrounding neonatal palliative care provision.

References

Acolet, D. (2008) *Perinatal Mortality 2006*, London: CEMACH.

Badenhorst, W., Riches, S., Turton, P. and Hughes, P. (2006) 'The psychological effects of stillbirth and neonatal death on fathers; systematic review', *Journal of Psychosomatic Obstetrics and Gynaecology* 27(4): 245–56.

Bowlby, J. (1973) *Attachment and Loss*, Vol. 2, *Separation*, New York: Basic Books.

Catlin, A. and Carter, B. (2002) 'Creation of a neonatal end-of-life palliative care protocol', *Journal of Perinatology* 22: 184–95.

De Frain, J., Martens, L., Stork, J. *et al.* (1991) 'The psychological effect of a stillbirth on surviving family members', *Omega* 22(2): 81–108.

Freud, S. (1957) 'Mourning and melancholia', in J. Strachey (ed. and trans.) *The Standard Edition of the Complete Psychological Works of Sigmund Freud*, London: Hogarth Press.

Gold, K.J. (2007) 'Navigating care after a baby dies: a systematic review of parent experiences with health providers', *Journal of Perinatology* 27(4): 230–7.

Klass, D., and Walter, T. (2001) 'Processes of grieving: how bonds are continued', in M.S. Stroebe, R.O. Hanson, W. Stroebe, and H. Schut (eds) *Handbook of Bereavement Research: Consequences, Coping and Care*, Washington, DC: American Psychological Association.

Klass, S., Silverman, P.R. and Nickman, S.L. (eds) (1996) *Continuing Bonds: New Understandings of Grief*, Washington, DC: Taylor & Francis.

Kübler Ross, E. (1970) *On Death and Dying*, London: Tavistock.

Lake, M., Knuppel, R.A., Murphy, J. *et al.* (1983) 'The role of a grief support team following stillbirth', *American Journal of Obstetrics and Gynecology* 146(8): 877–81.

Lang, A., Edwards, N. and Benzies, K. (2005) 'A "false sense of security" in caring for bereaved parents', *Birth* 32(2): 158–9.

Larson, D.G. and Hoyt, W. (2007) 'What has become of grief counselling? An evaluation of the empirical foundations of this new pessimism', *Professional Psychology: Research and Practice* 38(4): 347–55.

Leuthner, S.R. and Pierucci, R. (2001) 'Experience with neonatal palliative care consultation at the Medical College of Wisconsin – Children's Hospital of Wisconsin', *Journal of Palliative Medicine* 4(1): 39–47.

Lyon, A. (2004) 'Perinatal autopsy remains the gold standard (commentary)', *Archives of Disease in Childhood: Fetal and Neonatal Edition* 89: F89.

McHaffie, H.E. (2001) *Crucial Decisions at the Beginning of Life*, Abingdon: Radcliffe Medical.

McHaffie, H.E. and Fowlie, P.W. (1996) *Life, Death and Decisions: Doctors and Nurses Reflect on Neonatal Practice*, Cheshire: Hochland and Hochland.

Mekosh-Rosenbaum, V. and Lasker, J.N. (1995) 'Effects of pregnancy outcomes on marital satisfaction: a longitudinal study of birth and loss', *Infant Mental Health Journal* 16(2): 127–43.

Murray, J.A., Terry, D.J., Vance, J.C. *et al.* (2000) 'Effects of a program of intervention on parental distress following infant death', *Death Studies* 24: 275–305.

Neimeyer, R.A. (2000) 'Searching for the meaning of meaning: grief therapy and the process of reconstruction', *Death Studies* 24(6): 541–58.

Nuffield Council on Bioethics (2006) *Critical Care Decisions in Fetal and Neonatal Medicine: Ethical Issues*, London: Nuffield Council on Bioethics.

Oliver, L. (1999) 'Effects of a child's death on the marital relationship: a review', *OMEGA: Journal of Death and Dying* 39(3): 197–227.

Parkes, C.M. (1972) *Bereavement: Studies of Grief in Adult Life*, New York: International Universities Press.

Peppers, L.G. and Knapp, R.J. (1980) *Motherhood and Mourning: Perinatal Death*, New York: Praeger.

Rando, T.A. (1986) *Loss and Anticipatory Grief*, Lexington, MA: DC Heath and Company.

Royal College of Paediatrics and Child Health (2004) *Withholding or Withdrawing Life Saving Treatment in Children: A Framework for Practice*, London: RCPCH.

Royal College of Pathologists (2000a) *Examination of the Body after Death: Information about Post-mortem Examination for Relatives*, London: The Royal College of Pathologists.

Royal College of Pathologists (2000b) *Guidelines for the Retention of Tissues and Organs at Post-mortem Examination*, London: The Royal College of Pathologists.

Schott, J., Henley, A., and Kohner, N. (2007) *Pregnancy Loss and the Death of a Baby: Guidelines for Professionals*, 3rd edn, London: Stillbirth and Neonatal Death Society.

Turton, P., Hughes, P., Evans, C.D. and Fainman, D. (2001) 'The incidence and significance of post traumatic stress disorder in the pregnancy after stillbirth', *British Journal of Psychiatry* 178: 556.

Worden, J.W. (1991) *Grief Counselling and Grief Therapy: A Handbook for the Mental Health Practitioner*, 2nd edn, London: Springer.

Zeanah, C.H., Danis, B., Hirshberg, L. *et al.* (1995) 'Initial adaptation in mothers and fathers following perinatal loss', *Infant Mental Health Journal* 16: 80–93.

Chapter 20

Ethics and Neonatal Nursing

Helen Frizell

Contents

Introduction

Neonatal nursing has witnessed a level of technological change and development in recent years which has resulted in the survival of extremely premature infants. This has called for a simultaneous development in the theoretical and practical skills of neonatal nurses. It has also increasingly exposed them to the intriguing world of ethics and moral decision-making, involving fragile human beings, often at the edge of viability or with the prospects of facing some long-term disability.

Decision-making is common to us all, indeed, it is part of everyday life. For neonatal nurses, those decisions can have far-reaching consequences for others. Allmark (1992) examines the ethical component of the nature of nursing, suggesting that nurses make many ethical decisions in the course of their daily work. Not all of these decisions result from ethical or moral dilemmas: the decision may result from the nurse being faced with more than one option in a given situation and having to decide what is the most appropriate course of action to take. A moral or ethical dilemma arises when two or more of these courses of action could be appropriate and yet conflict with each other. Which ought the nurse to take? Beauchamp and Childress (2001) state that often these dilemmas can be resolved through reasoning and reflection. Some, however, may not. Jones (1997) provides further insight into the neonatal nurse as an autonomous practitioner who has to make choices. Whatever the situation, ethical decision-making is demanding and can lead us to explore our own attitudes and beliefs further (Tschudin 1994).

The aim of this chapter is not to provide answers to specific situations but rather to stimulate thought and awareness about some of the ethical issues within neonatal care. The words of Aristotle still ring true: 'In a practical science, so much depends on particular circumstances that only general rules can be given' and 'the agents are compelled at every step to think out for themselves what the circumstances demand' (Aristotle, *Nicomachean Ethics*, 1103b26–1104a11).

Ethical theories: an overview

According to Beauchamp and Childress (2001), there are several types of ethical theory. It is not possible within the confines of one chapter to provide an extensive exploration of these. For more detailed information, reference should be made to the work of Gillon (1986), Rumbold (1993), Tschudin (1994) and Beauchamp and Childress (2001). The partnership between ethics and the law as applied to medicine and nursing can be explored in the work of Tingle and Cribb (2007) and Herring (2008). A brief overview follows of four of the ethical theories.

Utilitarianism or consequentialism

This first theory adopts the belief that the act that leads to the best overall result is the right one to implement. If this were to be rigidly applied within neonatal nursing, then every nursing action would seek to result in the maximum benefit for every infant and family within the unit, all the staff and for society as a whole. There are, of course, occasions when a utilitarian-based decision may be the appropriate one to implement. An example of this would be where the maximum safety of all persons within the neonatal unit had to be ensured. A major criticism of utilitarianism is that it tends to be a more impersonal approach. It may even cause an immoral act to be committed against an individual while pursuing the maximum benefit for the majority of individuals (Beauchamp and Childress 2001).

Deontological or Kantian theory

This second theory results from the work of Immanuel Kant (1724–1804) and is obligation- or duty-based. Tschudin (1994) explains this as 'The action itself counts and has to be right, regardless of any consequences.' Rumbold (1993) provides an example of this, which could be applied to neonatal care, by citing the duty to preserve life. If this duty were to be rigidly adhered to in the purest deontological sense, decisions such as the withdrawal of treatment in the best interests of the infant would not be ethically possible. The duty is performed, irrespective of the consequences (Seedhouse 1998).

Virtue-based theory

Virtue ethics are concerned with the person who is required to make a choice and initiate the ensuing action. The morality of the action would be judged on the basis of whether or not this person is considered to be a good or virtuous person – that is, they demonstrate characteristics which are socially and morally valued. Although virtue ethics may influence one's perception of another, even virtuous people can make errors of judgement resulting in inappropriate action being taken. This creates a weakness in the sole use of this theory to try to determine the morally right course of action to take.

Rights-based theory

Rights, or justified claims, predominantly arise from legal and moral sources. They may also arise from documents such as the National Service Framework for Children, Young People and Maternity Services (Department of Health 2004), or from individual institutions. Some rights are absolute but generally they are *prima facie* (Beauchamp and Childress 2001). In other words, most rights are only obligatory if not overridden by competing rights. Infringement of a right occurs when another has justifiably overridden it; violation occurs when it has been unjustifiably overridden. Certain rights are enshrined within the Human Rights Act 1998. For neonatal staff, Articles 2, 3 and 8 are possibly the ones which are likely to have the greatest impact. These Articles are: the right to life, the right not to be subjected to inhuman or degrading treatment, and the right to respect for private and family life.

Herring (2008) identifies the impact that religious beliefs can have on individual people's choices and the fact that health care professionals can be faced with this added dimension influencing ethical decision-making. The case of the conjoined twins, *Re A (Children) (Conjoined Twins: Surgical Separation)* ([2000] 4 All ER 985), was a demonstration of how rights under Articles 2, 3 and 8 can apparently conflict and, for the parents, be strongly influenced by religious beliefs. This high-profile case generated much debate professionally and publicly and raised many questions about best interest decision-making in such complex circumstances. This particular case highlights the fact that best interest decision-making is by no means a straightforward issue. Further reading of articles relating to the case, such as that by Harris (2001), is recommended.

The introduction of the Mental Capacity Act 2005 has made best interest decision-making a more transparent process for adults who have been proven to lack capacity for making a specific decision. While only applicable to young people 16 years old and upwards, it does identify the types of considerations that must be made when acting in a person's best interests. It may be useful for staff acting in the best interests of neonates to consider the underlying principles reflected in the accompanying guidance (Department for Constitutional Affairs 2007) and consider how they aid interpretation of any professional guidance and that given by the Department of Health (2001a, 2001b). *F* v. *Berkshire HA* ([1989] 2 All ER 545) and *Re C* (medical treatment) ([1998] 1 FLR 384) provide legal examples of how doctors can, at times, have a common law duty to act on behalf of patients for their best interests. There have been more recent cases which show just how complex a process seeking to act in best interests continues to be and that the need for external, objective assessments of all the facts will never disappear (*Glass v. The United Kingdom* ([2004] ECHR 103; *Charlotte Wyatt Litigation* [2005] EWCA Civ 1181). One common theme that does seem to arise from some of these references is the issue of good communication between the various parties and highlights the importance of this essential skill for all staff concerned.

In complex decision-making, we may trust the decisions of our colleagues based on our perception of how good and knowledgable a practitioner they are. This is a form of virtue ethics. However, it is more likely that ethical decision-making will be founded on a combination of the other three theories. For ease of use, these can be succinctly summarised as being goal-, duty- or rights-based. Each has strengths as well as weaknesses but an awareness of the concepts should help neonatal nurses to be better advocates for the babies and families within their care. This can be enhanced if the nurses have an awareness of some of the wider issues affecting health care delivery and are able to seek out common principles that will inform and guide practice.

Ethical principles

Respect for autonomy

Autonomy suggests the ability of an individual to think and act freely, to be able to make decisions and to be responsible for the results of those decisions (Jones 1997). This is reflected in the principles of responsibility and accountability, as laid out in *The Code: Standards of Conduct, Performance and Ethics for Nurses and Midwives* (NMC 2008a). Respect for autonomy places a requirement on individuals to acknowledge the rights of others to act autonomously. Beauchamp and Childress (2001) develop this further and state that to do this requires more than just help. It also involves respectful attitude and action by one person or group of people to another. Obviously this does not necessarily mean promoting or respecting action that is illegal.

The neonate cannot exercise autonomy but parents can and, under the terms of the Mental Capacity Act 2005, they must be presumed to be competent to do so unless otherwise proven. If this is to be respected and parents are enabled to make truly informed choices, it is important that neonatal staff ensure that appropriate information is given and understood. This should include the consequences of any decisions made. It will not always be the duty of the neonatal nurse to give this information but, as a partner in care, there is a responsibility to ensure that parents have the opportunity to obtain it. They must also make every reasonable effort to ensure that, where necessary, parents have been helped to understand the information. An example of this is the use of interpreters or relevant commnication aids.

The principle of respect for autonomy can also be applied to the role of the neonatal nurse, particularly as role expansion and development continue to increase. Hunt (1994) states that nursing autonomy is far more than simply the gaining of further biomedical knowledge. While maintaining the close and cooperative inter-professional working relationships required when caring for neonates, neonatal nurses can exercise their authority to influence changes in policy and practice. This should be possible whether they have clinical, managerial or educational responsibilities. In order to do this, it is necessary that nursing knowledge must also increase. Using the four patterns of knowledge identified by Carper (1978), it can be seen that development would be required in the areas of aesthetics or the art of nursing, personal knowledge and ethics as well as empirically.

The Scope of Professional Practice (UKCC 1992) enabled nurses to develop more autonomous practice and this scope continues under the terms of *The Code* (NMC 2008a). There is a risk, perhaps, that increased nursing autonomy may be viewed as being a power struggle between medicine and nursing. The challenge to neonatal nurses is to develop their autonomy as suggested by Hunt (1994) in order to be respected by others as professional practitioners.

Non-maleficence

In essence, this principle is that of *primum non nocere*, or the duty to do no harm. Therefore, any known side-effects of treatment, for example, must be weighed against the anticipated benefits (Gillon 1986). It would be morally reprehensible to pursue a line of care where side-effects outweighed any benefits, particularly in the name of research. The duty to do no harm is a very clear underlying principle of *The Code* (NMC 2008a), identifying this responsibility for nurses. Inexperience may be excusable, as all neonatal nurses have had to learn their skills. Ignorance, however, is not an excuse when minimising or doing no harm to a vulnerable neonate is under consideration. Legally, the principle of a minimum level of competence is upheld in the findings of the case *Nettleship* v. *Weston* ([1971] 2 QB 691 (CA)) (Kennedy and Grubb 1994). All staff involved in patient care are held to a same minimum level of competence necessary for the safety of the patient. For nurses, this highlights the importance of appropriate delegation, ensuring that staff are not placed in the position of having to take responsibility beyond their level of competence. Equally, individuals need to recognise their personal limits of competence and not accept tasks or activities that they feel unable to perform competently. Lack of competence may arise from lack of confidence in admitting what is not known or through over-confidence. Therefore, it is the responsibility of more experienced neonatal staff to support and encourage staff development through appropriate exposure to learning opportunities.

To seek advice, when uncertain, from a more experienced colleague is good practice. It may also, as demonstrated by *Wilsher* v. *Essex AHA* ([1986] 3 All ER 801), prevent individual staff from being held liable in the event of a parental claim of negligence. In the event of medical/nursing staff facing litigation for negligence, standards of professional practice must be legally determined. This is done by the application of the Bolam principle in which staff are measured by the standard of practice deemed acceptable and reasonable by a responsible group of practitioners from the same specialty (Tingle and Cribb 2007).

In an ideal world, accidents would not happen. Unfortunately, this is not the case and even the most meticulous care cannot always prevent incidents such as extravasation injuries from occurring. Nursing responsibility is to ensure that any necessary help and advice are sought and care initiated to reduce any further risks to the infant. Provision of evidence-based care is a fundamental requirement of nursing practice, as can be witnessed from many clinical guidelines (NMC 2008a). Berragan (1998), in an exploration of how different ways of knowing influence nursing practice, appears to voice some caution about a total reliance upon evidence-based guidelines. The reason given is that it could exclude the use of areas of aesthetic or personal knowledge such as intuition. Professional accountability and the principle of non-maleficence bind all medical, nursing and paramedical staff. Knowledge and information, however gained, are not under the exclusive ownership of a minority of people but need to be shared and discussed for the benefit of all.

Beneficence

Essentially, the ethical principle of beneficence is about doing good and actively seeking to promote the patient's welfare (Gillon 1986; Rumbold 1993; Beauchamp and Childress 2001). As with non-maleficence, beneficence is also an underlying principle of *The Code* (NMC 2008a) and to exercise it is therefore a professional responsibility. Beauchamp and Childress (2001) divide beneficence into two further principles, those being positive beneficence and utility. The former is concerned with the provision of benefits while the latter asks that those benefits be weighed and balanced against any drawbacks. Provision of neonatal care facilities is obviously a benefit to many families, that is positive beneficence. Utility, on the other hand, requires that the provision of such facilities to every infant, irrespective of their condition at birth, be balanced against what is in the best interests of the infant. This is probably particularly pertinent with the birth of an extremely preterm infant.

Beneficence is inextricably linked with the other ethical principles of autonomy, non-maleficence and justice (Gillon 1986; Beauchamp and Childress 2001). The following example aims to apply this link to practice. Neonatal nurses seek to promote the welfare of the babies in their care and to take reasonable precautions to minimise any harm to those babies. Yet they must also respect individual parental autonomy while balancing the needs of all the families in the unit. Policies and protocols offer some degree of fairness and equality for all, although this may not always be readily understood by relatives and visitors, who can then start to place additional demands upon staff. The process of acting beneficently can become a juggling act for staff, but there can be little argument that the welfare of all the babies will inevitably be the greatest influence upon the nurse.

Justice

It is very clear from the cited texts that any attempt to define what justice means is far more complex than may at first be anticipated. A common consensus within the literature is that Aristotle's principle of justice as being that which is fair and lawful is widely accepted within other theories (Gillon 1986; Beauchamp and Childress 2001). Fairness and legality appear to be straightforward terms to understand, but they are, in fact, influenced by political, sociological and religious beliefs. This is apparent from Gillon's description of libertarian, utilitarian and Marxist theories of justice (Gillon 1986).

In order to focus on what justice is, it may help to consider what constitutes an injustice. It is also important to remember that rights not only bring benefits, but equally place responsibilities upon individuals. According to Beauchamp and Childress (1994), injustice occurs when failure to act or a misdoing by one person or a group of people prohibits others from experiencing the benefits of their rights. That same failure to act or misdoing could result in an unequal or unfair distribution of responsibilities, something which could also create an injustice.

Justice may be distributive, criminal or rectificatory (Beauchamp and Childress 2001). Distributive justice essentially refers to the appropriately fair and equal distribution of resources within society. It is influenced by the infrastructure of that society and involves areas such as civil and political rights as well as the more obvious ones of health care and education. Criminal justice is concerned with the maintenance of law and order and the punishment of those who break the criminal law. Rectificatory justice is generally applied via the civil law and can be seen to be effected through fair compensation for medical malpractice, for example.

For neonatal nurses, it is probably the principle of distributive justice that is of most concern. This can be viewed from different perspectives. *Re B* ([1981] 1 WLR 1421) demonstrates how the judicial system may have to be involved in order to ensure fair access to health care if this is deemed to be in the interests of the child. The case centred on a baby with Down's syndrome who also had a duodenal atresia, the question of whether or not surgery should be performed being the cause of referral to the courts (McHale 1998a). The decision of the court was that surgery should be performed, Down's syndrome not being a prohibitive factor. With increasing demands being placed upon the National Health Service to provide a vast range of general and specialist services, it is difficult to see how finite resources can be equally, fairly and appropriately distributed throughout the country. Many neonatal staff will be familiar with the scenario of a pregnant woman in premature labour having to be transferred to another hospital due to lack of resources, for whatever reason, at the local hospital. Although that may be considered by some as being unfair to that individual woman, those making the decisions must also take the needs of others into consideration. Given the need for informed decision-making, information obtained from studies such as EPICure (www.epicure.ac.uk) can provide valuable evidence to help clinical advice and decision-making. Decisions involving the issue of resource allocation are reflected in *R* v. *Secretary of State ex p Hinks* ([1980] 1 BMLR 93 (CA)) and *Re J (a minor)(wardship: medical treatment)* ([1993] Fam 15, [1992] 4 All ER 614 (CA)). In the latter case, Lord Donaldson identified that it is a reality of life that health authorities may, due to insufficient resources, have to make choices regarding treatment. In the former case, Lord Denning stated that consideration must be given as to how a service can be provided to the whole country, not just to a particular hospital (Kennedy and Grubb 1994). As with beneficence, justice is closely linked with the other three ethical principles and it is clear that there are no easy answers as to how it can be truly implemented within an imperfect society (Gillon 1986; Beauchamp and Childress 2001).

Despite this having been only a brief overview of ethical theories and principles, it can be seen how they can influence even the simplest day-to-day decisions within a neonatal intensive care unit. When allocating staff to infants at the beginning of a shift, consideration is given to the needs of the infants as matched against the skills of the staff and the overall needs of the unit. Surely this is an unconscious balancing of the needs of individuals against the whole and an effort to maximise benefits and minimise risk of harm within the given resources. The application of ethics and moral decision-making to practice is not just about life-and-death decisions or the provision of resources on a national scale. It is present in everyday life and neonatal nurses, as autonomous practitioners, should be encouraged to develop their awareness of the subject.

Fetal rights

The issue of fetal rights or maternal–fetal conflict is one that can provoke some controversy, judging by the amount of literature published on the subject in recent years (Carter 1990; Draper 1996; Flagler *et al*. 1997; Reid and Gillett 1997; Rhodes 1997; Mohaupt and Sharma 1998). Although this trend has mainly emanated from the United States of America, there have been cases involving the issue in Great Britain. Most notable was that of *Re S* ([1992] 4 All ER 671) in which a woman was admitted to hospital in labour with the post-mature fetus known to be in a transeverse lie (Kennedy and Grub 1994; Draper 1996). Despite the gravity of the situation and being given relevant information, she refused consent to delivery by Caesarean section on the grounds of religious belief. Application by the Health Authority to the courts for permission to perform the operation in order to save the life of Mrs S and the unborn baby was granted.

While this may be a fairly extreme case, the underlying issues are important to the subject of fetal rights. The concept of fetal rights has already become an issue within legal cases such as *Re F (in utero)* ([1988] 2 All ER 193) and *Re MB* ([1997] 2 FLR 426). *Re F (in utero)* questioned whether or not F could be made a ward of court while in utero. F's mother led a nomadic lifestyle and there was concern about the adverse effects that this might have upon the fetus if medical attention was not received. In this case, wardship was denied (McHale 1998b). *Re MB* [1997] involved a pregnant woman, overwhelmed by needle phobia, who refused consent to delivery by Caesarean section despite the fact that this decision could have an adverse effect upon the fetus. The courts could not declare such delivery as lawful if refused by a competent woman. In this case, however, surgical delivery was judged lawful, as the woman was deemed incompetent due to her needle phobia. Mason *et al*. (1999) and Harris (2001) provide valuable legal insight into this issue of fetal rights within the United Kingdom.

Fetal rights should also be important to paediatric and neonatal staff, as they are concerned with the welfare of the infant once born. An inappropriate choice of delivery could result in hypoxic damage to the infant, necessitating admission to the neonatal unit. To help facilitate informed decision-making, it is important that neonatal staff should be able to share their perspective in any debate about fetal rights.

Should fetal rights exist?

There seems a certain irony in the fact that, with one exception, the fetus is not a legal person before birth and therefore has no rights. Yet immediately after birth, the infant has legal and moral rights as a living person. The need for safeguard and care as well as legal protection for children before and after birth is acknowledged within the Convention on the Rights of the Child (General Assembly of the United Nations 1992).

The only legal rights afforded to the fetus under English law are contained within Section 59 of the Offences Against the Person Act 1861 and the Infant Life Preservation Act 1929 (Davies 1994). The former protects the fetus from death resulting from the unlawful causation of miscarriage. The latter makes it an offence to intentionally kill a fetus that is capable of being born alive, this being defined as a fetus with a gestational age of 28 weeks or more. Obviously the Abortion Act 1967, amended by the Human Fertilization and Embryology Act 1990, permits the legal termination of pregnancy. It was as a result of the last Act that the age of viability was reduced to 24 weeks.

The reason why there are no other fetal rights is because, legally, the fetus is not a person (Montgomery 1997). What constitutes being a person? Why should the fetus prior to birth not be regarded as a person and yet afterwards is? The arguments about what is a person and what is personhood are complex and contentious. They also appear to be strongly influenced by views on when life begins, when a human being is capable of self-consciousness or when they have had a biographical life (Brykczńska 1994; Harris 2001; Strong and Anderson 1994; Reid and Gillett 1997).

There has been some debate as to whether a newborn baby can truly be regarded as a person due to lack of self-consciousness (Boyd *et al.* 1997). According to Ivamy (1993), any human being who is capable of having rights is a person. This stand is supported by legislation such as the Children Act 1989 and the Human Rights Act 1998 which offer legal protection to children from the time of birth, irrespective of gestational age.

Neonatal nurses are well aware of the effect that technological advance has had within obstetric and neonatal care. The lives of infants of 24 weeks' gestation, occasionally less, can be saved and it is possible for some forms of fetal surgery to be performed. This may cause some people to question why the fetus should not have rights. Equally, the distress of caring for a baby suffering from severe drug withdrawal secondary to maternal addiction may prompt the same question. In order to try to find an answer, the wider issues involving the ethical principles must be considered.

If, for example, the fetus had the legal right to be protected from harmful substances what effect would this have upon the mother's moral right to act as an autonomous individual? Draper (1996) offers the example of women who smoke during pregnancy. The suggestion is made that if the fetus was given legal protection against exposure to passive smoking while in utero, then the resultant obligation placed upon the mother would also have to be placed upon society to protect all children from the effects of passive smoking. Such fetal rights could put society on a road towards prohibition of certain lifestyles. Conversely, to argue against action taken in the interests of the fetus because it is not a person could ultimately place society on a road towards infanticide (Draper 1996).

It is evident from the literature that there are no easy or quick answers to the controversies contained within the subject of fetal rights (Carter 1990; Draper 1996; Reid and Gillett 1997). Perhaps the legal system is correct in adopting the stance it does. On the other hand, technology enables infants to survive who may not have done so when the laws came into being. For parents who suffer the loss of a fetus of a viable age through no fault of their own, possibly as the result of accident or injury, there can be little comfort to realise that the law does not regard their 'baby' as a person. The time may be coming for the law to recognise 'potential personhood'. Will neonatal nurses be ready to advocate on behalf of the unborn child in a manner that supports and complements maternal rights?

Respecting parental autonomy: the giving of informed consent

Respect for autonomy is one of the four ethical principles and being autonomous is linked to the right to give or withhold consent to treatment (Carter 1990). The Children Act 1989 and Adoption and Children Act 2002 clarify who holds parental responsibility and therefore can give or withhold consent on behalf of a child. The nature of neonatal care means that staff do not always have time to seek parental consent before carrying out treatment in the best interests of the baby. However, parental autonomy must be respected and parents involved as much as possible in decision-making processes. It may cause conflict with staff if the parents refuse to consent to a procedure or treatment for their baby. An example of this is the refusal to allow blood products to be given on the basis of religious belief. However, it could simply be due to lack of understanding about what is being proposed. People need information to help them make choices. If they do not have the information, how can they understand the implications of their choice or the rationale for professional decisions? The importance of gaining informed consent has been recognised by the NHS Litigation Authority following the case of Chester v. Afshar ([2004] UKHL 41) (NHSLA 2004). Staff have a duty of care to the babies and parents; the use of informed consent forms part of that duty.

This raises the issue of how much information should be given and who should give it. Too much information may cause undue anxiety and distress while too little may give rise to an accusation of negligence (Harris 2001). Professional guidance is available from the Nursing and Midwifery Council, the Department of Health and the British Association of Perinatal Medicine and should be used to guide practice (BAPM 2004; DoH 2001a, 2001b; NMC 2008b).

Clearly, the nurse is responsible for giving information when that is what would be reasonably expected under the terms of the Bolam principle, but it is not always nursing responsibility to give the information. If, however, the nurse is concerned about the level of information given or the recipient's comprehension of it, personal accountability is primarily to the patient or client (NMC 2008b). This does not mean that the nurse should immediately provide further information; rather, the advice and help of an appropriate doctor and/or line manager should be sought in order to reduce the risk of legal proceedings being initiated against the nurse (McHale 1998c).

The importance of careful documentation following the giving of information cannot be over-stressed. In years to come, this is what will provide evidence to support or refute personal recollection of events. This is particularly important where practice in the neonatal unit may vary from information given to the public. One example could be the recommendation to place babies on their backs to sleep as a means of reducing cot death (Department of Health 1996). In neonatal units, it is not unusual to observe preterm babies being nursed prone as this contributes towards an improved respiratory status (Kurlak *et al.* 1994). This apparent conflict of practice may cause confusion for parents and it is therefore important that staff clearly explain the rationale for their actions and the parameters within which they work. Prior to the discharge of the baby, professional practice should be seen to be consistent with information given to parents.

It is possible, despite attempts to persuade otherwise, that parents may choose not to consent to or follow the professional advice given. This is their right as autonomous people but they must then also be willing to accept the responsibility for the consequences of that choice. *Re T (a minor) (wardship: medical treatment)* ([1997] 1 All ER 906) confirms that it may be legally permissible for a parent to make an autonomous decision not to consent to professional advice being carried out. This does not absolve staff from their duty of care. They may have to seek more experienced or specialist help and will have to continue to provide care within the parameters placed upon them. There must be documentation regarding the information given, which includes the consequences of a refusal and the reasons for the refusal (Brahams 1995; Montgomery 1997).

Ethics in practice

Throughout this chapter, it has been demonstrated that the use of ethical theories and principles has a very real place within clinical practice for neonatal nurses. Unfortunately, the application of ethics to practice does not always remove the interpersonal conflicts that can occur when staff hold different views that may all be equally justifiable. If professional ethics conflict with the law, clearly the legal guidance must be adhered to if there is not to be an accusation of breach of civil or criminal law levied. The blind following of a doctor's order will not be sufficient justification for the nurse who recognises an error but fails to exercise professional accountability and autonomy in seeking to correct it. The need for nurses to be guided by medical instruction, especially in areas such as neonatal intensive care, creates the paradoxical situation of the nurse being, yet not being, an autonomous professional. How can this be overcome and will it ever be overcome? Perhaps it requires nurses to reflect upon what is happening in both their practice and that of others. If the consequences of decisions made are considered using some form of ethical framework, this may aid nurses to feel sufficiently empowered to exercise their professional autonomy.

When reflecting upon situations and trying to find what the right answer may be, there is a very real risk that personal values and feelings may inhibit the adoption of an unbiased perspective (Johnstone 1988). Research by Hammerman *et al.* (1997) suggests that families, when involved in medical decision-making, are more strongly influenced by philosophical, moral and religious beliefs rather than specific life experiences. If such research were to be repeated with neonatal staff, it would be interesting to observe whether the same phenomenon appears. It can be difficult not to allow a blurring of the edges between professional and personal relationships with babies and their families, especially those who are longer term, but nurses must maintain clear professional boundaries at all times (NMC 2008a). An enhanced understanding of ethics can help staff to help maintain those boundaries when conflict between personal values and the need for objective ethical decision-making arises.

Reflective processes should be a familiar concept to most nurses. A useful tool is Gibb's reflective cycle (Gibbs 1988, cited in Bulman and Schutz 2004) which has been used as the basis of a reflective ethical decision-making cycle offered in Figure 20.1. By using a reflective process, nurses can explore

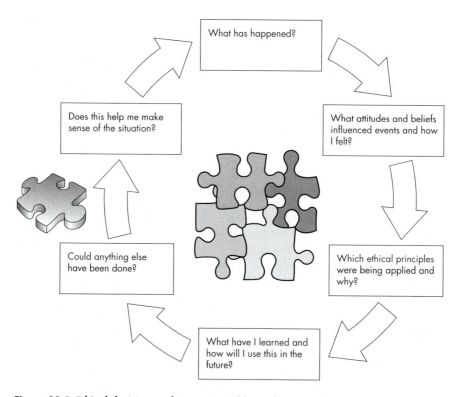

Figure 20.1 Ethical decision-making using Gibb's reflective cycle

Source: Seedhouse (1998: 209), with permission of John Wiley & Sons.

underlying issues, beliefs and attitudes to a given situation in a very personal way. It is from this process that further learning comes which influences personal practice and development. In many ways, it is like a jigsaw of development and ethical awareness that builds up piece by piece.

The difficulties encountered in reaching life-and-death decisions within neonatal care have been researched by McHaffie and Fowlie (1996). Staff must adhere to the laws of the country but balance decisions against risks and evidence around long-term outcomes. In the case study on p. 486, the baby was legally viable and, once born, had the right to life under the terms of Article 1 of the Human Rights Act 1998. This placed a direct legal responsibility on the paediatric and neonatal staff at the time of delivery. The ethical dilemmas arise when this right to life begins to conflict with another absolute right. Article 3 of the Human Rights Act gives the right not to be subjected to inhuman or degrading treatment and prolonged intensive and invasive care may be perceived as straying into this area depending upon specific circumstances. There are no straightforward answers in these situations and it is then that staff must utilise the appropriate legal and professional guidelines, for example, those produced by the Royal College of Paediatrics and Child Health (2004).

Conclusion

Ethical decision-making occurs on many occasions within neonatal units. It is not solely about dealing with difficult situations or dilemmas such as those presented within the case study. If the question 'what is the right thing to do in this situation?' is asked, then an ethical approach is required to answer it. In order to do this, neonatal nurses must have some understanding of the principles and theories that are involved.

Consideration should be given as to why a particular course of action is believed to be correct. An overview of four theories demonstrates the diverse approaches that can be taken and the fact that no one theory will always be the right approach for every situation. On some occasions it will be necessary to achieve the best outcome for all concerned. Other occasions will require pre-dominant consideration by staff of duty or the rights of an individual. It is prob-able that the majority of situations will require a combination of approaches.

Whichever theoretical stance is adopted for the problem-solving or decision-making process, the four ethical principles of respect for autonomy, non-maleficence, beneficence and justice must be adhered to. As neonatal nurses expand and develop their roles, so professional accountability and responsibility increase. An enhanced understanding of the ethical and legal framework within which nursing and medicine function will enable nurses to increase their professional autonomy.

Neonatal nurses should be aware of external factors that may impact upon their practice and be able and willing to respond to the opportunities and challenges that can result. Ethical decision-making is prevalent in day-to-day activities within neonatal units and, although the subject is complex and contentious, it is not beyond the reach of every member of staff. All staff should have an awareness of ethical principles and be involved in the ethical decision-making processes.

Case study: consideration of the ethical issues when there is conflict of opinion between health professionals

Mrs G has had two courses of IVF and is 25 weeks' pregnant with her first baby. She has been in her local district general hospital since her membranes ruptured at 16 weeks. The liquor volume has been steadily decreasing and is now minimal. Mrs G has had antibiotic therapy but became pyrexial and went into labour unexpectedly. Labour is advancing rapidly and the obstetric team believe that it is too risky to transfer Mrs G to the nearest hospital with level 3 neonatal facilities. They have estimated the fetal weight at 750g. Fetal monitoring shows evidence of fetal distress and the paediatricans have been called as delivery is imminent. A paediatric consultant and neonatal nurse attend the delivery suite. Before entering the delivery room, they are met by the obstetric consultant who gives them Mrs G's history. He states that, in his opinion, the fetus is unlikely to survive delivery and that it is pointless to consider resuscitation. The paediatric consultant inidcates that she will make that decision and is supported by the neonatal nurse. The baby is delivered in apparently poor condition but takes gasps and full resuscitation is initiated. By 10 minutes of age, the baby has been intubated, is being ventilated and has a good cardiac output. Once stabilised, the baby is transferred to the neonatal unit and subsequently moved to a tertiary unit. The case is raised at the next perinatal mortality meeting and the ethics influencing decisions by all parties were discussed. Consideration is given to the potential long-term impact for the baby and family.

Q.1. What personal values may be influencing the staff and whose needs were being considered?

Q.2. Compare these values against each of the ethical theories. Which was influencing the various opinions and decisions? Did these create any bias within individulas?

Once the bias that arises from personal values in situations such as this has been identified and acknowledged, it is important that those involved can try to place it to one side as the wider issues are discussed.

Q.3. How may each of the ethical principles be related to this situation?

Q.4. It is important that staff consider all the consequences of any decisions made. In this situation, the baby was of a viable age but in a very high-risk category.

- What were those risks?
- What legal obligations did the staff have?
- What moral obligations may they have felt?
- What evidence may have influenced their decisions?
- Did they have any other options?
- What can be learned from this?

Q.5. Would you have done anything different?

Legal references

All ER	All England Law Reports
BMLR	Butterworths Medico-Legal Reports
ECHR	European Court of Human Rights
EWCA	England and Wales Court of Appeal
Fam	Family Division Law Reports
FLR	Family Law Reports
QB	Law Reports, Queen's Bench Division
UKHL	United Kingdom House of Lords
WLR	Weekly Law Reports

Cases cited

Charlotte Wyatt Litigation [2005] EWCA Civ 1181
Chester v. *Afshar* [2004] UKHL 41
Glass v. *The United Kingdom* [2004] ECHR 103
F v. *Berkshire HA* [1989] 2 All ER 545
Nettleship v. *Weston* [1971] 2 QB 691
R v. *Secretary of State ex p Hinks* [1980] 1 BMLR 93
Re A (Children) (Conjoined Twins: Surgical Separation) [2000] 4 All ER 985
Re B [1981] 1 WLR 1421
Re C (medical treatment) [1998] 1 FLR 384
Re F (in utero) [1988] 2 All ER 193
Re J (a minor) (wardship: medical treatment) [1993] Fam 15, [1992] 4 All ER 614
Re MB [1997] 2 FLR 426
Re S [1992] 4 All ER 671
Re T [1992] 4 All ER 649
Re T (a minor) (wardship: medical treatment) [1997] 1 All ER 906
Wilsher v. *Essex AHA* [1986] 3 All ER 801

Statutes

- Adoption and Children Act 2002
- Children Act 1989
- Human Rights Act 1998

References

Allmark, P. (1992) 'The ethical enterprise of nursing', *Journal of Advanced Nursing* 17(1): 16–20.

Aristotle (1989) *The Ethics of Aristotle: The Nicomachean Ethics*, London: Penguin Books.

Beauchamp, T.L. and Childress, J.F. (2001) *Principles of Biomedical Ethics*, 5th edn, Oxford: Oxford University Press.

Berragan, L. (1998) 'Nursing practice draws upon several different ways of knowing', *Journal of Advanced Nursing* 7(3): 209–17.

Boyd, K.M., Higgs, R. and Pinching, A.J. (1997) *The New Dictionary of Medical Ethics*, London: BMJ Publishing Group.

Brahams, D. (1995) 'The critically ill patient: the legal perspective', in J. Tingle and A. Cribb (eds) *Nursing Law and Ethics*, Oxford: Blackwell Science.

British Association of Perinatal Medicine (2004) *Consent in Neonatal Clinical Care: Good Practice Framework*. Available at: www.bapm.org/media/documents/publications/staff-leaflet.pdf.

Brykczńska, G. (1994) 'Ethical issues in the neonatal unit', in D. Crawford and M. Morris (eds) *Neonatal Nursing*, London: Chapman & Hall.

Bulman, C. and Schutz, S. (2004) *Reflective Practice in Nursing*, 3rd edn, Oxford: Blackwell Publishing.

Carper, B. (1978) 'Fundamental patterns of knowing in nursing', *Advances in Nursing Science* 1(1): 13–23.

Carter, B. (1990) 'Fetal rights – a technologically created dilemma', *Professional Nurse* 5(11): 590–3.

Davies, A. (ed.) (1994) *Halsbury's Statutes of England and Wales*, 4th edn, vol. 12 reissue, *Criminal Law*, London: Butterworth.

Department for Constitutional Affairs (2007) *Mental Capacity Act 2005: Code of Practice*, London: TSO.

Department of Health (1996) *Reduce the Risk of Cot Death*, Wetherby: Department of Health.

Department of Health (2001a) *Reference Guide to Consent for Examination or Treatment*, London:TSO.

Department of Health (2001b) *Seeking Consent: Working with Children*, London: Department of Health.

Department of Health (2004) *National Service Framework for Children, Young People and Maternity Services Core Standards*, London: TSO.

Draper, H. (1996) 'Women, forced cesareans and antenatal responsibilities', *Journal of Medical Ethics* 22(6): 327–33.

Flagler, E., Bayliss, F. and Rogers, S. (1997) 'Bioethics for clinicians: 12. Ethical dilemmas that arise in the care of pregnant women: rethinking "maternal-fetal conflicts"', *Canadian Medical Association Journal* 156(12): 1729–32.

General Assembly of the United Nations (1989) *Convention on the Rights of the Child adopted by the General Assembly of the United Nations on 20th November 1989. Cm. 1976 Treaty Series 1992 no. 44*, London: HMSO.

Gillon, R. (1986) *Philosophical Medical Ethics*, Chichester: John Wiley & Sons.

Hammerman, C., Kornbluth, E., Lavie, O., Zadka, P., Aboulafia, Y. and Eidelman, A.I. (1997) 'Decision-making in the critically ill neonate: cultural background *v* individual life experiences', *Journal of Medical Ethics* 23(3): 164–9.

Harris, J. (2001) 'Human beings, persons and conjoined twins: an ethical analysis of the judgment in *Re A*', *Medical Law Review* 9 (Autumn): 221–36.

Herring, J. (2008) *Medical Law and Ethics*, 2nd edn, Oxford: Oxford University Press.

Hunt, G. (1994) 'New professionals? New ethics?', in G. Hunt and P. Wainwright (eds) *Expanding the Role of the Nurse*, Oxford: Blackwell Science.

Ivamy, H. (ed.) (1993) *Mozely and Whiteley's Law Dictionary*, 11th edn, London: Butterworth.

Johnstone, M. (1988) 'Law, professional ethics and the problem of conflict with personal values', *International Journal of Nursing Studies* 25(2): 147–57.

Jones, V. (1997) 'Professional and ethical issues in neonatal nursing: making choices', *Journal of Neonatal Nursing* 3(5): 23–7.

Kennedy, I. and Grubb, A. (1994) *Medical Law: Text with Materials*, 2nd edn, London: Butterworth.

Kurlak, L.O., Ruggins, N.R. and Stephenson, T.J. (1994) 'Effect of nursing position on incidence, type, and duration of clinically significant apnoea in preterm infants', *Archives of Disease in Childhood: Fetal and Neonatal Edition* 71(1): F16–F19.

Mason, J.K., McCall Smith, R.A. and Laurie, G.T. (1999) *Law and Medical Ethics*, London: Butterworth.

McHaffie, H.E. and Fowlie, P.W. (1996) *Life, Death and Decisions: Doctors and Nurses Reflect on Neonatal Practice*, Hale: Hochland & Hochland.

McHale, J. (1998a) 'The end of life', in J. McHale, J. Tingle and J. Peysner (eds) *Law and Nursing*, Oxford: Butterworth-Heinemann.

McHale, J. (1998b) 'Reproductive choice', in J. McHale, J. Tingle and J. Peysner (eds) *Law and Nursing*, Oxford: Butterworth-Heinemann.

McHale, J. (1998c) 'Consent to treatment 1: general principles', in J. McHale, J. Tingle and J. Peysner (eds) *Law and Nursing*, Oxford: Butterworth-Heinemann.

Mohaupt, S.M. and Sharma, K.K. (1998) 'Forensic implications and medical-legal dilemmas of maternal versus fetal rights', *Journal of Forensic Sciences* 43(5): 985–92.

Montgomery, J. (1997) *Health Care Law*, Oxford: Oxford University Press.

NHS Litigation Authority (2004) *Risk Alert Issue Number 4, Informed Consent*. Available at: www.nhsla.com.

Nursing and Midwifery Council (2008a) *The Code: Standards of Conduct, Performance and Ethics for Nurses and Midwives*, London: NMC.

Nursing and Midwifery Council (2008b) *Consent (Advice Sheet)*. Available at: www.nnmc-uk.org.

Reid, M.C. and Gillett, G. (1997) 'The case of Medea – a view of fetal–maternal conflict', *Journal of Medical Ethics* 23(1): 19–25.

Rhodes, A.M. (1997) 'Maternal vs. fetal rights', *MCN: American Journal of Maternal and Child Nursing* 22(4): 217.

Royal College of Paediatrics and Child Health (2004) *Withholding or Withdrawing Life Saving Treatment in Children: A Framework for Practice*, 2nd edn, London: Royal College of Paediatrics and Child Health.

Rumbold, G. (1993) *Ethics in Nursing Practice*, 2nd edn, London: Baillière Tindall.

Seedhouse, D. (1998) *Ethics: The Heart of Health Care*, 2nd edn, Chichester: John Wiley & Sons.

Strong, C. and Anderson, G.D. (1994) 'An ethical framework for issues during pregnancy', in R. Gillon (ed.) *Principles of Health Care Ethics*, Chichester: John Wiley & Sons.

Tingle, J. and Cribb, A. (2007) *Nursing Law and Ethics*, 3rd edn, Oxford: Blackwell Publishing.

Tschudin, V. (1994) *Deciding Ethically: A Pactical Approach to Nursing Challenges*, London: Baillière Tindall.

UKCC (United Kingdom Central Council for Nursing, Midwifery and Health Visiting) (1992) *The Scope of Professional Practice*, London: UKCC.

Website

www.epicure.ac.uk

Appendix

Normal values in the neonate

Listed below are the 'average' normal values expected in the first days of life. However, the infant's gestational age and day of life and clinical condition need to be considered before treatment is instigated.

	Term	Preterm
Temperature (°C)		
Rectal	36.5–37.5	36.5–37.5
Axillary	36.5–37.5	36.5–37.5
Abdominal skin	35.5–36.5	36.5– 37.0

* The toe core temperature gap should not exceed 2°C.

	Term	Preterm
Apex beat (per minute)	100–160	120–175
Blood pressure (mmHg)		
Systolic	50–72	47–57
Diastolic	25–45	22–35
Mean	30–55	25–47
Blood		
pH	7.3–7.4	7.3–7.38
PCO2 (kPa)	4.5–6.0	4.5–6.5
PO2 (kPa)	8.0–12	7.5–10
Bicarbonate mmol/l	18–25	18–25
Base excess	– 7 to + 3	– 5 to + 5

* To convert kPa to mmHg multiply by 7.5.

Blood (cont.)	Term	Preterm
Creatinine μmol/l	37–113	39–156
Calcium (corrected) mmol/l	2.1–2.7	1.9–2.6
Glucose mmol/l	2.6–6.0	2.6–6.0
Lactate mmol/l	0.5–2.0	0.5–2.0
Magnesium mmol/l	0.7–1.0	0.7–1.2
Phosphate mmol/l	1.8–2.6	1.8–2.6
Potassium mmol/l	3.6–5.5	4.5–6.0
Sodium mmo/l	135–146	135–146
Urea mmol/l	0.5–4.2	1.0–5.0
Haemoglobin g/dl	16.5–18.0	16.5–18
Packed cell volume	0.53–0.58	0.53–0.58
Platelets × 10^9/l	150–400	150–350
Prothrombin time (seconds)	10–16	13–16
White cell count × 10^9/l	9.0–30	9.0–35
Neutrophils	50–80%	50–80%
Lymphocytes	25–40%	25–40%
Monocytes	5–8%	5–8%
Urine		
Osmolality mosmol/l	100–300	50–300
Sodium mmol/l	1.0	1–15.0
Specific gravity	1006–1020	1006–1020
Cerebrospinal fluid		
Protein g/l	0.3–2.5	0.5–2.9
Glucose mmol/l	1.5–5.5	1.5–5.5

* CSF glucose should be approximately 80 per cent of the serum level.

Red cell count	0–50	0–70

Index

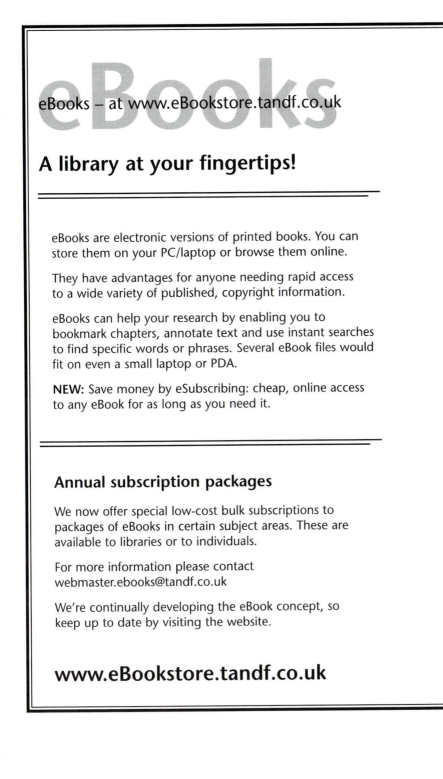